Find videos of the latest procedures and techniques from *Lasers and Light, Peels and Abrasions* online at MediaCenter.thieme.com!

	WINDOWS	MAC	TABLET
Recommended Browser(s)**	Microsoft Internet Explorer 8.0 or later, Firefox 3.x	Firefox 3.x, Safari 4.x	HTML5 mobile browser. iPad — Safari. Opera Mobile — Tabl
	** all browsers should have JavaScript enabled		
Flash Player Plug-in	Flash Player 9 or Higher * * Mac users: ATI Rage 128 GPU does not support full-screen mode with hardware scaling		Tabl
Minimum Hardware Configurations	Intel® Pentium® II 450 MHz, AMD Athlon™ 600 MHz or faster processor (or equivalent) 512 MB of RAM	PowerPC® G3 500 MHz or faster processor Intel Core™ Duo or faster proc 512MB o	
Recommended for optimal usage experience	Monitor resolutions: • Normal (4:3) 1024×768 or • Widescreen (16:9) 1280 • Widescreen (16:10) DSL/Cable internet of 384.0 Kbps o		

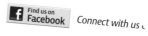

Lasers and Light, Peels and Abrasions

Applications and Treatments

William H. Truswell IV, MD
Clinical Instructor of Facial Plastic Surgery
Division of Otolaryngology–Head and Neck Surgery
University of Connecticut School of Medicine
Farmington, Connecticut
Private practice
Northampton, Massachusetts and Charleston, South Carolina

Thieme
New York • Stuttgart • Delhi • Rio de Janeiro

Thieme Medical Publishers, Inc.
333 Seventh Avenue
New York, New York 10001

Executive Editor: Timothy Y. Hiscock
Managing Editor: J. Owen Zurhellen IV
Editorial Assistant: Kate Barron
Director, Editorial Services: Mary Jo Casey
Production Editor: Sean Woznicki
International Production Director: Andreas Schabert
Vice President, Editorial and E-Product Development: Vera Spillner
International Marketing Director: Fiona Henderson
International Sales Director: Louisa Turrell
Director of Sales, North America: Mike Roseman
Senior Vice President and Chief Operating Officer: Sarah Vanderbilt
President: Brian D. Scanlan

Library of Congress Cataloging-in-Publication Data

Lasers and light, peels and abrasions : applications and treatments / [edited by] William H. Truswell.
    p. ; cm.
Includes bibliographical references and index.
ISBN 978-1-62623-001-9 (hardcover) – ISBN 978-1-62623-002-6 (eISBN)
I. Truswell, William, 1946- , editor.
[DNLM: 1. Skin Diseases–surgery. 2. Chemexfoliation–methods. 3. Dermabrasion–methods. 4. Dermatologic Agents–therapeutic use. 5. Laser Therapy, Low-Level–methods. 6. Rejuvenation–physiology. WR 670]
RL120.L37
617.4'770598–dc23   2015002882

Thieme Publishers New York
333 Seventh Avenue, New York, NY 10001 USA
+1 800 782 3488, customerservice@thieme.com

Thieme Publishers Stuttgart
Rüdigerstrasse 14, 70469 Stuttgart, Germany
+49 [0]711 8931 421, customerservice@thieme.de

Thieme Publishers Delhi
A-12, Second Floor, Sector-2, Noida-201301
Uttar Pradesh, India
+91 120 45 566 00, customerservice@thieme.in

Thieme Publishers Rio de Janeiro,
Thieme Publicações Ltda.
Edifício Rodolpho de Paoli, 25º andar
Av. Nilo Peçanha, 50 – Sala 2508
Rio de Janeiro 20020-906 Brasil
+55 21 3172 2297

Cover design: Thieme Publishing Group
Typesetting by Thomson Digital, India

Printed in India by Manipal Technologies Ltd.   5 4 3 2 1

ISBN 978-1-62623-001-9

Also available as an e-book:
eISBN 978-1-62623-002-6

Important note: Medicine is an ever-changing science undergoing continual development. Research and clinical experience are continually expanding our knowledge, in particular our knowledge of proper treatment and drug therapy. Insofar as this book mentions any dosage or application, readers may rest assured that the authors, editors, and publishers have made every effort to ensure that such references are in accordance with **the state of knowledge at the time of production of the book.**

Nevertheless, this does not involve, imply, or express any guarantee or responsibility on the part of the publishers in respect to any dosage instructions and forms of applications stated in the book. **Every user is requested to examine carefully** the manufacturers' leaflets accompanying each drug and to check, if necessary in consultation with a physician or specialist, whether the dosage schedules mentioned therein or the contraindications stated by the manufacturers differ from the statements made in the present book. Such examination is particularly important with drugs that are either rarely used or have been newly released on the market. Every dosage schedule or every form of application used is entirely at the user's own risk and responsibility. The authors and publishers request every user to report to the publishers any discrepancies or inaccuracies noticed. If errors in this work are found after publication, errata will be posted at www.thieme.com on the product description page.

Some of the product names, patents, and registered designs referred to in this book are in fact registered trademarks or proprietary names even though specific reference to this fact is not always made in the text. Therefore, the appearance of a name without designation as proprietary is not to be construed as a representation by the publisher that it is in the public domain.

Thank you, Lynn, my beacon and my anchor as I rush through my days.

Contents

Video Contents

Video 4.1 Fully ablative CO_2 resurfacing performed in conjunction with facelift and blepharoplasty.

Video 5.1 Full-face fractional CO_2 laser resurfacing.

Video 6.1 Full-thickness epidermal laser skin peel. Single-pass ablation of epidermal layer (forehead area, 53-year-old woman, Fitzpatrick skin type I) with dual mode erbium:yttrium aluminum garnet (Er:YAG) laser (Sciton, Palo Alto, California) using ablate mode set at 100 µm depth and 50% overlap.

Video 6.2 Intraepidermal laser skin peel. Google Glass (Google Inc., Mountain View, California) video of microablative laser skin resurfacing (51-year-old woman, Fitzpatrick skin type II) with the dual mode erbium:yttrium aluminum garnet (Er:YAG) laser (Sciton) using ablate mode set at 4 µm depth and 20% overlap.

Video 6.3 Laser ablation of skin lesion (LASL). Ablation of epidermal lesion (right temple area, 53-year-old woman, Fitzpatrick skin type I) with dual mode erbium:yttrium aluminum garnet (Er:YAG) laser (Sciton) using point beam (2 mm spot) and ablate mode set at 10 µm depth and repeat rate of 20 Hz.

Video 6.4 Noncontact low-frequency ultrasound (NCLF-US) treatment (UltraMIST, Celleration Inc., Eden Prairie, Minnesota) to face of 64-year-old woman (Fitzpatrick skin type II) one day after direct browlift, facelift, and full-face ablative fractional CO_2 laser skin resurfacing (Lutronic Inc., Freemont, California). Note the saline mist emanating from tip of the low-frequency ultrasound generator.

Video 9.1 Demonstrates the application of the CO_2 laser as a cutting and resurfacing tool for lower lid blepharoplasty.

Video 15.1 Nd:YAG laser hair removal procedure being performed on the left axilla.

Video 33.1 Treating Latino skin with lasers #1.

Video 33.2 Treating Latino skin with lasers #2.

Foreword

One of the most laudatory compliments one can make about any book is, "Once I started it, I couldn't put it down." This is what happened when I first read William H. Truswell's beautiful new book, *Lasers and Light, Peels and Abrasions: Applications and Treatments.* You are holding the most comprehensive, detailed, and informative contemporary book that I could have imagined. And notwithstanding the complexity and almost-infinite treatments and opinions covered, it is an enjoyable and easy read.

Dr. Truswell has selected a diverse, multispecialty group of leading experts who have each collated, distilled and refined their experience and wisdom. Each of the chapters is a treasure of pertinent basic science, clear and concise description of procedures, and clinical pearls. The chapters are well organized individually, each covering a specific clinical tool or condition. The subject matter is set out with specifically numbered titles and subtitles that enhance the reader's comprehension and ease of review.

Lasers and Light, Peels and Abrasions begins with a history of facial skin treatments and follows with a foundational knowledge chapter on skin anatomy, physiology, and pathology. It next describes the science of lasers, the various machines currently used, and how their power can be harnessed procedurally for maximal clinical benefit and minimal complications. A very helpful chapter describes how the reader might best select lasers for their own practice. There is an extensive discussion of current concepts of chemical peeling and dermabrasion. Of special interest are the sections on tattoo and hair removal, scar management, and the treatment of various skin pathologies. Adjunctive chapters discuss the role of light therapies, plasma skin resurfacing, and radiofrequency tightening: all providing indications, techniques, expected results, complications, and caveats. Several chapters focus on managing specific skin types associated with our globalized and multiracial demographic world. This book is completed with coverage of anti-aging products and a speculative, predictive and sometimes humorous look into the future. The 35 chapters admirably review the full breadth of this field, and insightfully delve into the details the reader wants and needs to know to be a superb practitioner of the art and science of lasers, phototherapy, peels, and abrasions.

The nascent facial plastic surgeon, plastic surgeon, otolaryngologist–head and neck surgeon, and dermatologist will appreciate and value the simple, detailed, and orderly description of the plethora of techniques and treatments available today. They will learn important scientific facts from the numerous clear and informative figures and tables. The text is richly augmented with representative patient results. Several chapters are supplemented with illustrative videos, and each chapter contains extensive references for the reader seeking even more information. This book will be an exceptional textbook from which to build a solid foundation of basic knowledge. Experienced clinicians, too, will benefit from the sophisticated, nuanced, and wise words of respected clinicians and teachers. It will cause them to reflect on their own practices, and perhaps modify or expand their repertoire of techniques. They will enjoy reading the pearls and perils. All scholars will appreciate the font and format, which as you can see are clear, crisp, and untiring on the eyes.

Lasers and Light, Peels and Abrasions stands as a unique, definitive and comprehensive resource to enhance one's cognitive abilities and technical skills. It manages to simplify and clarify a broad and complex subject. This collaborative effort of international experts, led by the experienced and wise Dr. Truswell, will be a signature literary treasure for years to come.

Peter A. Adamson, MD, FRCSC, FACS
Professor and Head, Division of Facial Plastic and Reconstructive Surgery
Department of Otolaryngology–Head and Neck Surgery
University of Toronto
Toronto, Ontario, Canada

Staff Surgeon, Toronto General Hospital, University Health Network
Consultant Surgeon, North York General Hospital
President, International Board for Certification in Facial Plastic and Reconstructive Surgery
Past President, American Academy of Facial Plastic and Reconstructive Surgery
Past President, American Board of Facial Plastic and Reconstructive Surgery
Past President, Canadian Academy of Facial Plastic and Reconstructive Surgery

Preface

Thousands of years ago, women in ancient Egypt bathed in sour milk to help keep their skin looking young and appealing. Little did they know that they were indulging in a primitive light chemical peel. When milk sours, lactose ferments and turns into lactic acid, an alpha hydroxy acid used today in many light chemical peels. Skin therapy may have been born in sour milk baths, but it has evolved into a multitude of sophisticated, somewhat confusing, and often very expensive treatments and procedures. Our purpose here is to instruct the reader about what methods are available today and how they are used in facial plastic surgery, plastic surgery, and dermatology.

This book has been written for medical professionals, residents, fellows, and practioners treating or beginning to treat skin with medical lasers, light therapy, chemical peels, and dermabrasion in health, beauty, and disease. It is comprehensive in its scope in that it includes all available modalities under one cover for the first time in many years and is authored by doctors of differing specialties. The great number of treatments available today and the great expense of the devices on the market make it a daunting challenge to decide how to proceed. The book is designed to guide the reader through the myriad devices and therapies for skin rejuvenation and skin pathology, to understand what can be done, how to do it, and even how to select the right device for his/her practice. It is equally important to have a thorough understanding of how the skin ages and how it reacts to various treatments applied to it.

The authors of the chapters of this volume are well known physicians in the specialties of facial plastic surgery, plastic surgery, and dermatology. They have all been in practice many years, are well published, and considered experts and leaders in their specialties. They are teachers and innovators of procedures and devices. I have also reached out to colleagues in a number of other countries for their expertise and perspectives.

The present is built on the past and is the foundation of the future. In medicine, it is important to learn how therapies have evolved to better understand why treatments are done today and how to develop newer and better modalities of therapy going forward. To this end, the book begins with an historical perspective of skin therapy. The subsequent chapters discuss the pertinent anatomy, physiology, and pathology of aging skin and laser physics with its application to the skin. The laser and light chapters follow and are inclusive of all modalities available today. Topics on skin rejuvenation from non- and minimally invasive therapies to fractional and ablative resurfacing are covered in chapters for specific lasers and light devices, the spectrum of chemical peels available, and abrasion techniques. Other topics include scar management, acne scarring, vascular malformations, tattoo and permanent makeup removal, acne rosacea, hair removal, and radiofrequency skin tightening. Two chapters discuss the use of the CO_2 laser in facelift surgery and in blepharoplasty. There are chapters on the complications of lasers and chemical peels. Perspectives of skin therapy in different ethnic populations are covered. Lastly there is a look to the future.

Acknowledgments

I wish to thank the American Academy of Facial Plastic and Reconstructive Surgery, the resource for education, guidance, support, and fraternity for facial plastic surgeons throughout the world, and the American Board of Facial Plastic and Reconstructive Surgery, our certifying board of the highest standards with over one thousand diplomats to date. I thank all the contributors to this book. I wish to also thank my talented son, Jason, who did illustrations for Chapters 8, 9, and 11. And to, you, Jody, my wonderful daughter who has worked in our office off and on since she was thirteen doing everything from filing to marketing.

Contributors

Manoj T. Abraham, MD, FACS
Clinical Assistant Professor
Department of Otolaryngology
New York Medical College
Valhalla, New York
Icahn School of Medicine at Mount Sinai
New York, New York

Macrene Alexiades, MD, PhD
Associate Clinical Professor
Yale University School of Medicine
New Haven, Connecticut
Director and Founder
Dermatology and Laser Surgery Center of New York
New York, New York

Jose E. Barrera, MD, FACS
Associate Professor
Uniformed Services University
Bethesda, MD
Clinical Associate Professor
University of Texas Health Sciences Center
Private practice, Texas Facial Plastic Surgery and ENT
San Antonio, Texas

Mark J. Been, MD
Facial Plastic and Reconstructive Surgeon
The Center for Facial Plastic Surgery
Barrington, Illinois

Stuart H. Bentkover, MD, FACS
Clinical Instructor in Otology and Laryngology
Harvard Medical School
Boston, Massachusetts
Associate in Otolaryngology
University of Massachusetts Medical School
Worcester, Massachusetts
Bentkover Facial Plastic Surgery and Laser Center
Worcester, Massachusetts and Stoneham, Massachusetts

Anthony E. Brissett, MD, FACS
Associate Professor and Director, Facial Plastic and Reconstructive Surgery
Co-Director, BCM Aesthetics
Bobby R. Alford Department of Otolaryngology–Head and Neck Surgery
Baylor College of Medicine
Houston, Texas

Paul J. Carniol, MD, FACS
Clinical Professor and Director of Facial Plastic Surgery
Department of Otolaryngology
Rutgers New Jersey Medical School
Summit, New Jersey

Irina Chaikhoutdinov, MD
Division of Otolaryngology–Head and Neck Surgery
Milton S. Hershey Medical Center
The Pennsylvania State University
Hershey, Pennsylvania

Donn R. Chatham, MD
Clinical Instructor
Department of Otolaryngology–Head and Neck Surgery
University of Louisville Medical School
Louisville, Kentucky
Chatham Facial Plastic Surgery
Louisville, Kentucky and New Albany, Indiana

Louis M. DeJoseph, MD
Clinical Instructor of Facial Plastic Surgery
Division of Otolaryngology–Head and Neck Surgery
Emory University School of Medicine
Premier Image Cosmetic and Laser Surgery
Atlanta, Georgia

J. Kevin Duplechain, MD
Laser Skin Care of Louisiana
Volunteer Faculty, Facial Plastic Surgery
Tulane University Medical Center
Lafayette, Louisiana

David A.F. Ellis, MD, FRCSC
Academic Professor
Division of Facial Plastic Surgery
Department of Otolaryngology–Head and Neck Surgery
University of Toronto
Medical Director
Art of Facial Surgery
Toronto, Ontario, Canada

Rafael Espinosa Delgado, MD
Department of ENT, Facial Plastic Surgery
Hospital San Jose de Hermosillo
Hermosillo, Sonora, Mexico

Fred G. Fedok, MD, FACS
Adjunct Professor
Department of Surgery
The University of South Alabama
Mobile, Alabama
Professor of Facial Plastic and Reconstructive Surgery
Division of Otolaryngology–Head and Neck Surgery
Milton S. Hershey Medical Center
The Pennsylvania State University
Hershey, Pennsylvania

Albert J. Fox, MD, FACS
Albert Fox Facial Plastic Surgery Center
Dartmouth, Massachusetts

David Galarza Lozano, MD
Department of ENT, Facial Plastic Surgery
Universidad Cuauhtemoc
San Luis Potosi, San Luis Potosi, Mexico

Frank G. Garritano, MD
Clinical Instructor
Department of Otolaryngology–Head and Neck Surgery
Columbia University Medical Center
Attending Surgeon
Harlem Hospital Center
New York, New York

Richard D. Gentile, MD, MBA
Facial Plastic and Aesthetic Laser Center
Youngstown, Ohio

Cynthia M. Gregg, MD, FACS
Gregg Facial Plastic and Reconstructive Surgery
Cary, North Carolina

Ariel B. Grobman, MD
Resident Physician
Department of Otolaryngology–Head and Neck Surgery
University of Miami Miller School of Medicine
Miami, Florida

Lisa D. Grunebaum, MD
Associate Professor of Facial Plastic and Reconstructive
  Surgery and Dermatology
University of Miami Miller School of Medicine
Miami, Florida

Mark M. Hamilton, MD, FACS
Clinical Assistant Professor
Department of Otolaryngology–Head and Neck Surgery
Indiana University School of Medicine
Indianapolis, Indiana

Sanaz Harirchian, MD
SH Facial Plastics
Houston, Texas

Jill Lynn Hessler, MD
Adjunct Clinical Assistant Professor
Stanford University School of Medicine
Stanford, California
Medical Director
Hessler Plastic Surgery
Palo Alto, California

Marcelo Hochman, MD
Hemangioma and Malformation Treatment Center
Charleston, South Carolina

J. David Holcomb, MD
Holcomb–Kreithen Plastic Surgery and MedSpa
Sarasota, Florida

Adam A. Ingraffea, MD
Clinical Assistant Professor and Associate Program Director
Department of Dermatology
University of Cincinnati
Cincinnati, Ohio

Joely Kaufman, MD
Voluntary Associate Professor of Dermatology
University of Miami Miller School of Medicine
Medical Director, Skin Associates of South Florida
Coral Gables. Florida

Sang W. Kim, MD
Private practice
Syracuse, New York

Bethany J. King, MD
Lakes Cosmetic Institute
Gilford, New Hampshire
Ear, Nose, and Throat Associates of New Hampshire
Laconia, New Hampshire

Theda C. Kontis, MD, FACS
Assistant Professor
Division of Facial Plastic and Reconstructive Surgery
Department of Otolaryngology–Head and Neck Surgery
Johns Hopkins Medical Institutions
Baltimore, Maryland

Carol H. Langsdon, RNP, BSN
The Langsdon Clinic
Germantown, Tennessee

Phillip R. Langsdon, MD, FACS
Professor and Chief, Division of Facial Plastic Surgery
Department of Otolaryngology–Head and Neck Surgery
University of Tennessee Health Science Center
Memphis, Tennessee

Tee Sin Lee, MBBS (S'pore), MRCS (Edin), MMed (ORL), FAMS (ORL)
Deputy Director and Consultant, Facial Plastic and
    Reconstructive Surgery Service
Department of Otolaryngology–Head and Neck Surgery
Changi General Hospital
Clinical Lecturer
Yong Loo Lin School of Medicine
National University of Singapore
Singapore

Sophie D. Liao, MD
Assistant Professor of Oculofacial Plastic and Orbital
    Surgery
Department of Ophthalmology
University of Colorado School of Medicine
Aurora, Colorado

Devinder S. Mangat, MD, FACS
Professor of Facial Plastic Surgery
Department of Otolaryngology–Head and Neck Surgery
University of Cincinnati
Cincinnati, Ohio
Private practice
Vail, Colorado

Ramsey F. Markus, MD, FAAD
Associate Professor of Dermatology
Director of Laser Surgery
Department of Dermatology
Baylor College of Medicine
Houston, Texas

Neha A. Patel, MD
Department of Otolaryngology–Head and Neck Surgery
New York Eye and Ear Infirmary of Mt. Sinai
New York, New York

Stephen W. Perkins, MD
Clinical Associate Professor
Department of Otolaryngology–Head and Neck Surgery
Indiana University
President
Meridian Plastic Surgeons
Founder and President
Meridian Plastic Surgery Center
Indianapolis, Indiana

Michael A. Persky, MD, FACS
Clinical Instructor
University of Southern California Medical School
Los Angeles, California
Private Practice
Encino, California

Dana K. Petersen, MD, DDS
Division of Otolaryngology–Head and Neck Surgery
University of Tennessee Health Science Center
Memphis, Tennessee

Amy Li Richter, MD
Department of Otolaryngology–Head and Neck Surgery
Baylor College of Medicine
Houston, Texas

Elizabeth F. Rostan, MD
Charlotte Skin and Laser
Charlotte, North Carolina

Daniel E. Rousso, MD, FACS
Assistant Professor
Department of Surgery
University of Alabama at Birmingham
Medical Director, Rousso Facial Plastic Surgery Clinic
Birmingham, Alabama

Ashley Rudnick, BS
Miami Dermatology and Laser Institute
Miami, Florida

Scott Shadfar, MD
Clinical Assistant Professor
Department of Otolaryngology–Head and Neck Surgery
Indiana University
Meridian Plastic Surgeons
Indianapolis, Indiana

James R. Shire, MD, FACS
Shire Facial Plastic Surgery
Chattanooga, Tennessee

Danny J. Soares, MD
Assistant Professor of Otolaryngology–Head and Neck
    Surgery
University of Central Florida College of Medicine
Orlando, Florida
Medical Director
Mesos Cosmetic and Laser Surgery
Lady Lake, Florida

Adam P. Stanek, MD
A.S.thetics Facial Plastic and Reconstructive Surgery
Hilden and Düsseldorf, Germany

Babar Sultan, MD
Sultan Facial Plastic and Reconstructive Surgery
Towson, Maryland

Miriam de la Torre Campos, MD
Department of ENT, Facial Plastic Surgery
Hospital San Jose de Hermosillo
Hermosillo, Sonora, Mexico

William H. Truswell IV, MD
Clinical Instructor of Facial Plastic Surgery
Division of Otolaryngology–Head and Neck Surgery
University of Connecticut School of Medicine
Farmington, Connecticut
Private practice
Northampton, Massachusetts and Charleston,
  South Carolina

Jill S. Waibel, MD
Miami Dermatology and Laser Institute
Chief of Dermatology
Baptist Hospital
Assistant Professor
Department of Dermatology and Cutaneous Surgery
University of Miami Miller School of Medicine
Miami, Florida

Danielle M. Waymire, MD
Chief Resident
Department of Dermatology
University of Cincinnati
Cincinnati, Ohio

Philip A. Young, MD
Aesthetic Facial Plastic Surgery PLLC
Bellevue, Washington

1 The History and Evolution of Skin Resurfacing

Bethany J. King

1.1 Introduction

Beauty of the face. Why should that matter? Why do so many people care? Why do some exert so much effort to achieve it or hold on to it? These are complicated questions to answer, and there will be a different answer from each person to whom you pose the question.

Beauty, as a philosophical concept, is an intangible element of human existence. You cannot measure it with a scientific instrument. Nevertheless, we know that it exists because we know it when we see it. Beauty is a component of our lives that affects each of us in varying degrees. Some care about it greatly—some not at all. For many of us, there is an undeniable urge to surround ourselves with beauty. Some choose to live in an environment where we see the beauty of the earth from every angle. We decorate our homes with colors and materials that stimulate an internal reaction that causes our own personal elation. We adorn our bodies with colors and fabrics that please us, make us feel confident, and hopefully please other human observers as well. We know that the perception of beauty pleases the one who perceives it. And human nature leads human beings to secure their own success. That is the impetus behind why human beings choose to amplify their own facial and body beauty.

Of all the elements of the body, the appearance of the face is the most critical to our success. The face is how a person sees the world and it is the first part of the body that is seen by the world. Therefore, it is the first part of us that is judged by the world. Communication begins without words. It begins with projection of intention by facial expression and body language. The interpretation of that projection is performed through the observer's eye. That is why when a human being communicates with another human being, they look into the eyes to do so. For that reason, the eye is the most important feature of the face. When an observer glances at another person, the observer instinctively and instantly assesses the age, health, and beauty of the person being observed by amassing a collection of subliminal judgments based upon shape of the face, shadows within the face, colors across the face, and quality of the skin. A heart-shaped face equals youth; a square face equals aging. Round cheeks equal youth; flat cheeks equal aging. Shadows under the eyes and in front of the jowls equal aging; no shadows in those areas equal youth. A light, rosy glow on round cheeks equals health; bright red across the cheeks and around the nose equals infirmity. Skin that is smooth in color, firm, and reflects light equals youth and health. Skin that is mottled with brown and red, loose, and unable to adequately reflect light equals aging disease.

There are many methods that human beings use to amplify their facial beauty. Long before there were means to supplement volume or to surgically remove or reconfigure tissue, people actively worked to augment their facial attractiveness. They did so by making their skin as beautiful as possible and by using cosmetics to create illusion. One of the goals when attempting to improve the appearance of skin was to make it "glow." Another objective was to make it look like "porcelain" (the goal of the geisha of ancient Japan). Thus, in our analysis of how we have come to accomplish these objectives over the centuries, it is appropriate to understand what changes happen histologically that result in an increase in glow and the achievement of a porcelain look.

Glowing, radiant, luminous skin. Each of these descriptions speaks in terms of light. The observer of such skin is appreciating some improvement in the way that light leaves the skin of the person being observed. Obviously, the person being observed does not have an internal light source that is emanating rays of visible light. Rather, the person with luminous skin is simply doing a better job of *reflecting* ambient light. When light is not trapped, absorbed, or scattered, it will more directly bounce off a surface. Imagine, if you will, that you are walking along a beach on a sunny day. The light reflected off the water surface can be blinding because it is bouncing off a surface that is not porous and does not diffuse light; however, the light coming off the sand is diffuse because so much of it is absorbed and scattered by the grains of sand. If you look at the skin of a 6-year-old child and compare it to the skin of a 70-year-old adult, you will immediately appreciate the difference in the ability of the younger skin to reflect light.

Porcelain skin. What does this mean? This descriptive term refers to skin that is homogenous in color (no brown or red spots) and smooth in landscape (not interrupted by large pores or depressed scars). The most effective way to accomplish this is by the illusion of makeup. However, makeup will do an even better job if the skin it is covering is closer to ideal. A child has not yet accumulated the effects of photodamage such as dyschromias or telangiectasias, or the large pores from teenage hypertrophic sebaceous glands, or the effects of scarring from acne. This is why, in the observer's quickly assessing, subconscious judgment, smooth skin of all the same color not interrupted by brown or red is a sign of youth and health—which goes hand in hand with beauty.

Human beings have learned that if you resurface the skin, that is, remove the outer layers of keratinized epithelium to produce a new-and-improved superficial surface, you can actually improve the reflectivity, color consistency, and microlandscape of the skin, thus improving the beauty of the skin. In this chapter, the history of how mankind has developed this art is reviewed.

1.2 Dermabrasion

Woodworking, stone sculpture. In an effort to adorn his world, ancient man worked with the materials in his environment and turned them into moments of beauty. He cut and polished wood, stone, and gems to turn them into pieces of art. He learned that rubbing them over and over again with an abrasive substance would file the surface down until it gleamed. This smooth surface was considered pleasing. A "polished" article was viewed as finished or complete. It wouldn't have taken long to learn that scrubbing the skin also made it shinier and smoother. There are references to a number of cosmetic rituals that have been passed down from antiquity and incorporate mechanical abrasion (exfoliation) to remove the outer surface of the skin to help it appear more beautiful.

It is said that for hundreds of years, Indonesian women would exfoliate their skin with coffee grinds. (The caffeic acid in coffee beans is a powerful antioxidant and may boost collagen.[1] Caffeine is often used in skin-tightening products today. Furthermore, caffeic acid is one of the main ingredients in argan oil, a popular antiaging oil used in many cosmetics today.) In India, cleansing the skin with milk mixed with wheat husk or gram flour was recommended (lactic acid and protein-infused mechanical exfoliation). An ancient Asian skin treatment was exfoliation by rubbing the skin with a mixture of cream, starch, and husk followed by an application of rosewater to tone (rose water is said to be a mild astringent, causing tightening of the skin that reduces pore size).

Egyptians also employed the techniques of dermabrasion by use of a mixture of pumice, alabaster, salts, and animal oils on the skin. They would also rub the skin with a mixture of animal oil, lime, and chalk (an abrasive).[2] In 1500 BC, Egyptian physicians attempted to improve scars with sandpaper. In India, women would use a mixture of urine and pumice to exfoliate their faces.[3] (Urine is mostly water followed by urea, which is neither acidic nor basic. Urea is included in many topical cosmetics for it is hydrophilic at low concentrations and is keratolytic at high concentrations [even used in products designed for wound débridement and for treatment of hyperkeratotic conditions].[4]) In ancient Japan, geishas would polish their skin with salt and cream scrubs. Masks of rice bran and cream would be scrubbed on the skin and allowed to remain for a period as a treatment (reported to have been used since 1100 AD. Rice bran is high in gamma oryzanol, which is a powerful antioxidant and collagen stimulator.[5]).

As the centuries went on and the Industrial Revolution blossomed, mechanical means of polishing were developed. At the turn of the 20th century, Kromayer made application of such a tool for use on the skin. He first described the means of resurfacing the skin by applying rotating burs to skin lesions.[6] Abner Kurtin, in the 1940s, modified this approach to develop the wire brush technique, adapting this to a powered dental tool.[7] In the 1950s, Burke modified the wire brush technique, leading to the techniques that are more likely to be used today.[8] Also in the 1950s, the term *dermabrasion* began to be used as the class of treatment used to plane irregularities of the skin.[9]

Over the next 20 years, dermabrasion was applied to many cutaneous conditions beyond just scars and acne pits, conditions that produce irregularities of the skin such as acne rosacea, rhinophyma, seborrheic keratoses, sebaceous hyperplasia, fibrous tumors of tuberous sclerosis, and discoid lupus erythematosus, just to name a few.[10,11,12,13,14] It was also widely applied in the removal of tattoos.[15] During this period, histological studies showed the significant dermal remodeling that takes place, an effect that is comparable to that seen in laser and deep peels.[16,17,18]

The primary application of dermabrasion has been to mechanically remove the epithelium and damage the papillary dermis to mid-dermis to induce restructuring and laying down of new type I and type III collagen in areas of hypertrophic scarring and depressions such as the sharp wrinkles around the mouth or acne scars—without creating new scars.[18,19] In general, any area of skin that has a sudden elevation or depression will cause light to be reflected (if the skin is elevated) or will cause shadow to be caught (if the skin is depressed), and the observer's eye will notice this unexpected attention-getter and will be drawn to it. The notice of this moment of deviation from "average skin" is perceived as a "flaw." One of the great powers of dermabrasion is to "level the playing field," to reduce the difference between high and low in terms of skin topography so that there is less material to induce inappropriate light reflection or shadow catching. However, dermabrasion has also been useful in resurfacing photodamaged skin as well, by removing the damaged epithelium and inducing dermal remodeling.[18,19]

Dermabrasion is an undeniably useful tool with predictable outcome. However, its application has become less frequently utilized in the last two decades because lasers have provided another means of inducing collagen re-conformation while at the same time accomplishing surface rejuvenation. Furthermore, the issue of blood splatter is another aspect of this technique that requires consideration. Dermabrasion produces a certain amount of splatter of blood and tissue particles. In the 1980s and 1990s, with blossoming awareness of the dangers of viruses such as the human immunodeficiency virus (HIV), the hepatitis B virus (HBV), and the hepatitis C virus (HCV), there naturally developed a heightened awareness of the need to protect the surgical staff from aerosolized, potentially infectious particles. There was a report of a possible transmission of HBV by contact with conjunctivae during dermabrasion.[20] Therefore, universal precautions are advisable during dermabrasion performance, and protection is easily accomplished for the surgical staff and patient with proper outfitting and proper room sterilization techniques. However, with the development of techniques that could produce similar results without the splatter of blood, attention turned toward the use of these other applications.

The ability of dermabrasion to effectively and soundly treat a wide number of conditions is as attractive as the low cost of the instrument (compared to the laser). Nevertheless, the laser has become the gold standard of resurfacing now, leaving fewer opportunities for facial plastic surgeons to master the art of dermabrasion.

1.2.1 Microdermabrasion

A subtler application of mechanical exfoliation to effect skin resurfacing is microdermabrasion, a technique first introduced by Tsai et al in 1995.[21] The initial technology incorporated applying a vacuum-suctioning device to the skin and then showering the suctioned skin with streams of aluminum oxide crystals to produce an exfoliation of the external stratum corneum. Studies have shown that there is a degree of dermal remodeling that takes place after this treatment (induction of procollagen I and III among other effects).[22] Modifications to the initial design include substituting sodium chloride crystals for aluminum oxide crystals, or substituting crystals entirely with a diamond fraise applied to the skin after it is sucked into the apparatus. It has been shown that there is improved absorption of topical medications (such as d-aminolevulinic acid for photodynamic therapy or topical anesthetic prior to laser resurfacing) after microdermabrasion.[23] For this reason, microdermabrasion as a resurfacing tool is often incorporated before other techniques to improve their performance.

1.3 Topical Agents and Chemical Peeling

In ancient Egypt, women would use sour milk (lactic acid) mixed with alabaster, animal oils, and salt to help remove the external surface of the skin and promote beauty.[24] There has also been found a vintage Egyptian recipe to combat wrinkles: senetjer resin (likely frankincense, one of the most antique anti-aging ingredients), wax, fresh balanos oil (a nut that grew on a native tree whose oil was considered fine and suitable for perfumery), and cyperus grass are to be ground and mixed with fermented plant juice (source of alpha hydroxy acid most likely) and applied to the face daily.[2] The Greeks and Romans were said to apply a poultice of sulfur, mustard, and a corrosive sublimate of limestone to the skin. They would use tree resins including frankincense and myrrh mixed with pumice to lighten the skin and remove wrinkles and freckles.[3] In the Middle Ages, women would treat their skin with old wine (with active ingredient tartaric acid, which is an alpha hydroxy acid) to accomplish rejuvenation. Lemon juice has been used as a brightening agent for as long as anyone can recall across multiple cultures. Also in the Middle Ages, women would use curdled milk (lactic acid) to treat acne, cucumber juice to remove freckles, and boiled nettles to produce a smooth, even complexion. In Japan, a mask of droppings from the nightingale bird has been used for hundreds of years. Initially, the droppings were used to bleach silk and then were later applied to the skin. A paste of the droppings is applied to the skin and then rinsed. The excrement was dried in the sun and then pulverized into a powder. (In modern times, the material is irradiated with ultraviolet radiation to kill bacteria.) Water was added to turn it into paste which was then applied to the skin. (These same ingredients are part of a geisha facial that is offered currently in some parts of the world. The primary ingredient, the droppings, is called *uguisu no fun*.)

Because man has known that certain chemicals on the skin can induce a change for the better, eventually prolonged application of these chemicals in a controlled fashion to produce a more profound effect was used. However, such historical references from antiquity are not available.

There are records of a Viennese dermatologist, Ferdinand Hebra, using various combinations of exfoliating chemicals to remove freckles and melasma in the mid-1800s. There were experiments by dermatologists with various compounds to lighten freckles and dyschromias with tinctures of iodine and lead, croton oil, and cantharides, as well as sulfuric, acetic, hydrochloric, and nitric acids. Lime-based compresses were applied to the skin for 4 hours, after which the ensuing blisters would be broken and treated with starch. Removal of the resultant crust was found to lighten the skin. In 1871, William Tilbury Fox mentioned using phenol to lighten the skin, and in 1881 croton oil as a compound that causes skin inflammation was recorded by Henry Piffard. In 1882, a dermatologist from Germany, P. G. Unna, described the use of trichloroacetic acid (TCA) as a peeling agent.

1.3.1 Phenol

Many peeling agents were experimented with in the late 1800s and early 1900s, but the one that garnered the most attention was phenol. The first American article on phenol was in 1917 by the dermatologist Douglass Montgomery. He described the use of phenol under bandages, using the agent as a "beautifier."[3] This was at the same period of time as the activities of the American lay "skinners" listed in Hetter's history described in a subsequent paragraph. Concomitantly, in Europe, it is said that Sir Harold Gillies was the first to use phenol for chemical surgery by applying it to lax lower eyelids.[25]

MacKee reported in 1952 his use of phenol to treat acne scars, beginning as early as 1903. He had a clinic at New York University through the 1940s, where he used phenol to treat acne scars and noticed the improvement in his patients' skin long term. His report was the first to attempt to correlate the histology of peeling with clinical results. He would apply phenol to the skin for a 30- to 60-second interval and then wash it off with ethanol. This would be repeated four to six times at 2-month intervals.[3,26]

However, a much more entertaining, fascinating, and rich history of the development of the phenol peel in America as a tool to achieve beauty can be acquired in Hetter's "An Examination of the Phenol-Croton Oil Peel: Part II. The Lay Peelers and Their Croton Oil Formulas."[27] This article provides a history gleaned from personal interviews and research of personal memoirs to uncover the development of a practice that was actually widely used in the first half of the 1900s by the starlets of Hollywood and the wives of wealthy Americans. The women who had the means to undergo this quietly held beauty treatment maintained skin that was more beautiful than their average contemporaries. The original practitioners were not physicians. They were lay peelers called "skinners." There were a select few of them in America who made quite a good living. They jealously guarded the recipes of their peels, which, of course, were eventually discovered. These were the sources of the phenol peels known today. It is said that, initially, use of phenol as a cosmetic peel originated in Europe and was learned by these lay peelers. These American skinners were also the same people who recognized that croton oil is the additive that produces a deeper effect than just phenol alone. Eventually, as plastic surgery became a specialty after World War II, and plastic surgeons realized that this was a tool their patients desired, they published articles against the lay peelers—many of whom had stumbled upon the complications of full thickness burns and hypertrophic scars in the necks of their clients. Plastic surgeons filed charges of inappropriate practice of medicine against some lay peelers, acquired their formulas, and began to take over that market.[27]

In 1941, Eller and Wolff described the use of a paste of resorcinol and phenol along with solid carbon dioxide (CO_2) cryotherapy to resurface the skin.[28] The first references in the medical literature regarding the addition of croton oil to phenol appeared in a suite of debuts beginning in 1959, when first Brown applied for a patent, then Litton presented a paper at a meeting in October 1961, and finally Baker and Gordon published their preliminary report in December 1961.[29] Each of these physicians, it has been discovered, independently learned of the addition of croton oil from one of the lay peelers of the time. We, as physicians, were all initially taught that phenol was the primary active ingredient in this peel. But it has since been learned that croton oil is also very important, inducing greater penetration of the phenol to produce a deeper effect. The greater the percentage of croton oil, the greater the penetration of phenol.[27]

In 1960, Ayres treated sun-damaged skin with phenol and then performed a histological analysis. His research showed that a new 0.3- to 0.4-mm thick subepidermal layer of organized, parallel collagen fibers was deposited superficial to the old elastotic collagen. Over the next three decades, there were other papers that verified the consistent enlargement of the papillary dermis after deep chemical peeling (as well as dermabrasion).[26,30]

The Baker and Gordon phenol recipe published in 1961 is a deep phenol peel composed of phenol, croton oil, tap water, and Septisol (a surfactant that allows a better mix of ingredients) (active ingredient **hexachloraphene**, VESTAL Labs, Toronto, Canada). In their original description, it was recommended to occlude the skin with waterproof tape.[30] This recipe and treatment became the standard for the next 20 years. McCollough and Hillman in 1980 demonstrated that a Baker-Gordon peel without tape was just as effective, more comfortable, and had fewer complications.[25] The phenol peel has been modified since to include lower concentrations of croton oil to reduce the risk profile. These modifications can be seen in the phenol peels developed by Hetter and Stone.[31,32,33]

1.3.2 Medium and Superficial Peels

Chemical exfoliation had been performed for decades to achieve deep peels. However, recovery was long and risk was sometimes high. Thus, effort was expended toward considering the benefit of lighter, more superficial peels. Alpha hydroxy acid (AHA) peels, salicylic acid (SA) peels, Jessner's peels (detailed later), and various strengths of TCA were used in various combinations.

Since its initial description by Unna, the use of TCA has been modified to include a variety of applications including different strengths and the addition of other components to achieve a greater depth of penetration—the addition of Jessner's solution, or use of CO_2, glycolic acid, or microdermabrasion just prior to application. TCA has also been used as a deep peel, but it has been found to carry a risk of scarring that is unacceptably high. Nevertheless, it is very valuable as a medium depth peel.[34]

Jessner's solution was created by Dr. Max Jessner and has been in use for more than 100 years. This peel is composed of resorcinol, SA, lactic acid, and ethanol. The solution reliably peels to the superficial papillary dermis, useful for conditions of hyperpigmentation and acne.[34]

AHAs typically come from fruits: glycolic acid from sugar cane, lactic acid from sour milk, tartaric acid from grape wine, malic acid from apples, and citric acid from citrus fruits. In terms of molecular size, glycolic acid is the smallest of these alpha hydroxy acids, which means that it can penetrate the skin more effectively and deeply. AHAs impact epithelium by reducing the cohesion between corneocytes. The AHAs that have greater bioavailability (glycolic, lactic, and citric) are able to reach the dermis. At that level, they have been shown to impact epithelium by increasing mucopolysaccharides and collagen

and increasing skin thickness. AHAs produce increased exfoliation based upon an influence in the cell's metabolism by interference with enzymatic processes that are supposed to increase cell adhesion. However, if used at high concentrations, the acidity itself will destroy the cells (toxicity), resulting in peeling.[35]

Initially, AHAs were thought to produce only a freshening effect. Some studies found that repeated applications could produce improvement in skin texture and dyschromias, if not wrinkles. Higher concentrations of 20% used for 3 months could elicit mild impact upon fine wrinkles.[36] Other studies found that levels of 25% AHAs could produce increased thickness of the dermis, increased mucopolysaccharides, improved quality of elastic fibers, and increased density of collagen.[37]

Beta hydroxy acids (BHAs) are not as strong as AHAs, but they do a better job of getting down into the pore. SA is the prime example; it is lipid soluble, which is why it is a better peel for people with comedonal acne. Urkov introduced SA in 1946. He added occlusion to amplify its effect.[34] SA is keratolytic and comedolytic (and is a primary ingredient in Jessner's peel, which is often recommended for treatment of acne).[35]

1.3.3 Tretinoin

It has been known since the 1930s that vitamin A (retinol) has antikeratotic effects. The following is Gunter Stüttgen's synopsis of how he discovered the effects of tretinoin on the skin.[38] Studor and Frey showed that retinyl palmitate (the ester of retinol) decreased the epidermal proliferation rate when given in large oral doses. This finding initiated the use of the drug to treat psoriasis. Psoriatic lesions would improve with dosages of 3 to 8 million units per day of retinyl palmitate. However, at these doses, the condition of hypervitaminosis A would develop and the use of retinyl palmitate for psoriasis was stopped. To avoid the systemic effects of retinyl palmitate, efforts were employed to develop a topical application. However, the beneficial antikeratotic effects of systemic retinyl palmitate on conditions such as psoriasis and ichthyosis could not be achieved topically. This led Stüttgen to consider that perhaps it was actually a metabolite of retinyl palmitate that was producing the therapeutic effect—a metabolite that could not be produced via topical application. Thus he, in collaboration with Hoffmann-La Roche, began to topically test the metabolites of retinyl palmitate, one of which was vitamin A acid, also known as retinoic acid (also known as all-*trans*-retinoic acid, or tretinoin), the major metabolite of retinol. Quickly, it was seen that there was improvement in patients with ichthyosis. However, there was also consistent redness and inflammation of the skin. In 1962, Stüttgen and Hoffmann-La Roche applied for a patent for tretinoin primarily for cosmetic application; however, they expanded their research applications to include other conditions such as actinic keratosis and basal cell carcinoma with promising results. Notwithstanding, the dermatology community was not encouraging because it felt that the dermatitis coinciding with the treatment was an undesirable side effect. Furthermore, at that time, it was believed by dermatology circles that the desquamation was simply a side effect of the irritation and not an indication of any therapeutic effect. However, in 1969 Kligman et al reported on the histological changes that resulted from the use of tretinoin, namely that acne was not improved upon simply because of inflammatory changes from tretinoin but rather that tretinoin resulted in rapid cell turnover and unplugging of the comedone.[39] Later histological studies by Plewig and Braun-Falco showed that shedding of desmosomes and tonofibrils is the change that leads to increased peeling action of the keratinized epithelium.[40] This discovery led to greater acceptance in the scientific community. And in 1971, the Food and Drug Administration (FDA) approved tretinoin for use in the treatment of acne. In 1975, the first international symposium of vitamin A acid was held, which helped to establish the clinical efficacy of tretinoin in the minds of the medical community.[38] Tretinoin became a mainstay in the treatment of acne from the 1960s on.

Later, in 1986, Kligman et al reported that tretinoin was seen to reverse some of the effects of photoaging such as dullness, hyperpigmentation, and wrinkling.[41] Over the following years, a great deal of research was undertaken to study the effects of tretinoin on sun-damaged skin. In multiple studies, tretinoin has been shown to improve sun-damaged skin both histologically (with thickness of the epithelial layer, increase in dermal collagen, and increase in mucin) as well as visually (with improvement in fine and coarse wrinkles, lentigines, and skin texture).[42,43,44,45] Although not a classic resurfacing agent, part of the therapeutic effect of tretinoin is due to increased stratum corneum exfoliation, which is the essence of resurfacing. Therefore, tretinoin is another of the tools at our disposal to accomplish this goal.

1.4 Laser Resurfacing

Light and heat, as well, have been used for the treatment of skin from ancient times. Turkish treatments involved the use of minimal fire to exfoliate the skin by lightly singeing it.[3] Egyptians are known to have treated many skin conditions with sunlight. Physicians in the 1700s and 1800s used sunlight to treat eczema and psoriasis. However, it wasn't until we developed the ability to harness the power of light energy, direct it, and use it for our own purposes that light as a tool became powerful in our hands. No chapter on lasers would ever begin without the explanation of where the word came from. L.A.S.E.R. is an acronym formed from "light amplification by stimulated emission of radiation." In 1917, Albert Einstein proposed that the application of a photon of electromagnetic energy to an atom in an excited state could induce the emission of an identical photon from the excited atom.[46] This concept was eventually realized, and in 1959, the first laser was created by Maiman as a ruby crystal that when stimulated released a red light of 694 nm wavelength.[47] Dr. Leon Goldman, in 1963, initiated the use of the laser for the medical treatment of skin by applying the ruby laser to a variety of cutaneous conditions.[48,49,50] Over the next 20 years, CO_2 and argon lasers were developed and were used as the primary means to treat skin conditions. Argon was able to address vascular lesions and CO_2 was used for tissue vaporization and destruction of skin pathologies; however, both had high rates of unacceptable scarring when used on the skin primarily because of the nonspecific, global, uncontrolled injury that was caused.[51]

The ability to harness the power of lasers with a decrease of adverse events was realized with the development of the theory of *selective photothermolysis* by Anderson and Parrish in the 1980s.[52] This theory postulates that complicating injury can be decreased by controlling the production of heat around the site of treatment. This is achieved by understanding two concepts: (1) the relationship between target tissue and laser type used, and (2) how to properly adjust laser parameters to achieve the desired result while reducing collateral damage. When we treat skin, we generally aim at brown spots, red spots, or global skin surface (in which water is the primary chemical component). Brown spots are caused by melanin. Red spots are caused by blood (hemoglobin). And water is pervasive throughout, as is the target when the goal is global resurfacing. The target tissue is called a chromophore (because it "likes" a certain color on the electromagnetic spectrum). Melanin is known to preferentially absorb light at lower wavelengths (600–1,100 nm). Hemoglobin absorbs sharply between the wavelengths of 514 to 590 nm. Water absorbs at much higher wavelengths than do the other chromophores, which is why CO_2 (whose laser vibrates at 10,600 nm) will be absorbed by water much more quickly than it will the other chromophores. The type of laser is chosen by the practitioner so that its wavelength will be strongly absorbed by the target chromophore. The more *absorption* takes place (rather than *transmission* or *scatter* of the laser energy), the greater the energy kept within the chromophore (and the higher the heat that builds up within the chromophore) and the less energy that escapes outside of the chromophore (so that surrounding tissues stay cooler and are less likely to burn). Having first taken advantage of this characteristic, the practitioner then adjusts the laser settings such that the time the chromophore is exposed to the laser energy (the *pulse duration*) is less than the *known thermal relaxation time* (a fixed, known characteristic of the chromophore—defined as the time it takes for the chromophore to cool down to half of the peak temperature it reached immediately after it was treated by the laser pulse). Finally, the amount of energy applied (the *energy density* or *fluence*) must be high enough to achieve destruction of the chromophore. Thus, putting it all together, if the practitioner chooses a laser that is preferentially absorbed by the tissue that needs to be treated, *and* the energy density is of adequate intensity to produce destruction, *and* if it is applied over a period of time that is *shorter* than the known thermal relaxation time of the target tissue, then the practitioner should feel confident that the risk of scarring should be low.[51] Having these new guidelines opened the doorway to widespread application of lasers.

As mentioned previously, the first CO_2 and argon lasers were applied by continuous wavelength (CW), which was without pauses. These emitted long exposures of energy that could result in nonspecific tissue injury (thus, the scarring that was seen). The industry expanded to accommodate the ability to harness the principles of selective photothermolysis. Multiple lasers were developed to target chromophores, and the instruments were altered to allow greater flexibility in not only the amount of energy emitted but in the timing of emission pulses to prevent the exceeding of the thermal relaxation times. Pulsed laser systems were developed that allowed pulses of increasingly high energy with greater pauses in between to allow for thermal relaxation. Categories of modifications of pulsing include long-pulsed lasers as seen in the pulse dye laser, short-pulsed lasers such as the quality-switched or Q-switched lasers of ruby, alexandrite, or Nd:YAG (neodymium:yttrium aluminum garnet), and superpulsed CO_2 lasers.[51]

In terms of the application of lasers to achieve resurfacing of facial skin (*ablative* removal of the outer layer to improve texture, wrinkles, pigmentation, and overall beauty), the superpulsed CO_2 laser became the gold standard, but still required a prolonged recovery. The short-pulsed, 1,940-nm Er:YAG (erbium:yttrium aluminum garnet) laser was developed after the CO_2 laser in an effort to limit the difficult recovery seen with the CO_2. Er:YAG is absorbed even more effectively by water (and the epithelium is composed of 90% water), meaning that the energy of the laser ultimately causes less collateral thermal injury. Because of this, there is less impact on the collagen of the dermis and there is also less hemostasis during the procedure. One of the benefits of the CO_2 laser is the long-term continued improvement in the collagen of the dermis, which improves the state of wrinkles. Therefore, although the Er:YAG laser does a good job of reversing the superficial signs of photoaging of the skin, it is not able to induce the collagen changes seen after CO_2 laser resurfacing.[18,51,53]

Once CW CO_2 lasers were updated to pulsed systems that controlled collateral damage, CO_2 laser resurfacing became the primary means of resurfacing for general skin rejuvenation, eventually surpassing the deep phenol peel in frequency of use. However, no single modality is perfect. Recovery was long and arduous, the risk of scarring was still uncomfortably high, and hypopigmentation was not suitable to many patients. Because of these reasons, the industry has continued to seek improvements in the application of the laser. CO_2 laser systems were designed to allow for single passes of the laser (as opposed to multiple passes) to allow for quicker recovery. Er:YAG systems were designed with longer pulse durations to produce more collateral thermal injury to achieve greater collagen contraction. Both of these modifications are also thought to decrease postinflammatory hyperpigmentation, making them more suitable for patients with more native pigment.[51,53]

The concept of fractionated photothermolysis (FP) was published by Dr. Dieter Manstein et al in 2004.[54] His model, developed in 2001, produced pixilated passes of laser contact that resulted in columns of thermal injury resulting in coagulative necrosis. This produced an effect of tissue tightening with mild improvement of superficial signs of photoaging. Although histologically, cell death in the microthermal zone (MTZ)—the zone directly associated with the column of treatment—is seen in the epidermis, the stratum corneum remains structurally intact; therefore, this technique has been named "nonablative." Hantash et al described how the epithelium rids itself of the necrotic debris through the column of treatment.[55] The regions of epithelial necrosis are healed over in around 24 hours; thus, there is a much quicker recovery than that seen in classical ablative laser resurfacing. Since the epithelium is not removed as it is in ablative laser treatment, there is no immediate reduction of dyschromic lesions. Nevertheless, there does seem to be a gradual reduction in these lesions after treatment with FP.[56] Because of the disparity in superficial improvement relative to classical ablative laser resurfacing as well as deep and medium peels, Hantash et al later developed an ablative fractionated model that provided collimated passes of energy that produced the surface ablation while maintaining the columns of thermal necrosis.[57] This technology had the benefit of improving surface irregularities and texture while tightening dermal collagen over the subsequent months of healing, all with a shorter immediate

postoperative recovery of 5 to 7 days and reduced risk of scarring, hypopigmentation, and prolonged erythema.[58,59,60]

1.4.1 Nonablative Laser and Light Treatments for Dyschromias

As more and more patients seek the interventions of facial plastic surgery, the pool of potential subjects increases. This growth has swelled the number of people who want improvement without sacrifice. For the sake of less sacrifice in terms of pain, time off from work, and unpleasant postprocedural appearance, patients are willing to undergo procedures that are designed to produce less dramatic results. The industry has been working to produce a wider array of laser and light-source options that satisfy this increasingly large subset of patients. The recovery process is undeniably quicker and more pleasant if the surface of the epithelium is left intact (*nonablative* treatments). Ablative technologies intentionally destroy the outer layer of the skin. Nonablative technologies intentionally bypass the epithelium to effect a change on the dermis only. The treatment goals for the subset of patients who would choose nonablative modalities include improvement in rhytids and atrophic scars with tissue tightening (techniques that are not technically part of the realm of resurfacing), and also reduction in dyschromias. The treatment of dyschromias is technically a resurfacing result. Laser energy is taken up selectively by melanin, which is heated and denatured within the epithelial cell, which then flakes off, carrying its pigment with it. This controlled processing of the necrotic epidermal debris leads to a gradual reduction in the appearance of the pigmented skin lesion. Typically, for this reason, a number of treatment sessions are required. However, the prolonged recovery with the ablative modalities is not seen.[18,59]

The laser modalities currently available for slow, nonablative resurfacing of skin dyschromias and tattoos include FP with CO_2 and Nd:YAG lasers among others. Tattoos have been seen to respond well when Q-switched pigment lasers are combined with fractionated devices. Other devices shown to be effective in reduction of dyspigmentation include the 1,550-nm erbium-doped fiber laser, the fractionated 1,927-nm laser, the use of low-fluence Nd:YAG, and intense pulsed light and pulsed dye lasers.[18,51]

1.5 Conclusion

The quest for beautiful skin is as old as mankind and is one of the primary reasons that facial plastic surgery exists as a specialty. Never before has such attention been directed toward stopping or turning back the clock in terms of facial aging. Such a driving force will surely maintain the impetus to push the envelope and uncover new facets of skin physiology and mechanics. We look forward to what is surely just beyond the horizon.

References

[1] Song HS, Park TW, Sohn UD, et al. The effect of caffeic acid on wound healing in skin-incised mice. Korean J Physiol Pharmacol 2008; 12: 343–347

[2] Manniche L. Sacred Luxuries: Fragrance, Aromatherapy, and Cosmetics in Ancient Egypt. Ithaca, NY: Cornell University Press; 1999: 134

[3] Brody HJ, Monheit GD, Resnik SS, Alt TH. A history of chemical peeling. Dermatol Surg 2000; 26: 405–409

[4] Castello M, Milani M. Efficacy of topical hydrating and emollient lotion containing 10% urea ISDIN® plus dexpanthenol (Ureadin Rx 10) in the treatment of skin xerosis and pruritus in hemodialyzed patients: an open prospective pilot trial. G Ital Dermatol Venereol 2011 Oct; 146: 321–325

[5] Muhammad SI, Maznah I, Mahmud R, Zuki AB, Imam MU. Upregulation of genes related to bone formation by γ-amino butyric acid and γ-oryzanol in germinated brown rice is via the activation of GABAB-receptors and reduction of serum IL-6 in rats. Clin Interv Aging 2013; 8: 1259–1271

[6] Kromayer E. Die Heilung der Akne durch ein Neues Narbenloses Operationsverfahren: das Stanzen. Illust Monatssehr Aerztl Poly Tech 1905; 27: 101

[7] Kurtin A. Corrective surgical planing of skin; new technique for treatment of acne scars and other skin defects. AMA Arch Derm Syphilol 1953; 68: 389–397

[8] Burke J. Wire Brush Surgery. Springfield, IL: Charles C. Thomas; 1956

[9] Blau S, Rein CR. Dermabrasion of the acne pit. AMA Arch Dermatol Syphilol 1954; 70(6): 754–766

[10] Rattner H, Lazar P. Dermabrasion for the improvement of acne scars. J Am Med Assoc 1959; 171: 2326–2331

[11] Arouète J. Treatment of diffuse blotchiness, erythrosis and acne rosacea with dermabrasion [in French] Bull Soc Fr Dermatol Syphiligr 1970; 77: 799–800

[12] Brown GR, Burks JW, Farber GA. Dermabrasion for showers of seborrheic keratoses. J Dermatol Surg 1976; 2(3): 258–259

[13] Earhart RN, Nuss DD, Martin RJ, Imber R, Aeling JL. Dermabrasion for adenoma sebaceum. J Dermatol Surg 1976; 2(5): 412–414

[14] Roenigk HH Jr. Dermabrasion for miscellaneous cutaneous lesions (exclusive of scarring from acne). J Dermatol Surg Oncol 1977; 3(3): 322–328

[15] Clabaugh W. Removal of tattoos by superficial dermabrasion. Arch Dermatol 1968; 98(5): 515–521

[16] Fitzpatrick RE, Tope WD, Goldman MP, Satur NM. Pulsed carbon dioxide laser, trichloroacetic acid, Baker-Gordon phenol, and dermabrasion: A comparative clinical and histological study of cutaneous resurfacing in a porcine model. Arch Dermatol 1996; 132: 469–471

[17] Giese SY, McKinney P, Roth SI, Zukowski M. The effect of chemosurgical peels and dermabrasion on dermal elastic tissue. Plast Reconstr Surg 1997; 100: 489–498, discussion 499–500

[18] Hanke CW, Moy RL, Roenigk RK, et al. Current status of surgery in dermatology. J Am Acad Dermatol 2013; 69: 972–1001

[19] Nelson BR, Metz RD, Majmudar G, et al. A comparison of wire brush and diamond fraise superficial dermabrasion for photoaged skin. A clinical, immunohistologic, and biochemical study. J Am Acad Dermatol 1996; 34: 235–243

[20] Cox AJ III, Cook TA, Wang TD. Decreased splatter in dermabrasion. Arch Facial Plast Surg 2000; 2: 23–26

[21] Tsai RY, Wang CN, Chan HL. Aluminum oxide crystal microdermabrasion. A new technique for treating facial scarring. Dermatol Surg 1995; 21: 539–542

[22] Karimipour DJ, Rittié L, Hammerberg C, et al. Molecular analysis of aggressive microdermabrasion in photoaged skin. Arch Dermatol 2009; 145: 1114–1122

[23] Katz BE, Truong S, Maiwald DC, Frew KE, George D. Efficacy of microdermabrasion preceding ALA application in reducing the incubation time of ALA in laser PDT. J Drugs Dermatol 2007; 6: 140–142

[24] Kaminer MS, Arndt KA, Dover JS, Rohrer TE, Zachary CB, Eds. Atlas of Cosmetic Surgery. 2nd ed. Philadelphia: Saunders Elsevier; 2009: 225

[25] McCollough EG, Hillman RA, Jr. Chemical face peel. Otolaryngol Clin North Am 1980; 13: 353–365

[26] Kligman AM, Baker TJ, Gordon HL. Long-term histologic follow-up of phenol face peels. Plast Reconstr Surg 1985; 75: 652–659

[27] Hetter GP. An examination of the phenol-croton oil peel: part II. The lay peelers and their croton oil formulas. Plast Reconstr Surg 2000; 105: 240–248, discussion 249–251

[28] Eller JJ, Wolff S. Skin peeling and scarification. JAMA 1941; 116: 934–938

[29] Baker TJ. The ablation of rhytides by chemical means: A preliminary report. J Fla Med Assoc 1961; 48: 451–454

[30] Perkins SW. Chemical peel. In: Cummings CW, ed. Otolaryngology-Head and Neck Surgery. 2nd ed. St. Louis: Mosby-Year Book; 1996: 588–607

[31] Hetter GP. An examination of the phenol-croton oil peel: part IV. Face peel results with different concentrations of phenol and croton oil. Plast Reconstr Surg 2000; 105: 1061–1083, discussion 1084–1087

[32] Stone PA. The use of modified phenol for chemical face peeling. Clin Plast Surg 1998; 25: 21–44

[33] Rullan PP, Lemon J, Rullan J. The 2-day light phenol chemabrasion for deep wrinkles and acne scars: a presentation of face and neck peels. Am J Cosmet Surg 2004; 21: 15–26

[34] Tosti A, Grimes PE, dePadova MP, eds. Color Atlas of Chemical Peels. 2nd ed. Heidelberg, Germany: Springer; 2012: 23–29, 33, 57

[35] Dewandre L, Tenenbaum A. The Chemistry of Peels: A Hypothesis of Action Mechanisms and a Proposal of a New Classification of Chemical Peelings. In: Tung R, Rubin M, eds. Procedures in Cosmetic Dermatology: Chemical Peels. 2nd ed. Philadelphia: Saunders Elsevier; 2011: 1–16

[36] Ridge JM, Siegle RJ, Zuckerman J. Use of alpha-hydroxy acids in the therapy for 'photoaged' skin. J Am Acad Dermatol 1990; 23: 932

[37] Ditre CM, et al. Effects of alpha hydroxy acids on photoaged skin: a pilot clinical, histologic, and ultrastructural study. J Am Acad Dermatol 1996; 34: 187–195

[38] Stüttgen G. Historical perspectives of tretinoin. J Am Acad Dermatol 1986; 15: 735–740

[39] Kligman AM, Fulton JE Jr, Plewig G. Topical vitamin A acid in acne vulgaris. Arch Dermatol 1969; 99: 469–476

[40] Plewig G, Braun-Falco O. Kinetics of epidermis and adnexa following vitamin A acid in the human. Acta Derm Venereol Suppl (Stockh) 1975; 74: 87–98

[41] Kligman AM, Grove GL, Hirose R, Leyden JJ. Topical tretinoin for photoaged skin. J Am Acad Dermatol 1986; 15: 836–859

[42] Weiss JS, Ellis CN, Headington JT, Tincoff T, Hamilton TA, Voorhees JJ. Topical tretinoin improves photoaged skin. A double-blind vehicle-controlled study. JAMA 1988; 259: 527–532

[43] Weinstein GD, Nigra TP, Pochi PE, et al. Topical tretinoin for treatment of photodamaged skin. A multicenter study. Arch Dermatol 1991; 127: 659–665

[44] Bhawan J, Olsen E, Lufrano L, Thorne EG, Schwab B, Gilchrest BA. Histologic evaluation of the long term effects of tretinoin on photodamaged skin. J Dermatol Sci 1996; 11: 177–182

[45] Sekula-Gibbs S, Uptmore D, Otillar L. Retinoids. J Am Acad Dermatol 2004; 50: 405–415

[46] Einstein A. Zur Quantentheorie der Strahlung. Phys Z 1917; 18: 121–128

[47] Maiman T. Stimulated optical radiation in ruby. Nature 1960; 187: 493–494

[48] Goldman L, Blaney DJ, Kindel DJ Jr, Franke EK. Effect of the laser beam on the skin. Preliminary report. J Invest Dermatol 1963; 40: 121–122

[49] Goldman L, Blaney DJ, Kindel DJ Jr, Richfield D, Franke EK. Pathology of the effect of the laser beam on the skin. Nature 1963; 197: 912–914

[50] Goldman L, Rockwell RJ Jr, Meyer R, Otten R. Investigative studies with the laser in the treatment of basal cell epitheliomas. South Med J 1968; 61: 735–742

[51] Tanzi EL, Lupton JR, Alster TS. Lasers in dermatology: four decades of progress. J Am Acad Dermatol 2003; 49: 1–31, quiz 31–34

[52] Anderson RR, Parrish JA. Selective photothermolysis: precise microsurgery by selective absorption of pulsed radiation. Science 1983; 220: 524–527

[53] Alexiades-Armenakas MR, Dover JS, Arndt KA. The spectrum of laser skin resurfacing: nonablative, fractional, and ablative laser resurfacing. J Am Acad Dermatol 2008; 58: 719–737, quiz 738–740

[54] Manstein D, Herron GS, Sink RK, Tanner H, Anderson RR. Fractional photothermolysis: a new concept for cutaneous remodeling using microscopic patterns of thermal injury. Lasers Surg Med 2004; 34: 426–438

[55] Hantash BM, Bedi VP, Sudireddy V, Struck SK, Herron GS, Chan KF. Laser-induced transepidermal elimination of dermal content by fractional photothermolysis. J Biomed Opt 2006; 11: 041115

[56] Laubach HJ, Tannous Z, Anderson RR, Manstein D. Skin responses to fractional photothermolysis. Lasers Surg Med 2006; 38: 142–149

[57] Hantash BM, Bedi VP, Chan KF, Zachary CB. Ex vivo histological characterization of a novel ablative fractional resurfacing device. Lasers Surg Med 2007; 39: 87–95

[58] Hantash BM, Bedi VP, Kapadia B, et al. In vivo histological evaluation of a novel ablative fractional resurfacing device. Lasers Surg Med 2007; 39: 96–107

[59] Tierney EP, Kouba DJ, Hanke CW. Review of fractional photothermolysis: treatment indications and efficacy. Dermatol Surg 2009; 35: 1445–1461

[60] Janik JP, Markus JL, Al-Dujaili Z, Markus RF. Laser resurfacing. Semin Plast Surg 2007; 21: 139–146

2 Anatomy, Physiology, and Pathology of the Skin

Ariel B. Grobman, Sanaz Harirchian, and Lisa D. Grunebaum

2.1 Introduction

Skin is an intricate organ, providing a protective outer layer that supplies insulation, mechanical protection, defense from pathogens, and temperature regulation. This chapter reviews skin anatomy, embryology, and physiology, as well as age-related changes focusing on photoaging.

2.2 Skin Embryology

The earliest stage of skin development is known as the specification stage, which occurs by the 4th week of gestation. During specification, ectoderm lateral to the neural plate is committed to become epidermis, and subsets of mesenchymal and neural crest cells are committed to form the dermis. Initially, a single layer of ectodermal cells covers the embryo's surface. In the 2nd month of gestation, this layer divides to form a superficial protective layer of simple, flattened squamous epithelial cells, the periderm. The cells of the periderm layer then undergo keratinization and begin to slough superficially to be replaced by cells arising from the basal layer. The framework of future layers and specialized structures of skin are now formed. Next, during the morphogenesis stage, these tissues begin to take their particular form: The dermis and hypodermis are delineated; vascular formation occurs; epidermal stratification and epidermal appendage formation also take place. By the 11th week, the basal layer (stratum germinativum) forms an intermediate skin layer. By the end of the 4th month, all the epithelial layers of the epidermis have acquired their definitive arrangement. Also by the 4th month, the mesoderm underlying the ectoderm has differentiated into the dermal layer, which begins to produce collagen and elastic fibers; blood vessel formation also takes place in this dermal layer. Hair follicle and sebaceous gland growth initiate in the growing fetus by the 5th month. During the first 3 months of development, neural crest cells infiltrate the epidermis and differentiate into pigment-producing melanocytes.[1]

2.2.1 Epidermis

The skin is divided into three main layers that vary in quality and appearance in different areas of the body: the epidermis, dermis, and superficial fascia. The epidermis is divided into five distinct layers and may range in thickness from 0.05 mm on the eyelids to 0.8 to 1.5 mm on the soles on the feet. The cellular layers of the epidermis from deepest to most superficial (▶ Fig. 2.1) include:

- Stratum basale (basal or germinal cell layer)
- Stratum spinosum (spinous or prickle cell layer)
- Stratum granulosum (granular cell layer)
- Stratum corneum (horny layer)
- Stratum lucidum (a thin layer of translucent cells seen in thick epidermis representing a transition from the stratum granulosum and stratum corneum)

The epidermis is mainly composed of keratinocytes, with smaller numbers of melanocytes, Langerhans cells, and Merkel cells. The Langerhans cells are dendritic cells responsible for capturing and presenting antigens within the epidermis to circulating lymphocytes. Merkel cells are somatic afferent sensory cells that provide light touch discrimination; they can become neoplastic in some cases and form Merkel cell carcinoma.

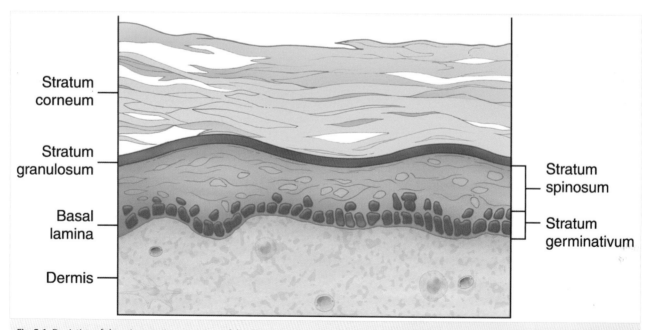

Fig. 2.1 Depiction of the microscopic appearance of the dermis and epidermal layers. Note the progression of the nucleated keratinocytes of the basal layer as they migrate superficially and differentiate into the anucleated, flattened corneocytes of the stratum corneum.

The stratum basale, the innermost layer, lies adjacent to the dermis and contains keratinocytes in various stages of division, attached to the basement membrane by hemidesmosomes. The basal layer also contains melanocytes, the pigment-producing cells. Through their dendritic processes, the melanocytes transfer pigmented melanin granules in vesicles named melanosomes to keratinocytes. The melanosomes accumulate atop the nucleus of the recipient cell protecting the deoxyribonucleic acid (DNA) from ultraviolet (UV) radiation damage. Melanin, a derivative of tyrosine, is an effective absorber of light; it is able to dissipate more than 99.9% of absorbed UV radiation. The number of melanocytes is the same in equivalent body sites in human beings of all skin pigments; however, the distribution and rate of production of melanin differ.

The cells of the stratum basale are anchored into a complex structure known as the basement membrane, or dermoepidermal junction. This poorly defined, eosinophilic staining structure provides nutrients and waste disposal for the epidermis, and acts as chemical and physical barriers. The basement membrane has strong anchoring collagen fibrils that secure it to the underlying dermis. In addition, the undersurface of the epidermis contains epithelial projections called rete ridges, or rete pegs, that extend between the papillae of the dermis and provide increased mechanical support.

Superficial to the stratum basale lies the stratum spinosum, or prickle cell layer that derives its name from the appearance of the intercellular desmosomes linking these keratinized polygonal cells. The next layer is the stratum granulosum, or granular cell layer. At this point the keratinocytes begin to lose their nuclei, exhibit coarse cytoplasmic granules, and appear basophilic. On the palms of the hand and the soles of the feet there is an intermediate, clear cell layer, the stratum lucidum; this represents a transition between the cells of the stratum granulosum and stratum corneum. The stratum corneum, the outermost layer, forms a protective barrier against infection, dehydration, chemicals, UV radiation, and mechanical stressors. Studies have determined this layer to be from 8.7 to 12.9 μm thick.[2] The cells of this layer, known as corneocytes, are anucleated keratinocytes that become flattened and stack up 10- to 30-cells thick at the skin surface. The palms of the hand and soles of the feet have the highest density of corneocytes at the skin surface. The corneocyte is enveloped in a proteinaceous covering and contains water-retaining keratin. In addition, the extracellular matrix surrounding these cells contains stacked, lipid bilayers providing a hydrophobic barrier.

2.2.2 Dermis

The dermis is found beneath the basement membrane and is composed of a supportive cell matrix. The dermis varies in thickness from 0.6 mm on the eyelids to 3 mm on the back, palms of the hands, and soles of the feet. Within the dermis lie cells such as fibroblasts, mast cells, and macrophages, as well as branches of the peripheral nervous system, blood vessels, and epidermal appendages. The two layers of the dermis are the papillary layer and the reticular layer.

The papillary dermis contains loosely organized collagen fibers, blood vessels, and fibroblasts. It is located below the dermoepidermal junction and is relatively thin in comparison with the reticular dermis. The fibroblasts are plentiful within the papillary dermis and are responsible for synthesizing collagen, elastin, and proteoglycans. During the wound-healing process they may become active collagen-producing cells and may transform into contractile cells during the contraction phase of wound healing. Experimental data suggest that this differentiation occurs after wound formation under the influence of transforming growth factor-beta (TGF-β1), mechanical tension, and exposed extracellular matrix components. Blockade of the contraction cascade and treatment of wounds with new dermal regeneration templates appear to prevent scar formation.[3]

The reticular dermis is composed of rigid, netlike, bundles of collagen that run parallel to the skin surface, extending from the papillary layer to the subdermis or superficial fascia. The structure of the dermis differs greatly at diverse anatomical sites. For example, the structure of facial dermis is highly influenced by abundant hair follicles and numerous large sebaceous glands in men. The high concentration of these appendages likely puts the connective tissue matrix of the dermis under added tension.

2.3 Skin Appendages

Hair follicles are most abundant on the scalp and the face, and are derivatives of the epidermis and dermis. Each hair follicle is lined by germinative cells that produce keratin and melanocytes that synthesize pigment. The hair shaft consists of an outer cuticle, a cortex of keratinocytes, an inner medulla, and a surrounding root sheath. An erector pili muscle is associated with the hair shaft and is innervated by the sympathetic nervous system.

Sebaceous glands are epidermal cell derivatives that are found in the hair-bearing regions of the skin. Sebaceous glands secrete a substance called sebum through holocrine secretion into the hair follicle. Sebum may help to maintain the epidermal permeability barrier, function in hormonal signaling, transport antioxidants, and provide added protection from UV radiation. Sweat glands are classified into two main types: apocrine and eccrine. Apocrine glands are found in the axillae and groin and produce an odorless, protein-rich secretion. When acted upon by bacteria, this secretion becomes odiferous. Eccrine sweat glands are found throughout the body, and in especially high density on the palms, soles, forehead, and axillae. In fact, the only cutaneous regions lacking eccrine glands are the mucocutaneous junctions and nail beds (▶ Fig. 2.2).

2.3.1 Superficial Fascia

This layer, also known as the subcutis, contains a mixture of fibrous and fatty tissue. The ratio of fibrous to fatty substance differs based on the following factors: bodily region, gender, and nutritional status (smaller fat deposits in more malnourished individuals). On the trunk and extremities the fatty substance predominates, allowing easier surgical undermining of the skin.[4] On the face the subcutaneous tissue plays quite an important functional role since it contains the tendon fibers of the facial muscles.[5] The superficial fascia of the face contains a mixture of fibrous septa and fatty tissue. On the lateral face, the fibrous septa attach to the dermis with vertical septa, forming the superficial musculoaponeurotic system (SMAS) that extends from the platysma to the galea aponeurotica. The SMAS

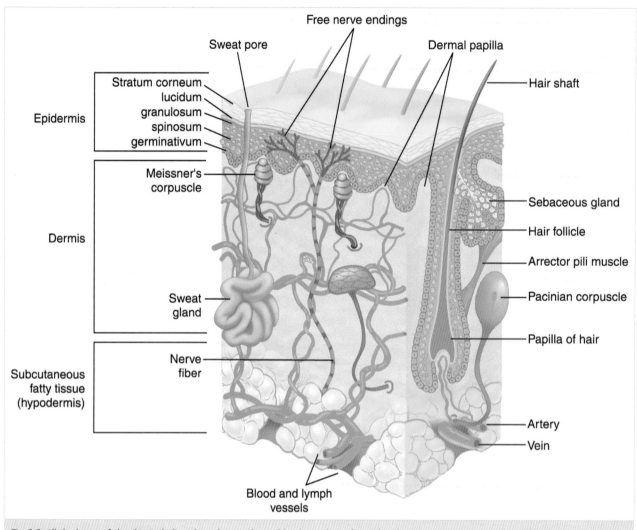

Fig. 2.2 All the layers of the skin including dermal appendages, blood vessels, and peripheral nervous structures are shown here.

constitutes a compartment through which vessels branch and connect before reaching the subdermal level.

2.3.2 Blood Vessels

The deep plexus is a vascular network that lies in the outer portion of the superficial fascia. From this deep network small arteries pass vertically to the papillary dermis becoming the superficial plexus. Branches of the superficial plexus give rise to ascending capillary loops that supply the dermal papillae before becoming venules in the superficial venous plexus. Due to the dilated arteriolar network concentrated in the face, telangiectasias of the facial skin respond well to lasers emitting wavelengths in the yellow portion of the spectrum.[4] Venous predominant telangiectasias respond better to sclerotic agents than to laser therapy.

2.3.3 Nerves

All cutaneous nerves have their cell bodies in the dorsal root ganglia. Free nerve endings in the dermis sense pain and temperature. Specialized receptors named Meissner corpuscles lie in the dermal papillae and receive light touch sensation. Pressure and vibration are detected by specialized structures named Pacinian corpuscles that are densely distributed throughout the superficial fascia of the palms and soles. The autonomic nervous system supplies the motor innervation of the skin—adrenergic fibers innervate blood vessels, erector pili muscles, and apocrine glands—whereas cholinergic fibers innervate eccrine sweat glands. The endocrine system regulates the sebaceous glands, which are not innervated by autonomic fibers.

2.4 Wound Healing

The wound-healing process consists of four highly integrated and overlapping phases[6]:
- Hemostasis
- Inflammation
- Proliferation
- Tissue remodeling

Tissue injury (e.g., abrasion, laceration, burn, or contusion) affecting the dermal blood vessels triggers an immediate 5- to 10-minute vasoconstrictive response. The exposed, injured endothelial cells activate the coagulation cascade initially triggering platelet aggregation and adhesion. Vasoconstriction is then followed by a period of vasodilation, due to mast cell-mediated release of histamine and serotonin. Vasodilation allows infiltration of platelets and leukocytes, which release cytokines, thereby initiating the inflammatory process—persisting for up to ~ 72 hours. Gross inflammation manifests as hyperemia and edema in and around the wound. Cytokine release by platelets, exposure to bacterial antigens, and the complementing activation cascade stimulate neutrophil influx into the wound. The inflammatory stage can be classified into two parts: In the early phase there is an influx of neutrophils followed by a late phase in which macrophages predominate. Cytokine release and the complementing activation stimulate neutrophil migration, an essential aspect of proper wound healing. The neutrophils migrate to the site of the wound and through phagocytosis remove bacteria and foreign debris from the wound. By the 3rd day after the injury, macrophages become the predominant cell type found in the healing wound. Macrophages stimulate wound healing through direct phagocytosis; activation of lymphocytes; and synthesis of potent growth factors such as transforming growth factor (TGF), fibroblast growth factor (FGF), platelet-derived growth factor (PDGF), and vascular endothelial growth factor (VEGF). These growth factors promote endothelial cell growth, fibroblast proliferation, and angiogenesis.

By the 3rd to 7th day of wound healing, the system focuses on covering the wound surface, forming granulation tissue, and restoring the vascular network. This is referred to as the proliferative stage. During this period fibroblasts migrate along the fibrin network laying down the matrix of connective tissue for wound closure and restoration of mechanical strength. Next, keratinocytes lying at the edge of the wound, as well as epithelial stem cells from hair follicles and sweat glands, migrate toward the center of the wound. This process occurs through enzymatic loosening of keratinocyte desmosomes and keratinocyte "shuffling" along the newly created fibrin network along a chemotactic network toward the center of the wound.[7]

The final wound-healing stage, known as neovascularization, deals with the restoration of the intricate vascular network of the fresh wound. Existing endothelial cells on intact neighboring vessels interact with newly synthesized growth factors from the wound and begin to proliferate and sprout new branches that connect with others, forming vascular loops. From this point, the new endothelial cells may recruit pericytes and smooth muscle cells in order to differentiate into venules and arterioles.

Next, granulation tissue forms through high density of fibroblasts, granulocytes, macrophages, capillaries, and loose bundles of collagen. It appears characteristically red and fragile due to disorganized, incomplete angiogenesis. The final stage of wound healing is tissue remodeling, which may last from 21 days up to 1 year after injury. The fibroblast is the workhorse of extracellular matrix formation and is responsible for wound strengthening by the conversion of type III collagen to the stronger type I collagen. Fibroblasts begin to differentiate into myofibroblasts, leading to wound contraction and closure. Wound myofibroblasts help decrease wound surface area through extracellular collagen fiber deposition and contraction by intracellular contraction and concomitant alignment of the collagen fibers by integrin-mediated pull on collagen bundles. Finally, wound blood flow declines and metabolic activity within the wound stops.

Multiple experimental models have demonstrated that skin damage caused in utero heals differently from nonfetal skin. Fetal skin injuries heal without scar formation and with preservation of dermal appendages such as hair follicles and sebaceous glands.[3] In nonfetal scar tissue the dermoepidermal junction is repaired without rete ridges and dermal skin appendages, which may contribute to the susceptibility of scar tissue to damage from shearing forces. Scar formation in skin wounds appears to be secondary to contraction during healing; this was demonstrated in studies that showed near abolishment of scar formation when skin wounds were manipulated with scaffolds that partially blocked contraction.[3]

2.5 Skin Aging

In the newborn, the skin is smooth, usually uniform in pigmentation, and lacks surface irregularities. During the aging process there are endogenous and exogenous causes of skin change. Endogenous or intrinsic aging proceeds in all organisms due to the interplay of predetermined genetic factors and the influence of time. Endogenous changes can be characterized by cellular or microscopic tissue changes or macroscopic and functional changes. Similar to cellular aging in other organs, endogenous aging is thought to involve decreased proliferative capacity leading to cellular senescence, and altered biosynthetic activity of skin-derived cells.[8] It is believed that the progression of keratinocytes from their beginnings in the stratum basale to the anucleated corneocyte in the stratum corneum takes ~ 2 weeks. This cellular maturation process of the epidermal keratinocytes is thought to progress more slowly as the human being ages, thereby diminishing the capacity for re-epithelialization after tissue insult. As a result, corneocytes are found to be larger due to delayed epidermal turnover. Loose adhesion of the corneocytes due to the delayed epidermal turnover rate may contribute to epidermal skin loss after repeat application and removal of adhesive tape in the older adult, as well as predispose to higher rates of contact dermatitis due to greater dermal permeability.

The aging skin is also characterized by a decrease in the number of basal keratinocytes per unit area, thinning/flattening of the dermoepidermal junction, a decrease in Langerhans cell population, and a decrease in active melanocyte population by 8 to 20% per decade.[9] This population decline affects epidermal and hair follicle melanocytes resulting in irregular skin pigmentation and hypopigmented hair. Thinning of the dermoepidermal junction is observed by the sixth decade and is attributed to a decrease in the number and size of dermal papillae. Studies have demonstrated a decrease from 40 papillae/mm^2 in young skin to 14 papillae/mm^2 in subjects age 65 and older. In older skin, this decrease in dermal papillae interdigitation leads to increased susceptibility to tissue damage from shearing forces.[10] Other changes include decreased cell populations of Meissner and Pacinian corpuscles, resulting in poorer discrimination of pressure and light touch.

Over time, changes to the dermis include: elastic fiber degradation, decrease in collagen synthesis, decrease in blood vessel and nerve ending distribution, and overall decrease in

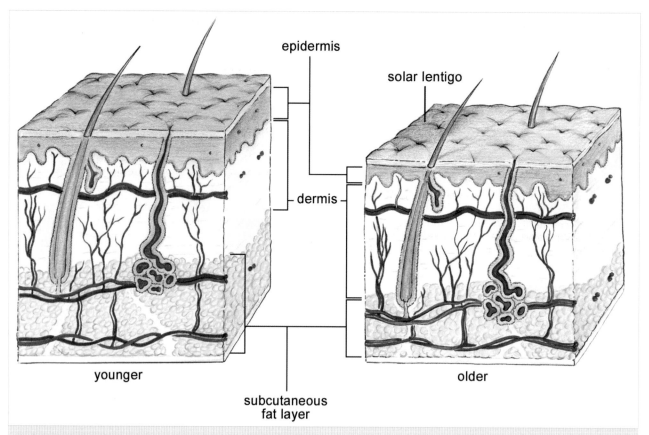

Fig. 2.3 Skin aging is characterized by endogenous and exogenous changes. Sun exposure mainly affects the epidermal layer of the skin, whereas age-related changes are found in each level. Epidermal pigment change in the aging skin, thinning of the epidermis and dermis, and atrophy of adipose tissue in the subcutaneous layer are displayed here.

cellularity. Rete pegs flatten in the aging human, causing increased susceptibility to shearing forces from minor trauma in the older adult.

In the human dermis the organization of collagen fibers determines the mechanical characteristics of the tissues and resistance to deformational forces. Elastin functions to recoil the stretched collagen fibers to their relaxed position. Fibroblasts and dermal dendrocytes produce proteoglycans, glycosaminoglycans, and glycoproteins that permeate the elastin network creating a structural steady state of connective tissue fibers.[11] As humans age there is a decrease in the elastic rebound properties of the skin with an increase in extensibility. This is likely due to increased degradation of dermal collagen by tissue matrix metalloproteinases over time. Collagen becomes more haphazardly oriented and loss occurs at around 1% per year throughout adult life.[12,13] There does not appear to be any relationship between gender and quantifiable change in human skin biomechanics over time.

One of the most ubiquitous and obvious skin changes with aging is reduction in skin thickness. Thinning of skin affects all cell layers, although dermal collagen and elastin losses account for most of the reduction in total skin thickness. This effect is most obvious in exposed areas such as the extensors, neck, upper chest, and face. The hypodermis and superficial fascia tend to undergo atrophy of fat deposits, contributing to volume loss; the basement membrane, however, is noted to increase in thickness over time (▶ Fig. 2.3).

On a macroscopic level, aging of facial skin takes place gradually over two to four decades. In its early stages, little clinical evidence is present with the exception of the mosaic, faint (subclinical) melanoderma. The characteristic clinical signs of facial aging usually begin to be recognized by individuals with the emergence of discrete furrows and wrinkles, together with a loss of firmness.[13] The skin thins, dries, wrinkles, and becomes unevenly pigmented. Skin may show a loss of tone and elasticity, increased fragility, areas of purpura caused by blood vessel weakness and benign lesions such as keratoses, telangiectasias, and skin tags. There is a loss of subcutaneous fat, and soft tissue ptosis and descent. Rhytids form due to a reduction in muscle mass and skin thickness, cross-linking of collagen and elastin in the dermis, and dehydration of the stratum corneum.

2.5.1 Photoaging

Extrinsic aging of skin changes occurs due to external factors, of which sun exposure is considered the most deleterious. Symptoms of photoaging, or *dermatoheliosis*, include rhytids, dryness, irregular pigmentation, loss of elasticity, telangiectasias, and purpura.[14] Extrinsically aged skin (such as that found on the face, hands, and chest) is wrinkled, sallow in color, and has areas of hyperpigmentation and hypopigmentation. The histological effect of photoaging on the epidermis has not been universal; some subjects report epidermal thickening, whereas others report thinning. Typically, photoaging results in

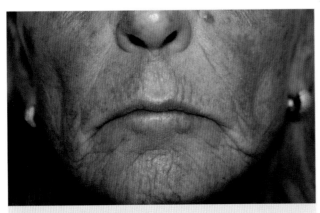

Fig. 2.4 This sun-exposed female patient exhibits signs of photoaging which include dermatoheliosis, rhytid formation, spotty pigmentation and telangiectasia.

epidermal thickening due to irregular growth of basal keratinocytes with cellular and nuclear atypia.[15] Dermal elastin also increases proportional to the amount of UV light exposure.[16] This elastosis and epidermal irregularity can result in a rough, dry, leathery texture with rhytids and deep furrows (▶ Fig. 2.4).

Specific histological changes characterize photodamaged skin. UV radiation is theorized to accelerate telomere shortening in sun-exposed skin and may induce expression of metalloproteinases that degrade dermal collagen and elastin.[11] In addition to a thickened epidermis, photoaged skin is characterized by an irregular, outer keratin layer,[17] fewer sebaceous glands, and increased water loss. Fibroblasts and inflammatory infiltrates in the dermis increase.[18] Heliodermatitis refers to this chronic inflammation seen in photoaged skin. The basement membrane is thickened; this reflects possible damage to basal keratinocytes.[19] Melanocyte distribution along the basement membrane becomes increasingly irregular, leading to dyschromias. In addition, elastosis occurs, developing at the junction of the papillary and reticular dermis.[20] Photodamage is primarily characterized by this elastosis, disorganization of collagen fibrils, and abnormal elastin-containing material.[18]

2.6 Conclusion

This chapter reviews skin anatomy, embryology, and physiology. Through understanding the clinical and histological changes seen with aging and photodamage, clinicians are better able to address cutaneous rejuvenation.

References

[1] Pansky B. Review of Medical Embryology. New York, NY: Macmillan; 1982

[2] Egawa M, Hirao T, Takahashi M. In vivo estimation of stratum corneum thickness from water concentration profiles obtained with Raman spectroscopy. Acta Derm Venereol 2007; 87: 4–8

[3] Yannas IV. Similarities and differences between induced organ regeneration in adults and early foetal regeneration. J R Soc Interface 2005; 2: 403–417

[4] Papel ID. Facial Plastic and Reconstructive Surgery. 3rd ed. New York, NY: Thieme Medical Publishers; 2009

[5] Ghassemi A, Prescher A, Riediger D, Axer H. Anatomy of the SMAS revisited. Aesthetic Plast Surg 2003; 27: 258–264

[6] Gosain A, DiPietro LA. Aging and wound healing. World J Surg 2004; 28: 321–326

[7] Reinke JM, Sorg H. Wound repair and regeneration. Eur Surg Res 2012; 49: 35–43

[8] Puizina-Ivić N. Skin aging. Acta Dermatovenerol Alp Pannonica Adriat 2008; 17: 47–54

[9] Rees JL. The genetics of sun sensitivity in humans. Am J Hum Genet 2004; 75: 739–751

[10] Südel KM, Venzke K, Mielke H, et al. Novel aspects of intrinsic and extrinsic aging of human skin: beneficial effects of soy extract. Photochem Photobiol 2005; 81: 581–587

[11] Pierard G, Henry F, Quatresooz P. Facial skin rheology. In: Farage MA, Miller KW, Maibach HI, eds. Textbook of Aging Skin. 1st ed. Berlin, Germany: Springer-Verlag; 2010:265–273

[12] Montagna W, Carlisle K. Structural changes in ageing skin. Br J Dermatol 1990; 122 Suppl 35: 61–70

[13] Lober CW, Fenske NA. Cutaneous aging: effect of intrinsic changes on surgical considerations. South Med J 1991; 84: 1444–1446

[14] Grunebaum LD, Murdock J, Hoosien GE, Heffelfinger RN, Lee WW. Laser treatment of skin texture and fine line etching. Facial Plast Surg Clin North Am 2011; 19: 293–301

[15] Rigel DS, Weiss RA, Lim HW, Dover J. Photoaging. Boca Raton, FL: CRC Press; 2004

[16] Draelos Z. Cosmetic Dermatology: Products and Procedures. Hoboken, NJ: John Wiley & Sons; 2011

[17] Pearlman SJ, Tadros M. Skin Rejuvenation. In: Truswell WH, ed. Surgical Facial Rejuvenation: A Roadmap to Safe and Reliable Outcomes. New York, NY: Thieme Medical Publishers; 2009: 113–130

[18] Rabe JH, Mamelak AJ, McElgunn PJ, Morison WL, Sauder DN. Photoaging: mechanisms and repair. J Am Acad Dermatol 2006; 55: 1–19

[19] Berneburg M, Plettenberg H, Krutmann J. Photoaging of human skin. Photodermatol Photoimmunol Photomed 2000; 16: 239–244

[20] Kligman AM. Early destructive effect of sunlight on human skin. JAMA 1969; 210: 2377–2380

3 The Science Behind Lasers: How the Physical Properties of Lasers Affect the Skin

Mark M. Hamilton

3.1 Introduction

Lasers have played an increasingly important role in facial plastic surgery as our understanding of how to harness their energy has grown. The initial concept of a laser started less than a century ago with Albert Einstein's paper on the quantum theory of radiation,[1] but it wasn't until 1954 that the first working model was built. The term *laser* was coined by Gordon Gould in 1958 for *l*ight *a*mplification by *s*timulated *e*mission of *r*adiation.[2] Just 2 years later, Theodore Maiman developed the first functioning laser, a flashlamp-pumped ruby laser emitting a 694-nm wavelength.[3]

The first reported use of lasers on skin by Leon Goldman et al was for tattoo removal.[4] Since that time, the applications for lasers in facial plastic surgery have grown exponentially. Lasers can be used in softening facial rhytids, improving skin texture, providing skin tightening, removing vascular and pigmented birthmarks, and disposing of unwanted hair. With this growth has come improved safety, reduced downtime, and improved effectiveness.

3.2 Laser Theory

All light travels in waveforms. The waveforms can be characterized by their wavelength, amplitude, and frequency (▶ Fig. 3.1). Ordinary light emits photons of varying wavelength, frequency, direction, and amplitude. Laser light is unique in that it is more uniform—the light is of a single wavelength (monochromatic), direction (collimated), and frequency (coherence).

Laser light development is based on Einstein's quantum mechanics. He first discovered the theory of stimulated emission within the framework of quantum theory, and all modern laser physics is based on this principle. Quantum mechanics states that if an atom is in an excited state, it is unstable and will seek to return to its lower energy, ground state. The atom will emit a photon in the process of returning to its ground state. However, if an incident photon strikes the already-excited atom, two photons will be emitted as it returns to its ground state. These two pathways for photon emission are referred to as spontaneous and stimulated emission, with the latter being the basis for laser physics.

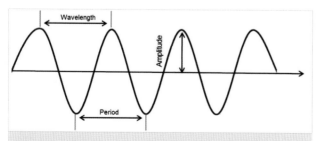

Fig. 3.1 Waveforms can be characterized by their amplitude, wavelength, and period.

Spontaneous emission of radiation occurs when an atom in excited state transitions to a state with a lower energy (ground state), and in the process emits energy in the form of a photon. A photon is a unit (or quanta) of light (▶ Fig. 3.2a).

Stimulated emission of radiation occurs when an incident photon strikes an atom already in an excited state. The atom again transitions to a lower energy state, but will emit two identical photons with the same wavelength, phase, frequency, and direction of the photon from the incident wave because it was struck in an excited state (▶ Fig. 3.2b).

3.2.1 Laser Components

A laser is constructed from three principal parts (▶ Fig. 3.3):
• An energy source (usually referred to as a pump source)
• A laser medium (can be a solid, liquid, gas, or semiconductive material)
• Two or more mirrors that form an optical resonator (also referred to as an optical cavity)

The laser medium is the component that determines the wavelength (and therefore the color) and frequency of the light

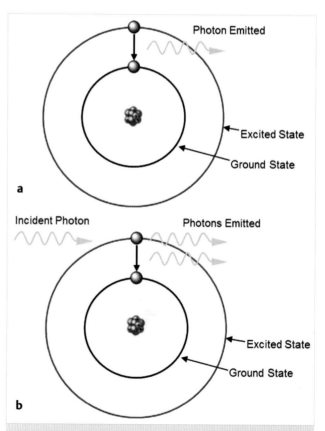

Fig. 3.2 Two pathways for photon emission. **(a)** Spontaneous emission. **(b)** Stimulated emission.

emitted. Lasers are most often categorized by their wavelength on the electromagnetic spectrum (▶ Fig. 3.4). Early lasers used gas as their laser medium: nitrogen (N), carbon dioxide (CO_2), helium (He), and neon (Ne). The lasers that followed used liquids, and were referred to as dye lasers. Dye lasers are capable of generating a wider range of wavelengths than other laser mediums. Solid-state laser mediums were the next iteration, with one of the earliest still being used today (neodymium: yttrium aluminum garnet [Nd:YAG] lasers).

The basic design of a laser is a laser medium placed within the reflective surfaces of the optical resonator. One of the surfaces is fully reflective and the other is partially reflective. Electrical current is the energy source for most clinical lasers, and provides the energy necessary to excite the laser medium. When the laser medium is in an excited state, the laser wavelength is amplified as it passes through the laser medium. The mirrors reflect the laser and ensure many passes of the laser light beam through the medium, allowing repeated amplification. The amplified light then escapes the partially reflective surface as a beam of light. This laser light is then transmitted to the intended treatment area by a delivery system.

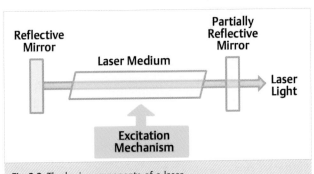

Fig. 3.3 The basic components of a laser.

Lasers are more organized, intense, and focused than ordinary light. Laser light is collimated, coherent, and monochromatic. All of these characteristics of laser light allow the focused, targeted use of light in clinical treatments.

3.3 Laser–Tissue Interactions

Laser light can have a variety of interactions with tissues. These include reflection, absorption, scatter, or transmission through the tissue.[5] There are a multitude of possibilities of overall interaction depending on the degree to which these four phenomena occur. The factors that determine the initial effect include the laser wavelength, laser power, laser waveform, tissue optical properties, and tissue thermal properties. In general, absorption controls to a great degree how much reflection, scatter, and transmission occur, and this is primarily determined by wavelength.

Energy is deposited in a tissue when absorption occurs. When light is either reflected, scattered, or transmitted, no energy is deposited and the laser has no effect. When absorption does occur, energy is deposited and molecules begin to vibrate. What occurs depends on how much energy is absorbed. At low energy levels, biological modifications can occur. These can include activation of biochemical reactions or stimulation of the tissues. Clinical examples of this include use of light-emitting diodes (LED) technology to provide skin rejuvenation and stimulate hair growth.

At higher energy absorption, thermal effects begin to occur. These can range from denaturation of biological proteins at lower energy levels to coagulation and vaporization of the tissues at higher energy levels. These are the effects for which lasers are most commonly used. Clinical examples include laser coagulation of bleeding tissues and skin rejuvenation by coagulation and vaporization of epidermal and dermal skin.

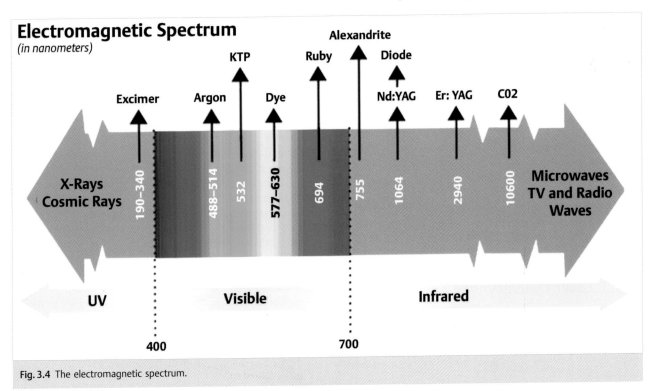

Fig. 3.4 The electromagnetic spectrum.

3.3.1 Selective Photothermolysis

Optimal use of lasers has been enhanced with understanding of the concept of selective photothermolysis.[6] Proposed by Anderson and Parrish in 1983, this theory refers to the precise targeting of a structure or tissue using a specific wavelength of light with the intention of absorbing light energy into that target tissue alone. The energy is directed into the target tissue in such a fashion as to damage the target while allowing surrounding tissue to remain untouched. Three components of this interaction are wavelength, intensity, and pulse duration.

The laser wavelength for the target in this theory is selected by its chromophore or substance that absorbs a particular wavelength. This is most obvious with tattoos, where a particular laser is chosen based on its absorption by the color of the tattoo ink (chromophore). With this, appropriate laser energy is absorbed more by the tattoo and less by the uncolored surrounding skin.

The laser energy must be of sufficient strength to either coagulate or vaporize the target. This energy level depends on the physical properties of the target. Laser parameters of power and spot size can be manipulated to reach this energy level.

A third component of selective photothermolysis is pulse duration. The pulse duration is the period of energy deposition. The pulse duration should be shorter than the time the target tissue is able to transfer heat (energy) to the surrounding tissues (thermal relaxation time). The shorter the pulse, the less energy dissipation and the more selectively the target is destroyed.

3.3.2 Laser Definitions

Using selective photothermolysis depends on understanding laser parameters that can be modified and the terms to describe them:

- Energy—basic physical quantitative property related to activity, measured in joules
- The capacity to do work—joules (J) = watts (W) × 1 second (s)
- Fluence—amount of energy (joules) that is applied to a surface area of tissue (cm^2)
- Power—amount of energy per period of time, measured in watts
- Power density—irradiance, rate of energy delivery per target area (W/cm^2)
- Wavelength—distance in waveform between two successive peaks
- Amplitude—height in waveform of peak, related to intensity
- Frequency—amount of time for one full wave cycle
- Chromophore—a part of a molecule responsible for its color
- Thermal relaxation time—the amount of time required for an object to dissipate one half of its heat
- Spot size—cross-sectional area of the laser beam

3.3.3 Laser Delivery

Lasers can be delivered in a variety of modes. In a continuous mode the laser is always on. Energy is dissipated to surrounding tissues and thus minimizes the chances for selective photothermolysis.

Pulsing of the laser can be performed to more selectively use laser energy. This allows for cooling of the tissues in between pulses. There are several ways to pulse laser energy.

In a shuttered or gated mode, laser energy is simply turned off between pulses. If the duration between pulses is less than the thermal relaxation time of the target tissue, there is less heat dissipation and less risk of injury to surrounding tissues. Typically, peak energy is unchanged from continuous mode.

In a superpulse mode, the laser energy is not merely turned off between pulses, but actually allowed to build up, allowing higher energy during the pulse. Thus, higher energy levels are achieved during superpulse than are achieved during continuous or shuttered.

An improvement on superpulse technology was ultrapulse. Ultrapulse technology allows for high peak energy levels for very short periods of time. Typically, it requires four to five superpulses to deliver the same energy as one ultrapulse. This allows for more precise removal of tissue with less heat dissipation. It is considered the standard for CO_2 laser resurfacing.

Q-switched or quality-switched lasers are another method of pulsing energy. Compared to shuttered, the pulse energies are much higher over a very short pulse width.

An alternative to pulsed systems was a scanning-type device. With a scanning of the system, the laser beam is swept across the tissue rapidly enough that the tissue dwell time is less than the thermal relaxation time. This can give the same effect as a pulsed device. Although this method was used by the Sharplan company in the early days of CO_2-laser resurfacing, this technology is no longer used today.

3.3.4 Fractional Resurfacing

Fractional lasers were developed to minimize downtime and lower the risk profile of resurfacing lasers. This technology depends on treating only a percentage of the skin surface at a microscopic level. This allows for bridges of untreated tissue that can assist with quicker healing. The areas of treated skin in fractional resurfacing are called microscopic treatment zones (MTZ), also called microthermal zones (▶ Fig. 3.5). The size and density of these can be varied depending on the device. The MTZ includes both the ablated tissue and any surrounding coagulated tissue.

The first fractional laser was a nonablative, 1,550-nm laser (Fraxel SR, Solta Medical, Hayward, California).[7] With time, ablative fractional laser devices such as CO_2 and erbium became available. Although these devices allowed better results than nonablative lasers, they also brought increased downtime and potential for risks.

Fractional lasers can be contoured to allow for extremely deep penetration. Some fractional CO_2 devices allow for treatment depths of 1,200 μm and with the erbium:yttrium aluminum garnet laser (Er:YAG) up to 1,500 μm. This is thought to be more effective for deep rhytids and acne scarring, but studies demonstrating their benefit are still lacking.

Fractionating lasers have allowed patients to get a portion of the benefit of nonfractional devices with less downtime and a lower risk profile. In addition, they allow for the treatment of a broader range of skin types. It is important for laser surgeons to recognize their limitations while discussing their benefits.[8]

Other laser variables to consider include laser spot size, laser tissue distance, and skin cooling. Given equal energy output, changes in spot size can have significant impact. In keeping the energy level constant while increasing spot size, there will be a decrease in thermal energy per centimeter of tissue and less response. On the flip side, decreasing spot size without decreasing energy will increase tissue effect as well as possible risk.

If a laser beam is truly collimated, changing the distance of the laser from the target should have little effect. Most lasers, however, are focused with a focal point for optimal treatment. If the laser tissue distance is increased, the resulting deposition of energy at the surface will be decreased. Most systems have an attached aiming arm for the appropriate laser tissue distance.

Skin cooling can also change the dynamics with laser energy. By cooling the top layers of skin to protect from thermal injury, higher energy levels can be delivered safely. A variety of cooling systems exist including forced cool air, cryogen sprays, and contact cooling (glass piece cooled by water or other coolant).

3.4 Laser Wavelengths

Lasers are most often first categorized by their wavelengths (▶ Fig. 3.4). In the sections that follow, the profiles of the main laser wavelengths utilized in facial plastic surgery are discussed.

3.4.1 Carbon Dioxide

The CO_2 laser is the most common type used for facial rejuvenation. Its high absorption by water makes it an excellent choice for resurfacing skin. Its 10,600-nm wavelength is in the infrared invisible range of the electromagnetic spectrum. Thus, it is often accompanied by a He-Ne beam for aiming. The laser medium is CO_2 gas and it is delivered through articulated arms that contain mirrors. Electricity is used for excitation.

The CO_2 laser is most often used for skin resurfacing with water as the chromophore. The critical threshold for tissue ablation with the CO_2 laser is 5 J/cm^2 in less than 1 second to achieve tissue vaporization.[8] Two methods were originally developed to achieve this goal—one, superpulsed technology, is primarily used today. Computer pattern generators (CPGs) were added to allow treatment of larger areas quickly. The other mode, scanning technology, has largely been abandoned.[9]

Laser resurfacing can be used to improve facial rhytids, dyschromias, and skin laxity (▶ Fig. 3.6a, b). The first effect of CO_2 lasers is vaporization of the tissue, just as it is achieved with chemical peels or dermabrasion. The depth of ablation varies depending on energy levels and number of passes. Typical treatments result in ablation depths in the same range as medium-depth trichloroacetic acid (TCA) peels or dermabrasion, but less than that of phenol peels.

In addition to ablation, the CO_2 laser produces a zone of irreversible thermal damage. This leads to visible tightening of the skin during treatment that is believed to be due to collagen

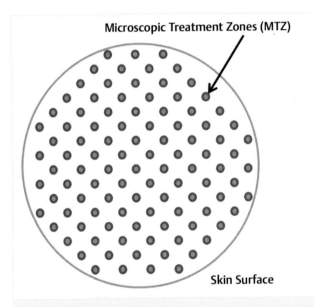

Fig. 3.5 Fractional laser technology.

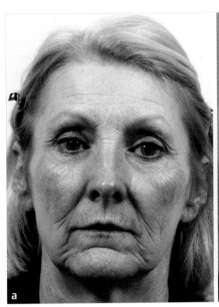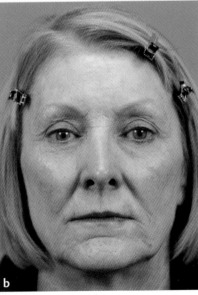

Fig. 3.6 CO_2 laser resurfacing can be used to improve facial rhytids, dyschromias, and skin laxity. (**a**) Before full-face procedure. (**b**) After full-face procedure.

shrinkage. Collagen fibrils are able to shrink by up to one third without a loss of structural integrity.[10] This gives the CO_2 laser a unique tightening effect as compared to other resurfacing methods including erbium resurfacing.

Controversy remains about the color of the skin after resurfacing and prediction for depth of penetration. That said, color can provide some guide.[11] A pinkish color would indicate ablation through the epidermis to the superficial papillary dermis. A chamois-colored appearance would be indicative of deeper papillary dermis and a cotton-threaded appearance would be the unsafe reticular dermal level. That said, beyond the papillary dermis, further laser pulses tend to leave more thermal injury resulting in a yellow-brown discoloration.

Histological studies on lasered skin will show a variety of effects. These include reversal of epidermal dysplasia and thickening of the Grenz zone with collagen deposition. Solar elastosis is noted to decrease with greater fibrillar content.

One unwanted phenomenon of CO_2 laser resurfacing is hypopigmentation. Whereas many resurfacing techniques create pseudohypopigmentation by way of removing sun-damaged, hyperpigmented skin, deep ablative CO_2 laser resurfacing may lead to an actual decrease in the presence of melanocytes. This true hypopigmentation is a delayed phenomenon and irreversible. It is one of the prime impetuses for the search for other resurfacing modalities such as erbium and fractional devices.

The CO_2 laser can also be used as a cutting or coagulating tool. In these modes, the laser has been used in blepharoplasty and rhinophyma removal.

3.4.2 Erbium

Erbium lasers include the 2,790-nm erbium:yttrium scandium gallium garnet (Er:YSGG) and the 2,940-nm Er:YAG. Lasers with wavelengths in this range have even higher water absorption than CO_2, with the 2,940-nm wavelength having 12 times the absorption. In addition, like CO_2 lasers, erbium devices provide an excellent tool for skin resurfacing. They can be used to reverse signs of aging such as rhytids, dyschromias, coarse skin texture, and skin laxity, as well as acne and traumatic scarring.

Because of erbium lasers' higher water absorption, they are associated with more ablation and less coagulation and thermal tightening. The ablation threshold is much lower for the erbium lasers than for the CO_2 lasers (1.6 vs. 5.0 J/cm²).[12] This has presented two issues—pinpoint bleeding after treatment and less thermal tightening than with CO_2 lasers. Newer devices have longer pulse options combined with lower fluences that allow for more coagulative effect when desired and at least partial correction of both of these issues.

Like CO_2 lasers, erbium can be delivered via a fixed spot, or a scanning or fractional handpiece. Like CO_2, the laser is in the invisible infrared region and thus requires an aiming beam. Erbium lasers use a flashlamp for excitation.

There are a variety of benefits to erbium's higher water absorption and less thermal effect. Recovery is typically shorter, being 1 week or less with ablative resurfacing versus 10 days to 2 weeks with CO_2. Erbium lasers in general can treat a broader range of skin types than CO_2—Fitzpatrick skin types III and IV can be safely treated with ablative erbium at appropriate settings. Lastly, the long-term risk of hypopigmentation is generally less than with traditional CO_2.

Although they have similar effects, the Er:YSGG can be seen as halfway between the Er:YAG and the CO_2 laser. It has less water absorption than the Er:YAG, but still 5 times that of CO_2. This gives it a more ablative effect than CO_2, but a more coagulative effect than Er:YAG.[13]

3.4.3 Argon Laser

The argon laser emits light at multiple wavelengths between 458 to 514 nm with high absorption by hemoglobin. It was one of the original lasers studied for the treatment of vascular lesions and produced results that made it the treatment of choice for several years.[14] The laser is used with shuttered pulse widths of 50 milliseconds to 0.3 seconds and with spot sizes of 0.1 to 1 mm. The laser was the first device to prove effective in lightening vascular lesions, with up to 75% showing improvement. Its shorter wavelength, however, was preferentially absorbed superficially preventing effective treatment of deeper lesions. In addition, scarring proved unacceptably high,[15] stimulating the search for a safer, more effective device.

3.4.4 Pulsed Dye Laser

The flashlamp-excited pulsed dye laser has been the gold standard for the treatment of vascular lesions for years.[16] At 585 nm, its wavelength is close to that of one of oxyhemoglobin's peaks at 577 nm, allowing preferential absorption by red blood cells.

This has allowed effective treatment of a variety of vascular pathologies, including telangiectasias, port-wine stains, and hemangiomas. The laser has also been used for the improvement of scars as well as improvement in postsurgical bruising.

The medium for the laser is rhodamine dye. The laser has been associated with a purpuric effect that persists for days to weeks after treatment (▶ Fig. 3.7). To minimize this as well as improve effectiveness, both wavelength and pulse width have been modified. Newer devices have up to a 1.5-ms pulse width (vs. 450 µs) that provides slower heating, less vessel rupture, and thus less purpura. Longer wavelengths (600 nm) have been used for deeper penetration and more effective treatment of larger, deeper lesions.

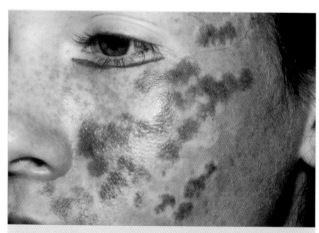

Fig. 3.7 Purpura is seen after treatment with short-pulsed pulsed dye laser.

3.4.5 Ruby Laser

The ruby laser is also a flashlamp-excited laser. With strong absorption by melanin, it was one of the first devices for laser hair removal. It was also one of the first devices utilized for tattoo removal and has proven effective for black, blue-black, and green ink. It is capable of treating pigmented lesions, with its longer wavelength allowing for deeper penetration.

The laser emits light at the 694-nm wavelength and is visible. It can be delivered as a Q-switched device used for tattoo and pigmented lesion removal or as a longer pulse width device for laser hair removal.

3.4.6 Alexandrite Laser

At 755 nm, the alexandrite wavelength is effective in treating green and black tattoos, unwanted hair, and pigmented lesions. Its longer wavelength allows deeper penetration into the skin. This, combined with high melanin absorption, has made it the most commonly used wavelength for hair removal. On the flip side, its high melanin absorption limits its use in darker skin types. It is a solid state device and being in the infrared region does require an aiming beam.

3.4.7 Diode Laser

Diode lasers are the most commonly manufactured laser type, with uses in everything from bar code scanners to laser pointers. They come in a variety of wavelengths depending on use. In medicine, the 810-nm wavelength is used for hair removal. It can be combined with a contact cooling system to allow use of higher fluencies without skin damage.

3.4.8 Nd:YAG Laser

The 1,064-nm wavelength has been used for a variety of purposes including the treatment of vascular lesions, laser hair removal, nonablative skin remodeling, and as a dissection tool. Its use in different areas is related to modifications in delivery, pulse width, and spot size.

3.4.9 KTP Laser

The KTP laser is an Nd:YAG laser where the 1,064-nm light is passed through an optical crystal composed of potassium titanyl phosphate (KTP) that changes the wavelength to 532 nm. This frequency-doubled Nd:YAG has proven effective at treating vascular lesions. Its ability to use longer wavelengths has allowed treatment of vascular lesions without purpura, as seen with traditional pulsed dye lasers (▶ Fig. 3.8a, b). One device has combined the 532-nm wavelength with a unique water-cooled glass piece to protect the skin. A Q-switched, 532-nm laser is available for effective treatment of pigmented lesions. In addition, the 532-nm wavelength can be utilized in a cutting, coagulating contact mode.

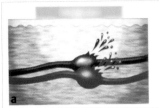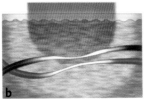

Fig. 3.8 Longer wavelengths allow treatment of vascular lesions without purpura, as seen with traditional pulsed dye lasers. (**a**) Short-pulsed, yellow-light treatment of vascular lesion with vessel rupture versus (**b**) longer pulsed, green-light treatment with vessel shrinkage and avoidance of purpura.

3.5 Summary

Better understanding of laser–tissue interactions has improved our ability to utilize this technology. We can look forward to future research exploring laser physics for improved outcomes, less downtime, and fewer risks.

References

[1] Einstein A. Zur Quantentheorie der Strahlung. Phys Z 1917; 18: 121–128

[2] Gould GR. The LASER, light amplification by stimulated emission of radiation. Paper presented at: Ann Arbor Conference on Optical Pumping; June 15–18, 1959; Ann Arbor, MI

[3] Maiman TH. Stimulated optical radiation in ruby. Nature 1960; 187: 493–494

[4] Goldman L, Blaney DJ, Kindel DJ Jr, Franke EK. Effect of the laser beam on the skin. Preliminary report. J Invest Dermatol 1963; 40: 121–122

[5] Ries WR, Wittkopf M. Lasers in facial plastic surgery. In: Papel ID, ed. Facial Plastic and Reconstructive Surgery. 3rd ed. New York, NY: Thieme Medical Publishers; 2009: 99–118

[6] Anderson RR, Parrish JA. Selective photothermolysis: precise microsurgery by selective absorption of pulsed radiation. Science 1983; 220: 524–527

[7] Manstein D, Herron GS, Sink RK, Tanner H, Anderson RR. Fractional photothermolysis: a new concept for cutaneous remodeling using microscopic patterns of thermal injury. Lasers Surg Med 2004; 34: 426–438

[8] Carniol PJ, Harirchian S, Kelly E. Fractional CO(2) laser resurfacing. Facial Plast Surg Clin North Am 2011; 19: 247–251

[9] Hamilton MM. Carbon dioxide laser resurfacing. Facial Plast Surg Clin North Am 2004; 12: 289–295

[10] Fitzpatrick RE, Goldman MP, Satur NM, Tope WD. Pulsed carbon dioxide laser resurfacing of photo-aged facial skin. Arch Dermatol 1996; 132: 395–402

[11] Goldman MP, Fitzpatrick RE. Cutaneous Laser Surgery: The Art and Science of Selective Photothermolysis, 2nd ed. St. Louis, MO: Mosby; 1999

[12] Holcomb JD. Versatility of erbium YAG laser: from fractional skin rejuvenation to full-field skin resurfacing. Facial Plast Surg Clin North Am 2011; 19: 261–273

[13] Smith KC, Schachter GD. YSGG 2790-nm superficial ablative and fractional ablative laser treatment. Facial Plast Surg Clin North Am 2011; 19: 253–260

[14] Dolsky RL. Argon laser skin surgery. Surg Clin North Am 1984; 64: 861–870

[15] Apfelberg DB, Maser MR, Lash H. Extended clinical use of the argon laser for cutaneous lesions. Arch Dermatol 1979; 115: 719–721

[16] Travelute Ammirati C, Carniol PJ, Hruza GJ. Laser treatment of facial vascular lesions. Facial Plast Surg 2001; 17: 193–201

4 Ablative Carbon Dioxide Laser Treatment

Michael A. Persky and J. Kevin Duplechain

4.1 Historical Perspective

Those who have used lasers in their medical training and practices will be able to relate to my thoughts the first time I used a laser: "How did anyone ever think of using light in such an extraordinary fashion?" Thankfully, as in many other aspects of our practices, we are the beneficiaries of the genius minds that came before us. We are fortunate to "stand on the shoulders of giants!"

Several decades ago the laser was used in science fiction as a death-ray machine. Today the laser has evolved to be a most useful tool in aesthetic medicine. Almost 60 years before the first actual laser was built, Albert Einstein developed the early theories essential to the development of the laser. His 1917 paper, "Zur Quantentheorie der Strahlung," was the first to discuss stimulated emission.[1] Gordon, Zeiger, and Townes built the first microwave laser, called a maser, in 1954.[2] The first theoretical calculations for a visible light laser were published by Schawlow and Townes at Bell Laboratories in 1958.[3]

The first laser used a ruby crystal and a lamp that produced weak flashes of red light. In 1960 Theodore Maiman at Hughes Aircraft made this first laser with pulses of light in the red spectrum at 694 nm.[4] Commercial lasers became available a year later. In 1961 a prototype ruby laser was the first laser used on a patient; it was used to destroy a retinal tumor. As lasers developed, medical experts considered further how lasers could help in patient care, particularly for surgical applications. Lasers quickly went from the laboratory to clinical use, with practitioners keeping in mind the potential occupational hazards, rather than repeating Madame Curie's slow realization of radiation hazards from radiographs (poor Madame Curie's hands!).

The expansion of laser use from ophthalmology to other medical fields was pioneered by Leon Goldman. In 1963 Goldman and colleagues described the pathological effects of the laser beam on the skin.[5] These authors also considered the potential use of lasers in medicine.

The carbon dioxide (CO_2) laser was developed in 1964 by Patel and coworkers;[6] however, it was not until 1968 when Polanyi[7] developed the articulated arm that more diverse specialized medical applications were possible. The CO_2 laser consists of a sealed tube of helium, nitrogen, and carbon dioxide gases. The gaseous mixture, called the gain medium, is stimulated either by high-voltage currents or radiofrequency discharge to produce an invisible infrared beam of 10,600-nm energy.[8] An "aiming" helium-neon laser that produces red light is used in conjunction with the CO_2 laser.

CO_2 laser ablation occurs when 10,600-nm energy is absorbed by tissue water, resulting in the production of heat and an ablative thermal effect. Once the temperature rises above 100°C, water in the tissue vaporizes. The steam expands and further tears open the tissue. Early medical lasers were used as light scalpels because they had simultaneous cutting and cauterizing capabilities. The early CO_2 lasers were continuous wave with a constant beam of energy delivered to the tissue. The CO_2 laser was used in head and neck surgery for tissue ablation, creating intense localized heat to effect vaporization of intracellular and extracellular water, leading to coagulative necrosis. Collateral heating of the zone adjacent to the area of vaporization is unique to CO_2 laser wounds. Otolaryngology was the first surgical specialty in which the CO_2 laser characteristics were recognized and successfully applied to large-scale clinical situations.

The ablative CO_2 laser held great promise as an aesthetic tool because of its unique ablative and thermal wound characteristics. It was not until the principle of selective photothermolysis was reported[9] that manufacturers began to develop lasers that reduced thermal injury by delivering energy in a series of short, repetitive bursts rather than a continuous, uninterrupted beam. When energy was delivered in pulses the lasered tissue had time to cool between pulses, a feature that gave rise to the use of CO_2 lasers for facial cosmetic applications.

During the 1990s these pulsed, ablative CO_2 lasers became very popular for skin resurfacing. Two CO_2 laser systems specifically designed for skin resurfacing were the Ultrapulse (Coherent Inc., Palo Alto, California) and the Silktouch (Sharplan Lasers Inc., Allendale, New Jersey). David and associates[10] were the first to report using the CO_2 laser for cosmetic correction of facial actinic damage, later expanding its use for purely cosmetic correction of surface wrinkling in the face and hands. The development of more sophisticated handpieces allowed the laser beam to be applied to human skin in many preprogrammed patterns and in a much shorter duration that prevented hot spots and bulk heating. Continuous wave lasers controlled depth of injury by the number of passes performed on a single area.

4.2 Rationale for Treatment

The rationale behind ablative CO_2 laser use for skin resurfacing is that it is still considered the best device for the correction of facial rhytids and remains the gold standard for facial skin resurfacing (▶ Fig. 4.1 and ▶ Fig. 4.2). It was extremely popular in the 1990s but, due to the very long healing times, prolonged erythema, lines of demarcation, and scarring, its use declined except in the hands of experienced and skillful surgeons.

4.3 Pertinent Anatomy

Knowledge of skin microanatomy, histology, physiology, and function are essential in all laser resurfacing procedures, particularly when using ablative CO_2 lasers. Skin is a dynamic organ and is continuously changing throughout life; outer layers are shed and replaced by inner layers. Skin also varies in thickness with age, anatomical location, and the gender of the individual. Skin consists of two layers (▶ Fig. 4.3), the epidermis and dermis, which lie above the fatty subcutaneous layer, the panniculus adiposus. The epidermis has pigment-containing melanocytes and does not contain any blood vessels. The dermis contains elastic fibers, collagen, blood vessels, nerves, and fibroblasts. The dermis has two layers, the more superficial papillary dermis, and the deeper reticular dermis.

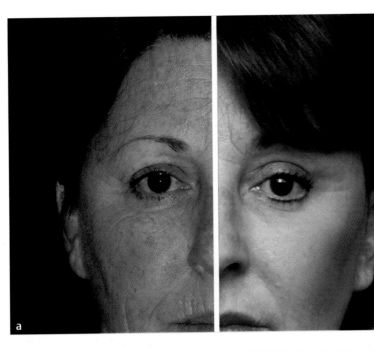

Fig. 4.1 (a, b) A 54-year-old woman who underwent fully ablative laser resurfacing with Lumenis ultrapulse CO$_2$ laser. She was treated at 100 millijoules (mJ), density of 5, at 250 Hz. The neck was treated at 80 mJ, density of 3, at 250 Hz. Note significant improvement in tone and texture with moderate wrinkle reduction.

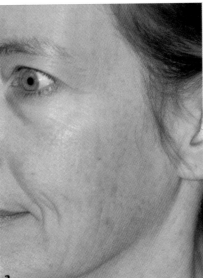
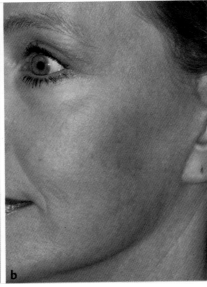

Fig. 4.2 (a) The effect of fully ablative CO$_2$ resurfacing combined with facelift surgery. **(b)** 3-month postoperative photograph.

The papillary dermis is made up of loose, connective tissue containing capillaries, elastic fibers, reticular fibers, and some collagen. The reticular dermis is a denser layer of connective tissue with larger blood vessels, bundles of collagen fibers arranged in layers parallel to the surface, and tightly interlaced elastic fibers. The reticular dermis also contains fibroblasts and epidermal appendages. The epidermal appendages of the reticular dermis are essential for proper skin healing following CO$_2$ laser resurfacing.[11]

Knowledge of the relative skin depth and thickness in various parts of the face is valuable to ensure that the laser does not penetrate too deeply, which could result in unnecessary skin injury and other complications. Histological studies of human skin[11] show that facial skin epidermis (forehead, nose, cheeks, chin) varies in depth from 110 to 126 μm (mean 120.2), whereas depth of the papillary dermis is more variable (75–110 μm, mean 94.2). The reticular dermis is deeper (mean 1,980 μm)

and facial areas are less variable (range 1700–2100 μm). Facial skin thicknesses, the sums of epidermal and dermal depths, range from 1,915 μm in the forehead to 2,360 μm in the medial cheek. The upper, middle, and lower neck skins are thinner (1,690, 1,552, and 1,330 μm, respectively) and more depleted of adnexa. Epidermal depths of the upper, middle, and lower neck areas are 115, 75, and 70 μm, respectively. The eyelids have much thinner skin, at 502 and 497 μm for the upper and lower eyelids, respectively.

When using ablative CO$_2$ lasers, it is essential that the laser operator is well aware of the depth of the laser effect. For many years the depth of penetration was visually assessed by the color of the treated area. Pink-lasered skin indicates epidermis; gray denotes papillary dermis; a yellow color reflects the reticular dermis. The absolute end point of the most aggressive ablative laser treatment is the yellowish, chamois-cloth color. In order to avoid permanent scarring, laser surgeons should not

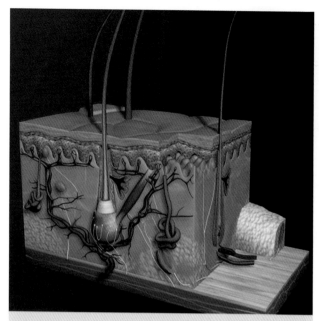

Fig. 4.3 Diagram of skin layers. (Courtesy of Lumenis Inc., Yokneum, Israel.)

proceed with further laser passes once the chamois appearance is present.

These early techniques of visually inspecting the skin during the treatment were likely among the causes of complications related to CO_2 resurfacing. Although clinical results were often outstanding, patients frequently endured several months of erythema, which frequently led to permanent hypopigmentation. Most laser companies now provide a depth of injury guide with a diagram identifying the depth of ablative and thermal injury so the treating physician can precisely plan and manage the level of injury. This advance in the treatment of patients in the authors' opinion has significantly reduced the incidence of complications.

4.4 Indications

Reduction of wrinkles and improvement of tone and texture are the most common indications for ablative CO_2 laser resurfacing. The fully ablative CO_2 laser is, after 20 years, still considered the gold standard by which all skin rejuvenation procedures are judged. Creating treatment protocols allows safe, fully ablative treatments and yields substantially better results than other treatment options. The versatility of the CO_2 device allows for fully ablative treatment options that significantly reduce the degree of wrinkles in a pan-facial manner. The laser can also be used more elegantly to simply remove a portion of the epidermis that will heal in 3 to 5 days (a "light CO_2 ablative peel").

CO_2 laser resurfacing can be combined with facial rejuvenation surgery including blepharoplasty, rhytidectomy, forehead lift, and neck rejuvenation surgery to enhance the appearance of the skin. In these instances, resurfacing limited to a portion of the epidermis can be performed safely and with satisfying results.[12]

There has been a significant resurgence in the use of the CO_2 laser in the treatment of postsurgical scars and, most recently, burn scars and scars related to battlefield wounds.[13] Ablative and nonablative lasers have demonstrated a resetting of the wound healing processes at a molecular level that involves matrix metalloproteinase, transforming growth factor-beta (TGF-β1), and messenger ribonucleic acid (mRNA) for collagen synthesis.[13,14]

The treatment of acne scars has received additional attention with the development of deep fractional CO_2 lasers. The combination of both a deep fractional treatment with a more superficial fully ablative treatment in the authors' experience has significantly improved outcomes. Fat grafting and subcision have also been combined simultaneously.[12] ▶ Fig. 4.4 shows a patient who underwent fat grafting in combination with CO_2 laser resurfacing.

A series of treatments may be required for hypertrophic scars and keloids, which are known to respond well to both ablative and nonablative treatments. Surgical resection of keloids with the CO_2 laser in conjunction with intralesional steroid injections were some of the earlier treatment options available for recurrent keloids.[15] Similar results were noted on sternal scars of patients who had undergone bypass surgery.[16]

Exophytic epidermal conditions that respond well to CO_2 laser include solar and actinic keratosis, sebaceous gland hyperplasia, lentigines, verruca vulgaris, and dermatosis papulosa nigra. Dermal exophytic lesions treated with the CO_2 laser tend to recur. These include xanthelasmas, syringomas, adenoma sebaceum, and angiofibromas. The CO_2 laser is a treatment of choice for rhinophyma. Bulky rhinophyma may require scalpel excision combined with CO_2 laser energy, whereas mild rhinophyma can be treated with laser alone. Actinic cheilitis responds permanently as long as sun protection is practiced after treatment.

4.5 Contraindications

Patients taking oral retinoids should not be treated with an ablative CO_2 laser for at least 12 months. A clinical guide to follow before treating those with a history of oral retinoids is to observe the return of oily skin or active acne lesions. Oral retinoids interfere with the function of sebaceous glands, preventing normal epithelial healing. Atypical hypertrophic scars may develop in patients treated too soon after oral retinoid therapy.

Active herpes simplex virus infection, skin infection, irradiated skin, and scleroderma are absolute contraindications for CO_2 laser treatment.

Patients who have had extensive electrolysis, deep chemical peel treatment, dermabrasion, or split thickness skin grafting may heal abnormally and should be treated with caution. Other relative contraindications include ongoing exposure to ultraviolet light and history of scarring or keloids, treatment of nonfacial areas, treatment despite a dark skin type (IV–VI), and collagen vascular disease. Patients with psychoneuroses (i.e., facial pickers) should not be treated.

The lower eyelids should be treated cautiously in patients with lower lid laxity and in patients with previous skin excision blepharoplasty. Excessive tightening of the delicate skin in this area may result in ectropion.

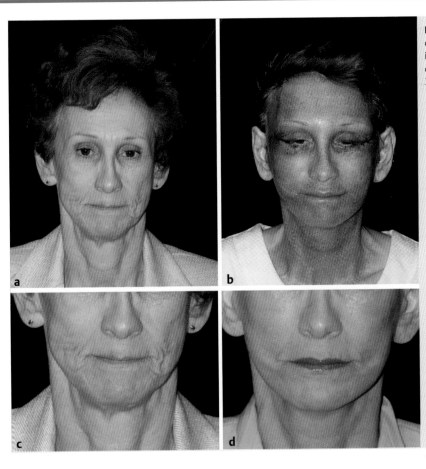

Fig. 4.4 A 70-year-old woman who underwent complete facial rejuvenation with laser resurfacing and fat grafting. (**a**) Before surgery. (**b**) One day after surgery. (**c**) Closeup before surgery. (**d**) 3 weeks after surgery.

Patients should be discouraged from smoking prior to and after laser surgery to avoid possible delayed or impaired healing. Excessive sun exposure is also a relative contraindication. Patients are typically counseled to avoid sun exposure for ~ 1 week prior to laser resurfacing and for a slightly longer period following the procedure. In many practices more ablative procedures are performed in the winter, since many patients are typically not able to avoid routine sun exposure during the summer months.

4.6 Advantages of Ablative Carbon Dioxide Laser

Any advantage offered by a device is often counteracted by a relative disadvantage. This is true of most resurfacing tools. For example, devices that offer shorter healing times and lower risk of complications typically yield less than stellar results. In contrast, devices such as the CO_2 laser, still the gold standard of resurfacing 20 years after its introduction, is considered by some a risky treatment with potential complications that may not warrant the risk. We believe this may have been true when CO_2 resurfacing was in its infancy, when treatment parameters and protocols were unclear and users were overly aggressive without giving enough thought to specific anatomical sites and depths of injury. Poor postoperative protocols also likely were responsible for bad outcomes. With the current ability to pinpoint the depth of injury and to manage the frequency, pulse width, and treatment density, CO_2 ablative resurfacing offers

many advantages when compared to other skin rejuvenation procedures.

CO_2 ablative laser treatment gives excellent results in the treatment of facial and neck rhytids, as well as the tightening of infraorbital skin in combination with transconjunctival blepharoplasty (► Fig. 4.5). The treatment of rhinophyma due to a coagulative effect results in less bleeding and better hemostasis.

4.7 Disadvantages of Ablative Carbon Dioxide Laser

As mentioned above, for every advantage, there is typically a coinciding disadvantage. In most cases of complications that occur as a result of CO_2 resurfacing, errors in treatment are most commonly the culprit. Attempts at "hitting a home run," despite good intentions, often result in complications that are avoidable if the surgeon adheres to more conservative treatment parameters. In almost every case we have been asked to investigate where a complication occurred, errors in judgment regarding treatment parameters were apparent. Despite adhering to these rules, complications can and still do occur, just not with the frequency of a decade ago. Some of the most common complications are slowly resolving erythema over months, temporary hyperpigmentation that may last for 6 to 9 months, and permanent hypopigmentation with lines of demarcation. Other adverse events include bacterial, yeast, and viral infections. Inherent thermal injury may result in collateral tissue damage and increased potential of skin scarring.

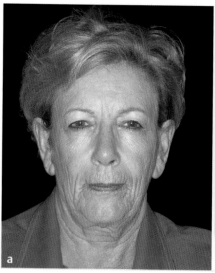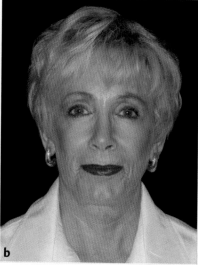

Fig. 4.5 (a) A 68-year-old patient is shown with severe solar damage, volume loss, and marked facial laxity. (b) Three months after undergoing combined facelift, blepharoplasty, browlift, fat grafting, and fully ablative laser resurfacing.

4.8 Preoperative Preparation of Patient

As with any aesthetic procedure, it is imperative for the physician to make absolutely sure that the patient has realistic expectations about ablative CO_2 laser resurfacing. For example, dynamic wrinkles will likely still be present after CO_2 treatment. There is the expectation that healing will be longer than with ablative fractional resurfacing, but in some cases healing times of epidermal fully ablative resurfacing can approach those of aggressive fractional resurfacing. The patient must be clearly informed of the arduous postoperative course. Patients should be shown clear examples of subjects who have been treated with ablative CO_2—not just before and after pictures, but photos taken immediately after treatment and every few days during the initial recovery period. Postoperative written instructions should be provided and reviewed prior to treatment. Patients are advised to follow the postoperative protocol precisely because often the introduction of unapproved compounds will irritate the skin during the immediate period following laser treatment. Patients are provided a 3-month postoperative protocol that will hopefully continue long after the treatment period. A comprehensive informed consent should be signed at the preoperative visit.

All patients begin antiviral medication 1 day prior to their treatment and continue for 7 days until the skin has re-epithelialized. There have been reports of patients denying history of herpetic infections, only to have widespread herpes infection after treatment. Commonly used regimens include famciclovir 250 mg orally twice daily, acyclovir 400 mg orally three times daily, or valacyclovir 500 mg orally twice daily for 7 days. We prefer valacyclovir due to its higher bioavailability.

Some laser surgeons use a broad spectrum antibiotic such as cephalexin 500 mg twice daily for 10 days, whereas studies by Alster[17] and a colleague (conversation with J. K. Duplechain, MD, February 2014) have demonstrated no benefit. Although we do not routinely prescribe oral steroids, some surgeons use both intravenous (IV) steroid intraoperatively followed by a methylprednisolone dose pack postoperatively. Ortiz and colleagues[18] reported a few infections after the use of steroid cream.

We do not use pretreatment skin care regimes because we have found no clinical benefit, although many others use tretinoin and hydroquinone preoperatively. Unless patients have experienced postinflammatory hyperpigmentation (PIH) in a previous treatment, the authors do not routinely recommend their use because of the inconsistency in results as part of a preoperative regimen. Often PIH can be minimized with proper density, frequency, and pulse duration settings.

Pretreatment with tyrosine inhibitors still remains controversial. Chan[19] recommended a 2-week course of hydroquinone and azelaic acid in Fitzpatrick skin types III and above; this was thought to possibly reduce the severity of PIH but not the incidence.

In considering any patient for fully ablative CO_2 laser resurfacing, the final question that is always asked at consultation and the preoperative visit is when the patient can resume normal activities. This is defined as being able to drive, return to work, or manage household duties. This final question helps determine the depth of injury associated with the treatment. As mentioned previously, epidermal fully ablative treatments can heal within 4 to 5 days and allow patients to resume day-to-day activities. It is the depth of ablation that is the limiting factor in the rate of re-epithelialization. Certainly a 50-μm, fully ablative epidermal injury will heal much more quickly than a 150-μm injury (Video 4.1).

4.9 Perioperative Care of the Patient

The skin is thoroughly prepped with a cleanser (we prefer chlorhexidine or Hibiclens [chlorhexidine gluconate 4%, Mölnlycke Health Care US, LLC, Norcross, Georgia]). A nonflammable degreasing agent should be used to avoid combustion such as may occur with solutions containing alcohol or acetone.

The patient should be upright when marking the cosmetic units of the face and carefully outlining the jawline. Markings should be made 1 to 2 cm above and below the jawline, where feathering should be performed to minimize lines of demarcation. Although with the new, shorter pulsed duration lasers, both the face and neck may be treated without hypopigmentation.

Fully ablative resurfacing is a painful procedure and is difficult to complete with topical anesthesia only. Local anesthesia is only used for small areas, and regional nerve blocks are useful for the perioral and forehead areas. Tumescent local anesthesia is useful for the cheeks and temples. IV sedation and general anesthesia are the mainstay anesthesia for full-face ablative CO_2. Plastic eye shields should never be used because they do not protect the globe. Nonflammable, sterile drapes must be used. Wet drapes and/or a reservoir of water must be immediately available at the treatment site in case of fire.

4.10 Postoperative and Home Care of the Patient

Immediately after the procedure the patient's face is covered with cool, moist compresses for 20 to 30 minutes. Despite the use of a topical or infiltrative anesthetic, most patients do notice a burning sensation for this period of time. Pretreatment or intraoperative treatment with ketorolac 60 mg does significantly improve the degree of discomfort, but a few minutes of burning sensation is expected. During the postoperative recovery period, patients are advised to use moist, cool compresses almost continuously, or at least as much as possible. The moist, cool compresses provide a level of comfort for patients, and most importantly provide essential moisture to the skin so that desiccation is minimized or prevented.

In fully ablative treatments, all of the stratum corneum has been removed. This essential layer prevents the skin from drying out. Its absence allows essential moisture to quickly evaporate, slowing the healing process. Although there are many options and documented home remedies, none seems to provide better moisture than cool compresses. Patients are allowed to shower twice daily on the day following treatment. The hair can be washed with a gentle baby shampoo, but cleansers are avoided on the face until re-epithelialization has occurred. The use of acetic acid soaks has not been adopted. As an adjunct to cool compresses, a perfluorodecalin product, Cutagenix (Cutagenesis Lafayette, Louisiana), has been utilized three to four times daily to help the skin remain soothed. This nonirritating product is discussed fully in Chapter 13 in this book. Significant reduction in complications has been observed while using this product, which has been well received by patients.

Patients are usually seen 1 week after treatment and skin care is reviewed. It is not unusual to hear from patients by phone during the first week. If there is any question about the course of healing, the patient is asked to e-mail a photo that is immediately reviewed. The most common reason for a call is that the skin may feel tight or swollen, both of which are expected and normal. Reassurance is provided and the use of moisture is reiterated.

The fully ablative CO_2 laser procedure removes the epidermis and heats the upper papillary dermis. Once re-epithelialization has occurred at 5 to 7 days, patients are allowed to use a simple cleanser such as Cetaphil (Galderma Laboratories, Ft. Worth, Texas) or CeraVe (Coria Laboratories, Ltd., Ft. Worth, Texas). Mineral makeup can be applied and a titanium and/or zinc-based sunscreen of sun protection factor (SPF) 50 (L'Oréal, Clichy, Hauts-de-Seine, France) must be utilized. No additional topical with the exception of the perfluorodecalin product is used. We have found this to provide the best outcomes and have experienced fewer minor or major complications than with any other therapy. Milia rate is 1% with this regimen and acneiform eruptions have not occurred in more than 500 patients.

Patients are again seen at 1 month after the procedure. Skin care is reviewed and it is not uncommon to consider the addition of an epidermal growth factor product or a low-dose retinol. If retinol is initiated, it is usually applied two or three times weekly for a period of 2 months. If evidence of hyperpigmentation is present, patients are placed on a kojic acid pad with 8% arbutin (Young Pharmaceuticals Inc., Wethersfield, Connecticut) or Trauma (Galderma, Ft. Worth, Texas)). We prefer the kojic acid pads because Trauma contains cortisone that has been shown to downregulate TGF-β1 and insulin-like growth factor 1 (IGF-1) when applied topically. Oral and topical corticosteroids reduce the levels of TGF-β1 and IGF-1.[20]

4.11 Complications

Fully ablative resurfacing is the mainstay of the type of skin rejuvenation that one of the authors (J. K. D.) performs with and without facial rejuvenation surgery. Over the years, he has found the procedure the most reliable of any resurfacing treatment available to his patients. Its precision is a true advantage in that depth of injury and density are absolutely controllable. The ability to regulate these two parameters with absolute accuracy makes this treatment extremely safe and predictable in expert hands.

The most common complications of ablative CO_2 laser are erythema, prolonged swelling, pruritus, contact dermatitis, PIH, hypopigmentation (▶ Fig. 4.6), acne flare up, milia, infection (herpetic, *Candida albicans*, *Staphylococcus aureus*), and hypertrophic scarring. Please see Chapter 13 for a more detailed discussion.

4.12 Counseling the Patient

Ablative CO_2 laser patients need to have appropriate and realistic expectations. Photographs are shown to patients at different intervals following treatment, including 1 day, 1 week, and 3 and 6 months. Understanding that early improvement is not the "endgame" and that healing will occur for about 6 months will help temper early disappointment if all wrinkles are not completely erased by the treatment. We manage all of the skin care for a period of at least 3 months, encouraging the use of products we believe will enhance collagenesis. Risks including scarring, failure to remove all the wrinkles, infection, and hyperpigmentation are discussed with the patient. We usually try to quantify a percentage of improvement for a particular area within the facial subunits. For example, if patients have deep perioral wrinkles, they are told that a 50 to 75% improvement may be expected, and that a second treatment will be necessary for better results. We explain that the skin simply can't withstand a more aggressive treatment than the one they are receiving without significantly increasing the risk of scarring. We have found this to be very helpful in preparing patients for the treatment and postoperative period.

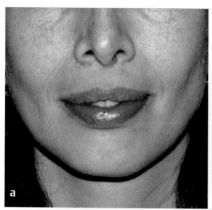
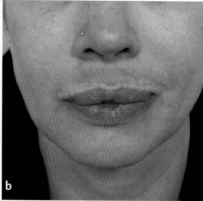

Fig. 4.6 Upper lip hypopigmentation at postablative CO_2 resurfacing.

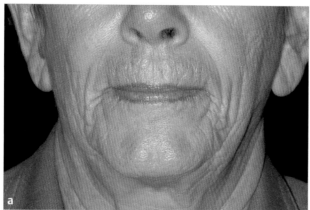
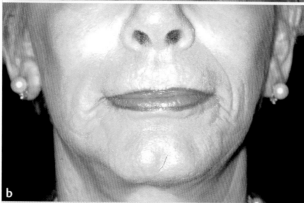

Fig. 4.7 A 68-year-old patient who underwent fully ablative CO_2 resurfacing of the perioral area in combination with facial rejuvenation surgery including facelift. The perioral area was treated with a double pass removing all of the epidermis and a portion of the papillary dermis. (**a**) Pre-treatment. (**b**) Post-treatment.

4.13 Pearls and Pitfalls

The greatest pearl that we can share is that when undertaking CO_2 ablative resurfacing, it is important—above all else—to know the laser you are using extremely well (▶ Fig. 4.7). Understanding density, frequency, thermal relaxation time of skin, and the energy required for skin ablation are the most important parameters in treatment planning to ensure success in helping your patients achieve their aesthetic goals in the safest and most efficient manner. Fully ablative CO_2 laser resurfacing is not a commodity; rather it is dependent on the dedication,

skill, and experience of the laser surgeon to help patients achieve excellent results. Understand and discuss with your patient the goals that are achievable during the time frame set by the patient. Realistic expectations are paramount! The last question we ask patients prior to starting therapy is: "How much time have you allowed for healing?" With this time period in mind, we can treat 100% of the epidermis at a depth that should allow the patient to heal successfully in the prescribed period.

A few final thoughts and pearls include the pretreatment use of onabotulinumtoxinA (Botox Cosmetic, Allergan, Inc., Irvine, California) in the forehead and crow's-feet areas. The two facial regions that deserve cautious attention to avoid hypertrophic scarring are the infraorbital area and the lower half of the mandibular ridge. Respect and do not cross aesthetic facial units when partially treating the face. Avoid charring by not overlapping pulses and flatten high points when possible.

Be prepared for the unexpected. As in any surgical procedure, prepare your patients well and listen to their complaints during the postoperative period. The laser surgeon must be cautious when using any laser; when using ablative CO_2 lasers, the surgeon must be extra cautious to ensure the best results in the safest manner.

4.14 Disclosure

Author J. Kevin Duplechain is a founder and stockholder of Cutagenesis, Lafayette, Louisiana.

References

[1] Einstein A. Zur Quantentheorie der Strahlung. Phys Z 1917; 18: 121–128
[2] Gordon JP, Zeiger HZ, Townes CH. Microwave amplification by stimulated emission. Physiol Rev 1954; 95: 282
[3] Schawlow AL, Townes CH. Infrared and optical masers. Phys Rev 1958; 112: 1940–1949
[4] Maiman TH. Stimulated optical radiation in ruby. Nature 1960; 187: 493–494
[5] Goldman L, Blaney DJ, Kindel DJ, Jr, Richfield D, Franke EK. Pathology of the effect of the laser beam on the skin. Nature 1963; 197: 912–914
[6] Patel CKN, McFarlane RA, Faust WL. Selective excitation through vibrational energy transfer and optical maser action in N2-CO2. Phys Rev 1964; 13: 617–619
[7] Polanyi TG. Laser physics. Otolaryngol Clin North Am 1983; 16: 753–774
[8] Wheeland RG. History of lasers in dermatology. Clin Dermatol 1995; 13: 3–10
[9] Anderson RR, Parrish JA. Selective photothermolysis: precise microsurgery by selective absorption of pulsed radiation. Science 1983; 220: 524–527

[10] David LM, Lask GP, Glassberg E, Jacoby R, Abergel RP. Laser abrasion for cosmetic and medical treatment of facial actinic damage. Cutis 1989; 43: 583–587

[11] Sasaki GH, Travis HM, Tucker B. Fractional CO2 laser resurfacing of photoaged facial and non-facial skin: histologic and clinical results and side effects. J Cosmet Laser Ther 2009; 11: 190–201

[12] Duplechain JK. Fractional CO2 resurfacing: has it replaced ablative resurfacing techniques? Facial Plast Surg Clin North Am 2013; 21: 213–227

[13] Qu L, Liu A, Zhou L, et al. Clinical and molecular effects on mature burn scars after treatment with a fractional CO(2) laser. Lasers Surg Med 2012; 44: 517–524

[14] Viera MH, Amini S, Valins W, Berman B. Innovative therapies in the treatment of keloids and hypertrophic scars. J Clin Aesthet Dermatol 2010; 3: 20–26

[15] Stucker FJ, Shaw GY. An approach to management of keloids. Arch Otolaryngol Head Neck Surg 1992; 118: 63–67

[16] Alster TS, Williams CM. Treatment of keloid sternotomy scars with 585 nm flashlamp-pumped pulsed-dye laser. Lancet 1995; 345: 1198–1200

[17] Walia S, Alster TS. Cutaneous CO2 laser resurfacing infection rate with and without prophylactic antibiotics. Dermatol Surg 1999; 25: 857–861

[18] Ortiz AE, Tingey C, Yu YE, Ross EV. Topical steroids implicated in postoperative infection following ablative laser resurfacing. Lasers Surg Med 2012; 44: 1–3

[19] Chan HH. Effective and safe use of lasers, light sources, and radiofrequency devices in the clinical management of Asian patients with selected dermatoses. Lasers Surg Med 2005; 37: 179–185

[20] Wicke C, Halliday B, Allen D, et al. Effects of steroids and retinoids on wound healing. Arch Surg 2000; 135: 1265–1270

5 Fractional Laser Skin Resurfacing

Paul J. Carniol and Louis M. DeJoseph

5.1 Introduction

Ablative skin resurfacing lasers were developed in the early 1990s. These resurfacing devices utilized high fluence, pulsed carbon dioxide (CO_2) lasers. They produced dramatic clinical results in the treatment of photodamaged facial skin, rhytids, lentigines, and dermal elastosis. However, this laser treatment frequently had a prolonged recovery with associated pinkness and risk of potential complications. These issues made laser resurfacing a less attractive skin rejuvenation option.[1]

This led to the development of other devices including fractional lasers. The first fractional lasers were nonablative. These were soon followed by ablative fractional lasers. These lasers provide clinically significant results with increased tolerability, lower risk of complications than ablative resurfacing, and a relatively minimal recovery.[2]

5.2 Background

Fractional photothermolysis has revolutionized laser skin resurfacing by providing significant improvement in clinical results with a relatively mild posttreatment recovery. There are also lower complication rates and associated morbidity.

The concept of fractional photothermolysis was first introduced by Manstein and colleagues in 2004.[3] Fractional lasers differ from ablative resurfacing lasers in that ablative lasers create microcolumns with intervening zones of untreated skin. Lasered columns are created in the epidermal and dermal layers to controlled depth, width, and spacing (▶ Fig. 5.1).

With these untreated areas there is additional cooling by heat dissipation through the unlasered area during treatment. Interestingly, bulk dermal heating occurs under the treated and untreated areas. This bulk heating creates a cascade of histochemical effects.

This is in contrast to devices that ablate the contiguous skin surface to a given depth. By ablating only columns of tissue, healing is more rapid and the potential for adverse effects such as new dyschromia, infection, scarring, and prolonged erythema is diminished. The adjacent untreated skin also allows for healing by epithelial migration from the adjacent unlasered areas. Thus, there is more rapid healing due to the benefits of the keratinocytes in the surrounding untreated skin.[4]

Ablative devices include the CO_2 (10,600-nm), erbium: yttrium scandium gallium garnet (Er:YSGG) (2,790-nm), and erbium:yttrium aluminum garnet (Er:YAG) (2,940-nm) lasers. The chromophore or target for these lasers is water in the epidermal and dermal skin layers. These high-energy lasers instantly heat the water causing vaporization of the treated tissue with each pulse. This creates wound columns.

Depending on the lasers, settings, and techniques during the first 24 hours, there can be minor bleeding, serous drainage, and/or swelling.

Time to initial recovery can range from a few days to 7 to 10 days. The duration of erythema postfractional ablative resurfacing varies but typically it lasts from 3 to 7 days. Uncommonly, depending on multiple variables including individual response to the procedure, postresurfacing pinkness can last for weeks.

Nonablative fractional lasers include 850- to 1,350-nm infrared, 915-nm, and 1,440-nm neodymium:yttrium aluminum garnet (Nd:YAG). These lasers are coagulative in nature, with no epidermal ablation. Recovery varies depending again on multiple variables and in general is shorter than ablative resurfacing.[5]

With these nonablative lasers, multiple treatments may be required to achieve the desired results and with present technology they may not be equivalent to the results of fractional ablative resurfacing. Longer wavelength, nonablative fractional lasers can be used to treat some conditions, such as scars, in patients with higher Fitzpatrick skin types (▶ Table 5.1).

5.3 Anatomy of Facial Resurfacing

The anatomical subunits of the face are an important concept in all cosmetic procedures of the face (▶ Fig. 5.2). Knowledge of these helps guide the physician when deciding on a segmental area of resurfacing versus a full-face procedure.

If a segmental resurfacing of the face is planned, such as rhytids in the perioral or periorbital regions, care must be taken to

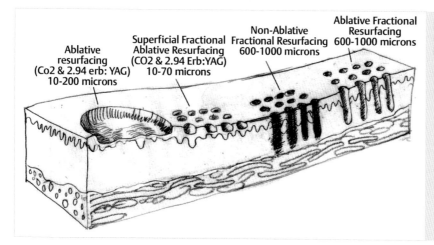

Ablative resurfacing (Co2 & 2.94 erb: YAG) 10-200 microns

Superficial Fractional Ablative Resurfacing (CO2 & 2.94 Erb:YAG) 10-70 microns

Non-Ablative Fractional Resurfacing 600-1000 microns

Ablative Fractional Resurfacing 600-1000 microns

Fig. 5.1 The evolution of resurfacing lasers leading to fractional ablation is demonstrated in this illustration.

Table 5.1 Fitzpatrick sun-reactive skin types and skin-color tanning response

Type I	White, always burns, never tans
Type II	White, usually burns, tans with difficulty
Type III	White, sometimes burns mildly, achieves average tan
Type IV	Brown, rarely burns, tans with ease
Type V	Dark brown, very rarely burns, tans very easily
Type VI	Black, never burns, tans very easily

resurface the entire subunit for proper blending. Also certain areas of the face can be more prone to scarring such as the malar prominence, and along the jawline. The subunits can be drawn on the face prior to resurfacing to help guide the practitioner. The authors prefer not to resurface individual facial subunits, but to perform a full facial resurfacing encompassing all subunits for balance and blending.

In general when an area is resurfaced, it has less photodamage and is smoother and tighter. Even with fractional ablative resurfacing, there may be a noticeable difference between the resurfaced area and an adjacent untreated area. Therefore, if segmental resurfacing is planned, we prefer to resurface at least the entire lower or upper two thirds of the face.

It is important to evaluate the characteristics of the skin when considering a resurfacing procedure.

Fitzpatrick skin typing groups a patient's skin based on sun reactivity and tanning response. Skin types I through III are usually considered resurfacing candidates because they have less pigmentation and hence less chance of dyschromia. It should be noted in patients with Fitzpatrick III skin type, if there are any olive tones to the skin there may be a greater risk of dyschromia. The authors do not routinely perform ablative fractional resurfacing on patients with Fitzpatrick skin types V and VI. Patients with Fitzpatrick skin type IV can have significant variation in skin tone. The authors only perform fractional ablative resurfacing on these patients if they have lighter skin tones. The Fitzpatrick skin type scale is listed in ▶ Table 5.1.

Another important skin characteristic is skin thickness. As patients get older their skin gets thinner. There is also a difference in skin thickness in different locations. For example, lower eyelid skin is significantly thinner than nasal skin.

The density and function of skin appendages are important and vary in different locations.

In general skin heals most rapidly and with a lower rate of complications where there is the greatest number of skin appendages and optimal blood supply. Medications such as isotretinoin reduce skin appendages and can cause a healing problem.

5.4 Patient Selection

One of the most important steps in the decision to perform a cosmetic procedure is proper patient selection. Several key points should be addressed in discussions with the patient prior to the procedure:
1. Patient concerns
2. Pertinent medical history (Hx)

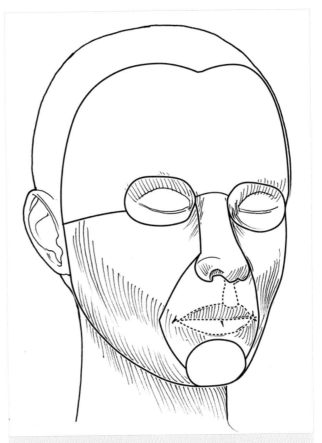

Fig. 5.2 Facial aesthetic subunits are shown in this drawing.

3. Physical examination
4. Treatment options
5. Patient expectations
6. Patient procedural experience
7. Complications, as well as after care

These obviously apply to every procedure we perform but some specifics to evaluation for laser resurfacing require discussion. The first step in the evaluation is patient concerns. Often it is helpful to have patients stand in front of a mirror with bright lighting, and point out the areas on the skin they would like addressed. This creates a general cosmetic skin "wish list" that really helps the practitioner understand patient desires. These commonly include rhytids, acne scarring, dyschromias, lentigines, rosacea, and actinic changes.

During this dialogue, a thorough evaluation of patient skin should be performed. This includes examination of elasticity, pigment, texture, laxity, thickness, scarring, actinic change, and of course neoplastic processes. All cosmetics should have been removed prior to this portion of the evaluation. In addition, a full facial examination should be undertaken with focus on areas of concern for laser resurfacing such as previous surgical and laser procedures, skin cancer resections, radiation therapy, Accutane (isotretinoin) usage in the last year, or Hx of scar or keloid formation. Radiation therapy, isotretinoin use, scleroderma, or Hx of burns can damage the adnexal structures of the skin that are vital to skin healing because re-epithelialization is initiated from within these structures. We recommend a 12-

month waiting period after cessation of isotretinoin before resurfacing. Attention should be placed on the periorbital region and Hx of blepharoplasty because even a slight lower ectropion or lid contraction can be greatly worsened by resurfacing. This can be evaluated by having the patient look upward while opening the mouth, which will reveal retraction or loss of lid elasticity.

The purpose of the initial patient evaluation is gaining a clear understanding of patient expectations, and managing them accordingly. We feel it is important to explain the expected result and that results vary from patient to patient. Photos of similar patients before and after the procedure help educate patients on expected changes. Showing staged photos of patients on days 1, 2, etc., demonstrating the healing and appearance during the postprocedure period have also proven helpful.

5.5 Preoperative Preparation

All patients are instructed to avoid sun exposure for 4 weeks prior to resurfacing and taught proper sun protection after the procedure. Preconditioning is accomplished with application of retinoic acid 0.025% cream 3 weeks prior to speed re-epithelialization.[6] Hydroquinone is used 3 weeks prior to decrease potential for postinflammatory hyperpigmentation, especially in darker skin types. Hydroquinone acts to block tyrosinase that decreases the formation and increases the destruction of melanosomes within the melanocytes.[7] Oral antibiotics are prescribed to start 2 days prior and continue 2 days after the procedure to diminish risk of superficial infection from skin bacterial organisms. Acyclovir is also started empirically 2 days prior at 800 mg twice daily and continued for a total of 5 days to help prevent herpes simplex virus (HSV) outbreak. Preoperative photographs are also obtained consisting of a front view and right and left three-quarter lateral views.

5.6 Procedure Technique

Patients are asked to cleanse their faces before coming in for the procedure and advised not to apply any makeup, moisturizer, or other topical skin products after cleansing. Because some patients will still apply moisturizer to their faces, we always ask when they arrive.

Further skin cleansing can be performed prior to the procedure with mild soap or glycolic wash. The type of anesthesia required for ablative fractional resurfacing can vary depending on the specific laser and the surgeon's preference.

The authors use a topical anesthesia regimen of 6% lidocaine and 6% tetracaine prior to the procedure. This is applied to the face and cervical region for 15 to 30 minutes. No occlusion of the topical anesthesia is used. This regimen provides a good level of anesthesia and patients are comfortable. It is then thoroughly removed. Because the lasers' chromophore is water, the face should be completely dry prior to starting the procedure.

During the procedure a chiller is used. This provides a comforting jet of cool air over the facial skin during the treatment. This increases patient comfort and helps to cool the surface of the unlasered portions of the skin.

We have not found a need for oral sedation for this technique or injection of any local anesthesia; however, there is no contraindication to either if needed for patient comfort. If sedation is utilized, patients should be carefully monitored.

Immediately prior to commencing the procedure, standard laser safety precautions are undertaken. These include but are not limited to: blocking out light from any windows, immediate availability of water, ease of access to a fire extinguisher, and eye protection. There should be eye protection for patient and staff. Staff eye protection should be designed for the type of laser that is being used. Patient eyes should be covered with metal eye shields. These can be external or corneal types of shields. Plastic eye shields are not used because there is a risk of melting if struck by the laser.

A multitude of lasers exist for fractional resurfacing today. As of this writing, there is no split-face study that clearly demonstrates the superiority of any one fractional resurfacing laser. The first author frequently uses a Cortex fractional CO_2 laser (Ellman International, Hicksville, New York). Some patients have extensive superficial actinic changes of their facial skin. These patients may derive greater benefit from combined laser treatment with a fractional CO_2 laser and superficial erbium laser treatment. Two separate laser devices can be used or both lasers may be available in the same laser device such as in the Cortex laser.

There are multiple fractional CO_2 lasers that are available. The settings used vary depending on numerous factors. First are physician laser experience and preference. Second are patient and physician goals for this treatment. Third are the time of recovery and the recovery experience that the patient is willing to undergo. Fourth are any potential risk factors for healing problems both systemic and local. Fifth are patient age and skin thickness. Although the authors rarely do this for fractional resurfacing, if there is any question about the effects of a planned laser treatment, test spots can be performed and complete treatment deferred until the results of the test spots are evaluated.

Another consideration is that if, at any time during the course of a laser procedure, either patient experience or effects of the laser vary from what was anticipated prior to the treatment, the procedure should be interrupted and an evaluation should be performed as to whether to continue.

The following settings are those used by the second author when treating patients with the Sandstone Matrix laser (Ellman). This laser has the capability of controlling many aspects of the laser process such as density, which is directly proportional to the percentage of skin surface area that is treated. The settings or techniques may be laser-specific and may not apply to any other device.

Before using a laser, check with the manufacturer for recommended settings and techniques. Pulse duration represents the pulse width or tissue ablation time. Laser power represented in watts (W) correlates directly with the laser fluence. All resurfacing is done in continuous wave mode for fractional ablation. The pattern is generated in the handpiece and can be used in differing sizes and shapes depending on the operator's preference and the area being treated.

The laser is positioned at the patient's side with the laser arm manipulated by the physician. The second author frequently uses a power of 21 to 23 W, density of ~ 30%, and duration of up to 2 ms. These settings are not universally used by all treating physicians on all patients. The second author treats each subunit with a uniformly, nonoverlapping, square-beam pattern beginning at the forehead. Care is taken to feather into the hairline for completeness. The first author does not treat by subunits. Rather he prefers to treat at least the lower two thirds of the face and, depending on the clinical findings, treat or omit treatment to the forehead region. An important consideration for any fractional laser is the dermal thermal effects. Excessive dermal heating can develop related to fluence, dermal density, and/or pulse duration. If the dermis is overheated there is a greater risk for scarring.

Most physicians use a smoke evacuator to remove the laser plume. Surgical masks with a 0.1-μm pore size are also frequently used by the physician and any other staff in the procedure room.

If resurfacing is performed in the periorbital area, milder settings should be used. The authors do not routinely resurface the skin of the upper eyelid below the upper eyelid fold. This is particularly important because fractional CO_2 laser resurfacing can have a significant penetration depth. Fractional CO_2 lasers can penetrate deeper than nonfractional resurfacing lasers.

The number of passes that are performed and the settings for each pass vary for each patient and among treating physicians. If a second pass is performed, it should be done starting over at the area that was first treated so that the dermis in this area has had time to cool while subsequent areas were treated. Furthermore, the fractional pattern of the second pass should not overlap the first pass to avoid double pulsing any area and thermal stacking.

The skin can have a patternlike appearance after fractional resurfacing. As long as excessive settings have not been used and there are no healing or infectious problems during the recovery period, this pattern is not visible after healing is completed. Pinpoint bleeding may also be noted in some areas immediately after the procedure or the evening after the treatment. This can occur when the fractional resurfacing extends into the level of the dermal plexus of vessels. The authors routinely discuss this possibility with their patients so it will not be a cause for concern.

Resurfacing will on occasion be extended into the neck and décolleté area. This can be done quite effectively with fractional resurfacing, but adjustment of the laser settings must be done. Patients should understand that as reduced settings are used, there will be a more limited result. Moving to a lower power (16 W), decreasing density to around 21%, and lowering duration to 0.8 ms have been proven safe and effective in this area for the second author. However, it should be remembered that the neck and décolleté area have a lower sebaceous unit (adnexal structure) count in comparison to the face, different blood supply, and a significantly greater tendency for scarring.

The lower settings are used to allow for these differences. Only one pass is made in these areas. These areas should be treated carefully because significant scarring has been reported in the cervical region after fractionated resurfacing.[8] The authors cannot guarantee the safety of these settings for any particular patient. Physicians must make their own judgments.

Two areas on the face that warrant further discussion and caution are the infraorbital and mandibular ridge regions. The skin of the infraorbital region is significantly thinner than the surrounding facial skin. This places it at higher risk for hypertrophic scarring and ectropion formation.[9] Care should be taken in this area with lowered passes or energy settings, especially when laxity or previous surgery is noted. Similarly, the skin of the mandibular ridge is prone to hypertrophic scarring; thus fewer passes, reduced energy, and/or lower density may be warranted in this area.

5.7 Postoperative Care

After the laser procedure is completed, as a comfort measure, the patient can be handed a chiller on a low setting to cool the treated surface. Aquaphor (Beiersdorf Inc., Wilton, Connecticut) or another petroleum-based ointment is then applied with a tongue depressor to all the treated areas. The first author has patients apply moist gauze compresses to the treated area with a mixture of white vinegar and water (1 tsp of white vinegar to 2 cups of water) at least three times a day and then reapply the Aquaphor. This vinegar and water mixture can be refrigerated to increase patient comfort.

The ointment can predispose the patient to milia or acneiform eruptions. Removing the ointment three times a day and applying the moist compresses helps to reduce this. Furthermore, the ointment use is reduced or discontinued when possible on the 4th day after the procedure. If a patient still has significant dry crusts after 3 days, it is continued for an additional 1 or 2 days.

In order to decrease the possibility of developing significant dyschromia after the procedure, it is important to avoid sun exposure. The authors start patients on daytime use of a sunscreen such as micronized zinc oxide that blocks ultraviolet A (UVA) and ultraviolet B (UVB), as soon as the Aquaphor use is diminished. In speaking with their patients, the authors emphasize the importance of the sunscreen. Many patients can start using a mineral-base foundation 5 to 7 days after the procedure. Typically, a mineral-base foundation also provides additional sun protection.

Patients may experience some pruritus during the 1st or 2nd week after treatment. If a patient scratches a resurfaced area, this can lead to hypertrophic scarring. Scratching can occur even while a patient is sleeping. Therefore it is important to discuss this with the patient after the procedure. The first author's standard postresurfacing instructions, in addition to advising the patient not to scratch, include taking an antihistamine such as diphenhydramine at bedtime, if there is even minimal pruritus. An antiscratching measure also discussed is the wearing of white cotton gloves while sleeping. The second author advises using a 1%-hydrocortisone cream once or twice daily for extreme itching. The first author does not routinely suggest this.

5.8 Expected Results

The results obtained from fractional CO_2 laser resurfacing can vary from patient to patient and with the problems being treated. Results can be quite dramatic when considering the reduced downtime associated with these lasers (▶ Fig. 5.3, ▶ Fig. 5.4, ▶ Fig. 5.5). After fractional resurfacing collagen stimulation occurs for at least 6 months. This is a gradual effect and is best seen comparing serial photographs. Because this is a gradual, progressive change, it may not be as obvious to patients who are checking their skin daily in the mirror. Therefore, the authors do not typically perform a second treatment until 6 months after the first treatment. This should be discussed in advance with patients so they are prepared for the gradual improvement.

Acne scars can be improved with minimal downtime with fractional resurfacing. As with other modalities and previous studies, different types of acne scars have a varied response to the laser treatments. The majority of patients will see a noticeable improvement. More than one treatment may be necessary to maximize the results. Patients should also be aware that acne scars cannot be completely removed.

Fractional and nonfractional CO_2 laser resurfacing have been shown to have similar histochemical effects. Reilly et al[10] demonstrated significant changes in the gene expression of several matrix metalloproteinases similar to full ablative resurfacing. Orringer et al found proinflammatory cytokine induction and an increase in type I collagen after fractional resurfacing.[11] Naouri et al demonstrated an increase in dermal thickness after fractional resurfacing.[12] Another study found greater deposition of type III collagen and neocollagen deposition on electron microscopy after fractional CO_2 laser resurfacing.[13]

Healing after CO_2 laser resurfacing appears to adhere to the well-established phases of wound healing.[14] The literature suggests a combination of collagen denaturation and contraction, and neocollagenesis as the most likely mechanism(s) of action for skin healing after laser resurfacing.[14,15,16]

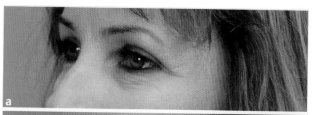
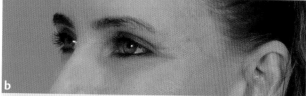

Fig. 5.3 Dramatic procedure results. (a) Before periorbital, segmental fractional CO_2 laser resurfacing. (b) 1 year after the treatment.

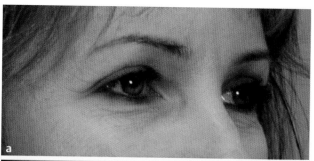
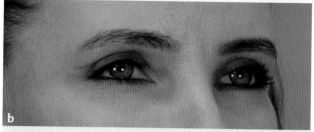

Fig. 5.4 Before and after photos of a particular modality. (a) Before periorbital, segmental fractional CO_2 laser resurfacing. (b) 6 months after the procedure.

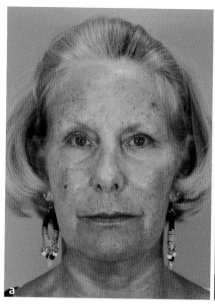
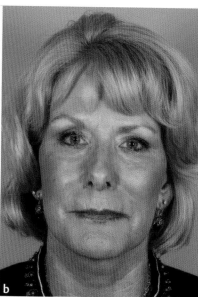

Fig. 5.5 Outcome of full-face technique combined with other modalities. (a) Before full-face fractional CO_2 laser resurfacing combined with facelift and upper lid blepharoplasty. (b) Results after the procedure.

5.9 Complications and Management

With any procedure there is an associated risk of complications. Careful preoperative planning and preparation reduce this risk but cannot eliminate it. Complications can occur. Early recognition and effective management can reduce but not completely eliminate the possibility of scarring or other undesirable sequelae. Some patients have a more challenging recovery than others. These challenges that may develop include but are not limited to pruritus, acneiform breakout, immediate posttreatment pinkness, minor bleeding, and edema. These should probably be considered minor complications. Other complications can be more significant (Video 5.1).

5.9.1 Prolonged Erythema

Prolonged erythema after fractional laser resurfacing has been reported in up to 7% of cases of ablative laser resurfacing at 3 months' posttreatment.[17,18] Traditional ablative resurfacing tends to carry a higher risk of prolonged erythema; however, fractional techniques that employ multiple passes, deep penetration, or pulse stacking (the authors recommend avoiding pulse stacking) also increase the incidence of prolonged erythema.[19] Treatment of this often consists of watchful waiting because most cases resolve within 3 months. Persistent pinkness should be differentiated from the erythema that can be associated with developing hypertrophic scars.

Treatment with 590-nm, light-emitting diode (LED) lasers has been reported to reduce the erythema intensity.[20] Flashlamp-pumped dye lasers and 532-nm, LED lasers can also be used to reduce this. If these modalities are used, it is important to use low settings so the erythema is improved and not worsened. Ascorbic acid applied topically has also been shown to decrease duration and intensity of erythema.[21]

5.9.2 Acne and Milia

Acne and milia are relatively common after fractional skin resurfacing, with 2 to 19% reported incidence.[22,23,24,25,26] They seem to relate to the use of occlusive ointment or moisturizers. In most cases, discontinuing occlusive moisturizers as early as possible postoperatively diminishes the risk of occurrence. As already described, removing the occlusive ointment at least three times daily and applying moist gauze compresses with a diluted white vinegar and water solution have almost completely eliminated these problems for patients of the first author. Occurrences usually respond well to discontinuing the occlusive moisturizer. If there appears to be an associated infection then antibiotic therapy should be initiated.

5.9.3 Pigmentary Changes

Postinflammatory hyperpigmentation (PIH) is uncommon after fractional skin resurfacing in comparison to nonfractional laser resurfacing. It has been reported ranging from 1 to 32%, depending on type of laser, intensity of treatment, and patient skin type.[17,23,27,28,29,30,31,32] It is more common in patients with higher Fitzpatrick skin types. Due to this risk, the authors do not routinely perform fractional ablative CO_2 resurfacing on patients with darker Fitzpatrick IV, V, and VI skin types.

All patients are instructed on sun-exposure avoidance for 4 weeks before and after the procedure to reduce PIH.[29,33] In general, patients with darker Fitzpatrick skin types (IV–VI) carry a higher likelihood of developing PIH.

In Asian patients, it's imperative that laser fluencies are reduced, lower densities used, and longer intervals between treatments utilized.[29,34] This hyperpigmentation usually is self-limited and resolves with time; however, it can be treated with strict sun precautions, topical lightening agents, and hydroxy acid skin peels. UVA and UVB sunscreens are also mainstays of treatment to reduce pigmentary melanocytic activity. Patients should be reminded to apply them each morning before leaving home for their regular activities.

At the other end of the spectrum is hypopigmentation, which is rare with fractional skin resurfacing. Delayed hypopigmentation occurs more frequently after multipass CO_2 laser resurfacing. Hypopigmentation after fractional resurfacing has been reported in two patients in an area of hypertrophic cervical scarring occurring in two patients.[8,9] This persisted for several months and eventually resolved.

When performing fractional resurfacing, care should be taken especially in the neck region where scarring can occur.[9]

5.9.4 Infection

Most infections associated with fractional skin resurfacing develop within the 1st week after treatment. This reinforces the need for close follow-up and evaluation so that expedient diagnosis and treatment can be established. HSV is the most common infection with fractional laser resurfacing, with incidence reported from 0.3 to 2%.[23,25,35] Most physicians favor pretreatment with antiviral prophylaxis to prevent this complication. The authors prefer acyclovir for this but have used other antiviral medications. This should be started 24 to 48 hours prior to the procedure.

If a patient has an active herpetic lesion, laser resurfacing should be postponed until complete resolution.

Bacterial infection is a rarely seen complication with 0.1% of cases developing impetigo superficial infection,[23] the common pathogens being *Staphylococcus aureus* and pseudomonas. If these infections develop, scarring may occur; thus treatment needs to be prompt. They present with increased pain, erythema, exudates, and erosions with crusts in the 1- to 3-day period posttreatment. Appropriate antibiotic therapy should be started along with wound culture and sensitivity tests. Fungal infection can also develop after laser treatment.[8,9] *Candida albicans* is the most common pathogen and can occur at a later postoperative period (7 to 14 days). Treatment is with appropriate antifungal medications because these infections have been shown to produce scarring.[8,9]

As previously noted, the first author has patients cleanse and soak with a dilute acetic acid solution consisting of 1 tsp of white vinegar mixed with 2 cups of water. This inhibits the growth of fungal and gram-negative organisms. He believes that this diminishes the risk of pseudomonas and fungal infections postresurfacing.

5.9.5 Scarring

The most feared complication of all resurfacing is scarring. It is relatively uncommon with traditional ablative resurfacing.[1,2] It is even less common with fractional resurfacing but it has been reported.[8,9,36] A literature review on the subject demonstrated that 9 of 10 published cases were from treatment on the neck area, resulting in vertical and horizontal hypertrophic scarring.[4]

They commonly present with areas of localized erythema and induration at 2 to 4 weeks posttreatment. Prompt diagnosis and treatment are important to decrease the scarring. It is theorized that the relative paucity of pilosebaceous units, as well as a different blood supply pattern in the neck in comparison to the face, lead to the increased risk of scarring.[37] Also, thin skin architecture adds to the susceptibility to thermal injury.

Care and caution must be applied when resurfacing the neck area. Cervical fractional resurfacing is not recommended for physicians who are just starting to use lasers. The indications for performing fractional resurfacing of this area vary among surgeons. Other areas of known concern are over the margin of the mandible and the lower eyelids. These areas should also be approached with caution because they are at risk for scar formation.[8] If a patient has a history of prior radiation therapy to an area for which laser treatment is being considered, there can be an associated risk of a healing problem. Radiation therapy to a different area (such as the breast or prostate) should not affect facial healing. Prior surgery to an area for which laser treatment is being considered may increase the risk of complications but is not a contraindication. With prior lower eyelid surgery there can be a greater risk of an ectropion. Surgery to the face or neck can increase the risk of a healing problem.

Problems with scarring can develop for multiple reasons. Depending on the reason this developed, a prior problem with scarring may not be a contraindication to a fractional resurfacing procedure. More recently, fractional lasers have been used to treat or prevent scarring.[38,39,40]

If hypertrophic scarring starts to develop, there are several treatment modalities available. These include vascular laser treatments, topical silicone gel products, and corticosteroids. The authors reserve intralesional corticosteroid injection for scars that do not respond to the prior three treatments.

5.10 Conclusion

Fractional ablative resurfacing has been a significant advance for skin rejuvenation. It bridges the gap that has existed between clinical results and postprocedure downtime. The first nonablative fractional laser treatment by Manstein et al in 2004 represented the step leading to a significant improvement in recovery compared to traditional resurfacing and the eventual development of fractional resurfacing.[3]

Fractional resurfacing has an easier, shorter recovery than traditional resurfacing. There is also a lower incidence of adverse events than with traditional CO_2 resurfacing.[5] Nonablative fractional modalities have been used to improve pigmentary[27] changes and skin texture. However for these conditions, fractional resurfacing laser results have been more notable.

These more outstanding results with their relatively high-safety profiles have led to increasing popularity for these procedures. Hantash et al[41] in 2007 published the first results of ablative fractional laser resurfacing, demonstrating promising results with skin-tightening comparable to ablative CO_2 and Er:YAG, but with shorter recovery periods of 7 to 14 days. These fractional lasers have been shown to be effective in the treatment of acne scarring[18] and facial rhytid reduction.[42]

Fractional resurfacing represents one of the most important and exciting discoveries in skin rejuvenation of the prior decade. The technology behind fractional resurfacing should continue to improve, as demand for cutting-edge treatments increases. The uses of this technology are already far-reaching, and will only magnify as research into the technology of fractional resurfacing delves deeper into improving results and defining new uses. It has become an effective and popular technology for the treatment of cutaneous photoaging, facial rhytids, dyschromia, acne scars, and other conditions.

References

[1] Aslter TS, Tanzi EL. Laser skin resurfacing: ablative and nonablative. In: Robinson JK, Hanke CW, Segelmann, RD, et al., eds. Surgery of the Skin. Philadelphia, PA: Elsevier; 2005: 611–624

[2] Alster TS, Tanzi EL. Complications in laser and light surgery. In: Goldberg DJ, ed. Lasers and Lights. Vol 2. Philadelphia, PA: Saunders Elsevier; 2008: 99–112

[3] Manstein D, Herron GS, Sink RK, Tanner H, Anderson RR. Fractional photothermolysis: a new concept for cutaneous remodeling using microscopic patterns of thermal injury. Lasers Surg Med 2004; 34: 426–438

[4] Metelitsa AI, Alster TS. Fractionated laser skin resurfacing treatment complications: a review. Dermatol Surg 2010; 36: 299–306

[5] Abbasi NR, Dover JS. Fractional laser resurfacing: why all the fuss? Dermatol Surg 2010; 36: 307–308

[6] Mandy SH. Tretinoin in the preoperative and postoperative management of dermabrasion. J Am Acad Dermatol 1986; 15: 878–879, 888–889

[7] Ortonne JP, Bose SK. Pigmentation: dyschromia. In: Baran R, Maibach HI, eds. Textbook of Cosmetic Dermatology. Boca Raton, FL: Taylor & Francis; 2005: 401–402

[8] Avram MM, Tope WD, Yu T, Szachowicz E, Nelson JS. Hypertrophic scarring of the neck following ablative fractional carbon dioxide laser resurfacing. Lasers Surg Med 2009; 41: 185–188

[9] Fife DJ, Fitzpatrick RE, Zachary CB. Complications of fractional CO2 laser resurfacing: four cases. Lasers Surg Med 2009; 41: 179–184

[10] Reilly MJ, Cohen M, Hokugo A, Keller GS. Molecular effects of fractional carbon dioxide laser resurfacing on photodamaged human skin. Arch Facial Plast Surg 2010; 12: 321–325

[11] Orringer JS, Rittié L, Baker D, Voorhees JJ, Fisher G. Molecular mechanisms of nonablative fractionated laser resurfacing. Br J Dermatol 2010; 163: 757–768

[12] Naouri M, Atlan M, Perrodeau E, et al. High-resolution ultrasound imaging to demonstrate and predict efficacy of carbon dioxide fractional resurfacing laser treatment. Dermatol Surg 2011; 37: 596–603

[13] Berlin AL, Hussain M, Phelps R, Goldberg DJ. A prospective study of fractional scanned nonsequential carbon dioxide laser resurfacing: a clinical and histopathologic evaluation. Dermatol Surg 2009; 35: 222–228

[14] Seckel BR, Younai S, Wang KK. Skin tightening effects of the ultrapulse CO2 laser. Plast Reconstr Surg 1998; 102: 872–877

[15] Orringer JS, Kang S, Johnson TM, et al. Connective tissue remodeling induced by carbon dioxide laser resurfacing of photodamaged human skin. Arch Dermatol 2004; 140: 1326–1332

[16] Ross EV, McKinlay JR, Anderson RR. Why does carbon dioxide resurfacing work? A review. Arch Dermatol 1999; 135: 444–454

[17] Rahman Z, MacFalls H, Jiang K, et al. Fractional deep dermal ablation induces tissue tightening. Lasers Surg Med 2009; 41: 78–86

[18] Chapas AM, Brightman L, Sukal S, et al. Successful treatment of acneiform scarring with CO2 ablative fractional resurfacing. Lasers Surg Med 2008; 40: 381–386

[19] Dierickx CC, Khatri KA, Tannous ZS, et al. Micro-fractional ablative skin resurfacing with two novel erbium laser systems. Lasers Surg Med 2008; 40: 113–123

[20] Alster TS, Wanitphakdeedecha R. Improvement of postfractional laser erythema with light-emitting diode photomodulation. Dermatol Surg 2009; 35: 813–815

[21] Alster TS, West TB. Effect of topical vitamin C on postoperative carbon dioxide laser resurfacing erythema. Dermatol Surg 1998; 24: 331–334

[22] Fisher GH, Geronemus RG. Short-term side effects of fractional photothermolysis. Dermatol Surg 2005; 31: 1245–1249, discussion 1249

[23] Graber EM, Tanzi EL, Alster TS. Side effects and complications of fractional laser photothermolysis: experience with 961 treatments. Dermatol Surg 2008; 34: 301–305, discussion 305–307

[24] Wanner M, Tanzi EL, Alster TS. Fractional photothermolysis: treatment of facial and nonfacial cutaneous photodamage with a 1,550-nm erbium-doped fiber laser. Dermatol Surg 2007; 33: 23–28

[25] Alster TS, Tanzi EL, Lazarus M. The use of fractional laser photothermolysis for the treatment of atrophic scars. Dermatol Surg 2007; 33: 295–299

[26] Gotkin RH, Sarnoff DS, Cannarozzo G, Sadick NS, Alexiades-Armenakas M. Ablative skin resurfacing with a novel microablative CO_2 laser. J Drugs Dermatol 2009; 8: 138–144

[27] Rokhsar CK, Fitzpatrick RE. The treatment of melasma with fractional photothermolysis: a pilot study. Dermatol Surg 2005; 31: 1645–1650

[28] Tanzi EL, Wanitphakdeedecha R, Alster TS. Fraxel laser indications and long-term follow-up. Aesthet Surg J 2008; 28: 675–678, discussion 679–680

[29] Chan HH, Manstein D, Yu CS, Shek S, Kono T, Wei WI. The prevalence and risk factors of post-inflammatory hyperpigmentation after fractional resurfacing in Asians. Lasers Surg Med 2007; 39: 381–385

[30] Hu S, Chen MC, Lee MC, Yang LC, Keoprasom N. Fractional resurfacing for the treatment of atrophic facial acne scars in Asian skin. Dermatol Surg 2009; 35: 826–832

[31] Walgrave SE, Ortiz AE, MacFalls HT, et al. Evaluation of a novel fractional resurfacing device for treatment of acne scarring. Lasers Surg Med 2009; 41: 122–127

[32] Rahman Z, Alam M, Dover JS. Fractional laser treatment for pigmentation and texture improvement. Skin Therapy Lett 2006; 11: 7–11

[33] Izikson L, Anderson RR. Resolution of blue minocycline pigmentation of the face after fractional photothermolysis. Lasers Surg Med 2008; 40: 399–401

[34] Kono T, Chan HH, Groff WF, et al. Prospective direct comparison study of fractional resurfacing using different fluences and densities for skin rejuvenation in Asians. Lasers Surg Med 2007; 39: 311–314

[35] Setyadi HG, Jacobs AA, Markus RF. Infectious complications after nonablative fractional resurfacing treatment. Dermatol Surg 2008; 34: 1595–1598

[36] Ross RB, Spencer J. Scarring and persistent erythema after fractionated ablative CO_2 laser resurfacing. J Drugs Dermatol 2008; 7: 1072–1073

[37] Goldman MP, Fitzpatrick RE, Manuskiatti W. Laser resurfacing of the neck with the Erbium:YAG laser. Dermatol Surg 1999; 25: 164–167, discussion 167–168

[38] Carniol PJ, Meshkov L, Grunebaum LD. Laser treatment of facial scars. Curr Opin Otolaryngol Head Neck Surg 2011; 19: 283–288

[39] Shumaker PR, Kwan JM, Landers JT, Uebelhoer NS. Functional improvements in traumatic scars and scar contractures using an ablative fractional laser protocol. J Trauma Acute Care Surg 2012; 73 Suppl 1: S116–S121

[40] Hedelund L, Haak CS, Togsverd-Bo K, Bogh MK, Bjerring P, Haedersdal M. Fractional CO_2 laser resurfacing for atrophic acne scars: a randomized controlled trial with blinded response evaluation. Lasers Surg Med 2012; 44: 447–452

[41] Hantash BM, Bedi VP, Kapadia B, et al. In vivo histological evaluation of a novel ablative fractional resurfacing device. Lasers Surg Med 2007; 39: 96–107

[42] Munavalli G. Single pass fractionated CO_2 laser resurfacing for improvement of lower eyelid rhytids. Abstract presented at: American Society for Laser Medicine and Surgery Conference; April 2008; Kissimmee, FL

6 Erbium:Yttrium Aluminum Garnet Laser Skin Resurfacing

J. David Holcomb

6.1 Background/History

The mid-1990s saw the publication of several initial reports regarding early experience with 2,940-nm erbium:yttrium aluminum garnet (Er:YAG) laser skin resurfacing.[1,2,3] The clinical allure of an alternative wavelength to the 10,600-nm carbon dioxide (CO_2) skin resurfacing laser was in part related to the desire to improve skin tone and texture while minimizing collateral thermal effects. The first Er:YAG skin resurfacing devices were low-power, narrow pulse width lasers with clinically limiting tissue ablation efficiency and minimal tissue coagulation effect. As a result, per-pass tissue ablation depth was shallow and multiple passes were required to reach the papillary dermis.[3] Whereas superficial dyschromia was greatly improved, the lack of a significant tissue coagulation effect resulted in bleeding upon reaching the papillary dermis and poor wrinkle effacement. The subsequent ability to modify the pulse duration (variable pulse vs. quasi-long pulse) and other energy delivery advances (e.g., optical multiplexing—see following text) with higher powered devices enabled laser surgeons to perform deeper treatments with less bleeding and improved rhytid reduction and tissue tightening.

The convergence of wavelengths for the Er:YAG skin resurfacing laser with the peak for water absorption in the near infrared spectrum (both ~ 2,940 nm) enables the defining characteristic photomechanical tissue interaction of this device. Extremely rapid and efficient absorption of radiant energy from the 2,940-nm Er:YAG skin resurfacing laser causes near instantaneous conversion of light energy into mechanical energy as the affected layers of the skin are photodisrupted, ejected, and partially vaporized; very little tissue coagulation occurs with the short pulse Er:YAG skin resurfacing laser. By comparison, with far less efficient water absorption (2,940-nm Er:YAG ~ 16 times greater), the 10,600-nm CO_2 skin resurfacing laser interacts with skin tissue primarily via a photothermal effect that creates extensive tissue coagulation and relatively less tissue ablation.[4]

Lengthening the pulse duration of the Er:YAG skin resurfacing laser through a series or train of subablative (laser fluence or energy below the threshold for maximum photomechanical effect and skin vaporization) pulses enabled laser surgeons to mimic the photothermal effect of the CO_2 laser. This new feature became known as "dual mode" or "variable pulse mode," wherein the Er:YAG laser was capable of delivering energy to the tissue via a short pulse (ablation) mode or a long pulse (coagulation) mode. Optical multiplexing—the use of a spinning

mirror assembly to integrate the photon energy output of two separate laser heads operating in either ablate or coagulate modes—was another significant and necessary tissue delivery advance that allowed laser surgeons to effectively harness the power of the new dual mode (ablation, coagulation) Er:YAG laser skin resurfacing systems for maximum flexibility and speed in treatment.[5] The ability to use either ablate or coagulate modes or both ablate and coagulate modes simultaneously while also controlling the depth of effect for each became known as "blending" or "tuning" the dual mode Er:YAG laser to meet specific treatment objectives.

6.2 Indications/Contraindications

Skin rejuvenation, the primary indication for Er:YAG laser skin resurfacing, encompasses improvement of coarse, dull surface texture, reduction of dyschromia and photodamage, along with wrinkle effacement and improvement of scarring (▶ Fig. 6.1, ▶ Fig. 6.2, ▶ Fig. 6.3 and ▶ Fig. 6.4). Whereas traditional full-field, dual mode Er:YAG deep laser skin resurfacing is most often performed in Fitzpatrick skin types I, II, and possibly III, a more superficial full-field, ablate mode–only Er:YAG laser skin resurfacing treatment may be preferred in darker Fitzpatrick skin types (III, IV, and V). Deeper dual mode treatments have been associated with prolonged erythema (more than 4 months) and a relatively high rate (nearly 40%) of postinflammatory hyperpigmentation (PIH).[6,7]

Several split-face (side-by-side) studies comparing modulated Er:YAG and pulsed CO_2 skin resurfacing lasers have determined that benefits from dual mode Er:YAG laser skin resurfacing of facial rhytids approach or match those of CO_2 laser skin resurfacing (treatment outcomes evaluated included wrinkle improvement, skin tightening, and improvement in photoaging scores), when similar immediate posttreatment end points are reached clinically and histologically.[8,9,10,11] Although similar clinical results may be achieved, tissue contraction may be mediated differently with heat-induced collagen tightening from the pulsed CO_2 laser with its significantly deeper residual thermal damage (e.g., 200 μm vs. up to 50 μm) and with wound contracture secondary to tissue healing following treatment with the Er:YAG laser.[12]

Photodamage and superficial dyschromia may be effectively treated with a single-pass intraepidermal peel (e.g., 50-μm depth) using ablate-only mode; however, when desired, the

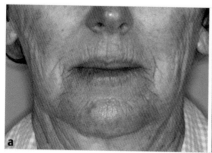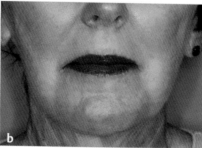

Fig. 6.1 (a) Before and (b) 7 months after close-up photographs of perioral area following dual mode erbium:yttrium aluminum garnet (Er:YAG) laser skin resurfacing (66-year-old woman, Fitzpatrick skin type II, four passes at 50% overlap with ablate/coagulate settings 120/0, 100/50, 140/50, and 50/100). Note: near complete effacement of perioral lines and wrinkles.

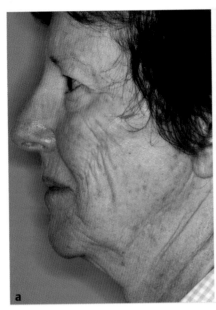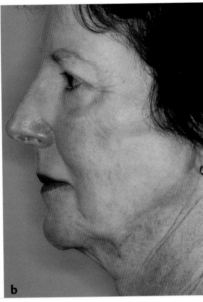

Fig. 6.2 (a) Before and (b) 7 months after left lateral photos following dual mode erbium: yttrium aluminum garnet (Er:YAG) laser skin resurfacing (66-year-old woman, Fitzpatrick skin type II, two passes on cheek areas at 50% overlap with ablate/coagulate settings 120/0 and 100/50). Note: effacement of rhytids, skin tightening, and increased contrast in skin tone between treated and untreated skin areas at jawline.

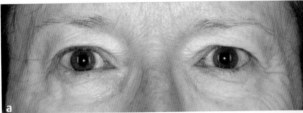
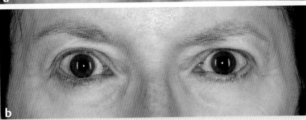

Fig. 6.3 (a) Before and (b) 7 months after close-up images of periorbital area following dual mode erbium:yttrium aluminum garnet (Er:YAG) laser skin resurfacing (66-year-old woman, Fitzpatrick skin type II, three passes at 50% overlap with ablate/coagulate settings 80/0, 60/50, and 60/50). Note: effacement of rhytids and skin tightening of the upper and lower eyelids.

related long-term structural change extending from the epidermis into the deep dermis (e.g., up to 1,000-μm depth) with just transient erythema (NFR) or limited downtime (AFR).

Although effective for removal of actinic keratoses and for nonmelanoma skin cancer prophylaxis, full-field laser skin resurfacing is not superior to other common treatment approaches including topical 5-fluorouracil (5-FU) or trichloroacetic acid (TCA) peels.[16] Various types of benign skin lesions (e.g., moles, seborrheic keratosis) may be effectively removed using a handpiece with a small spot (e.g., 2 mm) or point beam mode (Video 6.3). Skin layers covering deeper milia and small intradermal pseudocysts may be ablated, enabling mechanical extraction and/or laser ablation. In select cases large patulous pores or deep ice pick scars may be de-epithelialized and then allowed to close through cicatricial wound contracture or they may be closed with one or more small sutures. Whereas Er:YAG laser skin resurfacing has been employed for treatment of various types of scarring, newer approaches with NFR and AFR have become more prevalent and the de facto nonsurgical standard of care for these conditions.

Pretreatment considerations for Er:YAG laser skin resurfacing include absolute and relative contraindications that may require avoidance, delay, or modification of the proposed treatment. Patients who are deemed appropriate candidates for laser skin resurfacing must indicate willingness to accept downtime and responsibility for wound care during healing, as well as possible sequelae and attendant risks of complications. Absolute contraindications for laser skin resurfacing include active skin infection (bacterial, viral), isotretinoin use in the past 12 months, impaired immune function, suspicious skin lesion or skin cancer in treatment area, melasma, and unrealistic expectations regarding laser skin resurfacing benefits and outcomes.

Relative contraindications for laser skin resurfacing include collagen vascular disease, abnormal scarring, prior radiation therapy or deep burn in treatment area, diffuse hyperpigmentation, Koebnerizing skin conditions, inflammatory condition of skin, severe skin sensitivity, lower eyelid laxity, and prior lower eyelid surgery. Severe hyperpigmentation affecting the face, neck, and other areas of the body may lead to relative

entire epidermis may be removed and the upper dermis partially ablated with a single pass (e.g., up to 200-μm total depth in ablate-only mode) (Video 6.1). In addition to clinically evident improvement of skin tone, superficial or microablative (intra-epidermal, i.e., basement membrane remains intact) Er:YAG laser skin peels have also been shown to increase dermal matrix remodeling and to increase collagen types I, III, and VII as well as newly synthesized collagen (e.g., procollagen I and III) and tropoelastin.[13,14,15] Although microablative Er:YAG laser treatments (Video 6.2) initiate inflammatory and tissue regenerative responses that extend into the dermis and well beyond the depth of tissue injury, it appears that maintenance of these changes may require ongoing interval treatments with repeated stimulation of the skin. The advent of nonablative fractional resurfacing (NFR) and ablative fractional resurfacing (AFR) enabled thermal and/or mechanical microablative injury with

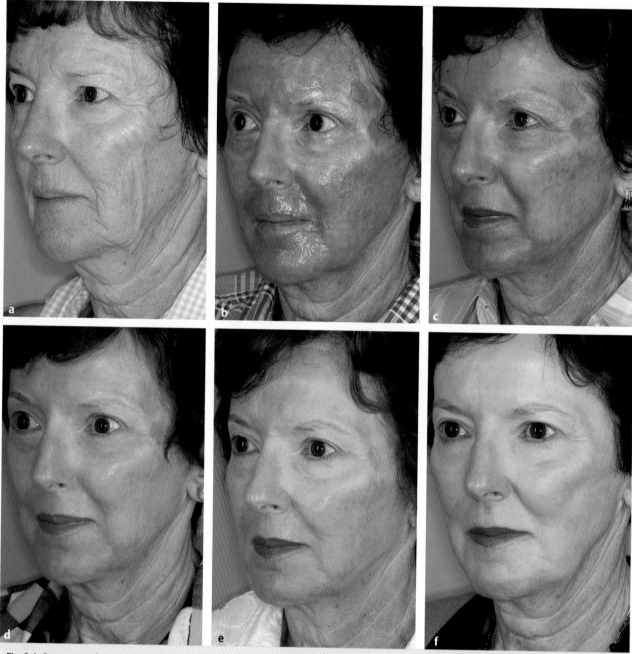

Fig. 6.4 Composite of six separate left oblique photographs documenting progression of erythema following dual mode erbium:yttrium aluminum garnet (Er:YAG) laser skin resurfacing (66-year-old woman, Fitzpatrick skin type II). (**a**) Before; (**b**) 7 days after; (**c**) 30 days after; (**d**) 60 days after; (**e**) 90 days after; (**f**) 210 days after. Note: persistent erythema 90 days following treatment and resulting moderate hypopigmentation at 210 days.

hypopigmentation of the treated skin with an unusually stark contrast between treated lower facial skin and untreated neck skin (▶ Fig. 6.2). Posttreatment camouflage with mineral make-up and/or adjunctive treatment(s) of the adjacent skin (e.g., intense pulse light photorejuvenation) may be beneficial. Patients with abnormal lower eyelid laxity are at higher risk for treatment-related lower eyelid malposition following deep laser resurfacing of the lower eyelid skin; therefore, preemptive (pretreatment or concurrent) lower eyelid tightening (e.g., lateral canthoplasty) should be considered. Paradoxically, patients with minimal lower eyelid skin laxity following transcutaneous

lower eyelid blepharoplasty may also be at higher risk for lower eyelid malposition after deep periorbital laser skin resurfacing—skin tightening achieved may exceed the ability of the lower eyelid to maintain its normal vector and apposition to the globe.

6.3 Advantages/Disadvantages

Compared to the CO_2 laser, healing time for re-epithelialization following dual mode Er:YAG skin resurfacing is slightly shorter; and posttreatment sequelae and complications are more favorable, with decreased posttreatment erythema intensity and duration, similar incidence but shorter duration posttreatment hyperpigmentation, and reduced risk of hypopigmentation.[17] The ability to precisely control tissue ablation depth (e.g., 4–200 μm) and the more limited depth of residual thermal damage with the dual mode Er:YAG skin resurfacing laser enable greater flexibility in treatment approaches over a wider range of skin types. Nevertheless, excellent correlation of chosen treatment depth and histological treatment depth (ablate or ablate plus coagulate) with the dual mode Er:YAG skin resurfacing laser is not well maintained beyond the initial pass.[18] The main disadvantages of the dual mode Er:YAG skin resurfacing laser lie in the more limited depth of residual thermal damage and the modest decrease in ability to efface the most severe rhytids when compared to the CO_2 laser.[19]

6.3.1 Clinical Treatment Approach

Preoperative considerations include establishing proper indications, absence of contraindications, and obtaining an appropriate informed consent for the proposed laser skin resurfacing procedure. Although studies have not generated a consensus on the benefit of pretreatment topical therapy (e.g., tretinoin, alpha hydroxy acid [AHA], bleaching agents) or on the use of perioperative antibiotics, herpes simplex virus (HSV) prophylaxis with antiviral therapy (generally starting the night before and continuing for 1 week after treatment) is clearly beneficial when treating the perioral skin regardless of HSV infection history.

Microablative laser skin resurfacing (micro peel or micro laser peel; ablate mode only, **Video 6.2**) may be performed with topical anesthesia if the ablation depth is very superficial. Regional nerve blocks, labial blocks, and oral medication(s) (e.g., anxiolytic and/or narcotic) may be desirable with deeper ablate mode–only intraepidermal peels. Deep laser skin resurfacing treatments require greater sedation and pain control (e.g., oral anxiolytic supplemented with intramuscular narcotic, intravenous sedation, and general anesthesia). Safety considerations during treatment under general anesthesia include ensuring use of a laser-safe endotracheal tube or laryngeal mask airway. For patients under other types of sedation, supplemental oxygen should be discontinued before use of the Er:YAG skin resurfacing laser. Many potential postoperative problems may be avoided by following a detailed laser skin peel treatment plan and by careful attention to execution of the technical aspects of the procedure. Additional passes and/or repeated overlap of adjacent scans may create excessive wound depth and lead to delayed healing, prolonged redness, and scarring.

Immediate postoperative care involves application of a hydrating, nonirritant, protective artificial barrier to help prevent contamination and desiccation as well as to provide an optimal environment for efficient re-epithelialization. Many different products have been used by the author including petrolatum-paraffin balm, aqueous gel, plant oil-based balm, and more recently a 3%-micronized sucralfate emulsion (Eau Thermale Avène, Cicalfate Post-Procedure Skin Recovery Emulsion, Pierre Fabre Dermo-Cosmetique, Parsippany, New Jersey) supplemented with hydrating water spray as needed (Eau Thermale Avène, Thermal Spring Water, Pierre Fabre Dermo-Cosmetique, Parsippany, New Jersey).

Early studies on chronic wounds have suggested that treatment of wounded skin with noncontact low frequency ultrasound (NCLF-US) may enhance skin healing through reduction of bacteria counts, mechanical cleansing, and stimulation of healing through multiple pathways.[20,21] We implemented NCLF-US in our clinic to facilitate acute wound healing after laser skin resurfacing several years ago. The NCLF-US device (MIST Therapy, Celleration, Inc., Eden Prairie, Minnesota) uses a disposable tip that is held approximately 1 cm offset from the skin's surface while a gentle saline mist or spray carries the low frequency (40 kHz) ultrasound energy to the wound (Video 6.4). Our nurses perform NCLF-US treatments at multiple intervals (e.g., postoperative days 1, 3, 5, and 7) following laser skin resurfacing. In addition to the benefits listed above, the protocol of periodically reevaluating each patient's progress during the critical initial healing period enables earlier recognition and intervention for unforeseen problems that may interfere with normal skin healing.

Follow-up after dual mode Er:YAG laser skin resurfacing should continue at regular intervals after initial healing is complete. During these subsequent intervals continued healing occurs with normalization of erythema, skin tone, texture, and sensitivity and with ongoing tissue contraction and dermal tissue remodeling. Common patient questions early on after treatment include: "What is the expected duration of erythema? When can I resume normal activity? When should I use sunscreen? When should I resume use of topical cosmeceuticals and/or medications? When will my skin itching stop?" And "why do I still have lines?"

In general, erythema intensity and duration is related to skin type and condition as well as depth of treatment and extent of thermal injury. Fair skin types, with preexisting redness, who undergo deep, multipass, dual mode laser skin resurfacing may have posttreatment erythema that lasts up to several months or longer. Posttreatment erythema may be exacerbated by skin sensitivity and contact dermatitis. Resumption of normal activity is permissible sooner (e.g., upon completion of re-epithelialization) with more superficial microablative laser skin resurfacing treatments. Deeper laser skin resurfacing treatments have the potential for relatively increased skin sensitivity for several weeks or longer after re-epithelialization is complete. Topical sunscreens, cosmeceuticals, and medications should not be introduced until erythema and peak skin-sensitivity have substantially abated. At that point, introduction of these substances to the newly resurfaced skin should be done individually so that assessment for irritation is accurate. Pruritus of newly resurfaced skin may indicate ongoing skin irritation and contact dermatitis and the need to remove the offending substance(s) from the skin care regimen. Pretreatment patient counseling regarding the expected benefits for wrinkles versus dynamic facial lines may reduce the potential for posttreatment concern about "nonresponsive" dynamic facial lines.

6.3.2 Treating Complications

Adequate pretreatment informed consent and education are essential to prepare patients for the possibility of treatment-related complications. Prolonged posttreatment erythema lasting more than 4 months may occur after aggressive dual mode

Er:YAG laser skin resurfacing (▶ Fig. 6.4). Prolonged erythema after Er:YAG laser skin resurfacing may precede hypopigmentation in patients with lighter (e.g., Fitzpatrick I or II) skin types (▶ Fig. 6.4), whereas temporary skin darkening may follow prolonged erythema after Er:YAG laser skin resurfacing in patients with darker skin types (Fitzpatrick III and higher). Although localized hypopigmentation may respond to a series of fractional laser skin resurfacing treatments, a modality for diffuse hypopigmentation is lacking. Epidermal PIH may respond to topical tyrosinase inhibition, retinoids, corticosteroids, or a series of light chemical (e.g., AHA) peels.

Delayed healing may be the result of desiccation, infection, overly aggressive treatment, secondary wounding, decreased activity of pilosebaceous units (e.g., isotretinoin, prior radiation therapy), or unknown factors. Delayed healing is more likely in areas of the face that may be less vascular (e.g., peripheral areas). Patients who have undergone prior facelift procedures wherein neck skin has been transposed up over the caudal margin of the mandible may be at higher risk for healing complications in these areas. Atrophic or hypertrophic scarring may occur following delayed wound healing (typically the result of excessively deep laser skin resurfacing treatment, wound desiccation, or infection). Appropriate treatment for hypertrophic scarring may involve corticosteroid or 5-FU injections, whereas both atrophic and hypertrophic scars may require surgical scar revision or AFR.

Although many studies have shown that concurrent facelift surgery and laser skin resurfacing may be performed safely,[22] typical deep dual mode Er:YAG resurfacing should not be performed over skin flaps. And whereas deeper resurfacing may be permissible over composite flaps, few rhytids are typically present over the posterior cheek after rhytidectomy. In the event that complete re-epithelialization has not occurred within 7 days after Er:YAG laser skin resurfacing, reevaluation of the current skin condition is warranted. Alternative topical therapy (e.g., silver sulfadiazine 1%, if not precluded by medication allergy) and meticulous wound care or promotion of natural tissue regeneration with porcine urinary bladder matrix (epithelial basement membrane extracellular matrix, MatriStem Wound Matrix, Acell, Inc., Columbia, Maryland) may help prevent an unsatisfactory outcome such as atrophic or hypertrophic scarring.[23]

Infection can lead to delayed wound healing and scarring. Whereas maintaining good hygiene may be second nature for health care workers, patients undergoing laser skin resurfacing procedures (and any responsible caregivers) should receive formal wound care instructions from nursing staff regarding the imperative of avoiding skin contamination during the initial healing process. Bacterial wound colonization invariably occurs during the initial healing process following laser skin resurfacing; nevertheless, bacterial counts may be affected by the particular wound care regimen implemented[24] and may be diminished with supplemental NCLF-US treatments. Despite the potential for bacterial and fungal wound infection following laser skin resurfacing and no consensus regarding prophylactic antibiotic and/or antifungal coverage, many laser surgeons nonetheless implement perioperative antibiotic coverage.[25]

With nearly ubiquitous potential for activation of latent HSV following perioral laser skin resurfacing (including patients with a negative history of HSV infection), consensus does exist for prophylactic antiviral coverage (e.g., acyclovir, famciclovir, and valacyclovir).[26] Although HSV activation following perioral laser skin resurfacing may begin as a mild, localized viral exanthem, progression to extensive involvement of the perioral and adjacent skin may occur. Uncontrolled HSV infection requires more aggressive therapy with intravenous antiviral medication to minimize the risk of delayed wound healing and scarring. With appropriate laser skin resurfacing treatment, antibiotic and antiviral prophylaxis (if indicated), and meticulous wound care, infectious complications are unlikely.

Dermatitis, milia, and unmet expectations are among the most common complications encountered following laser skin resurfacing. Despite best efforts, contact (allergic, irritant) dermatitis may occur prior to reformation of the normal skin architecture or following re-epithelialization. Manifestations may include edema, erythema, pruritus, and an apparent setback in the healing process. Supportive care generally includes changing the skin care regimen in an attempt to eliminate continuing irritation, oral antihistamines, and a burst and taper of systemic corticosteroids. Milia are keratin-filled pseudocysts that frequently occur during the early postoperative period. The use of occlusive topical medications to facilitate re-epithelialization or the subsequent use of topical moisturizers may contribute to the formation of milia. Although milia may resolve spontaneously, manual extraction may become necessary. Unrealized or unmet patient expectations should be preempted where possible through appropriate pretreatment patient counseling and education regarding alternatives, risks, and likely outcomes.

6.4 Pearls and Pitfalls

A thriving laser skin resurfacing practice must: (1) carefully select patients for procedures with extended downtime; (2) skillfully match indications with appropriate treatments; (3) provide thorough pretreatment patient education regarding related risks, alternatives, and anticipated benefits; (4) competently execute the planned treatment while avoiding overtreatment; and (5) supply compassionate and substantive postresurfacing skin care during initial healing and beyond, until the newly resurfaced skin reaches maximum improvement with respect to tone, texture, and sensitivity. Despite these efforts, patient expectations regarding downtime and outcomes may fail to align with the skin's response to treatment.

6.5 Conclusion and Future Directions

Full-field Er:YAG laser skin resurfacing remains both challenging and gratifying. The challenge lies in selecting effective therapies for particular skin types and conditions while avoiding undesirable outcomes. The flexibility of the dual mode Er:YAG skin resurfacing laser to meet diverse patient needs (e.g., removal of skin lesions, treatment of superficial photodamage and dyschromia, effacement of lines and wrinkles) provides repeated validation of the technology and gratification for the laser surgeon. So far, the "future"—that now includes both ablative and nonablative erbium-based fractional laser skin rejuvenation treatment approaches—has not significantly eroded the utility of traditional full-field Er:YAG laser skin resurfacing.

References

[1] Kaufmann R, Hibst R. Pulsed erbium:YAG laser ablation in cutaneous surgery. Lasers Surg Med 1996; 19: 324–330

[2] Teikemeier G, Goldberg DJ. Skin resurfacing with the erbium:YAG laser. Dermatol Surg 1997; 23: 685–687

[3] Perez MI, Bank DE, Silvers D. Skin resurfacing of the face with the erbium:YAG laser. Dermatol Surg 1998; 24: 653–658, discussion 658–659

[4] Holcomb JD. Versatility of erbium YAG laser: from fractional skin rejuvenation to full-field skin resurfacing. Facial Plast Surg Clin North Am 2011; 19: 261–273

[5] Sapijaszko MJ, Zachary CB. Er:YAG laser skin resurfacing. Dermatol Clin 2002; 20: 87–96

[6] Kim YJ, Lee HS, Son SW, Kim SN, Kye YC. Analysis of hyperpigmentation and hypopigmentation after Er:YAG laser skin resurfacing. Lasers Surg Med 2005; 36: 47–51

[7] Ko NY, Ahn HH, Kim SN, Kye YC. Analysis of erythema after Er:YAG laser skin resurfacing. Dermatol Surg 2007; 33: 1322–1327

[8] Khatri KA, Ross V, Grevelink JM, Magro CM, Anderson RR. Comparison of erbium:YAG and carbon dioxide lasers in resurfacing of facial rhytides. Arch Dermatol 1999; 135: 391–397

[9] Newman JB, Lord JL, Ash K, McDaniel DH. Variable pulse erbium:YAG laser skin resurfacing of perioral rhytides and side-by-side comparison with carbon dioxide laser. Lasers Surg Med 2000; 26: 208–214

[10] Ross EV, Miller C, Meehan K, et al. One-pass CO2 versus multiple-pass Er:YAG laser resurfacing in the treatment of rhytides: a comparison side-by-side study of pulsed CO2 and Er:YAG lasers. Dermatol Surg 2001; 27: 709–715

[11] Rostan EF, Fitzpatrick RE, Goldman MP. Laser resurfacing with a long pulse erbium:YAG laser compared to the 950 ms pulsed CO(2) laser. Lasers Surg Med 2001; 29: 136–141

[12] Fitzpatrick RE, Rostan EF, Marchell N. Collagen tightening induced by carbon dioxide laser versus erbium:YAG laser. Lasers Surg Med 2000; 27: 395–403

[13] Pozner JN, Goldberg DJ. Superficial erbium:YAG laser resurfacing of photodamaged skin. J Cosmet Laser Ther 2006; 8: 89–91

[14] El-Domyati M, El-Ammawi TS, Medhat W, Moawad O, Mahoney MG, Uitto J. Multiple minimally invasive erbium:yttrium aluminum garnet laser mini-peels for skin rejuvenation: an objective assessment. J Cosmet Dermatol 2012; 11: 122–130

[15] Orringer JS, Rittié L, Hamilton T, Karimipour DJ, Voorhees JJ, Fisher GJ. Intraepidermal erbium:YAG laser resurfacing: impact on the dermal matrix. J Am Acad Dermatol 2011; 64: 119–128

[16] Hantash BM, Stewart DB, Cooper ZA, Rehmus WE, Koch RJ, Swetter SM. Facial resurfacing for nonmelanoma skin cancer prophylaxis. Arch Dermatol 2006; 142: 976–982

[17] Tanzi EL, Alster TS. Side effects and complications of variable-pulsed erbium:yttrium-aluminum-garnet laser skin resurfacing: extended experience with 50 patients. Plast Reconstr Surg 2003; 111: 1524–1529, discussion 1530–1532

[18] Pozner JM, Goldberg DJ. Histologic effect of a variable pulsed Er:YAG laser. Dermatol Surg 2000; 26: 733–736

[19] Alster TS, Lupton JR. Treatment of complications of laser skin resurfacing. Arch Facial Plast Surg 2000; 2: 279–284

[20] Kavros SJ, Liedl DA, Boon AJ, Miller JL, Hobbs JA, Andrews KL. Expedited wound healing with noncontact, low-frequency ultrasound therapy in chronic wounds: a retrospective analysis. Adv Skin Wound Care 2008; 21: 416–423

[21] Yao M, Hasturk H, Kantarci A, et al. A pilot study evaluating noncontact low frequency ultrasound and underlying molecular mechanism on diabetic foot ulcers. Int Wound J 11-19-12 online publication

[22] Weinstein C, Pozner J, Scheflan M. Combined erbium:YAG laser resurfacing and face lifting. Plast Reconstr Surg 2001; 107: 586–592, discussion 593–594

[23] Kruper GJ, Vandegriend ZP, Lin HS, Zuliani GF. Salvage of failed local and regional flaps with porcine urinary bladder extracellular matrix aided tissue regeneration. Case Rep Otolargyngol; 2013: 917183

[24] Goldman MP, Roberts TL, III, Skover G, Lettieri JT, Fitzpatrick RE. Optimizing wound healing in the face after laser abrasion. J Am Acad Dermatol 2002; 46: 399–407

[25] Walia S, Alster TS. Cutaneous CO2 laser resurfacing infection rate with and without prophylactic antibiotics. Dermatol Surg 1999; 25: 857–861

[26] Alster TS, Nanni CA. Famciclovir prophylaxis of herpes simplex virus reactivation after laser skin resurfacing. Dermatol Surg 1999; 25: 242–246

7 Combining Different Lasers in the Same Session for Optimal Outcomes in Treating Aging Skin

Elizabeth F. Rostan

7.1 Introduction

Aging and sun damage of the skin results in skin laxity, rhytids, texture irregularities, dyspigmentation, and vascular changes. This book outlines the use of many different laser devices to correct these changes of age and photodamage. Vascular lasers such as the pulsed dye laser (PDL) are used to treat redness and telangiectasia; long-pulsed (LP) alexandrite and quality-switched or Q-switched (QS) lasers are used to treat pigment abnormalities including lentigines and melasma; and ablative and fractional skin resurfacing procedures stimulate collagen and treat all aspects of solar damage including deeper wrinkles. In this chapter, the author describes her experience in combining laser technologies—different wavelengths and applications—in the same treatment session in order to achieve better outcomes with fewer visits for the patient.

7.2 Pigment and Vascular Lasers

Even in young patients with early changes of sun damage, there are often several different aspects of photoaging present—lentigines, erythema and telangiectasia, and wrinkles or skin texture changes. The author has found that treatment outcomes and patient satisfaction are increased when these different aspects of photodamage are targeted using two or more different lasers in the same session. Patients get better results with fewer treatments—saving money and time with both visits to the office as well as periods of healing.

The PDL laser is an excellent choice for reducing redness and very fine telangiectasias. Larger telangiectasias are more effectively treated with a 1,064-nm neodymium:yttrium aluminum garnet (Nd:YAG) laser. The longer wavelength of 1,064 nm can penetrate more deeply to better reach the deeper vessels, and longer pulse widths can be matched to larger vessel sizes. In the treatment of redness and capillaries, such as is often seen in rosacea as well as sun damage, the author often combines both the 595-nm PDL (Vbeam Perfecta, Candela Corporation,

Wayland, Massachusetts) and the LP 1,064-nm Nd:YAG laser (GentleYag, Candela Corporation, Wayland, Massachusetts). The 1,064-nm wavelength is first used to treat the more visible and larger telangiectasias; then, immediately after treatment with the Nd:YAG, the PDL is used to treat the finer vessels and diffuse erythema (▶ Fig. 7.1). This combination is so frequently used together that the lasers are kept in the same room.

There are a number of lasers that can be used to target the dyspigmentation of photodamaged skin. LP alexandrite and QS lasers—including QS 532-nm Nd:YAG, QS ruby, and QS alexandrite—can target specific pigmented lesions such as freckles or lentigines. QS lasers emit very short pulses of light that match the thermal relaxation time of the small particles of melanin and melanin storage units—melanosomes. LP alexandrite lasers likely target the larger melanocytes or the diffuse melanin staining of keratinocytes that characterizes solar lentigines.

Intense pulsed light (IPL) is a nonlaser, light-based system that is used to treat photodamage as well as unwanted hair. The IPL has a spectrum of wavelengths with an output of noncoherent light ranging from 500 to 1,200 nm, depending on cutoff filters on the lower wavelength spectrum. These varied wavelengths include wavelengths that target erythema (hemoglobin) as well as wavelengths that target pigment (melanin), and even longer wavelengths that target water to induce dermal heating and collagen remodeling. Because the energy is spread over a range of wavelengths, no single wavelength is particularly focused or powerful. Thus, the IPL is best used for mild changes of sun damage, maintenance of results achieved from other procedures, or for those who desire a treatment with minimal downtime. With more significant changes of either a vascular or a pigmented nature, better results may be achieved using lasers whose wavelengths more specifically target the predominant issue. Additionally, in the treatment of more severely sun-damaged skin that has a significant amount of erythema or pigment, IPL can leave well-demarcated areas of clearance in the rectangular shape of the delivery crystal. Subsequent treatments with IPL can reduce the appearance of

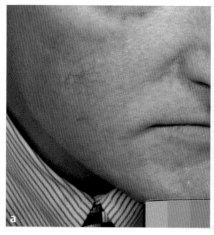
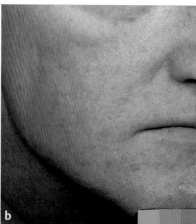

Fig. 7.1 Laser treatments for telangiectasias and erythema. **(a)** Prior to procedures. **(b)** Improvement shown after one treatment with combination long-pulsed (LP) dye laser and 1,064-nm neodymium:yttrium aluminum garnet (Nd:YAG) laser.

these areas but patient distress in between treatments can be significant.

Fractional resurfacing devices can treat dyspigmentation while globally improving photodamaged skin. Fractional photothermolysis (FP) creates microscopic columns of thermal injury referred to as MENDs or microscopic epidermal necrotic debris columns. As these MENDs heal, pigment can be pushed to the surface and subsequently exfoliated—resulting in improvement in unwanted pigment.

The author's selection of laser in the treatment of pigmented lesions depends on the clinical situation. In the case of a light-skinned patient with darker lentigines that are either diffusely spread over a large area or just a few larger lesions, the author prefers the LP 755-nm alexandrite laser (Candela GentleLase, Candela). This laser is used at a low fluence with no epidermal cooling (i.e., dynamic cryogen cooling turned off). Typically a spot size of 12 mm and an energy setting of 16 to 30 J/cm^2 are used, depending on patient skin type and darkness of the lesion. Higher fluence can be used in lighter skin types. Overlapping and multiple passes are done over the entire cosmetic unit (cheeks, forehead, or full face) until a slight change is noted in the pigmented lesions, which should turn darker with possibly a slightly dry appearance and redness at the periphery. No blistering or lifting of the skin should be seen. The efficacy of this treatment is best when the contrast between skin color and pigmented target is great (i.e., very fair skin and very dark spots are the most ideal situation). This observation has also been noted in a controlled study.[1] When there is very little contrast between skin color and pigmented lesion color, the author does not use this technique due to lack of efficacy and increased risk of unwanted side effects. The LP alexandrite is not used on tanned skin or any skin type darker than Fitzpatrick type IV. The lighter the lesion, the more energy is required to have an effect on the target. For darker lesions, lower energy is needed to achieve a clinical effect and to minimize side effects.

In the case of lighter lentigines, darker skin types, treatment location of arms or legs, or very little contrast between skin color and lesion color, the author chooses either QS 532-nm laser spot treatment or a nonablative fractional laser alone or in combination with an LP alexandrite or a QS laser. Desired end points of treatment with the QS laser are varying degrees of whitening or an ashy appearance—in lighter skin types a larger degree of whitening is appropriate and more effective; however, in darker skin types, a very slight whitening or only slight ashy appearance is preferred in order to minimize size effects of hypopigmentation and postinflammatory hyperpigmentation.

7.3 Combining Lasers in the Same Treatment Session

7.3.1 Background

A number of devices have built-in combinations of therapies. Radiofrequency (RF) energy has been combined in several devices with IPL and diode lasers. The goal of the combination of technology is to achieve skin tightening and improvement in the visible changes of sun damage in the skin, or enhancement of the improvement seen with the light-based device alone. Sadick[2] et al reported significant overall skin improvement

(75.3%) and significant patient satisfaction (92%) using the novel device of electro-optical synergy (ELOS) that combines RF and IPL energy in a single pulse. In 2006, Alexiades-Armenakas[3] evaluated the sequential combination use of two devices that combined bipolar RF with light-based energy—one device combined RF with a diode laser and the other mechanism combined RF with IPL. Blinded physician evaluation of improvement per category (rhytids, laxity, elastosis, dyschromias, erythema-telangiectasias, keratoses, and texture) after each treatment was mild (average improvement of 10.9% per treatment), but overall patient satisfaction was significantly higher (71.4%). Patient satisfaction was attributed to the combined effects of the technologies.

Several studies have investigated the combinations of different lasers in the same session for the cosmetic enhancement of facial skin. Berlin[4] et al reported successful combination of very light erbium followed sequentially by IPL. The number of patients who finished the study (12 out of 15) reported mild erythema lasting up to 1 week and mild scaling for 3 to 4 days after the treatment. Overall satisfaction at the 3-month follow-up was 63%. A study by Lee[5] compared the efficacy of the 532-nm, msec potassium titanyl phosphate (KTP) laser alone and the 1,064-nm, msec Nd:YAG laser alone as well as in combination for the treatment of skin changes of photoaging. The combination of the two wavelengths gave slightly better results than either alone. A similar study by Tan[6] et al was a split-face study that showed slightly greater improvement in the side that received combination treatment of 532-nm and 1,064-nm wavelengths. Studies by Goldman[7,8] et al have shown benefit in sequential use of ablative erbium immediately after ablative carbon dioxide (CO_2) laser in resurfacing to improve healing times and outcomes.

The combination of QS lasers—532 nm followed by 1,064 nm—was shown to be significantly more effective in the treatment of Hori's nevus than the 1,064 nm alone.[9] A higher incidence of postinflammatory hyperpigmentation was seen on the combination laser side but all resolved in 2 months. In treating giant congenital nevi, Funayama et al demonstrated effective and safe pigment lightening using sequential PDL followed immediately by QS ruby laser.[10] Trelles et al reported better results in leg vein treatment (blue veins and veins > 1 mm responded best) using a laser that combined a pulsed dye and Nd:YAG laser sequentially in the same pulse.[11] The sequential pulsed dye–1,064-nm Nd:YAG laser has also been reported to be an effective and safe treatment for venous malformation.[12]

Recently, investigators have shown safe, same-session combination of nonablative fractional lasers with other laser and light sources. Chan et al demonstrated the safety of combination IPL and nonablative fractional treatment on the same treatment day (either before or after nonablative fractional treatment).[13] A retrospective chart review detailed similar clinical outcomes after one treatment on the chest of either IPL or nonablative fractional combined with LP, PDL, and QS alexandrite. Safety was confirmed with the combination of devices and there was a trend toward greater wrinkle and texture improvement in the combination laser group, suggesting assessment after more treatments might reveal an advantage to the combination approach.[14]

In nonrejuvenation applications, lasers have been combined to treat tattoos as well as unwanted hair. Recently, Weiss and Geronemus reported more efficient tattoo removal with sequential QS ruby laser followed by ablative fractional resurfacing in the same session.[15] Not all studies have shown benefit in combining wavelengths in the same session. A private group in Iran reported a study of laser hair removal on the legs using either 755-nm alexandrite, 1,064-nm Nd:YAG, or a combination of both lasers.[16] There was greater pain and increased side effects in the area treated with the combination of the two wavelengths.

7.4 Personal Experience in Combining Lasers

7.4.1 Nonablative Lasers

As previously discussed, it is commonplace for this author to combine LP 1,064-nm Nd:YAG laser with PDL in the same session for more effective clearance of vascular conditions. There is also frequent combination of a vascular laser treatment (595-nm pulsed dye, 1,064-nm Nd:YAG, or both) with a laser treatment specifically to target the pigmented areas of concern. This approach is chosen by the author when it is felt that the vascular component is too great to get good results with IPL but there is also pigment present to treat. A good example would be a face with numerous larger telangiectasias as well as lentigines and freckles.

For larger areas of pigment or large patches of pigment such as seen in melasma, a nonablative fractional laser (1,550 nm or 1,927 nm) is used either alone or in combination with low energy LP alexandrite laser prior to the fractional laser. If there is any erythema or telangiectasia, it is treated with one or both of the vascular lasers prior to treatment with the nonablative fractional laser. There is a nominal charge for the additional laser treatments and patient satisfaction with the procedure is greatly increased because several different aspects of skin concerns are taken care of in one session. The series is as follows if all lasers are utilized: vascular lasers first, then LP alexandrite or QS 532-nm Nd:YAG laser, then fractional nonablative laser.

When there are more significant texture changes or rhytids from sun damage, the preference is to use a nonablative fractional device. In order to achieve the most consistent and quick results with pigment when a patient is having a series of fractional nonablative procedures, the LP alexandrite laser is often used, as described above, prior to the fractional laser on the same day. Similarly, erythema and telangiectasias are pretreated with a vascular laser before the fractional treatment

(▶ Fig. 7.2). Fractional nonablative lasers do effectively treat pigment but the response is enhanced with pretreatment with the alexandrite laser; and patients note immediate improvement with reduction of pigmented lesions, whereas the collagen remodeling takes several months to occur. Another frequently used combination is pretreatment with full-face IPL followed by fractional nonablative laser (▶ Fig. 7.3).

7.4.2 Ablative Lasers

It is well known that the combination of ablative CO_2 laser resurfacing with erbium resurfacing can yield better outcomes and improved healing times than ablative CO_2 laser resurfacing alone. The erbium laser can be used to blend edges of the treatment area, remove CO_2-charred tissue to improve healing, and can also be used to sculpt down edges of deep lines and scars. With the advent of fractional ablative lasers, the number of completely ablative resurfacing cases has declined for most practitioners. In very deep rhytids and severe elastotic changes from sun damage, the CO_2 laser remains the gold standard; however, often the fractional CO_2 is the selected modality due to its shorter healing time and reduced side-effect profile compared to ablative resurfacing.

In many cases, patients and this practitioner elect to do full-face fractional CO_2 except in regions of more severe rhytids, such as the glabella and perioral areas. In these locations, fully ablative CO_2 is done. The downtime and wound care for these localized areas are more manageable than for full-face ablative treatments.

This author first became interested in combining ablative and fractional ablative treatments by fate. A resurfacing case was planned with full-face fractional CO_2 and traditional ablative CO_2 laser in the perioral area for deeper lines and elastosis. During the case, the CO_2 laser malfunctioned and would not produce enough energy for resurfacing. It was decided to treat with high energy fractional CO_2 in the perioral area and follow that with ablative erbium resurfacing. The patient, who was a smoker, did very well and had excellent healing except in a few areas where this practitioner was more aggressive with the erbium laser—angled to carve down the edges of deep, vertical lip lines. The author felt that these areas healed with mild hypopigmentation; however, these were the areas the patient was most happy about because they were the smoothest. A second resurfacing procedure was done in the perioral area with ablative CO_2 and erbium 6 months after the initial treatment (▶ Fig. 7.4). Since that case, the author frequently treats the

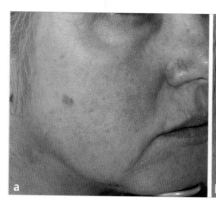
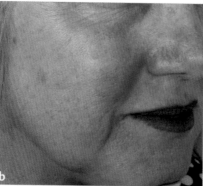

Fig. 7.2 Erythema and telangiectasias' combined pretreatment and treatment. (a) Image before utilization of modalities. (b) Benefits apparent 1 month after single, sequentially combined use of pulsed dye laser (PDL), long-pulsed (LP) alexandrite laser, and fractional nonablative laser.

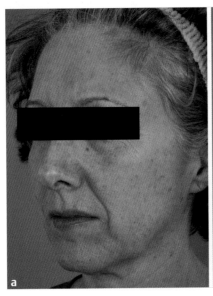
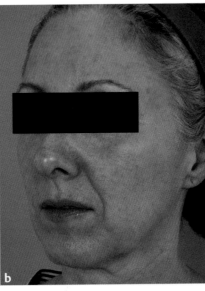

Fig. 7.3 Enhanced facial response following laser preprocedure and procedure. (a) Initial photo. (b) Dramatic difference 1 month after two combination treatments utilizing intense pulsed light (IPL) and then fractional nonablative laser.

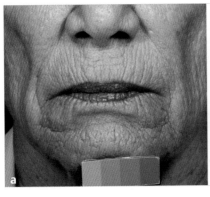
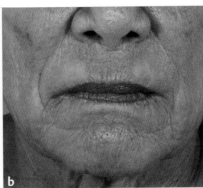

Fig. 7.4 More youthful appearance after two separate resurfacing procedures. (a) Before treatments. (b) 18 months after ablative fractional carbon dioxide (CO_2) immediately followed by erbium resurfacing and second ablative CO_2 and erbium laser treatment 6 months after initial treatment.

perioral area with full treatment of fractional CO_2 laser prior to ablative resurfacing and working the edges of rhytids with erbium laser.

Other lasers that are combined with fractional CO_2 include pretreatment of lentigines with the LP alexandrite and occasionally treatment of vascular lesions with the PDL or Nd:YAG laser. The nonspecific heat of the fractional CO_2 laser can reduce telangiectasias so that often the treatment of the telangiectasias, especially smaller diameter ones, is saved until after healing from the fractional laser.

7.5 Limitations and Precautions

Lasers deliver significant amounts of heat to the tissue. When different lasers are combined in the same session, caution must be used to avoid too much heat delivery to a confined area—a so-called "heat sink" issue. A short amount of time in between successive lasers is usually adequate to avoid overheating the tissue. During treatment, heat of the tissue is often checked subjectively by touching the skin. If the skin feels very hot, then the procedure is paused until the skin cools to the touch. Overheating the tissue may lead to blistering and even deep dermal damage that can lead to atrophic scarring. The risk for overheating the tissue is greatest when there is a significant amount of target such as in a deeply colored, port-wine stain.

Use of several lasers in one session may also increase the downtime for the patient. When vascular lasers such as the IPL or PDL are used, more edema is expected after the treatment. If lasers that specifically target pigment are used, there may be a slight increase in light crusting or dryness over the lesions and the treated lesions often appear slightly darker before peeling.

Additionally, even when combining lasers, often a series of procedures is needed for optimal results. Setting patient expectations and preparing the patient for the treatments is critical to success. Finally, the treatment of aging and photodamage requires attention to many different aspects of the aging face including treating laxity of skin and facial structures, addressing loss of volume in the face, and relaxing lines of muscle movement as well as addressing the visible changes of sun damage and aging in the skin with lasers, peels, and/or skin care.

7.6 Summary

Correction of sun damage of the skin can be achieved safely and efficiently using combinations of different lasers in the same session. Choice of laser treatments is customized to patient goals and the degree and type of changes that are present. Caution should be used when combining laser treatments, but careful attention to tissue reaction during treatment should avoid any untoward side effects. Using combinations of lasers that specifically target diverse aspects of photoaging in the same session can achieve better outcomes and greater patient satisfaction.

7.7 Key Points

- Different lasers can be safely and effectively combined in the same treatment session.
- Choice of lasers depends on skin type of patient, degree of sun damage, and goals of treatment.
- Frequently used combinations include the combination of vascular lasers with lasers to target pigment and the combination of one or both of these with fractional nonablative lasers.
- Laser treatments can be combined with fractional ablative lasers but with greater caution due to the amount of heat delivered to skin during fractional ablation.
- Combinations of lasers can achieve better outcomes in fewer sessions and lead to greater patient satisfaction.

References

[1] Trafeli JP, Kwan JM, Meehan KJ, et al. Use of a long-pulse alexandrite laser in the treatment of superficial pigmented lesions. Dermatol Surg 2007; 33: 1477–1482

[2] Sadick NS, Alexiades-Armenakas M, Bitter P, Jr, Hruza G, Mulholland RS. Enhanced full-face skin rejuvenation using synchronous intense pulsed optical and conducted bipolar radiofrequency energy (ELOS): introducing selective radiophotothermolysis. J Drugs Dermatol 2005; 4: 181–186

[3] Alexiades-Armenakas M. Rhytides, laxity, and photoaging treated with a combination of radiofrequency, diode laser, and pulsed light and assessed with a comprehensive grading scale. J Drugs Dermatol 2006; 5: 731–738

[4] Berlin AL, Hussain M, Phelps R, Goldberg DJ. Treatment of photoaging with a very superficial Er:YAG laser in combination with a broadband light source. J Drugs Dermatol 2007; 6: 1114–1118

[5] Lee MW. Combination 532-nm and 1064-nm lasers for noninvasive skin rejuvenation and toning. Arch Dermatol 2003; 139: 1265–1276

[6] Tan MH, Dover JS, Hsu TS, Arndt KA, Stewart B. Clinical evaluation of enhanced nonablative skin rejuvenation using a combination of a 532 and a 1,064 nm laser. Lasers Surg Med 2004; 34: 439–445

[7] Goldman MP, Manuskiatti W. Combined laser resurfacing with the 950-microsec pulsed CO2 + Er:YAG lasers. Dermatol Surg 1999; 25: 160–163

[8] Goldman MP, Marchell N, Fitzpatrick RE. Laser skin resurfacing of the face with a combined CO2/Er:YAG laser. Dermatol Surg 2000; 26: 102–104

[9] Ee HL, Goh CL, Khoo LS, Chan ES, Ang P. Treatment of acquired bilateral nevus of ota-like macules (Hori's nevus) with a combination of the 532 nm Q-Switched Nd:YAG laser followed by the 1,064 nm Q-switched Nd:YAG is more effective: prospective study. Dermatol Surg 2006; 32: 34–40

[10] Funayama E, Sasaki S, Furukawa H, et al. Effectiveness of combined pulsed dye and Q-switched ruby laser treatment for large to giant congenital melanocytic naevi. Br J Dermatol 2012; 167: 1085–1091

[11] Trelles MA, Weiss R, Moreno-Moragas J, Romero C, Vélez M, Alvarez X. Treatment of leg veins with combined pulsed dye and Nd:YAG lasers: 60 patients assessed at 6 months. Lasers Surg Med 2010; 42: 609–614

[12] Bagazgoitia L, Boixeda P, Lopez-Caballero C, Beà S, Santiago JL, Jaén P. Venous malformation of the eyelid treated with pulsed-dye-1064-nm neodymium yttrium aluminum garnet sequential laser: an effective and safe treatment. Ophthal Plast Reconstr Surg 2008; 24: 488–490

[13] Chan CS, Saedi N, Mickle C, Dover JS. Combined treatment for facial rejuvenation using an optimized pulsed light source followed by a fractional non-ablative laser. Lasers Surg Med 2013; 45: 405–409

[14] Wu DC, Friedmann DP, Fabi SG, Goldman MP, Fitzpatrick RE. Comparison of intense pulsed light with a 1,927-nm fractionated thulium fiber laser for the rejuvenation of the chest. Dermatol Surg 2014; 40: 129–133

[15] Weiss ET, Geronemus RG. Combining fractional resurfacing and Q-switched ruby laser for tattoo removal. Dermatol Surg 2011; 37: 97–99

[16] Davoudi SM, Behnia F, Gorouhi F, et al. Comparison of long-pulsed alexandrite and Nd:YAG lasers, individually and in combination, for leg hair reduction: an assessor-blinded, randomized trial with 18 months of follow-up. Arch Dermatol 2008; 144: 1323–1327

8 Subcutaneous Fiber Laser and Energy-Based Techniques for Facial Rejuvenation

Richard D. Gentile

8.1 Introduction

Less invasive procedures for facial rejuvenation are becoming more and more popular as prospective patients seek out treatment options that offer the best possible results with the least amount of downtime. As the demand for "quick-recovery" procedures increases and patients spend more time researching options, more informed choices are being made and many times patients opt for technologically advanced procedures. The interface of advanced technology and aesthetic surgery has been characterized by several different practice-altering technological innovations that have occurred. These recent advances are represented by the rapid introduction of a new aesthetic technology that has quickly and favorably been integrated into mainstream aesthetic practice. The first such innovation occurred in the early 1990s when laser skin rejuvenation was introduced for rhytids and actinic skin damage. Radiofrequency (RF) approaches to skin tightening in 2006 are considered another practice-altering technological innovation. The advent of fiber lasers for lipolysis and internal aesthetic surgery in 2007 is also a practice-altering technological advance. One might ask how the impact and potential benefit to patients from technological innovations are assessed. Although this has never been reviewed, the author would like to suggest parameters that would correlate with the significance of the technological innovation being introduced. As shown in ▶ Table 8.1, which details technology innovations and transformational change in aesthetic surgery, the criteria for assessing improved outcomes in technology-aided procedures should describe what the technology adds to current practice or conventional methods. Six criteria for assessing potential benefits of the use of a specific innovation are listed; it could be inferred that the more criteria the technological innovation fulfills, the more likely it will become an important innovation for clinical aesthetic practice. Likewise those innovations meeting few criteria will most likely not be long-lived in clinical aesthetic practice. Patients are now more informed about aesthetic technology than ever before and are more likely to undergo technology-aided procedures—especially if the tech-aided innovation is perceived to shorten the recovery period, reduce risk (e.g.,

anesthetic risk), or improve the outcome. One such technological option involves subcutaneous fiber laser and energy-based techniques for facial rejuvenation that center on interstitial laser lipolysis and skin tightening through tissue coagulation of the fibroseptal network (FSN) of skin, reticular dermis, and superficial soft tissues. These techniques for facial rejuvenation provide a revolutionary and minimally invasive procedure using a high-peak power laser to aid in tissue separation with simultaneous skin tightening through tissue coagulation and induced changes in the FSN and extracellular network of the hypodermis.

8.2 History of Subcutaneous Fiber Laser Techniques for Facial and Neck Rejuvenation

The history of laser lipolysis and energy-based soft tissue coagulation/contraction is a relatively brief one and has been summarized well by DiBernardo et al[1] who note Apfelberg[2] is credited for describing the laser–fat interaction in 1992. Publications by Blugerman, Schavelzon, and Goldman[3] followed where each demonstrated personal experience with lasers on adipose tissue. Badin et al[4] also highlighted the important tissue retraction observed with a technique of laser lipolysis. Ichikawa et al[5] published on the histological evaluation of tissue treated with laser lipolysis, showing the destructive changes of heat-coagulated collagen fibers and degenerated fat cell membranes with dispersion of lipids after laser irradiation of human specimens. These histological changes correlate with clinical changes seen by both physician and patient. Further, the hemostatic properties of the 1,064-nm wavelength have been well documented. The thermal effect produced by the neodymium: yttrium aluminum garnet (Nd:YAG) laser (1,064 nm) in the adipose tissue promotes better hemostasis resulting in less surgical trauma and wound healing with fewer adverse sequelae. In addition to the histological evidence, the clinical evaluation shows improved postoperative recovery, resulting in a more rapid return to daily activities with an excellent aesthetic result. The application of laser lipolysis to facial and neck rejuvenation in conjunction with the advanced facial rejuvenation techniques of SmartLifting were first studied by Gentile in 2007 and reported in 2008,[6] 2009,[7] 2010,[8] and 2011.[9,10] The initial procedures were performed with the SmartLipo (▶ Fig. 8.1) (Cynosure, Waltham, Massachusetts) 1,064-nm laser but on introduction of the SmartLipo MPX (Cynosure) (▶ Fig. 8.2) the 1,064/1,320-nm multiplexed laser was used. The SmartLipo Triplex (▶ Fig. 8.3) and, beginning in 2012, the Precision TX handpiece (▶ Fig. 8.4)—operating at 1,440 nm and delivered through an 800-μm fiber—have been utilized. The Cynosure SmartLipo laser was the first laser to be approved by the Food and Drug Administration (FDA) for laser lipolysis. In addition to the laser lipolysis indication the laser is approved for the surgical

Table 8.1 Criteria for assessing improved outcomes in aesthetic surgery resulting from technology innovations

Criteria	Reduces anesthetic requirements for procedure
	Reduces operating time for procedure
	Reduces complications or morbidity for procedure
	Reduces recovery time for procedure
	Facilitates new or improved technical approaches lacking in conventional or existing techniques
	More than one novel application is possible with new technology

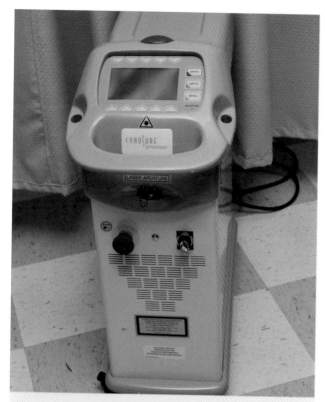

Fig. 8.1 Small Footprint SmartLipo 1,064-nm neodymium:yttrium aluminum garnet (Nd:YAG) laser. The SmartLipo laser was initially approved at 6 watts (W) and underwent power upgrades to 18 W prior to advancing to the MPX and now Triplex versions. (Reproduced with permission from Gentile RD, ed. Neck Rejuvenation. New York, NY: Thieme Medical Publishers; 2011:147.)

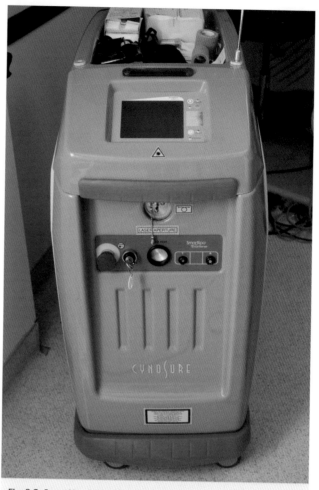

Fig. 8.2 SmartLipo MPX. The MPX or MultiPlex permits laser use in either the 1,064 or 1,320-nm mode or MultiPlex, which is sequential emission of 1,064 and 1,320 nm in three blends. (Reproduced with permission from Gentile RD, ed. Neck Rejuvenation. New York, NY: Thieme Medical Publishers; 2011:149.)

incision, excision, vaporization, ablation, and coagulation of soft tissue. All soft tissue is included—skin, cutaneous tissue, subcutaneous tissue, striated and smooth tissue, muscle, cartilage meniscus, mucous membrane, lymph vessels and nodes, organs, and glands. Since the 2006 advent of subcutaneous laser-based lipolysis techniques, many other laser companies have developed similar products and many have introduced different wavelengths for the specific indication of laser lipolysis. Other wavelengths for laser lipolysis include 980 and 1,444 nm. Since the introduction of these fiber laser techniques in 2007 many other authors including DiBernardo,[11] Sasaki,[12] Holcomb et al,[13] Goldman et al,[14] and Sarnoff[15] have described their experiences with subcutaneous fiber lasers in facial and neck rejuvenation procedures.

8.3 The Technology of Subcutaneous Fiber Laser Techniques for Facial and Neck Rejuvenation

The original SmartLipo laser (▶ Fig. 8.1) delivered 1,064 nm of optical energy through a 300-μm fiber at 6 W (▶ Fig. 8.5). Subsequently, next-generation Cynosure SmartLipo and SmartLipo MPX lasers utilized a 600-μm fiber (▶ Fig. 8.6) as well as a 1,000-μm fiber (▶ Fig. 8.7) for high-power laser lipolysis. The unit developed for dedicated facial and neck contouring known

as the Precision TX handpiece utilizes an 800-μm fiber. First-generation lasers operating at 6, 10, 12, and 18 W utilized a 600-μm optical fiber introduced through a 1-mm diameter stainless steel microcannula of variable length for facial laser-assisted procedures. The laser is fired through the distal end of the fiber that protrudes 2 mm beyond the tip of the cannula. The distal end of the fiber interacts with the facial and neck soft tissue. For visualization purposes, an aiming laser source is provided in the beam path providing the precise location of the fiber tip, indicating where the laser is working. For most facial and neck anatomical regions, a 6- to 12-W setting, 100-μs pulsed laser at 40 Hz and 150 mJ was used. The SmartLipo MPX laser, which is capable of blending both the 1,064- and 1,320-nm wavelengths, was used in subsequent years and in 2012 was replaced by the 1,440-nm laser available in the SmartLipo Triplex and is also used in the Cellulaze (Cynosure) system. The SmartLipo systems all utilize an Nd:YAG laser tuned to the desired wavelength that produces photomechanical and thermal effects. This facilitates dissection of tissues quickly and easily. In addition, the Nd:YAG laser's hemostatic properties allowed for the coagulation of small blood vessels in the subcutaneous plane with

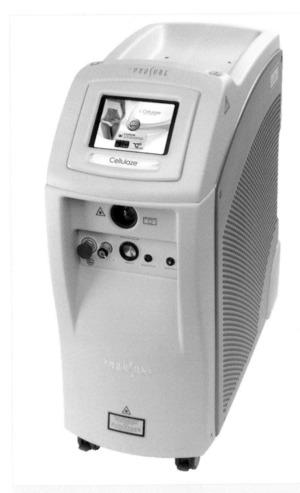

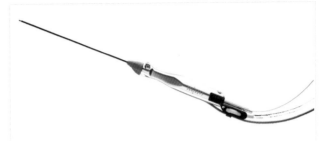

Fig. 8.4 The Precision TX fiber (SideLaze 800 3D) uses the same laser wavelength as Cellulaze but the fiber is smaller and is able to deliver less energy more precisely. The laser beam is split, just as is in Cellulaze, so that the energy can be directed toward the undersurface of the skin to achieve enhanced skin tightening. The Precision TX device was designed to treat small areas in the face such as the neck and jowls. (Courtesy of Cynosure, Westford, Massachusetts.)

preservation of the dermal plexus of vessels. Multiplexing the 1,064- and 1,320-nm wavelengths provides some unique advantages. SmartLipo with multiplex (SmartLipo MPX) (▶ Fig. 8.2) allows individual as well as sequential emission of 1,064- and 1,320-nm wavelengths. The sequential firing of these two wavelengths in combination maximizes the positive properties of both. The combination of these wavelengths increases the efficiency of fat lipolysis and offers a more evenly distributed laser energy profile that benefits superficial and deep treatment. These two wavelengths emitted sequentially offer a more efficient vascular coagulation through the conversion of hemoglobin to methemoglobin.[8] The 1,320-nm wavelength heats the blood, converting hemoglobin to methemoglobin. The 1,064-nm wavelength has a 3 to 5 times greater affinity for methemoglobin than for hemoglobin, thereby increasing absorption resulting in more efficient coagulation leading to enhanced skin tightening. SmartLifting permitted flap separation in typically difficult to reach areas such as the nasal labial folds (NLF) and the corner of the mouth and infracommissural folds, also known as marionette lines, when completing "full rhytidectomy." The wavelength characteristics and

Fig. 8.3 Introduced in 2011, the advancement of the SmartLipo Triplex allows the use of three laser wavelengths (1,064, 1,320, and 1,440 nm) to be utilized independently or uniquely blending the MultiPlex technology. The 1,440-nm wavelength alone has a 40 × greater absorption rate in fatty tissue than that of other diode lasers (924 and 980 nm) available. The Triplex also offers the Cellulaze platform for correction of cellulite. (Courtesy of Cynosure, Westford, Massachusetts.)

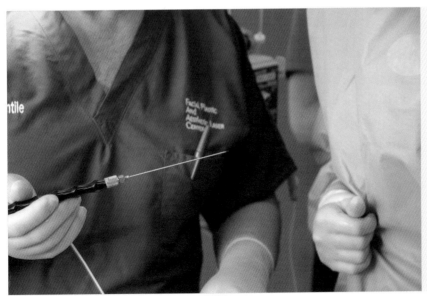

Fig. 8.5 The original 300-μm fiber used for lipolysis and tissue coagulation. (Reproduced with permission from Gentile RD, ed. Neck Rejuvenation. New York, NY: Thieme Medical Publishers; 2011:148.)

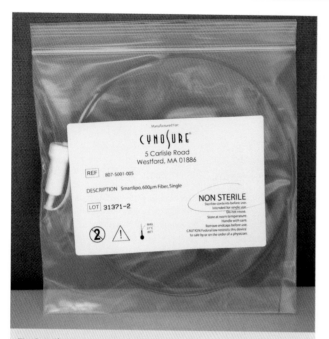

Fig. 8.6 The 600-μm fiber. (Reproduced with permission from Gentile RD, ed. Neck Rejuvenation. New York, NY: Thieme Medical Publishers; 2011:148.)

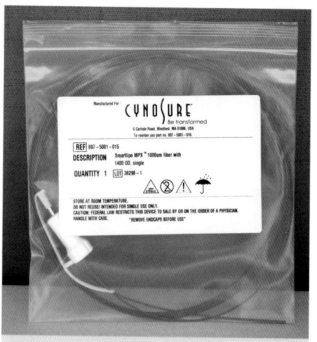

Fig. 8.7 The 1,000-μm fiber. (Reproduced with permission from Gentile RD, ed. Neck Rejuvenation. New York, NY: Thieme Medical Publishers; 2011:148.)

1064 nm Wavelength Characteristics

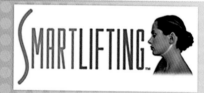

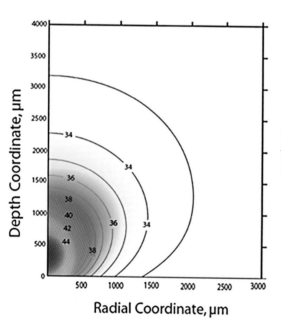

- ☐ 32 C
- ☐ 36 C
- ☐ 40 C
- ☐ 44 C
- ☐ 48 C
- ☐ 52 C
- ☐ 56 C

10W, 40Hz, 375ml per pulse, 1s energy delivery
Starting temperature is 32°C

- Broadly absorbed by Hb
- Energy delivered is distributed more **homogenously** into fat

- Enhanced hemostasis for less surgical trauma and faster recovery
- Broad area of adipocytes disrupted
- Enhanced skin tightening

Fig. 8.8 Wavelength characteristics in laser-assisted facial rejuvenation. Characteristics and photothermal footprint of 1,064-nm wavelength. (Reproduced with permission from Gentile RD. Neck Rejuvenation. New York, NY: Thieme Medical Publishers; 2011:150.)

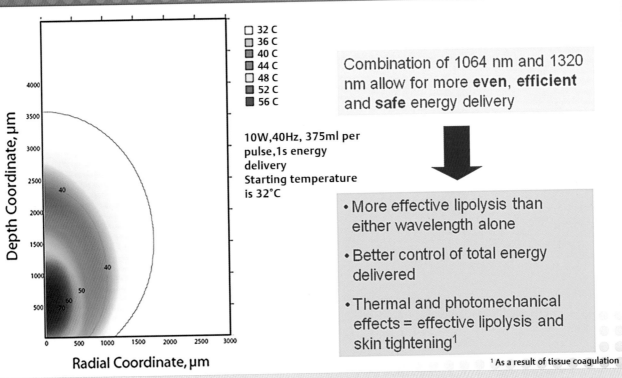

1064 nm and 1320 nm MPX Wavelength Characteristics

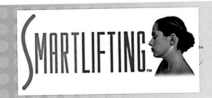

- 32 C
- 36 C
- 40 C
- 44 C
- 48 C
- 52 C
- 56 C

Combination of 1064 nm and 1320 nm allow for more **even**, **efficient** and **safe** energy delivery

10W,40Hz, 375ml per pulse,1s energy delivery
Starting temperature is 32°C

- More effective lipolysis than either wavelength alone
- Better control of total energy delivered
- Thermal and photomechanical effects = effective lipolysis and skin tightening[1]

[1] As a result of tissue coagulation

Fig. 8.9 Wavelength characteristics in laser-assisted facial rejuvenation. Characteristics and photothermal footprint of blended 1,064- and 1,320-nm wavelengths. (Reproduced with permission from Gentile RD. Neck Rejuvenation. New York, NY: Thieme Medical Publishers; 2011:152.)

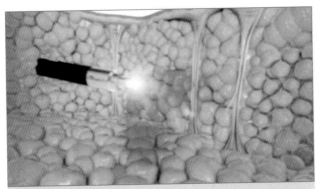

Fig. 8.10 The SideLaze 3D fiber permits the surgeon to aim the beam down, sideways, or up, which facilitates lipolysis, fibroseptal network (FSN) tightening, and dermal skin tightening.

thermodynamic photo spectrum of the 1,064-nm laser are shown in ▶ Fig. 8.8; and the properties of the blended 1,064/1,320-nm multiplexed laser are displayed in ▶ Fig. 8.9. With the advent of the SmartLipo MPX laser, several innovations were introduced to enhance patient safety in reducing the risk of thermal injury. One feature is the SmartSense motion control sensor that will stop laser emission when the laser is not being

moved. The second device is the ThermaGuide, a deep temperature sensor that gives the operator instant feedback on the temperature of the laser internally. The final technology innovation by Cynosure in the SmartLipo platform and a by-product of the Cellulaze research is the Precision TX (▶ Fig. 8.4 and ▶ Fig. 8.10) fiber utilized with the 1,440-nm laser also known as SideLaze 3D. Due to its unique structure and design it is able to fire in specific directions. This differs from the unidirectional firing of the earlier SmartLipo fibers. The operator changes hand position in order to change laser firing position from down to sideways to up. The laser also fires ahead as well as the other selected direction. A chevron marks the spot of directional firing for the Precision TX (▶ Fig. 8.11). The incorporation of the 1,440-nm wavelength offers increased benefits for laser lipolysis and tissue lifting for facial rejuvenation. The 1,440-nm wavelength achieves high thermal absorption within fat and collagen (water), leading to fat reduction and collagen denaturation, and progressive tissue lifting. The longer wavelength provides increased localized photothermal and vaporizing effects in front of the fiber on fatty tissue and collagen fibers (water), achieving 20 times more absorption in adipose tissue than the 1,064/1,320-nm (▶ Fig. 8.12) and 40 times more absorption than the 924/980-nm wavelengths. The combination of the 1,440-nm wavelength, side-firing fiber, and the

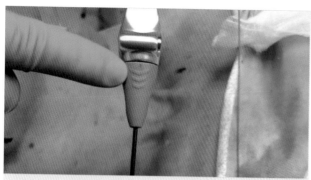

Fig. 8.11 The Precision TX handpiece and SideLaze 3D fiber are aimed by having the chevron on the handpiece positioned down, sideways, or up.

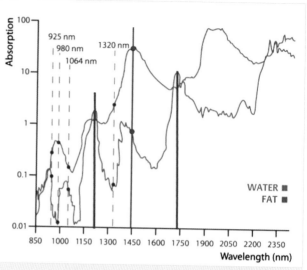

Fig. 8.12 The water and fat absorption graph shows peak absorption for fat at 1,210, 1,740, and 2,300 nm. The 1,440-nm wavelength alone has a 40 × greater absorption rate in fatty tissue than that of other diode lasers (924 and 980 nm) available.

thermal-control systems provided a safe and effective means for facial rejuvenation.

8.4 Classification of Energy-Based Fiber Laser Lifts for Facial and Neck Rejuvenation Techniques

As the technology powering the lipolysis lasers advanced over the past decade, the types of procedures being done in conjunction with interstitial laser lipolysis did so as well. As with other types of techniques, not every surgeon performs each procedure in quite the same way. For example, in performing "laser facelifting" or fiber laser lifting (FLL): is the surgeon only laser treating the face and neck subcutaneously? Or is the surgeon laser treating the face and neck, aspirating and placing sutures, or removing skin in conjunction with the interstitial laser lipolysis? As the number of reports of these procedures grew, the author wanted to develop a classification system of energy-based facial and neck rejuvenation procedures that would permit students and colleagues to understand exactly what was being done in conjunction with the interstitial laser lipolysis. It was decided to broaden the categorization to include as well energy-based neck treatments that do not puncture the skin and are delivered transcutaneously.

8.4.1 Type I: Superficial Noninvasive Transcutaneous Laser or Energy-Based Face/Neck/Skin Rejuvenation

There has been a very rapid progression of technologies that have facilitated our ability to provide moderate, minimally invasive, nonexcisional skin tightening with transcutaneous laser and energy-based devices. Many of these procedures have become important and sought after by our patient populations and are a centerpiece of consumer interest. Because patients desire effective procedures with decreased downtime, it behooves aesthetic physicians and surgeons to seek a nonsurgical approach to neck rejuvenation that centers on skin tightening. There has been an evolution of devices starting with near-infrared lasers operating in the 1,320- to 1,440-nm wavelengths, long-pulsed Nd:YAG lasers, and multiplexed lasers operating in the same infrared spectrum. These lasers were then replaced by various RF externally applied instruments that acted as efficient "bulk heaters" of the dermis. Monopolar RF and combined optical–bipolar RF mechanisms emerged and used procedures with multiple-pass, multiple-session protocols. These tools are static in nature and provide inadequate dermal stimulation, exposing dermal tissues to relatively low thermal stimulation due to short pulse duration. More recent developments in technology have produced devices that are not short pulse duration in design. These are continuous wavelength (CW) RF systems that are constantly moved along the surface of the skin. These dynamic systems have the ability to heat tissues to therapeutic temperatures relatively quickly, and to maintain these therapeutic temperatures for longer periods of time without significant patient discomfort or thermal-related skin complications. These transcutaneous, deep, dermal ablative devices include high frequency ultrasound (US) that acts by creating US-induced fractional thermal ablative zones in the deep dermis and in some cases the superficial aponeurotic system. These devices and their trade names are reviewed by Mulholland.[16]

8.4.2 Type II: Subcutaneous Laser or Energy-Based Interstitial Lipolysis/Liposculpture and the Fibroseptal Network

Type II procedures are focused on the subcutaneous and interstitial application of energy (laser or RF) via small portals on the face and neck. As this chapter goes to press several new devices have been introduced that utilize RF microneedling techniques such as the Syneron Profound and the Lutronic Infini. These devices will be classified as Type II A (▶ Fig. 8.42) as they perforate the skin aiming energy at the reticular dermis (the microincision laser or catheter-based devices are classified as Type II B). The interaction of the laser with the tissue is achieved by the absorption of the laser energy by the receptive

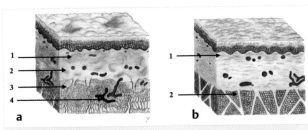

Fig. 8.13 Effects of subcutaneous laser and energy-based devices in dermis and hypodermis. (**a**) Short-term soft tissue effects in dermis and hypodermis are depicted: (1) nonablative papillary changes, (2) reticular dermal coagulation, (3) adipose coagulation, vascular coagulation, and (4) contracted fibroseptal network (FSN) bands. (**b**) Also shown are long-term reorientation of intermediate hypodermis and FSN, and (1) dermal neocollagenesis with remodeling; dermal remodeling 30% contraction; and (2) remodeled FSN bands.

chromophores, thus producing sufficient heat to cause the desired thermal damage. The heat acts on the fatty cell and the extracellular matrix including the fibrous septa (fibroseptal network [FSN]) to produce both reversible and irreversible cellular damage. Several studies have demonstrated that for low energy settings at different wavelengths a tumefaction of the adipocytes is observed leading to an increase of their diameter up to 100 μm.[4,5] The heat generated by the laser would alter the balance of sodium and potassium of the cellular membrane, allowing the free transport of extracellular liquid to the intracellular atmosphere. For higher energy settings, rupture of adipocytes and coagulation of collagen fiber and small vessels are observed.[3,5] Due to the rupture of the membrane, lipases liberated by the adipocyte are responsible for the liquefaction of the tissue, which further facilitates the subsequent aspiration. Through the liquefactive effect of the laser, the back and forth movement of the cannula is performed much more easily than when performing the conventional liposuction technique. The fact that heat also induces coagulation of small vessels in the fat tissue is very important; this phenomenon facilitates the liposuction through lesser trauma and bleeding. Liposculpture removes significant amounts of fat, serum, and blood. In cases where large amounts of fatty tissue are to be removed, a physiologically significant loss of blood can provoke metabolic alterations. In this way, laser-assisted liposculpture offers the advantage of removing larger volumes of fat without hemodynamic repercussions.[4] As with type I procedures, the thermic and athermic events induce deep reticular dermal collagen denaturization and a cascade to neocollagenesis of the deep reticular layer and remodeling of the FSN (▶ Fig. 8.13, ▶ Fig. 8.14, ▶ Fig. 8.15), which serve to help firm, tighten, tone, or lift the skin. In FLL type II the procedure description should include referencing whether or not aspiration was performed.

8.4.3 Type III: Concurrent Nonexcisional Surgical Neck Techniques (Submentoplasty or SMAS Procedures)

In the remainder of the energy-based facial and neck rejuvenation techniques, all procedures are preceded by a subcutaneous interstitial laser lipolysis and then a subsequent rhytidectomy procedure of the neck (FLL type III), face (FLL type IV), or both

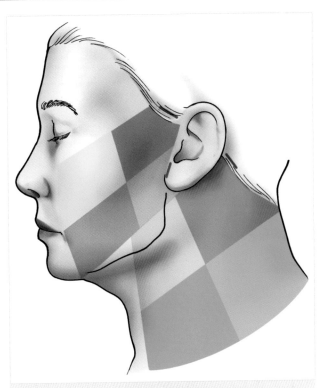

Fig. 8.14 The LaserFacialSculpting (LFS) treatment grids utilized for delineating the procedure areas in facial zones in midface, lower face, and lateral neck. (Reproduced with permission from Gentile RD, ed. Neck Rejuvenation. New York, NY: Thieme Medical Publishers; 2011:159.)

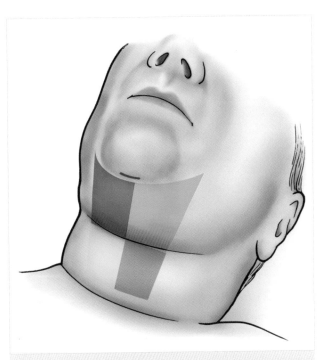

Fig. 8.15 The LaserFacialSculpting (LFS) central and lateral treatment zones for the middle neck. (Reproduced with permission from Gentile RD, ed. Neck Rejuvenation. New York, NY: Thieme Medical Publishers; 2011:159.)

Table 8.2 Gentile rhytidectomy classifications

Mini-lift (mini-lifts are designated by either being short flap or short scar including minimal-incision approaches.)	ML type I (short flap)	Flap length from tragus < 3–4 cm
	ML type II (short scar/minimal incision)	The incision(s) are limited, not extending beyond the retrotragal component. A series of small incisions are also classified as short scar.
	ML type III (combined)	Incorporates both short flap and short scar/minimal-incision components
Intermediate lift	IL type I	Flap length > 4 cm from tragus
	IL type II	Incision extends > 1 cm into posterior hairline
	IL type III	Incorporates both longer flap and longer incision
Full facelift	FFL type I	Incorporates IL with extended dissection past zygomatic or mandibular cutaneous ligaments or to the nasal labial fold (NLF)
	FFL type II	Incorporates IL with extended (side-to-side) neck dissection
	FFL type III	Incorporates both extended facial and neck dissection

Note: The use of terms to describe more limited rhytidectomy techniques should take into consideration: anesthesia requirements, operative time, complication risk, and recovery time.

face and neck (FLL type V) involving concurrent rhytidectomy techniques. In type III procedures, there are isolated nonexcisional platysmal or superficial musculoaponeurotic system (SMAS) procedures that may include surgical correction of platysmal banding that can be diminished by plication or division of the platysma muscle. Limited SMAS elevation can also be placed in this minimal incision non-excisional category. After identifying the medial platysmal edges, approximation is performed. An absorbable or nonabsorbable suture is used to create a muscle sling. The plication should extend from the submental incision to the thyroid cartilage. If a running suture is used, the plication should continue in a reverse direction, allowing for the plication of the lateral edges. A wedge excision of the medial border of the platysma at the cervicomental angle may also provide additional definition. Another technique for platysmaplasty is purse-string platysmaplasty.[17] At times in the performance of a laser neck lift the author will also place lateral sutures or a running suture along the inferior border of the mandible in order to define the mandible. In type III procedures, any nonexcisional neck rejuvenation procedure performed and preferred by the surgeon in completing an isolated submentoplasty or isolated neck lift can be performed, and it differs only by the antecedent laser irradiation/elevation of the neck flaps with or without concurrent laser lipolysis and liposculpture.

8.4.4 Type IV: Concurrent Facial Rhytidectomy Techniques (Mini-Lifts)

In FLL type IV procedures a platysmaplasty or submentoplasty is not performed but a facial rhytidectomy is performed. This rhytidectomy may include a lateral plication of the superficial musculoaponeurotic system (SMAS), but does not utilize midline surgical techniques other than laser lipolysis with or without liposculpture. In the event subplatysmal fat is treated, it would be classified as a type IV procedure provided medial suture techniques are not used. As with the FLL type III procedures, any type of rhytidectomy procedure may be performed as long as midline platysmaplasty techniques are not used. Most commonly in the author's practice a *mixed plane rhytidectomy*[18] is performed via an intermediate length incision and a short or intermediate flap elevation. In adding rhytidectomy techniques it is useful to know what exactly is done during the rhytidectomy, and there exists considerable confusion as to what different nomenclature means. Is the lift called a mini-lift short scar, short flap, or both? In order to be able to compare facelift results based on what actually was done, the author has proposed a classification of cervicofacial rhytidectomy that simplifies the nomenclature. Up until now the definition and classification of mini-lifts and other more extensive forms of rhytidectomy have been lacking in the plastic surgery literature. A classification listing the extent of rhytidectomy performed is shown in ▶ Table 8.2, referencing flap and incision length as the parameters of assessment.

8.4.5 Type V: Concurrent Surgery for both Face and Neck (Cervicofacial Rhytidectomy)

FLL type V patients are characterized by subcutaneous laser-assisted cervicofacial flap elevation with or without interstitial laser lipolysis and liposculpture, and the performance of rhytidectomy procedures of the face and neck including midline platysmal plication or platysmaplasty.

8.5 Subcutaneous Optical Energy and Laser–Tissue Interaction

8.5.1 Hemostasis

The clinical observation of hemostatic effect of the fiber laser treatment of the facial flap in an early patient in 2007 led to a small clinical study that compared the 980-nm CW diode laser to the pulsed 1,064 Nd:YAG SmartLipo and SmartLipo MPX that utilized both the 1,064 and 1,320 nm in single wavelength or multiplexed mode. Split-face studies were done utilizing the same 10-W setting with the following findings: The diode laser was much more effective in passing through the superficial soft tissues when compared to the SmartLipo laser, but the hemostatic effects observed with the SmartLipo were not present in the diode laser. This was true when comparing the 980-nm diode to the 1,064 and 1,320 nm, or blended multiplexed 1,064/1,320-nm wavelengths. A similar comparison with the 1,440-

nm wavelengths likewise demonstrated less hemostatic ability than the 1,064 or 1,064/1,320 nm blended. A quantitative comparison showed that the SmartLipo had roughly 5 times the hemostatic capability when compared to the diode laser based on sponge counts. An explanation of this is shown in the following illustrations. First when comparing the pulse characteristics of the SmartLipo laser, it is evident that high-peak powers are generated with each laser pulse. This is known as a gradient pulse (▸ Fig. 8.16). The high-peak energies are responsible for sealing off the blood vessels before the fiber laser divides the blood vessels, and the probability of vessel coagulation is related to the high-peak power of the pulsed laser (▸ Fig. 8.17). The 980-nm CW laser does not generate the high-peak power seen in the SmartLipo laser—whether the 1,064-nm or the 1,064/1,320-nm blended MPX unit or the Triplex or the 1,440-nm laser alone. When the laser is passed subcutaneously, it simply divides the vessel without cauterizing it (▸ Fig. 8.18), which leads to no advantage for the laser use if hemostasis is the desired end point. At meetings over the past several years, the author has seen clinical photos of fairly large hematomas during use of the 980-nm CW diode laser subcutaneously in the face. This is not surprising because, as demonstrated in the author's study, the fixed-pulse, 980-nm fiber laser operating at 10 W and used subcutaneously does not provide substantial hemostatic effects. The author would be concerned about using the 980-nm CW diode laser on lower orbital fat due to the fact

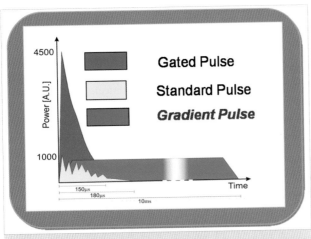

Fig. 8.16 Gradient pulse characteristics of SmartLipo and SmartLipo MPX. Wave configuration has much to do with the hemostatic properties of the investigated fiber lasers. The pulsed lasers generate higher peak powers for cauterization of facial blood vessels. (Reproduced with permission from Gentile RD, ed. Neck Rejuvenation. New York, NY: Thieme Medical Publishers; 2011:157.)

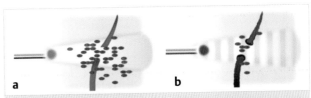

Fig. 8.18 Blood vessel interaction with continuous wavelength (CW) versus pulsed lasers. (a) CW lasers thermally lacerate blood vessels with little coagulation of the blood vessel. Red blood count (RBC) extravasation into the tissue increasing ecchymosis and edema. (b) High-energy pulsed lasers rapidly coagulate the blood vessel and divide it, sealing it off from RBC extravasation and reducing the sequelae of ecchymosis and edema.

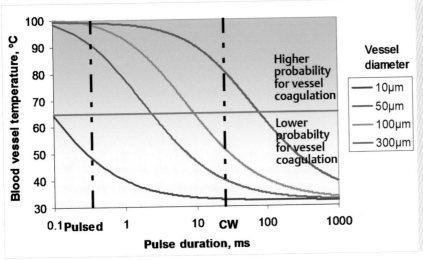

Fig. 8.17 Pulse characteristics, power, and the probability of vessel coagulation according to vessel size. CW, continuous wavelength. (Reproduced with permission from Gentile RD, ed. Neck Rejuvenation. New York, NY: Thieme Medical Publishers; 2011:158.)

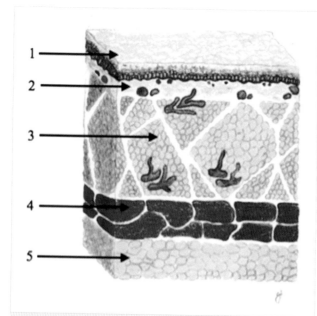

Fig. 8.19 The characteristics of an ideal youthful neck are shown: (1) epidermis, (2) dermis, (3) hypodermis (interstitial space), (4) platysma, and (5) deep platysmal fat.

that lack of effective hemostasis in orbital fat vessels could lead to catastrophic complications. Complications with skin burns and full-thickness necrosis have been reported with the 980-nm diode laser when used without temperature monitoring.[19]

8.5.2 Interstitial Lipolysis

A brief overview has already been presented of the laser–tissue interaction and the fundamental laser physics of interstitial laser lipolysis. To summarize, the laser–tissue interaction laser lipolysis works by a mechanism of photoacoustic ablation and selective photothermolysis of fibrous septa comprising the FSN. Different wavelengths have been selected for laser lipolysis in an attempt to specifically target fat, collagen (water), and blood vessels. According to the theory of selective photothermolysis, these chromophores will preferentially absorb laser energy on the basis of their absorption coefficients at specific wavelengths. Various wavelengths, including 924, 968, 980, 1,064, 1,319, 1,320, 1,344, and 1,440 nm, have been evaluated for interactions within the subcutaneous compartment. Whereas the debate over which wavelength is ideal for interstitial laser lipolysis continues on, research data suggest that the ideal wavelength peaks of 1,210, 1,440, and 1,720 nm are the peaks for fat absorption. Goldman et al[14] and McBean and Katz[20] have theorized that most of the purported mechanisms of action for interstitial laser lipolysis (photoacoustical, photomechanical, or photothermal effects) are either secondary to—or have been replaced by—the idea that heat generated on tissue is the primary mode of action in laser lipolysis. Khoury et al[21] proposed that photoacoustic ablation lends to thermal damage, although photoacoustic damage is difficult to evaluate histologically. Thus, the favored mechanism of action for laser lipolysis is a purely thermal effect.

8.5.3 Tightening of the Fibroseptal Network and Reticular Dermis (Skin Tightening)

The superiority of interstitial laser lipolysis over conventional lipolysis relies on the well-established and reviewed skin-tightening effect, and is perhaps the most significant advantage of laser lipolysis.[1,22] The basic premise of the skin-tightening ability of interstitial laser lipolysis is in targeting water as its chromophore—there is initial collagen contraction and destruction through both mechanical and biochemical pathways. As a result of the deep-delivered energy into the skin, collagen remodeling through a controlled wound-healing response occurs over time with associated neocollagenesis. This collagen remodeling also yields the desired tissue tightening that is seen with laser lipolysis. Early reports regarding the lack of efficacy of skin tightening in interstitial laser lipolysis may be related to the steep learning curve of the procedure, inadequate energy application, or insufficient heat accumulation. The emphasis in these procedures is to reach the goal internal temperature ranging between 48 and 50°C and external temperature of treatment location approximately 38 to 40°C. Reaching therapeutic temperature end points is facilitated by the use of internal temperature monitoring as well as external temperature sensing devices. Thermal stimulation results in deep reticular dermal collagen denaturization and a cascade to neocollagenesis of the deep reticular layer that serves to help firm, tighten, tone, or lift the skin. Surgeons and patients should also remember that skin tightening continues to improve several months and perhaps as long as a year after subcutaneous laser treatment due to the delayed nature of neocollagenesis (▶ Fig. 8.13).

8.6 Results of Subcutaneous Laser and Energy-Based Facial and Neck Rejuvenation

8.6.1 Type I Procedures and Results

Facial and nonfacial skin laxity has traditionally been treated using surgical lifting procedures. Over the past two decades, a wide range of noninvasive treatments such as ablative and non-ablative laser skin resurfacing—usually infrared light devices and RF or US energy—have been introduced as alternative therapies to achieve variable degrees and depths of tissue tightening through controlled dermal tissue heating.[3,4,5,6,7,8,9,10] In essence, these treatments deliver infrared light, RF energy, or US energy to induce controlled thermal injury as deep as 2 to 4 mm in the dermis.[11,12] Volumetric tissue heating causes immediate collagen contraction and delayed neocollagenesis over a period of 6 months, which leads to clinical skin tightening. Although tightening has been shown with these devices, several shortcomings exist; these include inconsistent clinical outcomes, need for multiple treatment sessions, and associated pain and costs. Treatment protocols vary for these devices but most do rely on repeated sessions of treatment. Advantages of these types of energy-based treatments are in the limited downtime and reduced costs when compared to excisional surgery. Type I transcutaneous energy-based lifting of a patient

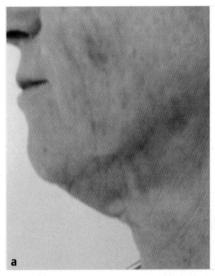
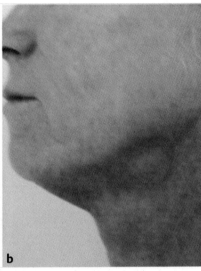

Fig. 8.20 (**a, b**) Results from an energy-based type I treatment, which is noninvasive, nonexcisional, and utilizes transcutaneous radiofrequency (RF) treatment of lower face and neck.

undergoing facial and neck-firming procedures is shown in ► Fig. 8.20.

8.6.2 Type II Procedures and Results

Interstitial Laser Lipolysis Technique

Until late 2007, most in-office procedures, which included SmartLipo techniques, were completed by using the laser for laser lipolysis, some liposuction, and the concurrent tightening of the facial soft tissues through tissue coagulation and the thermal and athermal effects that follow laser lipolysis. The first procedures usually did not have external temperature monitoring, so it is likely that the tissue tightening that was obtained was less than possible now; thermal end points have been introduced that bring the skin temperature to the highest possible temperature without inducing skin necrosis. These studies were first completed by DiBernardo,[1] who demonstrated that epidermal necrosis was associated with skin temperatures approaching 48 to 52°C. DiBernardo later published his results showing the degree of skin tightening available with subcutaneous laser irradiation with the thermal end points not exceeding 42°C.[1] The techniques for fiber laser or SmartLifting procedures have evolved, and the various techniques from the most fundamental to the more extensive are presented here. The subcutaneous technique without any concurrent rhytidectomy techniques is referred to as interstitial laser lipolysis or LaserFacialSculpting (LFS)[8] and is categorized as a type II fiber laser lift (FLL). Most of the procedures with concurrent rhytidectomy techniques utilized the initial subcutaneous LFS techniques prior to elevating the skin flaps and performing various deep tissue lifting maneuvers. These include the LaserNeckLift[10] (FLL type III), UltraMiniLift (FLL type IV), and the LaserSmartLift (FLL type V). The UltraMiniLifts are minimal-incision techniques without significant skin excision and utilize self-retaining sutures. The protocol for LFS procedures includes facial and neck patient marking into grids depicting the subcutaneous laser treatment zones of the lateral and midface as well as the lateral and central neck. The grids for the lateral and midface are shown in ► Fig. 8.14 and ► Fig. 8.15. The treatment zones for the lateral and central neck are shown in ► Fig. 8.19. After

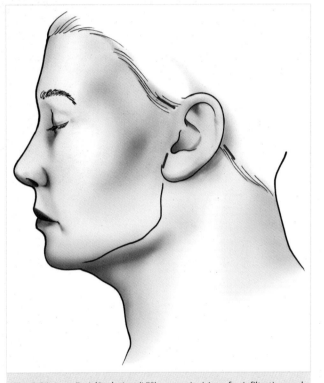

Fig. 8.21 LaserFacialSculpting (LFS) access incisions for infiltration and treatment. Three small incisions (red lines) are made for both infiltration of tumescent anesthetic fluid as well as fiber laser introduction. (Reproduced with permission from Gentile RD, ed. Neck Rejuvenation. New York, NY: Thieme Medical Publishers; 2011:160.)

marking, the access ports for both the tumescent anesthesia and the laser access are drawn (► Fig. 8.21). As shown, these small incisions are located in the temple, anterior to the lobule, and in the posterior hairline. A modified Klein's tumescent solution is then infiltrated. The composition of the modified Klein's solution infiltrated is shown in ► Table 8.3. Just prior to the tumescent infiltration 20 mL of 0.5% Xylocaine with 1:200,000 parts epinephrine is infiltrated into the grids. The tumescent solution is infiltrated with the use of a compression

Table 8.3 Modified Klein's solution

Component	Amount
Normal saline	1,000 mL
Xylocaine	500–1,000 mg
Epinephrine	0.5–0.65 mg
Sodium bicarbonate	10 mEq
Triamcinolone (optional)	10 mg

Abbreviation: mEq, milliequivalent.

sleeve on the liter bag of tumescent fluid dispensed through an infiltration cannula attached to a control cannula. After about 8 to 10 minutes the laser is inserted and treatment of each grid is accomplished. Because superheating a treatment area can lead to thermal necrosis, the more distal grid is always treated first before passing into the grids adjacent to the portals. This reduces the laser exposure to the more proximal grids and prevents the overtreatment of the sites closest to the insertion points. The treatment end points for FLL type II procedures (LFS) are 47 to 50°C internally and 38 to 40°C for those procedures that are not elevated. In skin flaps that will be elevated and skin placed under tension, 36°C is used as the end point

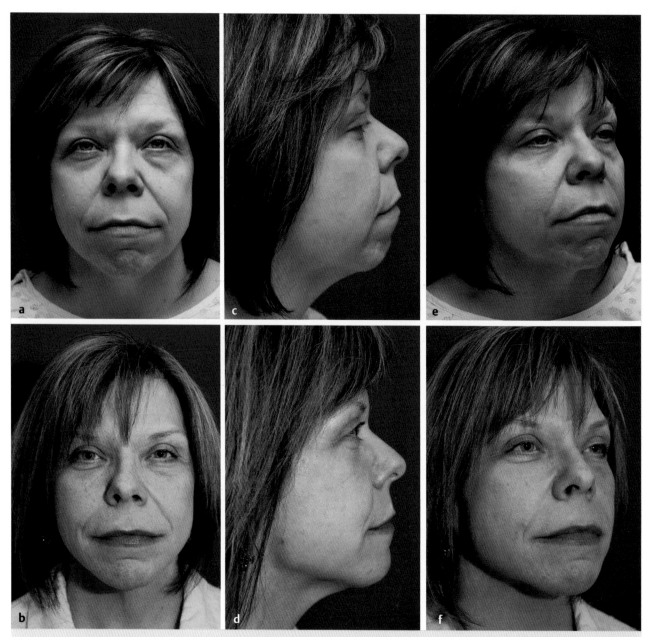

Fig. 8.22 A 50-year-old woman undergoing LaserFacialSculpting (LFS) fiber laser lift (FLL type II). This patient is shown (**a, c, e**) before and (**b, d, f**) 9 months after LFS with chin augmentation and microablative skin rejuvenation. The noticeable thinning of her face is evident with contour enhancements of the mandibular border. (Reproduced with permission from Gentile RD, ed. Neck Rejuvenation. New York, NY: Thieme Medical Publishers; 2011:161.)

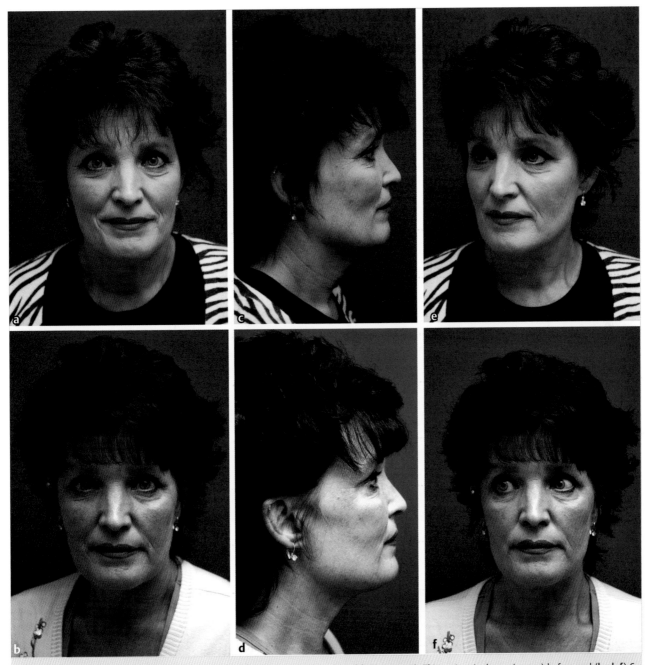

Fig. 8.23 A 52-year-old woman undergoing LaserFacialSculpting (LFS) fiber laser lift (FLL type II). This patient is shown (**a, c, e**) before and (**b, d, f**) 6 months after LFS with microablative skin rejuvenation. She demonstrates an almost complete correction of her midline fullness without any skin excision whatsoever. (Reproduced with permission from Gentile RD, ed. Neck Rejuvenation. New York, NY: Thieme Medical Publishers; 2011:162.)

because there is less need to try to achieve maximal skin contraction and skin excisional techniques are also being employed. The typical patient undergoing FLL type II techniques (LFS) has early laxity of the face and neck with fatty deposition and associated jowling that is not significantly ptotic. As jowling and facial and neck laxity increases, different rhytidectomy techniques rely on SMAS repositioning to achieve a satisfactory aesthetic result. Patients who desire facial firming and do not want incisions or a rhytidectomy are also good candidates for the procedure. Several FLL type II (LFS) patients undergoing

firming and sculpting procedures are shown in ▶ Fig. 8.22, ▶ Fig. 8.23, ▶ Fig. 8.24.

8.6.3 Type III Procedures and Results
LaserNeckLift Surgical Technique

The process of consultation with patients about their interest in facial rejuvenation involves a complete understanding of what the patients expect, and also what they believe is possible with

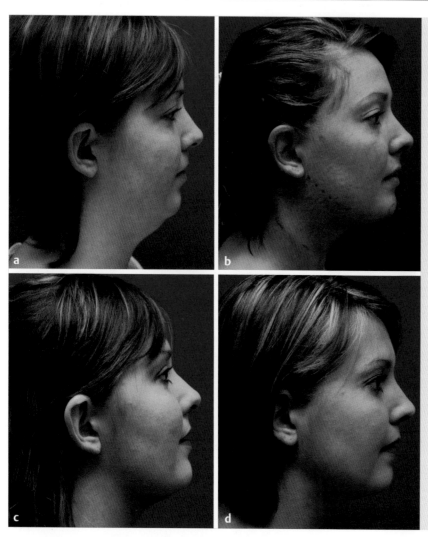

Fig. 8.24 A 26-year-old woman undergoing interstitial laser lipolysis fiber laser lift (FLL type II). This patient had a significant excess of cervical fat and was an excellent candidate for a FLL type II procedure consisting predominantly of interstitial laser lipolysis. She is shown (**a**) preoperatively, (**b**) 24 hours postoperatively, (**c**) 1 month postoperatively, and (**d**) 4 months postoperatively.

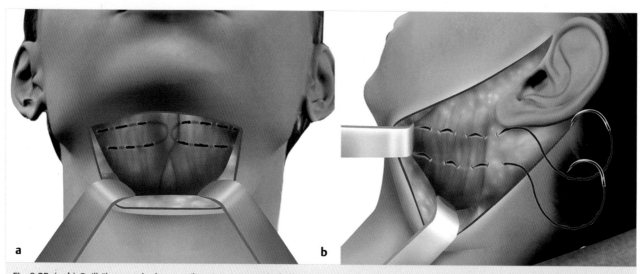

Fig. 8.25 (**a, b**) Quill "hammock platysmaplasty" or LaserNeckLift fiber laser lift (FLL type III). The LaserFacialSculpting (LFS) procedure may be enhanced by minor platysmal surgery. In patients undergoing LFS the surgical field in the central neck is very hemostatic and permits platysmal modification to be accomplished with minimal bleeding. (Reproduced with permission from Gentile RD. Neck Rejuvenation. New York, NY: Thieme Medical Publishers; 2011:165.)

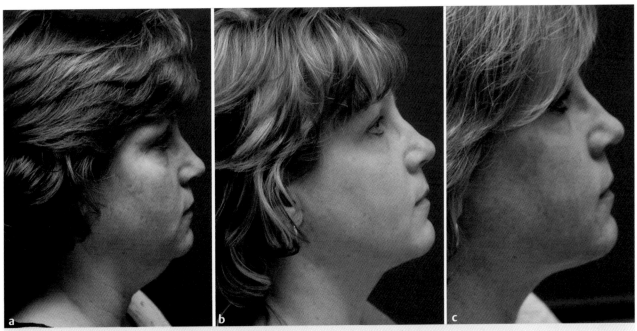

Fig. 8.26 A 50-year-old woman undergoing LaserNeckLift fiber laser lift (FLL type III). This patient underwent nonexcisional neck lift with isolated medial and lateral platysmaplasty with minimal incisions. She is shown (**a**) preoperatively, (**b**) 4 months postoperatively, and (**c**) 1 year postoperatively. Previously it had been thought that this result would require a full excisional rhytidectomy. No skin was excised in this patient.

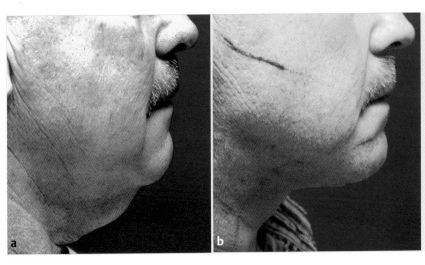

Fig. 8.27 A 57-year-old man 2 days after Laser-FacialSculpting (LFS) with LaserNeckLift fiber laser lift (FLL type III). Quick-recovery characteristics of the LaserNeckLift are seen in this patient shown (**a**) preoperatively, and (**b**) 3 days after surgery, with minimal bruising and swelling. (Reproduced with permission from Gentile RD, ed. Neck Rejuvenation. New York, NY: Thieme Medical Publishers; 2011:168.)

advances in facial rejuvenation procedures. In developing quick-recovery methods, there are several discussions that must be completed during this process. The fact that smaller incisions or less invasive methods can be utilized in a patient's treatment plan does not always mean that this will result in the best overall aesthetic outcome for the patient. Also in some minimal-incision techniques, the bruising and swelling may be on par with what may be seen in some mini-lift procedures. So patients must be counseled in such a way that gives them a complete understanding of what the final result can or will be and what the recovery time should be. In some of the LFS procedures and minimal-incision lifts the "maturation" phase of the result can take as long as 6 months to finalize, and the patient must be made to understand that quick recovery is not equated with the quick achievement of postoperative results. In attempting to bridge the results obtainable with LFS techniques

and mini-lifts, we started to implement some platysmaplasty techniques through very limited incisions with no skin excision. After following these patients for up to 6 months it became evident that platysmaplasty techniques via minimal-incisional approaches did contribute to enhanced neck results in certain patients. This has been especially evident in men with significant midline laxity and who would be thought to benefit only from facial and neck lift combined procedures. The technique for these patients includes performing LFS prior to focusing on the neck via the midline and posterior neck incision. We utilize a "hammock platysmaplasty" or midline platysmal overlap approach that was first described by Fuente del Campo.[23] In our modification of the overlap technique, we utilize Quill self-retaining sutures (SRS) (Angiotech Inc., Vancouver, British Columbia, Canada) and then purse-string the lateral component to the mastoid periosteal. The technique is shown in ▶ Fig. 8.25.

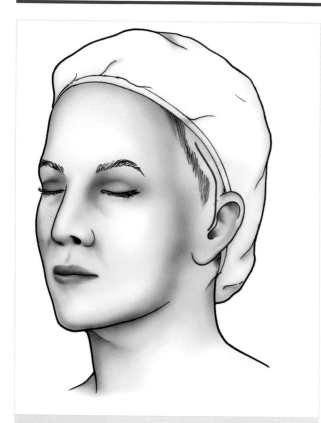

Fig. 8.28 Temporal tragal incision (red line) used for UltraMiniLift fiber laser lift (FLL type III). The UltraMiniLift is performed through a very limited superior-based temporal tragal incision. The incision may occasionally extend just past the lobule if necessary for contouring the skin. Minimal skin is excised with this technique. (Reproduced with permission from Gentile RD, ed. Neck Rejuvenation. New York, NY: Thieme Medical Publishers; 2011:163.)

Patients undergoing LaserNeckLift procedures are shown in ▸ Fig. 8.26 and ▸ Fig. 8.27.

UltraMiniLift Surgical Technique

A significant benefit of subcutaneous laser dissection is that it readily separates the skin from the deeper subcutaneous tissues with significant hemostasis. This permits the surgeon to consider lifting procedures and suture techniques for the SMAS performed through a very limited incision. Due to a very controlled dissection with little bleeding, the surgeon can be less concerned about having access to bleeding sites that would require the passage of cautery devices. The ability to obtain hemostasis frequently requires wide access and a larger skin incision. The UltraMiniLift was developed to permit a vertical elevation of the jowl via a small temporal-tragal incision (▸ Fig. 8.28 and ▸ Fig. 8.29). The procedure involves performing LFS as described via the three portals, making the larger incision, and elevating a facial skin flap of 5 to 5.5 cm through the limited or short-scar incision. Liposculpture of the jowl is frequently performed after LFS especially in the heavier jowl or face. Buccal fat may be contributing to large jowls and must be considered when completing the surgery, and in those patients buccal fat reduction may be completed. Next the midface and jowl are elevated with the Quill SRS technique of the mixed plane rhytidectomy

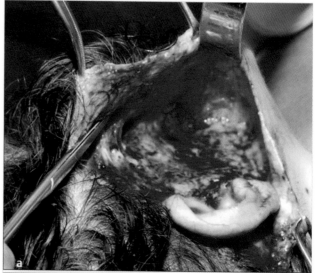

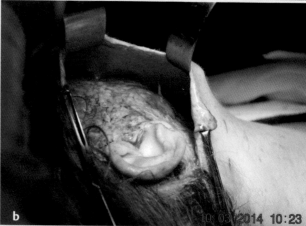

Fig. 8.29 Complications of LaserSmartLift fiber laser lift (FLL type IV). (a) Epidermal and (b) dermal necroses. (Reproduced with permission from Gentile RD, ed. Neck Rejuvenation. New York, NY: Thieme Medical Publishers; 2011:154.)

(▸ Fig. 8.30). This technique does not include the lower face or neck sutures. After the plication is completed, redundant skin is excised from the temporal-tragal incision (▸ Fig. 8.31). In some patients, repositioning of the temporal hair tuft is necessary to avoid an elevated hairline. The UltraMiniLift can be combined with limited-access platysmaplasty, due to the ability of the surgeon to widely undermine the midline and lateral neck skin through a very small incision. If midline platysmaplasty is performed, the procedure would be classified as an FLL type V procedure. Results of UltraMiniLift procedures can be enhanced with the use of ablative fractional skin rejuvenation. A patient undergoing UltraMiniLift is shown in ▸ Fig. 8.32.

8.6.4 Type IV and Type V Procedures and Results

LaserSmartLift Surgical Technique

The LaserSmartLift is the most frequently performed FLL or SmartLifting procedure and represents the combination of an LFS procedure with a mixed plane rhytidectomy (type IV)

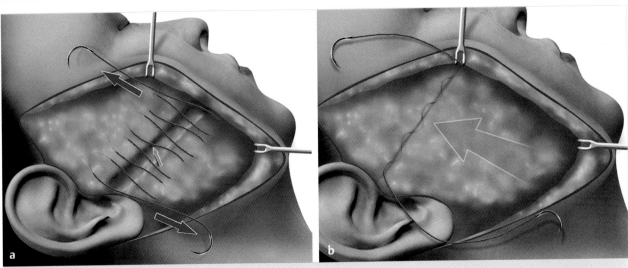

Fig. 8.30 Jowl lift in UltraMiniLift fiber laser lift (FLL type III) and LaserSmartLift (FLL type IV). This mixed plane rhytidectomy technique utilizing (**a**) Quill self-retaining suture (SRS) is employed to elevate the jowl in patients who may need extra elevation to contour the mandibular border. Small green arrow: starting point of double-ended suture. Purple arrows: direction of malar and cervical suture plication/imbrication. (**b**) Lift of the jowl also lifts the superior platysma in the neck. Suture continues down the neck for lateral platysmal tightening. Gray arrow: strong vertical vector lift achieved when completed. (Reproduced with permission from Gentile RD. Neck Rejuvenation. New York, NY: Thieme Medical Publishers; 2011:163.)

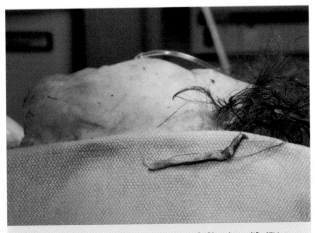

Fig. 8.31 Limited skin excision in UltraMiniLift fiber laser lift (FLL type III). In the UltraMiniLift a limited amount of skin is removed. The technique relies on skin contraction via tissue tightening to achieve its end points. (Reproduced with permission from Gentile RD, ed. Neck Rejuvenation. New York, NY: Thieme Medical Publishers; 2011:164.)

including platysmaplasty (type V). In the procedure, LFS is first performed prior to marking and elevating a 5- to 6-cm intermediate facial flap. The incision is depicted in ▶ Fig. 8.33 and is variable in the posterior neck, reflecting the skin redundancy or lack thereof. In some patients a very limited posterior incision is made. Certain patients will have an intermediate extension into the hairline, and for severe neck-skin redundancy the incision will extend well into the hairline. After elevating the skin flap, the upper and lower Quill SRS are placed consistent with the mixed plane rhytidectomy technique and the skin is redraped and trimmed of excess (▶ Fig. 8.29, ▶ Fig. 8.30, ▶ Fig. 8.34). In most patients, we reposition the temporal hair

tuft by excising a burrow's triangle and moving the hairline downward, as is done with a classic Hamra deep plane rhytidectomy. Patients with low temporal hair tufts may not require repositioning. It is rare for us to perform midline medial platysmaplasty procedures unless there is extensive subplatysmal fat or very heavy medial platysmal bands that need to be addressed. Patients undergoing LaserSmartLift procedures are shown in ▶ Fig. 8.29, ▶ Fig. 8.35, ▶ Fig. 8.36, ▶ Fig. 8.37, ▶ Fig. 8.38.

LaserSmartLift Extended and Ancillary Surgical Techniques

In some circumstances the flap elevation is longer than 6 cm to permit certain adjunctive procedures. In patients with extremely deep NLF, we will perform an upper face dissection along the zygomatic major muscle extending past the NLF and crease. One of the newer applications in laser-assisted facelifting is the use of the fiber laser (FL) to undermine the superior NLF, as shown in ▶ Fig. 8.39 and ▶ Fig. 8.40. By freeing the dermal cuticular ligaments, a more significant correction of the NLF is accomplished than would be possible in rhytidectomy procedures lacking this release. In these patients a portal and FL dissection are done through a small stab incision in the nasal labial crease (▶ Fig. 8.39). In some circumstances, the mouth has pronounced melolabial folds and in these patients, the author will dissect past the depressor anguli oris and release the mandibular cutaneous ligaments. The author may section the depressor anguli oris in these patients. Some patients will have prominent buccal fat (▶ Fig. 8.41), and when the mixed plane plication is performed excessive fullness in the midface may result. In these patients a subtotal excision of the buccal fat pad is accomplished. A patient undergoing extended LaserSmartLifting techniques is shown in ▶ Fig. 8.40.

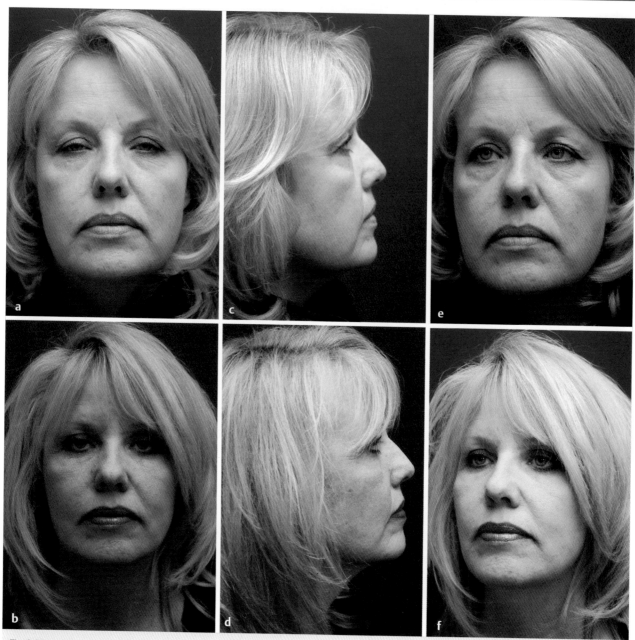

Fig. 8.32 A 53-year-old woman undergoing UltraMiniLift fiber laser lift (FLL type III). This patient is shown (**a, c, e**) preoperatively and (**b, d, f**) 1 year postoperative UltraMiniLift with upper and lower blepharoplasty. The reduction in vertical height of the face is demonstrated with a more youthful contour. (Reproduced with permission from Gentile RD, ed. Neck Rejuvenation. New York, NY: Thieme Medical Publishers; 2011:164.)

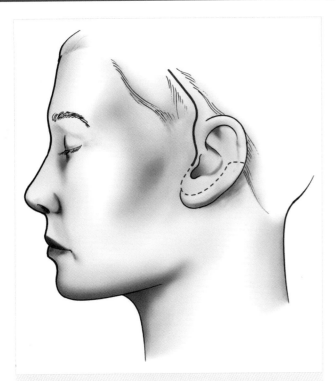

Fig. 8.33 Incision for LaserSmartLift fiber laser lift (FLL type IV). The incision for the LaserSmartLift (red line) is similar to other rhytidectomies but the posterior limb is adjusted to account for the amount of neck skin expected to be removed. (Reproduced with permission from Gentile RD, ed. Neck Rejuvenation. New York, NY: Thieme Medical Publishers; 2011:168.)

Other Energy-Based Devices and Subcutaneous Interstitial Techniques

With the advent of internal laser aesthetic plastic surgery encompassing subcutaneous techniques after the FDA approval of the original SmartLipo laser, other technologies have been introduced that also work in the interstitial layer that is intermediate to the deep reticular dermis and the hypodermis. Most of the subcutaneous devices introduced employ RF and include the ePrime system from Syneron (Yokneam, Israel) (▶ Fig. 8.42) and the ThermiRF devices (▶ Fig. 8.42b and ▶ Fig. 8.43) by ThermiAesthetics (Southlake, Texas). Although the delivery methods differ in the type of delivery interface (e.g., needles vs. blunt cannula), the technology is RF energy delivered subcutaneously into the fibroseptal network (FSN). Temperature-controlled subcutaneous RF enables three-dimensional (3D) structural lifting and tightening of tissue, and many primary investigators of this device now have more than 1-year clinical follow-up.[24] Thermistor-controlled subdermal skin tightening via percutaneous RF provides controlled thermogenesis to subcutaneous collagenous tissue, which includes the papillary and reticular layer of the dermis, the fascia layer between muscle and skin, and the septal connective tissue segmenting fat lobules. Treating the interstitial layer may be possible with other technologies that aim to bypass the epidermis and dermis in the delivery of thermogenic energy. ThermiRF is the first temperature-controlled RF device for general subcutaneous use in applications for soft-tissue tightening. One useful treatment

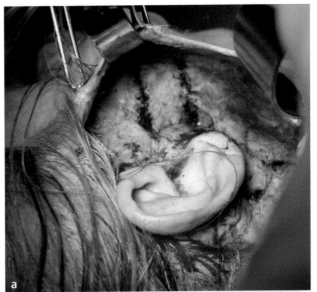

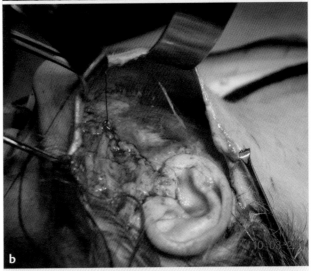

Fig. 8.34 (a) Grid for SMAS-Platysma Plication. (b) The SMAS Plication of the malar segment has been completed.

protocol of the Thermi procedure is the use of a thermal imaging camera during the treatment (▶ Fig. 8.44). The combination of internal thermal sensors and external thermal monitoring makes this a very useful procedure, assuring that therapeutic temperatures are reached subcutaneously and are maintained at the level of the epidermis. It is estimated that significant skin tightening occurs with subcutaneous temperature in the interstitial layers of 65°C, and with adequate temperature control to not elevate epidermal temperatures to above 46 to 48°C because this is the threshold for skin blistering and full-thickness burns.

8.7 Complications of Fiber Laser and Energy-Based Techniques

Since 2007 the author has utilized subcutaneous FL and energy-based techniques in close to 1,500 procedures and has

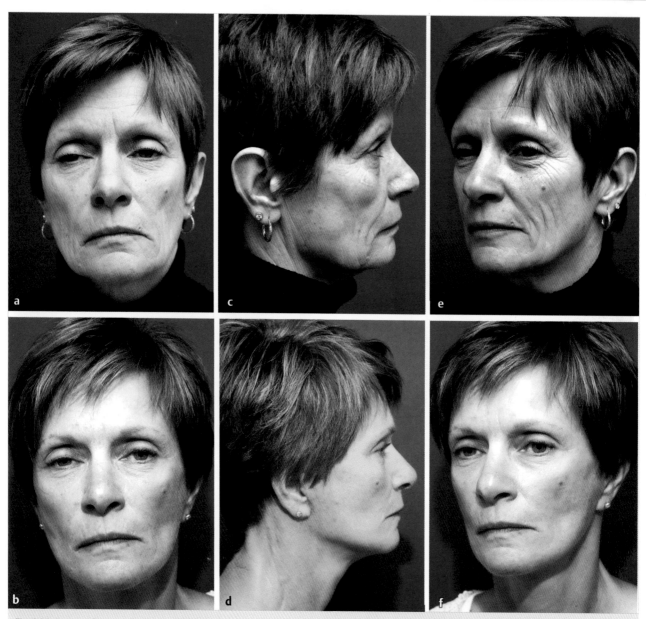

Fig. 8.35 Patient after LaserSmartLift fiber laser lift (FLL type IV). A 54-year-old woman with facial, perioral, and neck laxity is shown (**a, c, e**) preoperatively, and (**b, d, f**) 6 months postoperative LaserSmartLift, which is LaserFacialSculpting (LFS) followed by mixed plane rhytidectomy. Used with permission from Gentile RD, ed. Neck Rejuvenation. New York, NY: Thieme Medical Publishers; 2011:169.

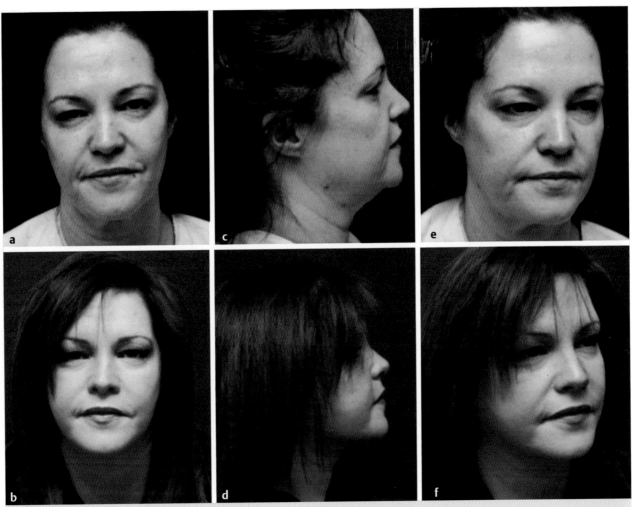

Fig. 8.36 Patient after LaserSmartLift, platysmaplasty. Following weight loss, a 48-year-old woman is shown (**a, c, e**) preoperatively and (**b, d, f**) 6 months after LaserSmartLift with platysmaplasty.

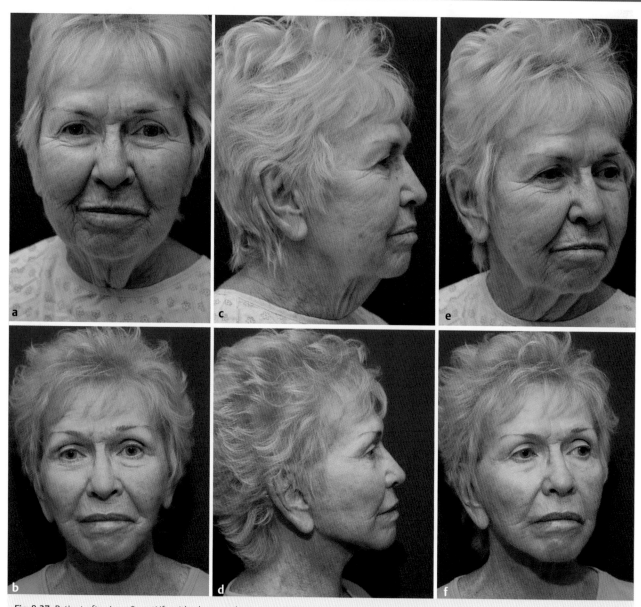

Fig. 8.37 Patient after LaserSmartLift with platysmaplasty, extended to encompass extensive laxity of face and neck. Patient is shown (**a, c, e**) preoperatively and (**b, d, f**) 9 months after extended LaserSmartLift, upper blepharoplasty, and fractional laser skin rejuvenation of lower eyelids and upper lip. (Reproduced with permission from Gentile RD, ed. Neck Rejuvenation. New York, NY: Thieme Medical Publishers; 2011:172.)

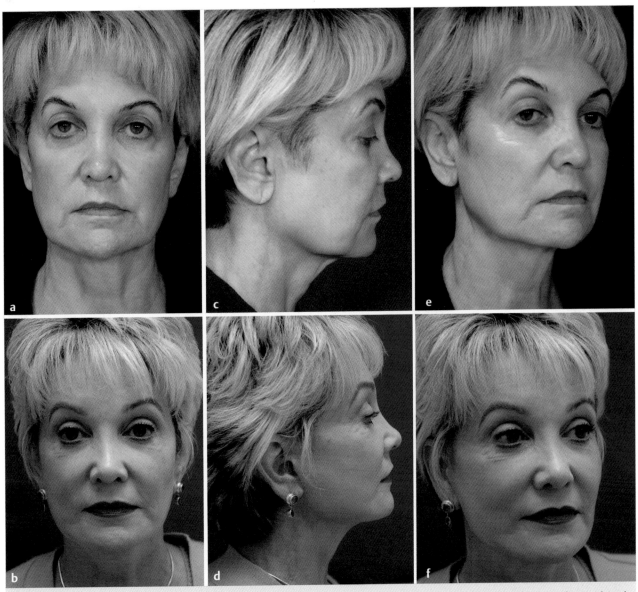

Fig. 8.38 Patient before (**a, c, e**) and after (**b, d, f**) LaserSmartLift fiber laser lift (FLL type IV). (Reproduced with permission from Gentile RD, ed. Neck Rejuvenation. New York, NY: Thieme Medical Publishers; 2011:170.)

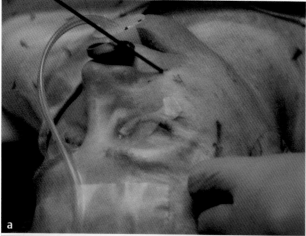

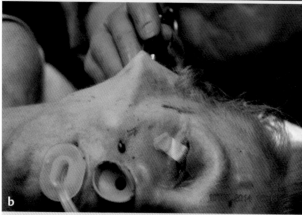

Fig. 8.39 Nasal labial fold (NLF) dissection. **(a)** The fiber laser is used to undermine the NLF, releasing the dermal cuticular attachments. **(b)** Undermining extends past the NLF, which facilitates correction of the excess.

seen very few complications. The complications encountered could have occurred with or without the use of the laser to undermine the facial skin flaps—hematomas, or seroma, or other complications typically associated with facial and cervical rhytidectomy. Whereas the specific data do not exist to prove or disprove a lower hematoma rate or bruising or swelling reduction, the author's observations are that these are all generally lower in patients treated with the subcutaneous laser prior to rhytidectomy. One benefit of laser-flap elevation is that the laser tends to elevate the flap with a flap thickness that is ideal for flap viability. With laser-flap undermining, there is very little variability in flap thickness. This is especially useful in revision rhytidectomy and the laser's ability to easily penetrate scar tissue during the flap separation.

8.7.1 Epidermal and Dermal Necroses

Although laser-flap elevation may be suspect of increasing the incidence of flap necrosis, this has not been a finding in many case procedures. Unlike trunk and extremity laser lipolysis, the energy settings for the SmartLifting are very low—rarely exceeding 9 to 12 W. With these lower energies and a selective slow heating of the flap, the author has not seen dermal and epidermal necroses in these patients that would exceed the expected incidence of 3%. As in non–laser-assisted flap elevation these can and do occur but are extremely rare. There were four episodes of minor blistering, one of which involved a necrosis near the lateral canthal area that most likely occurred due to the laser being used without the benefit of enough tumescent fluid; these also occurred prior to using extensive thermal monitoring of the regions (▶ Fig. 8.45 and ▶ Fig. 8.46). One of the patients with thermal injury most likely had dermal involvement due to electrocautery use but this occurred during a LaserSmartLift. The author finds it unnecessary and inadvisable to do extensive laser undermining inside the limits of the orbital rim. There were two episodes of full-thickness cervical blistering and skin necrosis despite thermal monitoring, and this was most likely due in part to using more than 15 W to perform the neck elevation. When using higher energies, the rate of temperature elevation is more unpredictable and overshooting the upper limit for skin safety can occur. With the advent of thermal guides and better appreciation of the thermodynamics of the skin heating process, fewer of these complications have been observed. All complications reported as a result of thermal injury and skin necrosis have responded well to conservative treatment. The patients underwent a limited scar revision with good aesthetic results. With thermal monitoring there have not been any thermal-related complications.

8.7.2 Neural Injury

It is recognized that the greatest fear of utilizing lasers subcutaneously in the face is that the energy will be uncontrolled and facial motor nerve injury will occur. Again, with hundreds of successful SmartLifting procedures this is not a documented complication, providing the laser and surgical guidelines are followed. It is very important to always see the aiming beam of the laser when elevating the skin flap, and if the laser is passed too deeply it is possible to cause neural injury. There were some short-term marginal mandibular neurapraxias in several

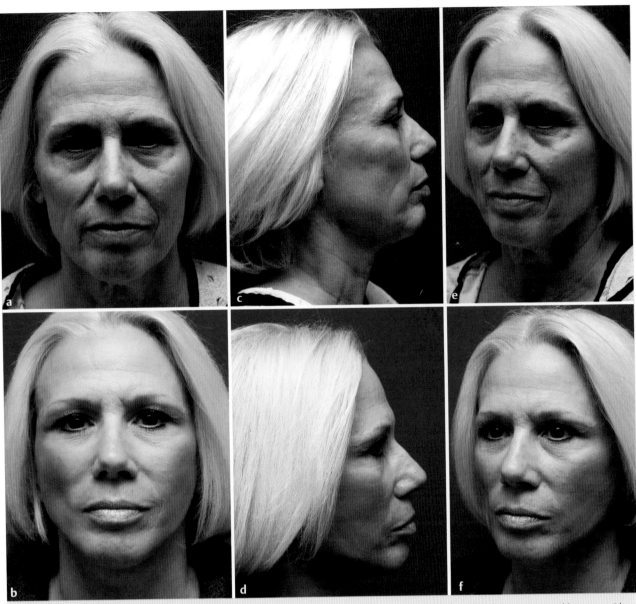

Fig. 8.40 Patient after LaserSmartLift, platysmaplasty fiber laser lift (FLL type V, with nasal labial fold [NLF] extension). A 58-year-old woman with extensive facial and neck laxity and deep NLF is shown (a, c, e) preoperatively, and (b, d, f) 3 months after LaserSmartLift with extended dissection into the NLF. (Reproduced with permission from Gentile RD, ed. Neck Rejuvenation. New York, NY: Thieme Medical Publishers; 2011:171.)

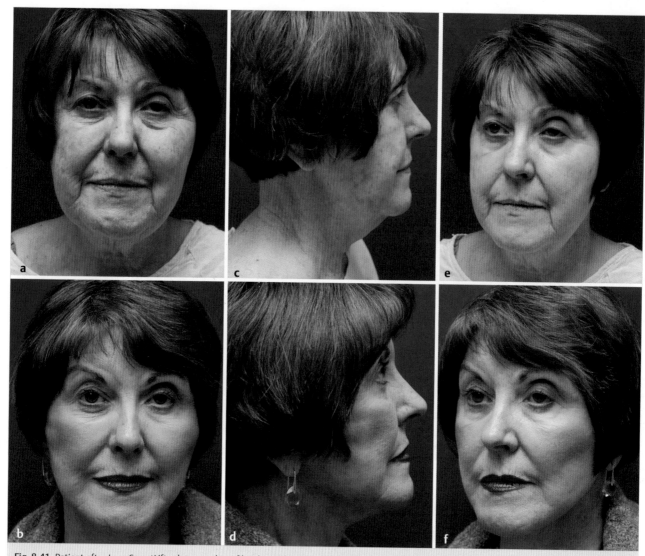

Fig. 8.41 Patient after LaserSmartLift, platysmaplasty fiber laser lift (FLL type V, with buccal fat removal). A 75-year-old woman undergoing extended LaserSmartLift to remove excess buccal fat. In this patient, intraoral excision was not performed and the buccal fat was removed via external approach. Patient is shown (**a, c, e**) preoperatively, and (**b, d, f**) 9 months after extended LaserSmartLift with platysmaplasty and buccal fat extraction.

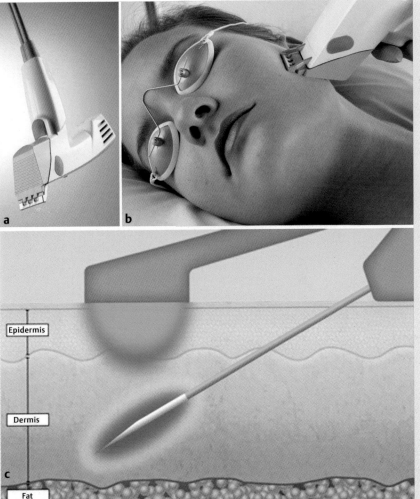

Fig. 8.42 ePrime from Syneron. The ePrime system (**a**) utilizes a minimally invasive micro-needle electrode array (**b**) to deliver bipolar radiofrequency (RF) energy directly into the (**c**) deep reticular dermis, without thermal impact to the epidermis. Clinical use: targets deep reticular dermis with fractionated RF energy. (Courtesy of Syneron-Candela, Yokneam, Israel.)

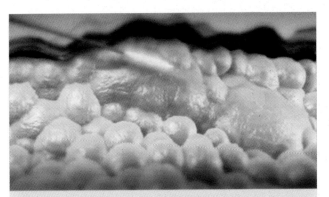

Fig. 8.43 ThermiTight from ThermiAesthetics is a new approach for stimulating the development of collagen. It is a nonsurgical procedure that introduces radiofrequency (RF) energy beneath the skin to stimulate the production of collagen to tighten and smooth the skin on the face, neck, and body. (Courtesy of ThermiAesthetics, Southlake, Texas.)

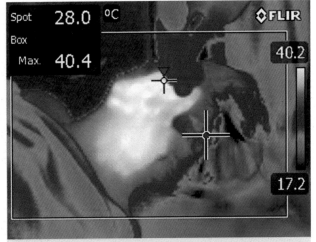

Fig. 8.44 Infrared thermal imaging. ThermiTight precisely monitors skin temperatures using an advanced infrared imaging camera that contributes to the overall safety of the device. The precise level of external and subsurface tissue monitoring enables medical professionals to deliver controlled heat to targeted tissues, without risking epidermal damage and helping patients reach their cosmetic goals.

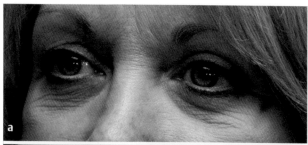

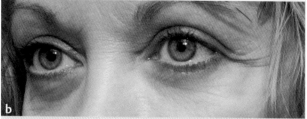

Fig. 8.45 Lateral canthal hyperpigmentation after LaserSmartLift. This patient had minor thermal injury due to either laser energy or most likely electrosurgical collateral injury. (**a**) Hyperpigmentation of the skin occurred. (**b**) Successful treatment with pulsed light treatment and filler to dermis. (Reproduced with permission from Gentile RD, ed. Neck Rejuvenation. New York, NY: Thieme Medical Publishers; 2011:173.)

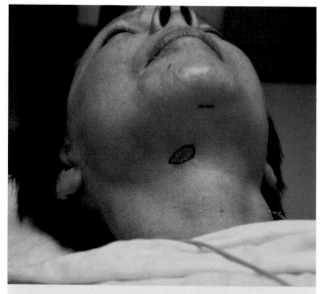

Fig. 8.46 Thermal neck injury after LaserSmartLift. Patient also had full-thickness injury due to either laser energy or electrosurgical collateral damage. This was treated with Kenalog injection followed by scar revision with a satisfactory aesthetic outcome. (Reproduced with permission from Gentile RD, ed. Neck Rejuvenation. New York, NY: Thieme Medical Publishers; 2011:173.)

patients—all of which resolved within weeks. The author occasionally sees these neurapraxias in nonlaser-elevated rhytidectomy patients, and attributes these temporary neurapraxias to liposuction trauma more than thermal trauma. There have been no permanent nerve injuries in any patient undergoing SmartLifting procedures. As with traditional rhytidectomy, there is temporary interruption of cutaneous sensory nerves during the flap elevation and repositioning phases of the rhytidectomy, and the resolution of the temporary sensory deficits is identical to the resolution of nonlaser-elevated rhytidectomies.

References

[1] DiBernardo BE, Reyes J, Chen B. Evaluation of tissue thermal effects from 1064/1320-nm laser-assisted lipolysis and its clinical implications. J Cosmet Laser Ther 2009; 11: 62–69

[2] Apfelberg D. Laser-assisted liposuction may benefit surgeons and subjects. Clin Laser Mon 1992; 10: 259

[3] Goldman A, Schavelzon D, Blugerman G. Laser lipolysis: liposuction using Nd:YAG laser. Rev Soc Bras Cir Plast 2002; 17: 17–26

[4] Badin AZ, Gondek LB, Garcia MJ, Valle LC, Flizikowski FB, de Noronha L. Analysis of laser lipolysis effects on human tissue samples obtained from liposuction. Aesthetic Plast Surg 2005; 29: 281–286

[5] Ichikawa K, Miyasaka M, Tanaka R, Tanino R, Mizukami K, Wakaki M. Histologic evaluation of the pulsed Nd:YAG laser for laser lipolysis. Lasers Surg Med 2005; 36: 43–46

[6] Gentile RD. Smartlifting™–A technological innovation for facial rejuvenation. Cynosure white paper. Available at: www.dcanavan.com/PDFS/Collateral/Compendium.pdf. Accessed April 24, 4014

[7] Gentile RD. Smartlifting™ A technological innovation for facial rejuvenation. Lasers Surg Med 2009; 41; (: Suppl 21:)

[8] Gentile RD. LaserFacialSculpting™ Minimally invasive techniques for facial rejuvenation utilizing the Smartlipo™ Nd:YAG laser. February 1, 2010. Available at: http://66.36.229.213/live/cynosureapp/Smartlipo_MPX_TP/smartlook_smartlifting/921-0187-000_r2_LaserFacialSculptingWP.pdf. Accessed April 27, 2014

[9] Gentile RD. SmartLifting fiber laser-assisted facial rejuvenation techniques. Facial Plast Surg Clin North Am 2011; 19: 371–387

[10] Gentile RD. Laser-assisted neck-lift: high-tech contouring and tightening. Facial Plast Surg 2011; 27: 331–345

[11] DiBernardo BE. The aging neck: a diagnostic approach to surgical and nonsurgical options. J Cosmet Laser Ther 2013; 15: 56–64

[12] Sasaki GH. Early clinical experience with the 1440-nm wavelength internal pulsed laser in facial rejuvenation: two-year follow-up. Clin Plast Surg 2012; 39: 409–417

[13] Holcomb JD, Turk J, Baek SJ, Rousso DE. Laser-assisted facial contouring using a thermally confined 1444-nm Nd:YAG laser: a new paradigm for facial sculpting and rejuvenation. Facial Plast Surg 2011; 27: 315–330

[14] Goldman A, Wollina U, de Mundstock EC. Evaluation of tissue tightening by the subdermal Nd:YAG laser-assisted liposuction versus liposuction alone. J Cutan Aesthet Surg 2011; 4: 122–128

[15] Sarnoff DS. Evaluation of the safety and efficacy of a novel 1440 nm Nd:YAG laser for neck contouring and skin tightening without liposuction. J Drugs Dermatol 2013; 12: 1382–1388

[16] Mulholland RS. Nonexcisional, minimally invasive rejuvenation of the neck. Clin Plast Surg 2014; 41: 11–31

[17] Gentile RD. Purse-string platysmaplasty: the third dimension for neck contouring. Facial Plast Surg 2005; 21: 296–303

[18] Gentile RD. Mixed plane rhytidectomy: the superior vertical-vector approach to rejuvenation of the neck. In: Gentile RD, ed. Neck Rejuvenation. New York, NY: Thieme Medical Publishers; 2011: 56–81

[19] Yu D, Biesman B, Khan JA. Bilateral eyelid dermal burn from subcutaneous diode laser lipolysis blepharoplasty. Lasers Surg Med 2009; 41: 609–611

[20] McBean JC, Katz BE. A pilot study of the efficacy of a 1,064 and 1,320 nm sequentially firing Nd:YAG laser device for lipolysis and skin tightening. Lasers Surg Med 2009; 41: 779–784

[21] Khoury JG, Saluja R, Keel D, Detwiler S, Goldman MP. Histologic evaluation of interstitial lipolysis comparing a 1064, 1320 and 2100 nm laser in an ex vivo model. Lasers Surg Med 2008; 40: 402–406

[22] DiBernardo BE, Reyes J. Evaluation of skin tightening after laser-assisted liposuction. Aesthet Surg J 2009; 29: 400–407

[23] Fuente del Campo A. Midline platysma muscular overlap for neck restoration. Plast Reconstr Surg 1998; 102: 1710–1714, discussion 1715

[24] Key DJ. Integration of thermal imaging with subsurface radiofrequency thermistor heating for the purpose of skin tightening and contour improvement: a retrospective review of clinical efficacy. J Drugs Dermatol 2014 Dec; 13: 1485–9

9 Laser-Assisted Lower Lid Blepharoplasty

William H. Truswell

She walks in beauty, like the night
Of cloudless climes and starry skies
And all that's best of dark and bright
Meet in her aspect and her eyes...
—Lord Byron, English Romantic poet, 1788–1824

9.1 Introduction

Poets have extoled the beauty of women's eyes in countless ways and over all of time. When we first meet someone and when we converse we look into the person's eyes.

The eyes are the facial feature we spend the most time observing in human intercourse. Women spend millions of dollars each year on eyeshade, mascara, Latisse (Allergan, Inc., Irvine, California), brow waxing, neuromodulation, and surgery to make their eyes more attractive and alluring.

When describing their perception of how they look, patients often use negative terms describing how their character or personality is projected vis-à-vis the appearance of their eyes. At the more youthful end of the aging spectrum, a patient will often complain of looking tired or unhappy. Whereas at the opposite end of this continuum, an older individual's vision may be obscured by redundant upper lid skin, and laxity of the lower lid may cause ectropion with chronic inflammation and irritation.[1]

Patients, wishing to have a more youthful appearance of the lower eyelid, most often speak of "my bags," wrinkles, and "dark circles." The lower lid, with its own senescent changes to the surrounding anatomical structures of the midface, necessitates a broader discussion with the patient. In youth, the actual demarcation between the lower lid and cheek is blurred. As a person passes through the late 30s and early 40s the malar fat pad and suborbicularis oculi fat (SOOF) pad descend. This enhances the separation of lower lid and cheek and draws increased attention to aging changes in the lower lid.[2,3] The goal of most patients is to have the "bags" reduced and the wrinkles softened. The procedure this author favors is a transconjunctival approach to the fat and fractional or ablative carbon dioxide (CO_2) laser resurfacing of the eyelid skin. If needed, fat repositioning can be done at the same time. When the lid needs tightening, a concomitant "pinch" technique will gain access for canthoplasty, canthopexy, tarsal strip, or other lid-supporting techniques.

The numerous techniques for lower lid surgery, midface elevation, and volume restoration are beyond the scope of this chapter. The focus of this chapter is on the application and rationale of using the CO_2 laser in rejuvenation of the lower eyelid. All the ancillary procedures for lid tightening, midface lifting, and volume restoration can be done, if indicated, concomitantly.

9.2 Anatomy of the Lower Eyelid

The lower eyelid extends from medial to lateral canthus and downward from its free upper edge to the orbital rim. There is a crease near the inferior border of the tarsal plate associated with fibers from the anterior layer of the capsulopalpebral fascia extending to the skin.[4] The lower lid consists of three lamellae. The description of these lamellae is not universal in the literature; however, the concept is useful in surgical approaches to the lower eyelid. The anterior lamella is made up of the skin and orbicularis oculi muscle.

The thinness of the skin of the lower eyelid is unmatched on the human body. The subcutaneous fat is meager and lies over the orbicularis oculi muscle. This muscle has three distinct parts, the pretarsal, palpebral or preseptal, and the orbital. Their points of origin are the inferomedial orbital rim, the frontal process of the maxilla, and the medial palpebral ligament.[5,6,7] The medial canthal ligament attaches to the frontal process of the maxilla and the posterior lacrimal crest. The lateral canthal tendon attaches to the Whitnall tubercle. The tendons form thickened attachments to the tarsal plate, and together they support the eyelid (▶ Fig. 9.1).[5,7]

The middle lamella is the orbital septum. The orbital septum is a dense extension of the orbital periosteum arising at the arcus marginalis. The orbital septum retains the orbital fat. The fat is divided into three pads. The inferior oblique muscle lies between the medial and middle pads. The arcuate expansion of the Lockwood ligament delineates the middle fat pad from the lateral pad. This particular division usually becomes visible in the aging lower lid.[5,6,8]

The posterior lamella consists of the tarsus, the lid retractors, and the conjunctiva. The capsulopalpebral fascia of the inferior rectus muscle splits to encompass the inferior oblique muscle before reuniting and forming a dense band that joins with the orbital septum to become the Lockwood ligament. The Lockwood ligament inserts into the inferior edge of the tarsal plate. The lid retractors are composed of the capsulopalpebral fascia and the tarsal muscle. On the surface of the lower lid conjunctiva is a vertical array of blood vessels.

9.3 How the Lower Eyelid Ages

The complex anatomical components of the lower eyelid age at different times and different rates. Like the entirety of the aging face, the lower lid will mature basically in three separate ways. The first to age is the skin, followed by laxity and loosening of structures, and volume loss of the tissues. When one is a teenager and is in the 20s and early-to-mid 30s, the skin shows that "glow of youth." It is smooth without rhytids, discoloration, and visible pores. The keratinocytes form at the basement membrane and rise upward forming the various dermal layers and the epidermis until they become the stratum corneum, cells without nuclei and organelles. At this point washing the face sheds them. In youth, washing cleans the lost cells away.[9] As age moves one into the later 30s and beyond, this layer becomes more adherent and the glow of youth surrenders to the flat and dull look of maturity. Extrinsic factors influence the rate and degree of aging skin. Sun exposure and tobacco use notoriously damage the skin. With time, the architecture of the

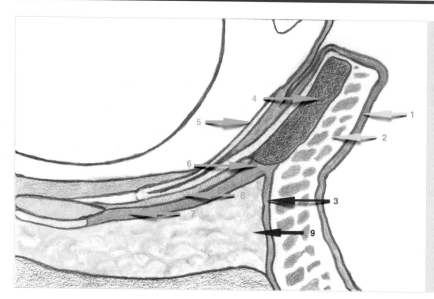

Fig. 9.1 Cross-sectional anatomy of the lower eyelid. Blue arrows are the outer lamella: 1, skin; 2, orbicularis oculi muscle. Red arrow is the middle lamella: 3, orbital septum. Green arrows are the inner lamella: 4, tarsal plate; 5, conjunctiva; 6, Lockwood ligament; 7, capsulopalpebral fascia; and 8, tarsal muscle. Purple arrow: 9, orbital fat.

dermis and epidermis alters. The skin becomes dry and flakey as the vascular supply diminishes and the tissue dehydrates. The epidermis no longer adheres firmly to the dermis with attenuation of the rete ridges. The various dermal glands and hair follicles lessen in number. Rhytids appear and deepen and elongate.[9,10] Photodamage lends greatly to the appearance of lesions such as lentigines, actinic keratoses, seborrheic keratoses, and skin cancers. ▶ Fig. 9.2a shows a 60-year-old woman before surgery. ▶ Fig. 9.2b is a computer-generated depiction of a Wood lamp view of her face. This highlights the photodamage and marked rhytids of her face. ▶ Fig. 9.2c,d are the postoperative pictures of the same woman after undergoing an endoscopic forehead lift, upper and laser-assisted lower eyelid blepharoplasty, facelift, and full face and neck fractional laser resurfacing including the eyelids. Note the marked rejuvenation of her skin with considerable softening of her rhytids and improvement of her photodamage secondary to the laser resurfacing. A lifetime of smiling coupled with thinning periocular skin produces visible "crow's-feet." These are seen at first in the younger patient only with a smile. As time advances and aging changes accelerate, these rhytids remain visible at rest.

The relation of the lower eyelid to the midface testifies to the youth or senescence of the face. In the young face, the skin descends from the lower edge of the tarsus in one smooth curve, a single convexity, to the mandible. This curve also extends smoothly from the nose, nasolabial fold, and corner of the mouth laterally across the cheek. The integrity of the lid structures is firm and supportive of lid position. Many events occur with aging in all the associated anatomical structures and contribute to the evolution of an older eye. Alterations in the appearance of the lower lid become evident about the start of the 5th decade of life. The orbital structures weaken and attenuate leading to descent of the globe within the orbit.[5,11] This pushes the inferior orbital fat against the weakening orbital septum. The laxity of the orbital septum, the attenuation of the orbicularis oculi muscle, and the downward pressure of the globe force the fat pockets to move forward as a pseudoherniation and create the lower lid "bags." The orbital septum is firmly attached to the orbital rim at the arcus marginalis. This prevents the lid structures from descending below the orbital rim.[12]

As the intrinsic changes of the lid occur, the malar fat pad and the suborbicularis oculi fat pad descend and pull away from the rim, which becomes skeletonized. Thus the single convexity of youth morphs into the double convexity of age. A depression is seen along the orbital rim between the pseudoherniated orbital fat and the lowering malar fat pad and SOOF, and the nasojugal groove or tear trough deformity develops. As the midface descent progresses and the lid structures continue to weaken, there is elongation of the lower eyelid. With time, senile ectropion may develop with all its attendant consequences of dry eye, chronic inflammation, and meibomian gland dysfunction (▶ Fig. 9.3).[2,3,5,13]

The aging changes occurring in the lower eyelid and periorbita and the descent of the malar and SOOF fat pads are further exacerbated by the alteration of the facial skeletal structure. As the soft tissues of the midface lower, volume is lost in the muscles, fat, and bone. The mature adult facial skeleton has a balance among the horizontal thirds of the face. As the face transitions to one of old age, the bony changes in the orbits manifest as an enlargement of the circle of the rims, and a lateral downward teardrop appearance occurs. This creates a more infantile shape where the upper third dominates the shape of the face and head (▶ Fig. 9.4).[9,13] The eyes appear sunken.

9.4 Clinical Assessment

Proper patient selection for lower eyelid blepharoplasty will be accomplished by conducting a complete and systematic consultation. As in all things medical, a total, detailed history is taken. The first things to be established are: Why is the patient seeking lower eyelid surgery? Are the patient's expectations realistic? This process involves a give-and-take between surgeon and patient. An ophthalmic history is taken along with general medical queries. The doctor must also educate the patient on the findings of the eye examination, on what can be accomplished and how it will be done, on what the patient should expect the outcome to be, on the preoperative and postoperative course, and on the likely sequelae and possible complications of the procedure.

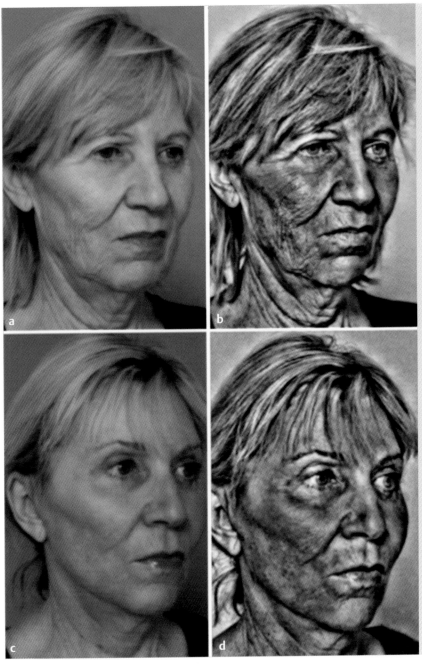

Fig. 9.2 (a) A 60-year-old woman before surgery. (b) Patient in a computer-generated Wood lamp depiction demonstrating the marked rhytidosis and photodamage of her skin. (c, d) Patient after an endoscopic forehead lift, upper and laser-assisted lower eyelid blepharoplasty, facelift, and full face and neck carbon dioxide (CO_2) laser fractional resurfacing. (Reproduced with permission from Truswell WH, IV. Combining fractional carbon-dioxide laser resurfacing with face-lift surgery. Facial Plast Surg Clin North Am 2012; 20: 201–213, vi.)

It is essential to note the general health of the patient, what prescriptive and over-the-counter medicines and supplements are taken, and what surgeries the patient may have had. Note if there is a bleeding or easy-bruising tendency. It is important to include history of alcohol and tobacco use. Record when the last ophthalmic examination was done, what the patient's vision is, and if there is a history of dry eye. The surgeon should ask the patient about itchy eyes or a sensation of something in the eye. Are over-the-counter eye drops used? Positive responses would suggest a developing dry eye syndrome and may warrant an ophthalmology consultation. Record the presence or absence of glaucoma, cataracts, recurring conjunctivitis, previous ophthalmic surgery, or trauma.[1,5]

It is also important to find out a history of skin disorders that could affect healing of lasered skin. Contraindications to resurfacing include skin diseases like scleroderma, sarcoidosis, psoriasis, eczema, irradiated skin, vitiligo, and a history of keloid or hypertrophic scarring. Is there a history of previous resurfacing of the skin? What cosmeceuticals does the patient use? Has the patient been on isotretinoin, which delays healing?[10,14]

The physical examination focuses on the structures to be addressed and the face as a whole. The Fitzpatrick or Glogau skin type, the amount of photodamage, and the degree of rhytids should be recorded. Determine the state of hydration. It is important to recognize telangiectasias and the presence of rosacea. Ascertain if there are any skin lesions such as lentigines, actinic keratoses, seborrheic keratoses, basal cell carcinomas, squamous cell carcinomas, and suspicious nevi. Determine how much asymmetry of the face is present and point it out to the

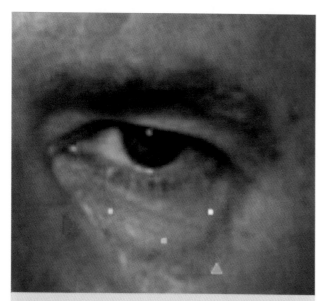

Fig. 9.3 The aging eye. Note: rhytids, photodamaged skin, eyebrow ptosis, upper eyelid dermatochalasis and hooding, laxity and rounding of the lower eyelid, elongation of the lower eyelid, nasojugal groove (red arrowhead), and skeletonization of the orbital rim (green arrowhead). There is also pseudoherniation of the medial, middle, and lateral fat pads (blue, green, and yellow dots, respectively).

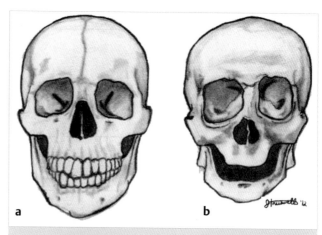

Fig. 9.4 The transition from the (a) adult to the (b) senescent facial skeleton. (Reproduced with permission from Truswell WH, IV. Aging changes of the periorbita, cheeks, and midface. Facial Plast Surg 2013; 29: 3–12.)

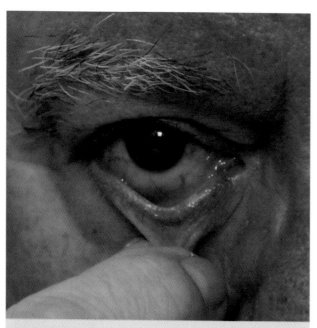

Fig. 9.5 The snap back test.

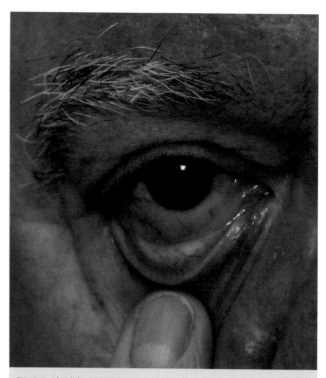

Fig. 9.6 The lid retraction test.

patient. Pay particular attention to asymmetries of the periorbita and be certain the patient acknowledges them.

The eye examination is done with the head and gaze in the neutral position. The lower lid margin will sit just touching the lower limbus. If the white of the sclera can be seen, it indicates possible lid laxity. Checking for lid laxity is done with the snap back test and the retraction test. To perform the snap back test (▶ Fig. 9.5), the lower lid is drawn gently forward from the globe and released. If it drifts back slowly it is an indicator of laxity. The lid retraction test (▶ Fig. 9.6) is done by drawing the lower lid downward. The test is positive if the puncta can be retracted more than 3 mm beyond the medial canthus. If so, a medial canthopexy may be necessary. If both or either of these tests is positive, the surgeon must consider performing a horizontal lid tightening procedure at the time of surgery. The integrity of the medial and lateral tendons is also determined. The medial canthal tendon is drawn laterally and released and the lateral canthus is, likewise, drawn medially and released. If either is easily pulled or stretched, a canthal tendon tuck procedure may be indicated.[15] If lid laxity goes unrecognized and addressed, it can lead to scleral show or ectropion.

The lower lid fat pads are evaluated in the neutral gaze and with the patient looking upward without moving the head. The lateral fat pads are best seen when the patient looks upward and to the opposite side of the eye being examined. Gentle pressure on the globe with the eyes closed will also delineate the pads.

Photographic documentation is an essential part of the recording process. Photographs of the face and neck in the neutral position (the Frankfort horizontal plane), forward, lateral, and 45-degree oblique positions are routine. Pictures should be taken in these positions with the face expressionless as well as smiling. A frontal photograph with the patient in upward gaze should be included, as well.

Once the patient's concerns have been heard and the examination is completed, it is time to review the options with the individual. Part of the education process is how the person's concerns can be addressed and what results are likely, given the physical findings. The patient must understand what the limitations are, as well as the certain sequelae and possible complications. Often an individual may worry about the "dark circles" under the eyes. These are often shadows under the protruding pseudoherniated fat. Sometimes they are from pigmentation that could be superficial or deep. The former may be helped by laser resurfacing. If they are deep, the patient must understand that they will persist. In some very fair-skinned people, the color of the orbicularis oculi can "bleed through." Another common concern is the wrinkled skin. This will be addressed with CO_2 laser resurfacing.

It is important to distinguish between the wrinkles seen at rest and the hyperdynamic crow's-feet. Whereas the laser will address the former, the latter will require neuromodulation. Lastly, patients often do not distinguish between the lower lid pseudoherniated fat and malar bags. When malar bags are present, it is imperative to point these out to the patient so there is comprehension that these will remain posttreatment.

9.5 Rationale

The transconjunctival approach to lower lid blepharoplasty with CO_2 laser resurfacing is the preferred technique for this author. The most common complications of transcutaneous lower eyelid blepharoplasty are lid retraction and ectropion. Scarring of the orbital septum causes postoperative retraction of the lower lid. The transcutaneous approach necessitates incising the orbital septum to reach the orbital fat. Scar tissue forms in the septum and adjacent tissues. As the scar tissue contracts over time, rounding of the canthus and scleral show occur. Excessive removal of skin from the lower lid will cause cicatricial ectropion.[16,17]

The transconjunctival incision allows direct access to the orbital fat without violating the orbital septum. Many studies have demonstrated that this approach all but eliminates these complications. Westfall et al analyzed 1,200 transconjunctival blepharoplasties and reported only 1 case of ectropion. The rate of ectropion on a number of studies ranges from 12 to 42%.[18] Often, other maneuvers are necessary to correct the problems with the aging lower eyelid. All the lid tightening and supportive procedures, orbital fat repositioning, and the pinch technique can be done without incising the orbital septum.

It is essential to understand that skin excision will not eliminate wrinkles or the crepelike appearance of the lid skin. The rhytids are a result of the intrinsic aging changes in the lid skin as described earlier. Attempts to eliminate or lessen the rhytids by putting tension on lid skin will increase the risk of ectropion. Skin resurfacing by chemical peels or laser is the most effective procedure to rejuvenate the skin. The fractional CO_2 laser is safe and effective and can be used to treat all types of skin. Fractional laser resurfacing allows quicker healing time with rapid return to normal skin color. The incidence of pigment alterations is lower than with ablative techniques.[14] The fractional laser allows the operator to choose what percentage of tissue is necessary up to full ablation. Full ablation should be restricted to Fitzpatrick skin types I through III.[19]

9.6 Technique

Once surgery has been scheduled, the patient meets with a nurse 3 weeks ahead of time for preoperative instructions. Prescriptions for an antibiotic, antiviral, and antifungal are given to the patient. At this visit a light chemical peel is performed consisting, in our protocol, of Sensi Peel (Physician's Choice of Arizona Inc. [PCA], Scottsdale, Arizona)—active ingredients: 12% lactic acid, 6% trichloroacetic and 3% kojic acids, and a single layer of 10% retinol.

The procedure is carried out with monitored anesthesia care (Video 9.1). ▶ Fig. 9.7 shows the instrumentation used. Once the patient is medicated, the face is prepped and draped. The lower lid is everted and the globe protected with a spatula-shaped shield. The conjunctiva is infiltrated with 1% lidocaine with a 1:100,000-epinephrine ratio. Time allowed to elapse for vasoconstriction to occur is 10 minutes. The surgical technician protects the globe with the spatulate shield. The lid is everted manually. Using the laser as a cutting tool, an incision is made (▶ Fig. 9.8a, b) in the conjunctiva through the middle of the vertical vascular arcade and carried through the lid retractors. The eyelid retractor holds the incision open. This allows a direct approach to the orbital fat. The fat is teased up with forceps and

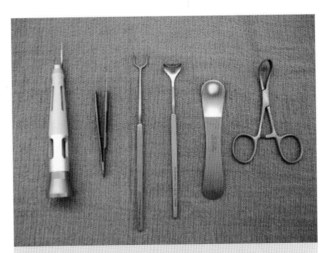

Fig. 9.7 Left to right: Cutting handpiece for the Ultrapulse Encore (Lumenis, Inc., Palo Alto, California) carbon dioxide (CO_2) laser, ophthalmic forceps, double-ball retractor, lid retractor, spatulate globe shield, and towel clip. All are burnished for laser safety.

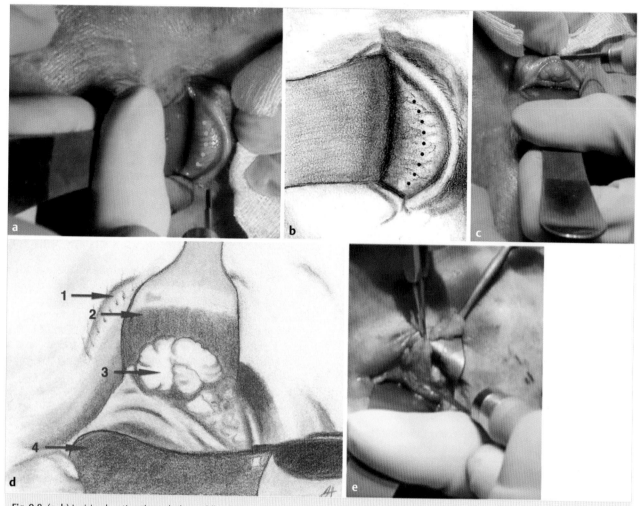

Fig. 9.8 (a, b) Incision location through the middle of the vertical vascular arcade on the conjunctival side of the lower eyelid (nose to right). **(c, d)** Fat pads exposed. In **(d)** red arrows and numbers: 1, lower lid everted; 2, lower lid retractor; 3, fat pad exposed; and 4, spatulate retractor protecting the globe. **(e)** Laser excision of fat pads using the lid retractor as a "backstop" (nose to right).

either excised (using the eyelid retractor as a protective "backstop") or repositioned as the situation dictates (▶ Fig. 9.8c–e). After the pads are removed, the laser beam is defocused and the fat is vaporized to the level of the inferior orbital rim. The incision is not sutured. The cut conjunctiva edges oppose directly when the lid is returned to position. If another lid procedure is indicated, it will be carried out at this juncture.

Once the surgical procedure(s) is done, the skin of the lower eyelid and crow's-feet area is resurfaced. Laser beam density and energy are chosen according to the degree of rhytidosis and skin type present. The deep beam, Deep FX (Lumenis, Inc., Palo Alto, California), is used over the periocular areas being treated but not over the lid skin. The settings the author employs for this beam are: energy, 17.5 to 20.0 mJ; power, 350 Hz; and density, 15. The superficial beam, Active FX (Lumenis, Inc., Palo Alto, California), is then applied. The density settings for Active FX with their respective percentages of surface ablation are: 1 (55%), 2 (68%), 3 (82%), and 4 and greater (100%) or total ablation. In Fitzpatrick skin types IV through VI, the density is not set higher than 3 and total ablation is never done. The energy settings for Active FX are 80 to 90 mJ directly on the lids to within 1 mm of the ciliary margin and the periocular skin

for skin types I through III, and 60 to 70 mJ for skin types IV through VI.

When done, Aquaphor (Eucerin, a division of Beiersdorf, Inc., Wilton, Connecticut) is applied to the lasered skin. If full ablation was carried out, platelet gel is sprayed over the skin and Silon-TSR dressing is applied (Bio Med Sciences, Bethlehem, Pennsylvania). The author's laser experience has been with the Lumenis UltraPulse 5000c CO_2 (Lumenis, Inc., Palo Alto, California) laser since 1995, and the Lumenis UltraPulse Encore CO_2 laser since January 2009. ▶ Fig. 9.9 shows the platelet gel and Silon-TSR dressing in place on a postoperative lower eyelid blepharoplasty patient. The patient is recovered in the postanesthesia recovery unit with cold compresses until discharge.

The patient is seen on postoperative days 1, 4, and 8, and then weekly for 2 or 3 weeks to check on the lasered skin. Patients treated with the fractional beam will wash their faces with tepid water several times a day. The skin will peel heavily. On the 4th-day postoperative visit, the nurse washes the remaining desquamating epithelium from the patient's face and applies Restorative Ointment (SkinMedica, Carlsbad, California). From the 5th day forward, the patient is instructed to wash the face with tepid water twice a day. The patient then begins using

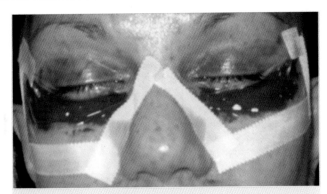

Fig. 9.9 Platelet gel and Silon-TSR dressing (Bio Med Sciences, Bethlehem, Pennsylvania) in place after a laser-assisted lower eyelid blepharoplasty and endoscopic brow lift. (Reproduced with permission from Truswell WH, IV. Combining fractional carbon-dioxide laser resurfacing with face-lift surgery. Facial Plast Surg Clin North Am 2012; 20: 201–213, vi.)

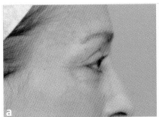
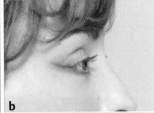

Fig. 9.11 Before (a) and 3 months after (b) endoscopic forehead lift and fractional laser-assisted lower lid blepharoplasty.

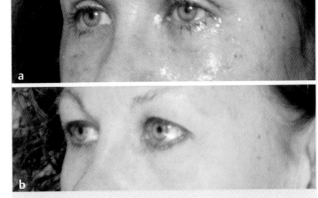

Fig. 9.10 Before (b) and 10 days postoperative (a) following an upper and laser-assisted lower eyelid blepharoplasty with total ablation, demonstrating the effectiveness of platelet gel and Silon-TSR dressing (Bio Med Sciences, Bethlehem, Pennsylvania) to hasten normalization of posttreatment color.

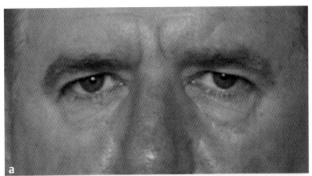
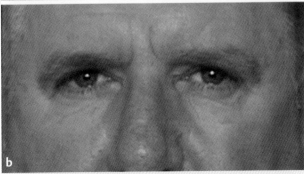

Fig. 9.12 (a) A man with dermatochalasis and hooding of the upper eyelids, lower eyelid laxity with rounding of the lid margin, pseudoherniation of fat in all three compartments, with rhytids and photodamage of the lower eyelids. (b) The photo was taken 6 months following upper lid and fractional laser-assisted lower lid blepharoplasty with a tarsal strip procedure.

TNS Recovery Complex (SkinMedica) and TNS Ceramide Treatment Cream (SkinMedica) twice a day, with a minimum sunblock of sun protection factor (SPF) 30. At this point makeup can be applied. The skin color is at or near normal in 7 to 10 days. Where the Deep FX was used, pinkness may persist for another few weeks.

Patients who had full ablation will be applying eye pads soaked in acidulated water (1 tsp white vinegar in 1 cup cool water) 6 times a day. On the 4th postoperative day, the Silon-TSR dressing is removed and any remaining platelet gel washed away. The same regimen as above proceeds forward from here. The platelet gel decreases the duration of pinkness to about 10 days.

▶ Fig. 9.10 shows before (bottom) and 10 days after (top) full ablative laser resurfacing and the use of platelet gel and Silon-TSR dressing. ▶ Fig. 9.11 displays a patient before (left) and 3 months after (right) endoscopic forehead lift and fractional laser-assisted lower lid blepharoplasty. ▶ Fig. 9.12 is a man (top) with dermatochalasis and hooding of the upper eyelids, lower eyelid laxity with rounding of the lid margin, pseudoherniation of fat in all three compartments, and rhytids and photodamage of the lower eyelids. The bottom photo was taken 6 months following upper lid and fractional laser-assisted lower lid blepharoplasty with a tarsal strip procedure. The patient in ▶ Fig. 9.13 is shown before (left) and 1 year after (right) an endoscopic forehead lift, rhinoplasty, facelift, and fractional laser-assisted lower lid blepharoplasty. ▶ Fig. 9.14 depicts before (top) and 1-year-after (bottom) results of an endoscopic forehead lift and fractional laser-assisted lower lid blepharoplasty.

9.7 Personal Experience with Laser-Assisted Lower Lid Blepharoplasty

The author has been using this technique for 8 years as of this writing. During that time period, 482 patients (419 women and 63 men) were treated with this procedure. Of the total number

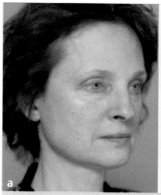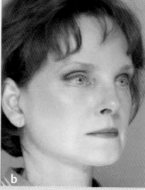

Fig. 9.13 Before (**a**) and 1 year after (**b**) an endoscopic forehead lift, rhinoplasty, facelift, and fractional laser-assisted lower lid blepharoplasty.

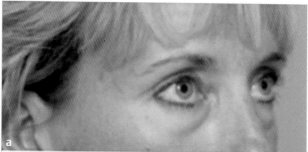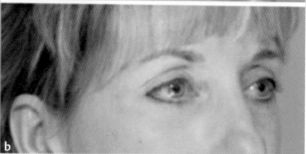

Fig. 9.14 Before (**a**) and 1-year-after results (**b**) of an endoscopic forehead lift and fractional laser-assisted lower lid blepharoplasty.

of patients, 16% also underwent ancillary lid procedures. The complication rate in this series was 12% (▶ Table 9.1). Prior to 2009 all patients underwent full ablative resurfacing. Thereafter, all had fractional CO_2 laser resurfacing. The overall complication rate was 12%. Pigmentary changes numbered 19 (~ 4%)—14 postinflammatory hyperpigmentation (PIH) cases and 5 patients with hypopigmentation. All of the PIH cases resolved with topical treatment. Hypopigmentation occurred in Fitzpatrick skin types I and II only, was spotty, and permanent. None of the pigmentation problems were seen in patients undergoing fractional CO_2 laser resurfacing. It is important to note that in the author's practice more than 90% of all the patients treated were Fitzpatrick skin types I through III, and the majority of them were type I or II. There were 39 (~ 8%) patients with prolonged erythema, all occurring with total ablation. There were no incidences of infection, lid retraction, or ectropion.

9.8 Conclusion

It is this author's opinion that the approach described above is safe with a lower rate of complications. The results are reliable and reproducible. When indicated, lid tightening and other ancillary procedures can be done in addition to this approach. Fractional laser resurfacing is a far more directed and effective way to treat rhytids of the lid than skin resection. Many patients undergoing lid surgery have concomitant cutaneous photodamage of the lid and periocular area. Considerable reduction or elimination of this problem greatly enhances the rejuvenation results achieved with blepharoplasty.

References

[1] Lee AS, Thomas JR. Lower lid blepharoplasty and canthal surgery. Facial Plast Surg Clin North Am 2005; 13: 541–551, vi

[2] McCann JD, Pariseau B. Lower eyelid and midface rejuvenation. Facial Plast Surg 2013; 29: 273–280

[3] Yeh CC, Williams EF, III. Midface restoration in the management of the lower eyelid. Facial Plast Surg Clin North Am 2010; 18: 365–374

[4] Shams PN, Ortiz-Pérez S, Joshi N. Clinical anatomy of the periocular region. Facial Plast Surg 2013; 29: 255–263

[5] Wong TD, Ross AT. Periorbital rejuvenation. In: Truswell WH IV, ed. Surgical Facial Rejuvenation. New York, NY: Thieme Medical Publishers; 2009:54–62

[6] Collar RM, Lyford-Pike S, Byrne P. Algorithmic approach to lower lid blepharoplasty. Facial Plast Surg 2013; 29: 32–39

Table 9.1 Complication rates in 482 patients between 2006 and 2014

Complication	Number of patients	Notes	Outcome
Postinflammatory hyperpigmentation (PIH)	14 (~ 3%)	All with total ablation	100% resolution with topical treatments
Hypopigmentation	5 (~ 1%)	All with total ablation	Permanent
Prolonged erythema	39 (~ 8%)	All with total ablation	Over time
Infection	0	0	0
Lid retraction	0	0	0
Ectropion	0	0	0

[7] Haddock NT, Saadeh PB, Boutros S, Thorne CH. The tear trough and lid/cheek junction: anatomy and implications for surgical correction. Plast Reconstr Surg 2009; 123: 1332–1340, discussion 1341–1342

[8] Most SP, Mobley SR, Larrabee WF, Jr. Anatomy of the eyelids. Facial Plast Surg Clin North Am 2005; 13: 487–492, v

[9] Truswell WH, IV. Aging changes of the periorbita, cheeks, and midface. Facial Plast Surg 2013; 29: 3–12

[10] Grunebaum LD, Murdock J, Hoosien GE, Heffelfinger RN, Lee WW. Laser treatment of skin texture and fine line etching. Facial Plast Surg Clin North Am 2011; 19: 293–301

[11] Shaw RB, Jr, Kahn DM. Aging of the midface bony elements: a three-dimensional computed tomographic study. Plast Reconstr Surg 2007; 119: 675–681, discussion 682–683

[12] Bergin D. Anatomy of the eyelids, lacrimal system, and orbit. In: McCord CD, Tannenbaum M, Nunery WO, eds. Oculoplastic Surgery. 3rd ed. New York, NY: Raven Press; 1995:8–10

[13] Grant JR, Laferriere KA. Periocular rejuvenation: lower eyelid blepharoplasty with fat repositioning and the suborbicularis oculi fat. Facial Plast Surg Clin North Am 2010; 18: 399–409

[14] Truswell WH, IV. Combining fractional carbon-dioxide laser resurfacing with face-lift surgery. Facial Plast Surg Clin North Am 2012; 20: 201–213, vi

[15] Putterman AM. Evaluation of the oculoplastic surgery patient. In: Putterman AM, ed. Cosmetic Oculoplastic Surgery. Philadelphia, PA: W.B. Saunders Company; 1999:11–22

[16] Bayliss HI, Goldberg RA, Groth MJ. Complications of lower blepharoplasty. In: Putterman AM, ed. Cosmetic Oculoplastic Surgery. Philadelphia, PA: W.B. Saunders Company; 1999:429–456

[17] Whipple KM, Korn BS, Kikkawa DO. Recognizing and managing complications in blepharoplasty. Facial Plast Surg Clin North Am 2013; 21: 625–637

[18] Westfall CT, Shore JW, Nunery WR, Hawes MJ, Yaremchuk MJ. Operative complications of the transconjunctival inferior fornix approach. Ophthalmology 1991; 98: 1525–1528

[19] Carniol PJ, Harirchian S, Kelly E. Fractional CO(2) laser resurfacing. Facial Plast Surg Clin North Am 2011; 19: 247–251

10 Simultaneous Full-Face Laser Resurfacing in the Setting of Facelift Surgery

Scott Shadfar and Stephen W. Perkins

10.1 Introduction

Facial rejuvenation and contouring procedures have evolved with a host of techniques aimed at addressing clinical aging. Patients often present with concerns regarding laxity, rhytids, and fat accumulation. As discussed in Chapter 2, the skin's unique anatomy and physiology result in specific pathological changes giving an aged appearance to the face and neck. Photoaging, for example, is a consequence of primarily sun-induced damage from ultraviolet (UV) irradiation and, like chronological aging, is a cumulative process. Patients with this cumulative damage present with moderate to severe rhytids of the cheeks, perioral region, and periocular crow's-feet, with overlying diffuse actinic damage and solar lentigines.

Whether using lasers, scalpels, or the combination of various new instruments and tools, the principal techniques in facial rejuvenation include surgical and nonsurgical therapies designed to refresh, contour, and resuspend those tissues. Sagging, lax skin is generally treated surgically with facial rhytidectomy; however, this does not address the fine wrinkles from aging or the photodamage from sun exposure. Conversely, laser resurfacing is used to address the cutaneous rhytids and actinic changes, and although some collagen contraction and remodeling can be seen with the carbon dioxide (CO_2) or erbium: yttrium aluminum garnet (Er:YAG) lasers, the tightening effects are not as long lasting, and cannot address severe laxity to the extent of a rhytidectomy. Therefore, the combination of rhytidectomy with simultaneous full-face laser resurfacing has emerged as a viable option in facial rejuvenation, allowing a dual cosmetic benefit with consolidation of the anesthetic and recovery times for patients.[1,2]

10.1.1 Historical Perspective

Historically, simultaneous resurfacing and surgical undermining in rhytidectomy was advised against because of reported skin necrosis seen after treatments with deep chemical peels.[3,4,5] Over the past few decades, isolated use of CO_2 and various lasers for full-face ablative resurfacing has shown beneficial effects with wide acceptance in aesthetic practices. More recently with fractional ablative resurfacing platforms, patients have enjoyed skin rejuvenation with less downtime than traditional ablative resurfacing, and potentially fewer risks.[6,7,8] Further details into the history, mechanisms, and the benefits of various laser therapies and systems are discussed throughout other chapters within this text.

Due to advances in resurfacing platforms, as well as improvements and better understanding of rhytidectomy techniques, the outcomes of simultaneous flap elevation and skin exfoliation have shown excellent results without an increased risk to the undermined skin flaps.[1,2] Different areas of the face often require varying levels of laser treatment, whether or not a simultaneous procedure is performed. The pertinent technical details are outlined to guide those physicians with a similar patient population wishing to implement this combined modality in their practice.

10.2 Patient Selection

Evaluation of the patient begins with a complete medical history with special attention to, and documentation of, medication use, skin sensitivities, and allergy history. Patients should be screened for conditions that may increase their risk of complications, or diseases that might prolong the postoperative healing time. These conditions include diabetes, peripheral vascular disease, collagen vascular diseases, and some autoimmune disorders that could compromise the microvasculature of the tissues.[9]

Another segment of patients who are very important to identify include patients who are actively smoking. Smoking greatly compromises the vascularity of the skin flap, increasing the likelihood of postoperative necrosis and sloughing with rhytidectomy alone. Therefore, the authors deem active tobacco use as a contraindication to simultaneous rhytidectomy with laser resurfacing.

Pertinent medications include previous or current use of powerful retinoids such as isotretinoin (Accutane, Roche Pharmaceutical, Basel, Switzerland) that can lead to increased scarring in patients undergoing facial resurfacing.[10,11] This medication can blunt regrowth of epithelial appendages that are essential for postoperative re-epithelialization.[11] The authors recommend waiting 6 to 12 months after use of isotretinoin before undergoing any type of ablative resurfacing procedure.

Patients with a history of head and neck radiation should also be approached cautiously when resurfacing because this subset of patients can have microvascular compromise even more severe than that of smokers. Radiation can decrease the blood supply as well as the number of pilosebaceous subunits, further delaying healing and potentially increasing the risk of scarring. Individuals who have active autoimmune diseases such as scleroderma, lupus, or Sjögren syndrome similarly carry a higher risk of skin flap compromise, and the decision to operate on these patients should be considered a relative contraindication. Discussions with a patient's rheumatologist should be initiated given the poor and unpredictable healing that can occur, as well as the risks of reactive cutaneous flares that can occur in these disease processes with laser treatment.

As always in the setting of aesthetic surgery, the motivations of the patient are of paramount importance. The surgeon should ensure the patient has realistic expectations and a firm understanding of the potential complications. This allows the patient and surgeon to choose the appropriate treatment and ensures that the patient understands the associated risks of combined modality treatment. The surgeon should not hesitate to defer treatment, and then schedule a second consultation to explore the patients' motives and ensure their expectations are realistic and align with the proposed intervention.

Table 10.1 Glogau photoaging classification

Group I	No wrinkles	No keratoses	20 s to late 30s
Group II	Wrinkles in motion	Keratosis palpable but not visible	Late 30 s to 40s
Group III	Wrinkles at rest	Obvious dyschromias, telangiectasias, and keratoses	50 s and older
Group IV	Only wrinkles	Actinic keratoses with or without skin cancers	70 s and older

(Adapted with permission from Glogau RG, Matarasso SL. Chemical face peeling: patient and peeling agent selection. Facial Plast Surg 1995; 11: 1–8.)

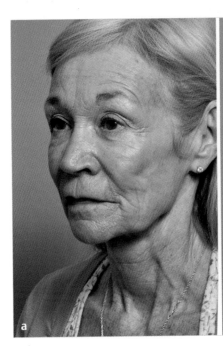 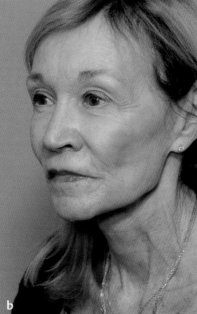

Fig. 10.1 (a) A 69-year-old woman with preoperative facial aging and severe photodamage. (b) Results 12 months postoperative following simultaneous rhytidectomy, full-face laser resurfacing, endoscopic forehead lift, and upper and lower eyelid blepharoplasty.

Considerations for psychological consultation should be raised in a patient who continues to have unrealistic expectations.[9]

Classification of the patient's skin type is essential before proceeding with a resurfacing procedure. The Fitzpatrick classification uses the skin's response to sun exposure and the person's baseline skin color as a means of categorizing patients (▶ Table 5.1).[12] Patients with darker complexions undergoing deep resurfacing procedures carry an increased risk of pigmentary changes, and therefore the ideal candidate for deep resurfacing would be a person of Celtic or northern European descent with Fitzpatrick skin type I or II.[13] Glogau further classifies the skin according to the amount of clinical photodamage (▶ Table 10.1), which guides the physician in choosing the appropriate level of resurfacing.[14] Most patients necessitating and undergoing CO_2 or deep Er:YAG ablative procedures would fall into the higher groups, such as III or IV (▶ Fig. 10.1).

10.3 Preoperative Care

Preoperative topical therapies are used by most treating physicians with several preoperative skin treatment regimens available to help maximize resurfacing techniques.[15,16] Tretinoin and glycolic acid are the most commonly used agents preoperatively, and are utilized for their exfoliative and rejuvenating effects to improve the skin's response to ablative wounding.

Additionally, a preoperative course of topical hydroquinone or hydroquinone mixtures (e.g., tretinoin, hydroquinone, and hydrocortisone) can help to reduce the risk of postoperative hyperpigmentation in those patients with darker complexions.[15,17]

The authors advocate for prophylactic treatment of all patients, with or without a known history of herpes labialis, with a regimen of acyclovir 800 mg orally three times a day. This course is started 2 days preoperatively and continued for 10 to 14 days after the resurfacing procedure, or until re-epithelialization is complete.

10.3.1 Anesthesia

Although rhytidectomy can be performed under local anesthetic, the addition of simultaneous laser resurfacing is advised against because many patients may still experience discomfort from areas that could not be fully anesthetized, as well as further discomfort from being supine for several hours while awake. Intravenous sedation in addition to a local anesthetic could be considered in the correct patient population; however, the authors prefer the use of a general anesthetic for patient comfort. Precautions should be taken with the use of lasers in the setting of an inhaled anesthetic or oxygen, given the known risk of airway fires.

10.4 Rhytidectomy Technique

Rhytidectomy begins with proper incision placement and concludes with meticulous closure resulting in well-hidden scars without changes in hairline position. This is central to achieve long-term patient satisfaction, by giving patients the freedom to style their hair without concerns of their scars showing.[9] The senior author's technique for the extended superficial muscular aponeurotic system (SMAS) rhytidectomy, including incision planning, has previously been described in detail, and relevant points are now highlighted.[9]

Utilizing a submental incision, the rhytidectomy begins by addressing the problematic areas within the neck. This may include submental, submandibular, and jowl liposuction, as well as anterior cervical platysma plication using the senior author's previously described Kelly-Clamp technique.[9] The neck skin is undermined completely in a subcutaneous plane using facelift scissors freeing the platysma from the overlying skin.

Using a no. 15 scalpel blade, the postauricular incision is started at the earlobe and continued along the posterior surface of the concha (not in the postauricular sulcus). At the level of the helical insertion or eminence of the concha, the incision is continued posteriorly with a gentle curve into the hairline but not parallel to the hairline. The incision should be beveled in the hair-bearing region, and the posterior skin flap is partially elevated maintaining the plane of dissection in the hair-bearing region deep to the roots of the hair follicles and superficial to the fascia of the sternocleidomastoid muscle. Postauricular skin flaps should then be elevated in the immediate subcutaneous plane and connected with the neck skin elevation.

From a preauricular aspect, beginning at the level of the helical insertion, dissection is carried forward in the subcutaneous plane and continued into the malar region just above the zygomatic arch in the subcutaneous plane extending just inferior to the orbicularis oculi muscle. This allows the dermal ligamentous attachments to the malar eminence to be released. Subcutaneous dissection is continued approximately 4 to 6 cm medially in the preauricular region connecting down to the elevated neck and postauricular flap allowing visualization of the neck–face interface at or below the mandibular margin into the neck (▶ Fig. 10.2).

An incision is then made in the SMAS extending from the inferior border of the zygomatic arch at the malar eminence diagonally down to the level of the earlobe and then continuing inferiorly 1 cm in front of the anterior border of the sternocleidomastoid. Dissection should then be carried out underneath the platysma muscle at approximately 3 to 4 cm. The first centimeter of SMAS elevation is performed with horizontal scissor dissection overlying the parotid gland. Further elevation of the SMAS is performed by spreading the scissors in a more vertical fashion, forming tunnels and bridges as the dissection is carried anteriorly.[9]

Just above the mandibular margin, dissection is continued anteriorly superficial to the masseter muscle over the premasseteric fascia in a deep sub-SMAS plane. The marginal mandibular nerve often is easily visualized in this transition from the neck up and over the mandibular inferior border.

When indicated, elevation should then extend superficial to the level of the zygomaticus muscle into the midcheek region. At this point there is a significant amount of skin elevated in

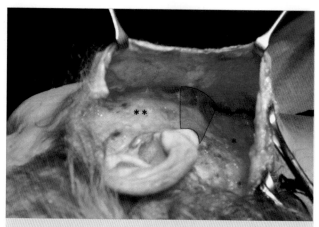

Fig. 10.2 Demonstration of the neck–face interface (highlighted area), or junction of SMAS (**) with the platysma (*), following elevation and connection of facial and neck subcutaneous dissections.

addition to the SMAS, creating two separate flaps for biplane vector suspension and redraping.[9]

The suspension of the midface and jowl tissues is accomplished by advancing the SMAS–subcutaneous skin unit in a posterior-superior fashion toward the helical insertion. The superior triangular portion of the SMAS is advanced, and the redundant preauricular portion excised. This is suspended with a buried 0 polyglactin 910 suture (Vicryl, Ethicon Inc., Somerville, New Jersey) at the level of the helical insertion and the postauricular mastoid fascia. Then 3–0 poliglecaprone 25 sutures (Monocryl, Ethicon) are used to reinforce the platysma-SMAS unit in the mastoid, infra-auricular, and preauricular areas.

The skin is advanced in a more posterior vector with 2 to 3 cm of undermined skin in the preauricular region remaining. The skin from the neck is also advanced toward the posterior mastoid hairline, and rotated superiorly. A single suspension staple is then placed high in the postauricular incision. The hair-bearing portions are approximated with staples allowing maintenance of the postauricular hairline and avoiding step-off deformities. A drain attached to a closed suction bulb system is placed in the neck portion of the wound on either side. The skin in the preauricular and tragal region is trimmed judiciously, with care taken to ensure that the earlobe is supported in a superior fashion to avoid a Satyr's ear deformity. The periauricular skin should be redraped and tailored so that there is no tension on incision line closure. Two simple interrupted 6–0 nylon sutures are used to reapproximate the ear lobule and remain in place for 10 days. The remaining incision lines are sutured with running interlocking 5–0 plain catgut sutures, and after 1 week, if they have not already dissolved, they are removed.[9]

10.5 Laser Resurfacing Technique

10.5.1 Carbon Dioxide Laser

Preoperatively all patients undergo facial cleansing and washes with Septisol (Sandent Co., Murfreesboro, Tennessee). The authors use a Lumenis Encore Ultrapulse 5000 (Coherent Inc.,

Table 10.2 Carbon dioxide (CO_2) laser settings by facial aesthetic unit: Part I

Treatment areas	Pulse energy (mJ)	Fluence (J/cm²)	Pulse width (Hz)	Power (W)	Density
Initial pass					
Perioral, lips, chin	80	6.0	600	48	5
Cheeks	80	6.0	600	48	5
Forehead	80	6.0	600	48	5
Eyelids	70	5.3	600	42	4
Additional pass*					
Glabella, crow's-feet	70	5.3	600	42	4
Perioral, lips, chin	70	5.3	600	42	4
Cheeks	70	5.3	600	42	4
Additional pass**					
Previously treated areas	60	4.5	600	36	4

Note: *Reserved for treatment of moderate to severe rhytids. **Reserved only for the most severe rhytids; rarely performed by the authors.

Table 10.3 Carbon dioxide (CO_2) laser settings by facial aesthetic unit: Part II

Treatment areas	Pulse energy (mJ)	Fluence (J/cm²)	Pulse width (Hz)	Power (W)	Density
Initial pass					
Preauricular undermined skin	70	5.3	600	42	4
Inferior mandibular border	70	5.3	600	42	4
Additional pass*					
Preauricular undermined skin	60	4.5	600	36	4
Inferior mandibular border	60	4.5	600	36	4

Note: *Not routinely performed by the authors.

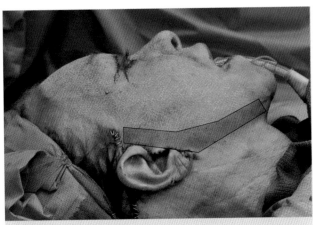

Fig. 10.3 Patient intraoperatively following rhytidectomy and full-face resurfacing sparing 2 cm of preauricular undermined skin and along the inferior mandibular border (highlighted area).

performed at an energy of 80 mJ, fluence of 6.0 J/cm², power of 48 W, and a density of 5, with a square pattern to move along the face expeditiously while maintaining control over the portions of the flap that are treated with the laser.

Once the first pass is made, the surface char should be gently wiped and removed with wet and dry gauze. The second pass is directed to areas of deeper wrinkles, such as the glabella, crow's-feet, and perioral region, and should be performed at an energy of 70 mJ, fluence of 5.3 J/cm², power of 42 W, and a density of 4. Similarly, the first treatment of the eyelids and preauricular area should be at the same settings. This is performed with an appropriate rectangular pattern to address each anatomical area (e.g., smaller for the eyelids). A 2- to 3-cm area of preauricular skin is left untreated by the senior author; however, if desired the surgeon may "taper" over the area corresponding to the subcutaneous skin elevation (▶ Fig. 10.3). Tapering involves decreasing the density to 4, while decreasing the fluence from 70 mJ to 60 mJ, which allows the surgeon to safely go over the 2- to 3-cm area of undermined skin in the preauricular region and jawline for blending and feathering (▶ Table 10.3).

Once again the surface char should be removed. Occasionally, a second pass can be made over the eyelids at an energy of 60

Palo Alto, California) for full-face CO_2 laser resurfacing. The most commonly used settings by the senior author are depicted in ▶ Table 10.2 and ▶ Table 10.3. The first laser pass on the face, excluding the upper and lower eyelids and preauricular area, is

Table 10.4 Erbium:yttrium aluminum garnet (Er:YAG) laser settings by facial aesthetic unit

Treatment areas	Depth (μm)	Fluence (J/cm^2)	Overlap (%)	Coag	Density
Resurfacing settings					
Full face	100	25.0	50	0	–
Eyelids	80	20.0	50	0	–
Preauricular undermined skin	50	12.5	50	0	–
Inferior mandibular border	50	12.5	50	0	–
Fractionated settings					
Full face	250–350	62.5–87.5	0.7	0	22
Eyelids	80	20.0	1.3	0	11
Preauricular undermined skin	Not treated	–	–	–	–
Inferior mandibular border	Not treated	–	–	–	–

mJ, fluence of 4.5 J/cm^2, power of 36 W, and a density of 4. If necessary, this setting is also used for feathering the jawline and for selected deep rhytids of perioral, glabella, and forehead regions. This additional pass is solely reserved for the deepest and most severe rhytids and is rarely used by the authors.

Immediately there will be visible tightening secondary to desiccation of the skin from heating of the subdermal vasculature. Punctate dermal bleeding can be visualized; however, this is often minimal with the CO_2 laser. If the chamois color is obtained in any areas, this marks the absolute deepest to carry treatment and should signal the end point to the surgeon.

10.5.2 Erbium:Yttrium Aluminum Garnet Laser

Patients undergoing simultaneous Er:YAG treatment are prepared preoperatively in an identical fashion to the CO_2 patients described above. The most commonly used settings for the Er:YAG laser are depicted in ▶ Table 10.4. Using a variable pulsed Er:YAG system (Contour, Sciton, Palo Alto, California), our technique begins with a 4-mm scanner resurfacing handpiece calibrated to a 100-μm depth and a 50% spot overlap. This initial resurfacing pass is used to treat the perioral region including vermilion border and chin, as well as the cheeks and forehead. Lower settings are used for the eyelids and preauricular region as depicted in ▶ Table 10.4.

The handpiece is then changed for vertical wounding using an erbium profractional scanner to treat all areas with the settings as dictated in ▶ Table 10.4; however, the preauricular area is spared. Although the preauricular area can be treated, and has been described as treated to within 2 mm of the incision line by Alster et al,[2] the senior author prefers to leave the immediate 2 to 3 cm of undermined tissue untreated. By doing so there is an attenuation of energy dispersed over the lateral aspects of the cheeks and jawline.

A major distinction between use of the CO_2 and Er:YAG lasers is the lack of hemostasis with the Er:YAG treatments. Any oozing should be wiped clear before treating an area. By maintaining a clean field the surgeon can avoid missing any untreated

regions, ensuring a more comprehensive treatment and achieving a more cohesive final result. Additionally, by recognizing previously treated regions, the surgeon can confidently avoid stacking pulses over any one area.

10.6 Postoperative Care and Home Care

The authors counsel patients to expect 2 weeks of downtime before they may feel comfortable being seen in public following full-face ablative resurfacing. Patients must commit preoperatively to an intense postoperative skin care routine, and support from family and friends is encouraged. Additionally, because there is a line of demarcation early after treatment between the untreated preauricular area and the treated cheek tissue, patients often need frequent reassurance that these areas will blend without sequelae.

Immediately postoperative when the CO_2 laser is used, a Silon-TSR dressing (Bio Med Sciences, Bethlehem, Pennsylvania) is applied to the full face. An Aquaphor-coated (Beiersdorf Inc., Wilton, Connecticut), nonadherent, single-layer dressing is applied over the periauricular areas and secured with a light, compressive, facial-gauze head wrap overnight (▶ Fig. 10.4).

All dressings and drains are removed the following morning on postoperative day 1, with exception of the Silon dressing. The Silon dressing, if used, should remain in place until postoperative day 3, after which time the patients begin their local wound care regimen. Our standard wound care regimen consists of water-soaked gauze cleanses and reapplication of an Aquaphor barrier 5 to 6 times a day to avoid any drying of the treated areas. This above-described regimen is also used for Er:YAG laser-treated areas immediately postoperative, however, without use of the Silon dressing. The wound care regimen is continued until re-epithelialization has been achieved, usually at the 10-day mark. If there is evidence of refractory crusting, then dilute acetic acid soaks as well are performed several times a day to loosen the crusts.

Once complete re-epithelialization has occurred, application of anti-inflammatory cream should be initiated with a

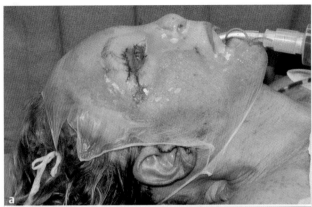

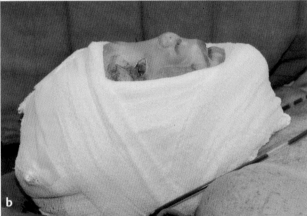

Fig. 10.4 (a) Postoperative facial dressing with Silon-TSR wound contact layer dressing (Bio Med Sciences, Bethlehem, Pennsylvania) and (b) light, compressive wrap.

nonfluorinated steroid, such as mometasone. For areas of delayed healing an occlusive hydrocolloid dressing may be left in place for 48 to 72 hours until epithelialization is complete. A skin care and makeup consultation is done on postoperative day 10, and the patient is allowed to resume normal daily activities, with reasonable discretion. Postoperatively it is imperative that the patient avoids direct sun exposure, and the regular use of sunscreen with a sun protection factor (SPF) of 45 or higher is mandatory to avoid compromising results. Preoperative and postoperative photos of a patient are shown in ▶ Fig. 10.1.

10.7 Complications

Complications related to isolated laser resurfacing include pigmentary changes, prominent lines of demarcation, prolonged erythema, and scarring, with the latter being related to unpredictable extended thermal damage previously seen with the use of older continuous wave and superpulsed CO_2 laser platforms. Simultaneous rhytidectomy and full-face laser resurfacing do not carry any further increased risk of hypopigmentation or hyperpigmentation than either treatment alone, when the patient-selection process as discussed earlier is followed. The complications listed below pertain more to those adverse conditions associated with surgical rhytidectomy alone. Please refer to Chapter 19 of this book for discussions of complications secondary to laser resurfacing, which could also be seen as part of this concurrent treatment regimen.

10.7.1 Flap Necrosis

Skin slough after rhytidectomy alone has historically been reported at a rate of 1.1 to 3.0%.[18] Various animal models have shown flap necrosis and deleterious effects of laser treatment; however, those studies used higher settings with multiple passes.[19,20,21] Consequently, the authors advocate the settings as described in the text and ▶ Table 10.2, ▶ Table 10.3, and ▶ Table 10.4. When combining rhytidectomy with CO_2 or Er:YAG laser resurfacing, there is a potential risk of irreversible injury to the delicate undermined tissue. In a meta-analysis, Koch and Perkins[1] as well as several other authors reported the percentages of complications in simultaneous modalities were no different from those of rhytidectomy alone with regard to flap loss and skin slough.[22,23] Similarly, Alster et al[2] and Weinstein et al[24] compared various ablative modalities with up to six passes with the Er:YAG laser in the setting of concurrent rhytidectomy without an increase in complications or skin slough.

10.7.2 Delayed Healing

Delayed healing occurs when a treated area persistently fails to re-epithelialize for more than 14 days. Care should also be taken to prevent some of the causes of delayed healing, such as management of patient comorbidities, infections, herpetic outbreaks, poor postoperative care, or secondary tissue injury, which may occur as a result of overaggressive cleansing, picking, or scratching the freshly wounded tissues.[11] The mainstay of treatment in cases of delayed healing is to apply an occlusive hydrocolloid dressing or ointment that protects the area and that allows for better epithelial cell migration.[15]

10.7.3 Infection

Resurfacing procedures by definition violate the protective epidermal barrier, exposing the skin to environmental factors that may make the skin more susceptible to infection. The patients' comorbidities can also reduce immune function—especially patients who are taking immunocompromising medications or patients with diabetes.

Superficial infections associated with laser resurfacing alone, whether bacterial, fungal, or herpetiform, have a reported incidence of 2 to 7%, despite prophylactic therapy.[1,25] The authors' perioperative routine includes prophylactic antibiotic dosing with a first-generation oral cephalosporin, as well as an antiviral prophylactic dose of acyclovir 800 mg three times daily prior to the laser treatment, which is then continued until epithelialization. As previously reported, the rates of superficial infection using the combination treatment do not differ, highlighting the robustness in the underlying vascularity even in the face undergoing concomitant rhytidectomy.[1,2]

10.7.4 Hematoma

Hematoma is the most common complication following rhytidectomy, and more common in men. The incidence in the literature varies from 2 to 15%, with the senior author's experience ranging from 1 to 2% incidence of hematoma with the use of closed-suction bulb system drains postoperatively.[9,26] When patients present with a postoperative hematoma, management includes observation or needle drainage for minimal to small hematomas; conversely, surgical evacuation and exploration are necessary for large, rapidly expanding hematomas.

10.7.5 Nerve Injury

Sensory and motor nerve injuries are rare, with a reported incidence of 0.7 to 2.5%.[27] The great auricular nerve, which provides sensation to the periauricular region, is the most frequently injured nerve. If injury is noted during surgery, primary repair is deemed the best practice because it can result in the return of sensation within 12 to 18 months usually.[28]

The temporal branch of the facial nerve is the most frequently injured motor nerve in most series, with a reported incidence of 0.8% temporary injury and of 0.1% permanent injury in a review of more than 12,000 rhytidectomies.[27] With meticulous dissection and the use of the modified SMAS elevation described earlier, surgeons should be able to prevent any injury to the facial nerve during rhytidectomy.[9]

10.8 Conclusion

Simultaneous rhytidectomy and full-face laser resurfacing continues to evolve with technological advances in laser platforms allowing precise control of thermal dispersion, while minimizing the number of passes necessary to treat actinic changes and static rhytids that may not be addressed with rhytidectomy alone. Simultaneous rhytidectomy and full-face laser resurfacing can safely provide an excellent cosmetic benefit for aesthetic rejuvenation of the face, while consolidating the anesthetic and recovery times for patients without an increase in complications.

References

[1] Koch BB, Perkins SW. Simultaneous rhytidectomy and full-face carbon dioxide laser resurfacing: a case series and meta-analysis. Arch Facial Plast Surg 2002; 4: 227–233

[2] Alster TS, Doshi SN, Hopping SB. Combination surgical lifting with ablative laser skin resurfacing of facial skin: a retrospective analysis. Dermatol Surg 2004; 30: 1191–1195

[3] Baker TJ. Chemical face peeling and rhytidectomy. A combined approach for facial rejuvenation. Plast Reconstr Surg Transplant Bull 1962; 29: 199–207

[4] Baker TJ, Gordon HL. Chemical face peeling: an adjunct to surgical facelifting. South Med J 1963; 56: 412–414

[5] Litton C. Chemical face lifting. Plast Reconstr Surg Transplant Bull 1962; 29: 371–380

[6] Taghizadeh F, Leibowitz A, Ellison T, Griego M, Traylor-Knowles M, Ramirez P. Short flap rhytidectomy and fractional CO2 laser rejuvenation of the aging face. J Cosmet Dermatol 2013; 12: 49–56

[7] Ortiz AE, Tremaine AM, Zachary CB. Long-term efficacy of a fractional resurfacing device. Lasers Surg Med 2010; 42: 168–170

[8] Brightman LA, Brauer JA, Anolik R, et al. Ablative and fractional ablative lasers. Dermatol Clin 2009; 27: 479–489, vi–vii

[9] Perkins SW, Patel AB. Extended superficial muscular aponeurotic system rhytidectomy: a graded approach. Facial Plast Surg Clin North Am 2009; 17: 575–587, vi

[10] Bernstein EF. Chemical peels. Semin Cutan Med Surg 2002; 21: 27–45

[11] Perkins SW, Castellano R. Use of combined modality for maximal resurfacing. Facial Plast Surg Clin North Am 2004; 12: 323–337, vi

[12] Fitzpatrick TB. The validity and practicality of sun-reactive skin types I through VI. Arch Dermatol 1988; 124: 869–871

[13] Brody HJ. Variations and comparisons in medium-depth chemical peeling. J Dermatol Surg Oncol 1989; 15: 953–963

[14] Glogau RG, Matarasso SL. Chemical face peeling: patient and peeling agent selection. Facial Plast Surg 1995; 11: 1–8

[15] Gibson FB, Perkins SW. Complications of Chemical Peels, Dermabrasion, and Laser Resurfacing. In: Eisele DW, Smith RV, eds. Complications in Head and Neck Surgery. 2nd ed. Philadelphia, PA: Mosby/Elsevier; 2009: 655–669.

[16] Apfelberg DB American Society for Aesthetic Plastic Surgery. American Society of Plastic and Reconstructive Surgeons. Summary of the 1997 ASAPS/ASPRS Laser Task Force Survey on laser resurfacing and laser blepharoplasty. Plast Reconstr Surg 1998; 101: 511–518

[17] Sensöz O, Nazmi Baran C, Sahin Alagöz M, Cağri Uysal A, Unlü RE. Long-term results of ultrapulsed carbon dioxide laser resurfacing of the Mediterranean face. Aesthetic Plast Surg 2004; 28: 328–333

[18] Baker DC. Complications of cervicofacial rhytidectomy. Clin Plast Surg 1983; 10: 543–562

[19] Guyuron B, Michelow B, Schmelzer R, Thomas T, Ellison MA. Delayed healing of rhytidectomy flap resurfaced with CO2 laser. Plast Reconstr Surg 1998; 101: 816–819

[20] Babovic SB, Bite U, Bridges AG, Clay RP. Laser resurfacing of skin flaps: an experimental comparison of three different lasers. Acta Med Acad 2011; 40: 4–9

[21] Adcock DP, Paulsen S, Katzen T, et al. Simultaneous cutaneous flap elevation and skin resurfacing in the rabbit model. Aesthet Surg J 1999; 19: 375–380

[22] Achauer BM, Adair SR, VanderKam VM. Combined rhytidectomy and full-face laser resurfacing. Plast Reconstr Surg 2000; 106: 1608–1611, discussion 1612–1613

[23] Fulton JE. Simultaneous face lifting and skin resurfacing. Plast Reconstr Surg 1998; 102: 2480–2489

[24] Weinstein C, Pozner J, Scheflan M. Combined erbium:YAG laser resurfacing and face lifting. Plast Reconstr Surg 2001; 107: 586–592, discussion 593–594

[25] Alster TS, Lupton JR. Treatment of complications of laser skin resurfacing. Arch Facial Plast Surg 2000; 2: 279–284

[26] Perkins SW, Williams JD, Macdonald K, Robinson EB. Prevention of seromas and hematomas after face-lift surgery with the use of postoperative vacuum drains. Arch Otolaryngol Head Neck Surg 1997; 123: 743–745

[27] Matarasso A, Elkwood A, Rankin M, Elkowitz M. National plastic surgery survey: face lift techniques and complications. Plast Reconstr Surg 2000; 106: 1185–1195, discussion 1196

[28] Chaffoo RA. Complications in facelift surgery: avoidance and management. Facial Plast Surg Clin North Am 2013; 21: 551–558

11 Nonablative Laser and Light Devices

Joely Kaufman and Sophie D. Liao

11.1 Introduction

The development of laser and light therapy for skin resurfacing has revolutionized the treatment of photodamage, wrinkles, scars, and a variety of pigmented lesions. The earliest lasers used for this purpose were ablative and included carbon dioxide (CO_2) and erbium: yttrium aluminum garnet (Er:YAG) devices. Treatment with these ablative lasers results in coagulation and vaporization of the entire epidermal unit with the goal of improving the quality of treated skin. Downtime is in the range of 5 to 14 days, and over this period of time patients can experience edema, oozing, and discomfort. Erythema can last for months to years and dyspigmentation, including depigmentation, can appear at any time after treatment—including years later. These complications are of particular concern for patients of higher Fitzpatrick skin types, and limit the use of these lasers to Fitzpatrick types I through III. Infection and scarring can occur as well due to prolonged compromise of the epidermal barrier unit. Results are dramatic for reversal of photoaging, but the side-effect profile is a deterrent for some patients and physicians and has limited the use of fully ablative laser resurfacing.[1,2,3]

Nonablative technologies were developed to allow for faster postprocedure skin recovery, targeting the deep dermis to remodel collagen. Although these lasers have the benefit of shorter downtime, more sessions are required to achieve results similar to the ablative lasers, often requiring five or six monthly treatments. These devices are also typically paired with a cooling tip that allows for cooling of the epidermis and selective treatment to the dermis. The damage induced by nonablative devices is by definition "not ablative" and does not result in disruption of the epidermis or vaporization of tissue. Characteristic histology includes coagulation of dermal components. The term *nonablative* is broad in nature, and can include any device that does not cause ablation. However, for true practical purposes, and for this chapter, the nonablative devices are those that are moderately absorbed by water with wavelengths ranging from 1,064 to 2,000 nm. Other devices, which deliver nonspecific thermal energy and are by definition nonablative such as radiofrequency and ultrasound technologies, are not discussed here.

11.2 Nonablative Nonfractionated Lasers

The 1,320-nm neodymium:yttrium aluminum garnet (Nd:YAG) laser (CoolTouch, ICN Pharmaceuticals, Costa Mesa, California) was the first exclusively nonablative laser developed. Energy penetration occurs to a depth of 1,600 µm, a potentially effective treatment depth. Safety was optimal, yet studies showed only minimal clinical improvement in rhytids and photoaging.[4,5,6] The Smoothbeam laser (Candela Corp., Wayland, Massachusetts) emits coherent light at 1,450 nm. This device also uses water as the chromophore and results in thermal injury to the dermis and dermal components. The epidermis is protected via dynamic cryogen cooling. In 2003, Tanzi et al reported a mild to moderate clinical improvement of wrinkles after a series of four treatments with the 1,450-nm diode laser. Biopsies showed an increase in collagen production in the dermis.[7] Although originally designed and cleared for wrinkle reduction, the clinical results for photoaging are modest, and now the device is more commonly used for the treatment of acne. Heating of the sebaceous glands results in improvement of acneiform lesions. Reports of mild improvement in atrophic acne scarring are also published, with the 1,450-nm diode laser outperforming the 1,320-nm laser. Nearly all subsequently developed nonablative lasers, including various Nd:YAG, 1,450-nm diode, 1,540-nm Erbium:glass (Er:glass), and 1,550-nm fractional nonablative lasers, have utilized fractionated delivery systems.

11.3 Broadband Light

Broadband light devices, also known as intense pulsed light (IPL), emit noncoherent, noncollimated polychromatic light in the 550- to 1,200-nm range. Since they can target melanin, hemoglobin, and water chromophores, they are useful particularly for removal of pigmented and vascular lesions, but have also been found to be useful for photoaging. Studies demonstrate new collagen formation 6 months posttreatment, and moderate subjective and objective improvement in rhytids and dyspigmentation can be seen.[8,9]

The current nonablative lasers in wide use utilize fractional photothermolysis (FP). The development of the concept of FP has completely changed the manner in which skin resurfacing is performed. In 2004, Manstein et al published a pivotal article describing this novel concept that focuses on the treatment of a *fraction* of the skin's surface. Tiny microscopic beams heat small columns of skin, leaving adjacent areas completely intact. The treated columns are termed microthermal treatment zones (MTZs). These MTZs vary in diameter and depth depending on the wavelength used and the energy employed, but are generally less than 400 µm in diameter.[10] In addition, the number of columns per square centimeter of skin, a parameter termed treatment density, can be changed in order to adjust the aggressiveness of a treatment. Treatment densities vary among devices, with average density ranging from 6 to 40%. A treatment density of 100% would be equivalent to the previously described full-face traditional ablative resurfacing and is generally not used in fractional devices. Producing tiny columns of damage surrounded by intact tissue allows the healing process to proceed at a much faster rate. In healing after fractional resurfacing, intact viable cells are able to migrate over the treated MTZs. In contrast, the healing process in traditional fully ablative resurfacing requires full differentiation. The process of healing in fractional resurfacing can take anywhere from 24 hours to 3 or 4 days.[11] The decrease in epidermal compromise has resulted in a decrease in downtime and complication rates, while maintaining an acceptable efficacy rate.

The introduction of fractional resurfacing has revolutionized laser treatment of photodamage. Devices can be divided into

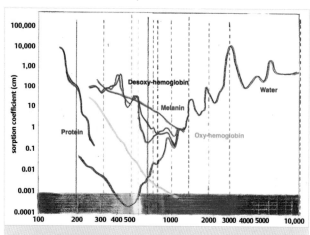

Fig. 11.1 All nonablative lasers use wavelengths that are moderately well absorbed by water (shorter than 2,000 nm). The ablative lasers use wavelengths that are highly absorbed by water (longer than 2000 nm).

Table 11.1 Ablative devices

Ablative Devices	Wavelength
CO2 (Fraxel re:pair)	10,600 nm
Er:YAG (Sciton ProFractional)	2,940 nm
Er:YSGG (Cutera Pearl)	2,790 nm

Table 11.2 Nonablative devices

Nonablative devices	Wavelength
CoolTouch	1,320 nm
Smoothbeam	1,450 nm
Emerge	1,410 nm
Clear and Brilliant	1,440 nm
Fractional XF	1,540 nm
Fraxel restore	1,550 nm
Titan	1,100–1,800 nm
Permea	1,927 nm
Fraxel Dual	1,550/1,927 nm

nonablative and ablative types. The first fractional device introduced by Manstein and colleagues was a nonablative device––meaning that the dermis is targeted—leaving the epidermis entirely intact.[10] Fractional ablative devices were introduced a few years later. All resurfacing devices, including fractional resurfacing devices, use water as their target chromophore. All of these wavelengths are in the infrared range, since this is where water is able to absorb light most efficiently (▶ Fig. 11.1). Ablative devices produce wavelengths that are highly absorbed by water, resulting in rapid heating of water and vaporization of tissue. Nonablative devices employ wavelengths that are only moderately or mildly absorbed by water, which results in low, slow heating and resultant coagulation of tissue. Both are used in fractional resurfacing and confer different risks and benefits. Ablative fractional devices include the CO_2 laser, Er:YAG laser, and erbium:yttrium scandium gallium garnet (Er:YSGG) laser (▶ Table 11.1). The nonablative lasers include the Er:glass and Nd:YAG lasers with wavelengths of 1,410, 1,440, 1,540, and 1,550 nm, as well as the Titan infrared light device, which utilizes wavelengths between 1,100-1,800 nm (Cutera, Brisbane, California). The 1,927-nm fractional device functions like a combination of the ablative and nonablative lasers. Each wavelength has its place in the armamentarium of fractional devices for photorejuvenation.

The parameters used in fractional resurfacing are somewhat different from those of traditional lasers. Most lasers operate by varying fluence (the amount of energy delivered to a certain surface area). Fractional resurfacing allows the amount of laser energy and treatment density to be adjusted independently. The energy chosen determines the depth of penetration of the treatment column. For low-energy settings, the penetration will be superficial. The converse is also true; higher energy settings allow for deeper dermal penetration. The energy should be chosen based on the condition being treated. For superficial lesions, a lower energy is needed; for deeper dermal conditions, a higher energy is required. The treatment density can vary depending on the wavelength used but, in general, the higher the density the larger the area of treatment and the more aggressive the treatment. Density settings may need to be reduced when treating darker skin types because lower

densities result in fewer side effects, such as dyspigmentation.[12] A higher treatment density may require fewer sessions to reach clinical efficacy. As energy settings are increased, MTZs will also increase due to the boost in heat delivered. The spot size from the light device itself does not change but the size of the MTZs will increase as energy rises. Furthermore, a larger diameter MTZ will step up the treatment density. Some devices on the market adjust for this and others do not. It is important to remember this when using a stamp technique device.

11.4 Nonablative Fractional Lasers

The nonablative fractional lasers were the first fractional devices to be introduced. The first nonablative fractional device was cleared by the Food and Drug Administration (FDA) in 2003. This original instrument is a 1,550-nm laser and was called the Fraxel laser (Solta Medical, San Francisco, California). Since its introduction, numerous fractional nonablative tools using multiple wavelengths have become available. All of these wavelengths (▶ Table 11.2) are only moderately well absorbed by water and result in tissue coagulation and not vaporization. The microscopic spot size, along with the relatively low affinity for water, allows the nonablative wavelengths to have deep penetration. The depth of penetration depends on the device, wavelength, and energy used. On average, a classic, nonablative fractional laser of 1,540 or 1,550 nm can deliver tissue coagulation to a dermal depth of up to 700 µm to 1 mm,[10,13,14] although proprietary data from one company claims to reach a depth of 1,400 µm (Fraxel Dual 1,550/1,927 nm). The ability to reach deep into the dermis and cause tissue remodeling while maintaining a very attractive side-effect profile is revolutionary for the field of laser medicine. Whereas a depth of 1 mm may not be needed in many clinical situations, deep penetration is desirable in some instances. Dermal conditions, such as deep wrinkling and scarring, respond best to treatment in the deep dermis, whereas superficial conditions, such as pigmentation, may not require such energy.

Recently, nonablative lasers that deliver light at wavelengths of 1,410 and 1,440 nm with relatively low densities have been introduced. These were designed for a "no downtime" procedure that can gradually improve skin texture and pigmentation with repeated treatments. Depth of penetration is up to 390 μm, reaching the dermis, although still relatively superficial when compared to the 1,540- and 1,550-nm instruments. One group presented findings with the 1,440-nm system on pore size and skin texture at the April 2012 American Society for Lasers in Medicine and Surgery meeting.[15] A group of 20 patients (Fitzpatrick I–VI) received 6 full-face treatments spaced 2 weeks apart using the company-recommended 8 passes at different preset levels. Using the VISIA-CR Imaging System (Canfield, Fairfield, New Jersey), a pore score was quantitatively evaluated, and a significant reduction was observed. On average, it was a 17% reduction in size. Patients can expect up to only a few hours of erythema. Treatments should be repeated for optimal results.

11.5 Histology of Nonablative Laser Treatment

Histological results of treatment with a nonablative fractional laser have been well studied. We briefly review findings here. Directly after treatment with nonablative FP, four characteristic features are seen: (1) a columnlike denaturation of the epidermis and dermis that represents the MTZ, (2) an intact stratum corneum, with (3) subepidermal clefting, and (4) adjacent vital, unharmed tissue. This viable tissue serves as a reservoir for healing of the treated sites. Within the first 24 hours, keratinocytes from the surrounding untreated skin migrate to replace the coagulated areas of epidermis. By the end of 24 hours, the epidermis is already fully re-epithelialized and the continuity of the epidermal basal cell layer is restored.[11,16] A button-shaped structure that is located below the intact stratum corneum over each MTZ and has been shown to contain necrotic tissue becomes evident as early as 1 day after FP. It therefore has been named microscopic epidermal necrotic debris (MENDs). This is a collection of coagulated dermal structures that are shuttled out of the skin. Melanin, elastic tissue, and other dermal contents can be found within this structure. These MENDs eventually get eliminated transepidermally through the stratum corneum. This process has been called the MEND-shuttle because it literally "shuttles" dermal content out of the skin. These MENDs are represented clinically by the bronzing of the skin that takes place from days 3 to 7 posttreatment. By day 7 most of these MENDS are completely shed and the skin returns to normal color. Introduction of thermal damage and coagulation of epidermis and dermis triggers the histological cascade of the wound healing process. Heat shock protein 70 is induced and collagen production is stimulated. Collagen remodeling in the dermis continues for 3 to 6 months in each MTZ site.[10]

11.6 Clinical Indications and Pearls

The original nonablative fractional device, as noted earlier, received FDA clearance in 2003 for the coagulation of soft tissue.[10] After further studies in 2004, this 1,550-nm fractional device obtained further approval for the treatment of pigmented lesions on and off the face and for periorbital wrinkles. Currently, the nonablative devices are also authorized for the treatment of melasma, acne scars, surgical scars, and actinic keratoses.

11.7 Clinical Data on Use of Nonablative Fractional Resurfacing for Photoaging

Changes associated with photoaging—including solar lentigines, actinic keratoses, dyspigmentation, poor skin texture, pore enlargement, and fine and moderate rhytids—respond well to nonablative FP. Procedures can be spaced 1 or more weeks apart and typically require several sessions. Unlike ablative laser resurfacing, which is safest used on the thicker skin of the face due to complications such as scarring and hyperpigmentation, nonablative fractional laser resurfacing can be used both on and off the face, including on the chest, back, neck, and extremities.[17,18,19,20,21,22,23] In one study of 50 women with photodamage to the face, neck, and chest, 73% of women with facial photodamage and 55% of women with nonfacial photodamage experienced at least 51 to 75% clinical improvement in dyspigmentation, skin irregularities, and rhytids at 9 months as assessed by masked investigators. Three treatments spaced 3 to 4 weeks apart were given using a 1,550-nm erbium-doped fiber laser (Fraxel, Solta Medical, San Francisco, California). Facial skin was treated with a fluence of 8 mJ/cm^2 and density of 250 MTZ/cm^2 to a total of 2,000 MTZ/cm^2. Nonfacial skin was treated with the same fluence and similar total density.[23] Other investigators have found similar results with significant improvements in skin texture and rhytids of the face[10,22,24]; perioral rhytids[22]; actinic keratoses[21]; and skin texture and rhytids of the hands,[20] back, and extremities.[22] Energies and densities vary depending on the device manufacturer and the wavelength employed.

11.8 Clinical Data for Acne and Surgical Scarring

Extensive data also support the utility of nonablative FP in treating acne, surgical, and burn scars. Improvement in acne scar appearance and objective scar volume assessed by topographic imaging, ranging from 22 to 66%, was noted in one study.[22] Several other studies have reported success in the subgroup of atrophic acne scars, achieving up to 95% improvement in 90% of patients after serial monthly treatments.[25,26] Unlike conventional ablative therapies, nonablative fractional lasers can be used to treat patients of higher Fitzpatrick skin types, who usually have a greater risk of postinflammatory hyperpigmentation (PIH). Although the threat of PIH still remains, reducing the number of passes and total treatment density were found to decrease the risk of PIH significantly in one study of 47 Asian patients treated for acne scarring.[27] Other investigators have reported successful use of this technology with darker phototypes.[12,22,28,29]

Hypertrophic surgical scars—which practitioners have attempted to treat by multiple modalities including intralesional steroid or 5-fluorouracil injections, massage, topical silicone, surgical excision, or pulsed dye and Nd:YAG lasers—have also been successfully treated with nonablative fractional lasers. Lin et al performed nonablative fractional laser resurfacing for 20 patients with surgical hypertrophic scars in a randomized controlled trial. The linear scars were split into a treatment side and a control side and subjects were also randomized into a low-density treatment arm, with 14% coverage, and a high-density treatment arm, with 26% coverage. Therapy was performed four times with treatments separated every 2 weeks. Of the 20 patients, 17 noted subjective improvement on the treated portion of their scars. Blinded observers rated scar appearance including pigmentation, erythema, and texture, all of which were improved compared to the untreated side.[30] Successful outcomes in other studies of postsurgical scar treatment have been reported.[31,32] Beneficial results have been documented in hypopigmented surgical and poststeroid injection scars as well.[33] In one small study, 7 patients with long-standing hypopigmented scars were treated with a 1,550-nm nonablative fractional device up to four times, and all experienced significant subjective and objective improvement.[34] In other research of 14 patients, 85% of the individuals experienced greater than 50% improvement in hypopigmented scars with the use of two or more 1,550-nm nonablative fractional resurfacing (NAFR) treatments with adjunctive topical bimatoprost and tretinoin or pimecrolimus.[35] Pham et al also found that postsurgical scars treated with four sessions of NAFR utilizing a 1,550-nm laser resulted in subjective improvement in 13 patients' ratings of color, stiffness, thickness, and irregularity as well.[36]

Burn scars, which also have been difficult to treat historically, were shown in one randomized controlled study to respond with improved skin texture after treatment with a nonablative fractional laser. Three monthly treatments were performed with a 1,540-nm instrument and blinded evaluations were performed 1 and 3 months after the final procedure. Of the total number of patients, 47% reported moderate or significant improvement, and another 47% reported mild improvement.[37]

11.9 Striae

Striae distensae, which may be found in all genders and races, may present with atrophic or depressed violaceous or white linear plaques. Erythematous striae have traditionally been treated with the pulsed dye laser with good results. However, striae alba, or hypopigmented lesions, had been difficult to treat until the nonablative fractional laser mechanisms were developed. A study by Stotland et al[38] assessed 20 patients with striae distensae treated with nonablative fractional laser, and found 26 to 50% improvement overall in 63% of patients. Of the 20 individuals, 50% had an improvement in texture of up to 50%. Improvement of striae distensae has also been reported by others.[22,39] Several procedures are needed to obtain the maximum benefit. A new deep-penetrating, pronged handpiece for the 1,540-nm tool has been helpful in our practice for the treatment of striae.

11.10 Clinical Data on Periorbital Resurfacing or Tightening

Periorbital tightening of lateral rhytids was first assessed by Manstein et al in 2004 on 30 patients with Fitzpatrick skin types II through III. Four treatments were given 4 to 7 days apart. At 1 month, 54% of test subjects demonstrated moderate to significant improvement in the appearance of wrinkles, 30% showed noticeable improvement, and 53% displayed moderate improvement in skin texture. These results were somewhat attenuated at 3 months postprocedure, with 34% of subjects exhibiting moderate improvement in wrinkles and 47% with moderate improvement in skin texture.[10] Other investigators have found improvement in periorbital skin laxity and rhytids, with one study showing greater than 50% eyelid tightening in 55% of test subjects and widening of the palpebral aperture in 56% of patients.[30] In another study, 55% of patients displayed moderate to excellent improvement after three serial treatments.[40] Because eyelid skin is very thin, high energies are not required to achieve effective skin tightening in this area, even with a nonablative device. A series of treatments is recommended for optimal results.

11.11 Clinical Data on Melasma

Melasma predominantly affects women, but is also seen in a minority of men. It can be very difficult to treat. Due to a high incidence of PIH, only modest success has been achieved with conventional ablative lasers. Tannous and Astner published the first case report using a nonablative fractional laser to treat a patient with melasma. Two treatments 3 weeks apart resulted in significant resolution of the subject's melasma, with only mild erythema for 2 days and mild bronzing lasting 3 days. Resolution of the melasma was maintained 6 months after the last procedure.[41] One group followed eight patients treated for melasma who had failed multiple prior treatments. Patients were pretreated and posttreated with a bleaching agent to reduce the risk of PIH, then given two to seven treatments separated by 4 to 7 weeks. Long-term follow-up to 3 years found that five of the eight patients had no or minimal recurrence of melasma, whereas three experienced some recurrence.[42] Others have reported successful use of nonablative fractional laser procedure in Asian patients with melasma with careful pretreatment and posttreatment adjunctive use of sunblock and bleaching agents for several months.[27,28] As exhibited in the above-referenced publications, treatment of melasma with any heat-based device can be problematic. Although some patients improve, others do not; in still others, the disease can worsen. Care must be taken to pretreat and posttreat these patients with hydroquinone, sun protection, and in many cases topical steroids for prolonged erythema. Patients with melasma should be treated as one would treat Fitzpatrick darker skin types, including the use of cooling and low-density treatments to avoid complications. Patients should be counseled on the possible risks of procedures. Fractional nonablative resurfacing for melasma is not a first-line treatment; however, it may be useful for those cases resistant to other procedure modalities or in those with dermal melasma for which there is no other effective strategy. Extreme caution should be used when treating melasma patients with any heat-based device, and the possible risks should be clearly explained to patients.

11.12 Miscellaneous Conditions

NAFR has been reported in a small number of cases to benefit several other conditions, including nevus of Ota, poikiloderma of Civatte, minocycline-induced hyperpigmentation, and others. Kouba et al reported one case of an Asian man with a nevus of Ota treated twice with a 1,440-nm fractionated Nd:YAG laser. The treatments were spaced 1 month apart, and by 6 weeks after the second treatment the lesion was completely resolved.[43] Behroozan and colleagues reported a case of poikiloderma of Civatte of the neck treated with the 1,550-nm Fraxel laser. After a single treatment complicated by only mild postoperative edema for 24 hours, improvement in the telangiectatic component of the lesion was noted within 2 weeks with persistence of the results at a 2-month follow-up visit.[44] Izikson and Anderson reported one case of a patient with minocycline-induced facial hyperpigmentation treated with serial Fraxel resurfacing. Four treatments spaced several months apart were given, with reported near-complete resolution of the pigment.[45] Karsai and colleagues reported one case of a patient with granuloma annulare of the arm treated with a 1,440-nm nonablative fractional Nd:YAG laser. Two treatments given 3 weeks apart resulted in significant improvement in the hyperpigmentation of the treated lesions within 10 days after the second treatment, complicated only by edema of the treated areas lasting 6 hours and erythema lasting up to 4 weeks. The patient subsequently underwent three total procedures for multiple lesions of the trunk and arms with complete clearance reported within 8 months.[46] One case of glabellar wrinkling with poor skin texture and scarring after prior excision and ablative laser treatment of a congenital hemangioma was reported to have excellent results after two procedures with a 1,440-nm erbium-doped fiber laser (Fraxel, Solta Medical, San Francisco, California).[47] Glaich and colleagues reported one case of a patient with matted telangiectasias of the thigh treated with a 1,550-nm nonablative fractional device. The patient was treated five times in a monthly fashion, and was reported to have significant improvement in the lesions 6 months after the final process.[48] A single case of a patient with facial colloid milium was also reported by Marra and colleagues to resolve successfully after five treatments using a 1,550-nm fractional photothermolysis device, with treatments separated by 2 to 3 weeks. Long-term follow-up in this case was not reported.[49] Although no complications such as hyperpigmentation, hypopigmentation, or scarring were noted in any of these cases, more data regarding use of NAFR for these and other conditions would be helpful in determining the effectiveness of treatment. Given the small number of cases treated, caution should be exercised in utilizing nonablative fractional lasers for any of these conditions.

11.13 Side Effects and Complications

FP is well tolerated with few serious side effects. In contrast to the complete loss of the epidermis that is seen in traditional ablative laser resurfacing, in NAFR the stratum corneum remains intact. Despite the preserved function of the epidermis, side effects and complications can still occur. In the immediate postoperative period, patients may report erythema, edema, flaking, xerosis, pruritus, bronzing, and acneiform eruptions.[50,51] Rarer side effects include hyperpigmentation and hypopigmentation, herpes simplex viral reactivation, and bacterial

infection. In a retrospective evaluation of 961 treatments for patients with Fitzpatrick skin types ranging from I through V, an overall complication rate of 7.6% was seen. Of these complications, 1.9% were acneiform and 1.8% were herpes simplex viral outbreaks. None of the complications resulted in long-term sequelae or scarring.[51] In other studies, short-term complications such as erythema and edema of the treated areas were noted to last an average of 2 to 3 days, and bronzing lasted 5 days.[39] Another study that utilized physician-administered questionnaires to 60 patients during follow-up visits after FP found that all patients reported transient posttreatment erythema, with more than 50% of the subjects experiencing transient facial edema, dry skin, and flaking. Of the 60 patients, 47% reported small superficial scratches, 37% had pruritus, and 27% had bronzing, all of which resolved. Only 10% of patients reported acneiform eruptions, and there were no patients with scarring, hyperpigmentation or hypopigmentation, infection, or herpetic outbreaks.[37] Of special note, treatment of higher skin types carries a risk of PIH. As previously mentioned, this threat may be mitigated by reducing the number of passes performed and hence the treatment density.[19] Furthermore, modifying treatments by decreasing the fluence as well as reducing the density has been shown to be well tolerated and efficacious in such patients.[21]

11.14 Conclusion

In summary, nonablative treatments refer to those devices emitting energy that is mildly or moderately absorbed by water. This results in heating of the dermis while maintaining the integrity of the epidermis. This category can include laser and light devices and also radiofrequency and ultrasound technology that result in thermal injury without vaporization of tissue. However, in clinical practice, most nonablative devices in use are nonablative fractional lasers. FP is a relatively new idea that has revolutionized treatment options for skin resurfacing. Since Manstein and colleagues' pivotal 2004 paper, centers around the world have found nonablative fractional lasers to be of great utility in the current armament of laser technology. These devices have FDA clearance for soft tissue coagulation, treatment of pigmented facial and nonfacial lesions, periorbital rhytids, melasma, acne scars, surgical scars, and actinic keratoses; and they have been found to be useful in the improvement of striae distensae, burn scars, and multiple other lesions. Furthermore, treatment across all skin types has been found to be feasible, without undue elevation of the risk of PIH in higher skin types. Although results may not be as rapid or dramatic as those seen with conventional ablative lasers or even ablative fractional lasers, nonablative FP offers expanded options for treatment of a wide variety of conditions with minimal downtime and an excellent side-effect profile.

References

[1] Hruza GJ, Dover JS. Laser skin resurfacing. Arch Dermatol 1996; 132: 451–455

[2] Dover JS, Hruza GJ. Laser skin resurfacing. Semin Cutan Med Surg 1996; 15: 177–188

[3] Waldorf HA, Kauvar AN, Geronemus RG. Skin resurfacing of fine to deep rhytides using a char-free carbon dioxide laser in 47 patients. Dermatol Surg 1995; 21: 940–946

[4] Bhatia AC, Dover JS, Arndt KA, Stewart B, Alam M. Patient satisfaction and reported long-term therapeutic efficacy associated with 1,320 nm Nd:YAG laser treatment of acne scarring and photoaging. Dermatol Surg 2006; 32: 346–352

[5] Goldberg DJ. Full-face nonablative dermal remodeling with a 1320 nm Nd:YAG laser. Dermatol Surg 2000; 26: 915–918

[6] Goldberg DJ. Non-ablative subsurface remodeling: clinical and histologic evaluation of a 1320-nm Nd:YAG laser. J Cutan Laser Ther 1999; 1: 153–157

[7] Tanzi EL, Alster TS. Side effects and complications of variable-pulsed erbium: yttrium-aluminum-garnet laser skin resurfacing: extended experience with 50 patients. Plast Reconstr Surg 2003; 111: 1524–1529, discussion 1530–1532

[8] Goldberg DJ. New collagen formation after dermal remodeling with an intense pulsed light source. J Cutan Laser Ther 2000; 2: 59–61

[9] Goldman MP, Weiss RA, Weiss MA. Intense pulsed light as a nonablative approach to photoaging. Dermatol Surg 2005; 31: 1179–1187, discussion 1187

[10] Manstein D, Herron GS, Sink RK, Tanner H, Anderson RR. Fractional photothermolysis: a new concept for cutaneous remodeling using microscopic patterns of thermal injury. Lasers Surg Med 2004; 34: 426–438

[11] Stumpp OF, Bedi VP, Wyatt D, Lac D, Rahman Z, Chan KF. In vivo confocal imaging of epidermal cell migration and dermal changes post nonablative fractional resurfacing: study of the wound healing process with corroborated histopathologic evidence. J Biomed Opt 2009; 14: 024018

[12] Kono T, Chan HH, Groff WF, et al. Prospective direct comparison study of fractional resurfacing using different fluences and densities for skin rejuvenation in Asians. Lasers Surg Med 2007; 39: 311–314

[13] Bedi VP, Chan KF, Sink RK, et al. The effects of pulse energy variations on the dimensions of microscopic thermal treatment zones in nonablative fractional resurfacing. Lasers Surg Med 2007; 39: 145–155

[14] Khan MH, Sink RK, Manstein D, Eimerl D, Anderson RR. Intradermally focused infrared laser pulses: thermal effects at defined tissue depths. Lasers Surg Med 2005; 36: 270–280

[15] Saedi N, Petrell K, Arndt K, Dover J. Evaluating facial pores and skin texture after low-energy nonablative fractional 1440-nm laser treatments. J Am Acad Dermatol 2013; 68: 113–118

[16] Laubach HJ, Tannous Z, Anderson RR, Manstein D. Skin responses to fractional photothermolysis. Lasers Surg Med 2006; 38: 142–149

[17] Tierney EP, Hanke CW. Review of the literature: treatment of dyspigmentation with fractionated resurfacing. Dermatol Surg 2010; 36: 1499–1508

[18] Cohen SR, Henssler C, Johnston J. Fractional photothermolysis for skin rejuvenation. Plast Reconstr Surg 2009; 124: 281–290

[19] Tierney EP, Kouba DJ, Hanke CW. Review of fractional photothermolysis: treatment indications and efficacy. Dermatol Surg 2009; 35: 1445–1461

[20] Jih MH, Goldberg LH, Kimyai-Asadi A. Fractional photothermolysis for photoaging of hands. Dermatol Surg 2008; 34: 73–78

[21] Lapidoth M, Adatto M, Halachmi S. Treatment of actinic keratoses and photodamage with non-contact fractional 1540-nm laser quasi-ablation: an ex vivo and clinical evaluation. Lasers Med Sci 2013; 28: 537–542

[22] Geronemus RG. Fractional photothermolysis: current and future applications. Lasers Surg Med 2006; 38: 169–176

[23] Wanner M, Tanzi EL, Alster TS. Fractional photothermolysis: treatment of facial and nonfacial cutaneous photodamage with a 1,550-nm erbium-doped fiber laser. Dermatol Surg 2007; 33: 23–28

[24] Rahman Z, Alam M, Dover JS. Fractional laser treatment for pigmentation and texture improvement. Skin Therapy Lett 2006; 11: 7–11

[25] Glaich AS, Goldberg LH, Friedman RH, Friedman PM. Fractional photothermolysis for the treatment of postinflammatory erythema resulting from acne vulgaris. Dermatol Surg 2007; 33: 842–846

[26] Alster TS, Tanzi EL, Lazarus M. The use of fractional laser photothermolysis for the treatment of atrophic scars. Dermatol Surg 2007; 33: 295–299

[27] Chan NP, Ho SG, Yeung CK, Shek SY, Chan HH. The use of non-ablative fractional resurfacing in Asian acne scar patients. Lasers Surg Med 2010; 42: 710–715

[28] Chan HH. Effective and safe use of lasers, light sources, and radiofrequency devices in the clinical management of Asian patients with selected dermatoses. Lasers Surg Med 2005; 37: 179–185

[29] Lee HS, Lee JH, Ahn GY, et al. Fractional photothermolysis for the treatment of acne scars: a report of 27 Korean patients. J Dermatolog Treat 2008; 19: 45–49

[30] Lin JY, Warger WC, Izikson L, Anderson RR, Tannous Z. A prospective, randomized controlled trial on the efficacy of fractional photothermolysis on scar remodeling. Lasers Surg Med 2011; 43: 265–272

[31] Cohen SR, Henssler C, Horton K, Broder KW, Moise-Broder PA. Clinical experience with the Fraxel SR laser: 202 treatments in 59 consecutive patients. Plast Reconstr Surg 2008; 121: 297e–304e

[32] Behroozan DS, Goldberg LH, Dai T, Geronemus RG, Friedman PM. Fractional photothermolysis for the treatment of surgical scars: a case report. J Cosmet Laser Ther 2006; 8: 35–38

[33] Gan SD, Bae-Harboe YS, Graber EM. Nonablative fractional resurfacing for the treatment of iatrogenic hypopigmentation. Dermatol Surg 2014; 40: 87–89

[34] Glaich AS, Rahman Z, Goldberg LH, Friedman PM. Fractional resurfacing for the treatment of hypopigmented scars: a pilot study. Dermatol Surg 2007; 33: 289–294, discussion 293–294

[35] Massaki AB, Fabi SG, Fitzpatrick R. Repigmentation of hypopigmented scars using an erbium-doped 1,550-nm fractionated laser and topical bimatoprost. Dermatol Surg 2012; 38: 995–1001

[36] Pham AM, Greene RM, Woolery-Lloyd H, Kaufman J, Grunebaum LD. 1550-nm nonablative laser resurfacing for facial surgical scars. Arch Facial Plast Surg 2011; 13: 203–210

[37] Haedersdal M, Moreau KE, Beyer DM, Nymann P, Alsbjørn B. Fractional nonablative 1540 nm laser resurfacing for thermal burn scars: a randomized controlled trial. Lasers Surg Med 2009; 41: 189–195

[38] Stotland M, Chapas AM, Brightman L, et al. The safety and efficacy of fractional photothermolysis for the correction of striae distensae. J Drugs Dermatol 2008; 7: 857–861

[39] Kim BJ, Lee DH, Kim MN, et al. Fractional photothermolysis for the treatment of striae distensae in Asian skin. Am J Clin Dermatol 2008; 9: 33–37

[40] Wattanakrai P, Pootongkam S, Rojhirunsakool S. Periorbital rejuvenation with fractional 1,550-nm ytterbium/erbium fiber laser and variable square pulse 2,940-nm erbium:YAG laser in Asians: a comparison study. Dermatol Surg 2012; 38: 610–622

[41] Tannous ZS, Astner S. Utilizing fractional resurfacing in the treatment of therapy-resistant melasma. J Cosmet Laser Ther 2005; 7: 39–43

[42] Katz TM, Glaich AS, Goldberg LH, Firoz BF, Dai T, Friedman PM. Treatment of melasma using fractional photothermolysis: a report of eight cases with long-term follow-up. Dermatol Surg 2010; 36: 1273–1280

[43] Kouba DJ, Fincher EF, Moy RL. Nevus of Ota successfully treated by fractional photothermolysis using a fractionated 1440-nm Nd:YAG laser. Arch Dermatol 2008; 144: 156–158

[44] Behroozan DS, Goldberg LH, Glaich AS, Dai T, Friedman PM. Fractional photothermolysis for treatment of poikiloderma of civatte. Dermatol Surg 2006; 32: 298–301

[45] Izikson L, Anderson RR. Resolution of blue minocycline pigmentation of the face after fractional photothermolysis. Lasers Surg Med 2008; 40: 399–401

[46] Karsai S, Hammes S, Rütten A, Raulin C. Fractional photothermolysis for the treatment of granuloma annulare: a case report. Lasers Surg Med 2008; 40: 319–322

[47] Blankenship CM, Alster TS. Fractional photothermolysis of residual hemangioma. Dermatol Surg 2008; 34: 1112–1114

[48] Glaich AS, Goldberg LH, Dai T, Friedman PM. Fractional photothermolysis for the treatment of telangiectatic matting: a case report. J Cosmet Laser Ther 2007; 9: 101–103

[49] Marra DE, Pourrabbani S, Fincher EF, Moy RL. Fractional photothermolysis for the treatment of adult colloid milium. Arch Dermatol 2007; 143: 572–574

[50] Fisher GH, Geronemus RG. Short-term side effects of fractional photothermolysis. Dermatol Surg 2005; 31: 1245–1249, discussion 1249

[51] Graber EM, Tanzi EL, Alster TS. Side effects and complications of fractional laser photothermolysis: experience with 961 treatments. Dermatol Surg 2008; 34: 301–305, discussion 305–307

12 Lasers for Vascular Anomalies

Marcelo Hochman

12.1 Introduction

There are numerous vascular lesions that affect the skin and mucosa of the head and neck and they constitute some of the most common indications for the use of lasers. This chapter uses the accepted nomenclature to describe vascular anomalies as detailed by the International Society for the Study of Vascular Anomalies.[1] The discussion is limited to the most common of these anomalies and other frequently encountered facial vascular conditions for which laser therapy is appropriate.

The concept of selective photothermolysis by laser energy is detailed throughout this book and applies to treatment of vascular lesions as well. The target chromophore in the vascular lesion is oxyhemoglobin, with absorption peaks at 18, 542, and 577 nm. The thermal relaxation time is the cooling time of oxyhemoglobin and is proportional to the vessel diameter squared. By keeping the pulse duration equal to or less than the thermal relaxation time, thermal injury to the surrounding tissues is minimized. Devices with adjustable pulse durations allow for treatment of vessels of different sizes. Melanin has a broad absorption spectrum (250–1,200 nm) that unfortunately overlaps the peaks of oxyhemoglobin. This makes it difficult to treat vascular lesions in dark-skinned or tan individuals and needs to be taken into account in the parameters used. In addition, in order to see continued improvement in some anomalies, it is often necessary to employ high energy levels that exceed the calculation of the thermal relaxation time for blood vessels. In order to address this problem and the problem of heat accumulation by the energy absorption of melanin, cooling mechanisms have been added to the laser devices. By simultaneously cooling the skin before, during, and after the laser pulse, the unwanted heat accumulation is minimized and, additionally, patient comfort is increased. Laser spot size is another determinant of laser depth penetration. Larger spot sizes allow for greater penetration of larger fluences (energy per unit area, J/cm^2). Thus devices with adjustable spot sizes allow for treatment of vessels at different depths. The dynamic cooling devices increase the safety of using larger spot sizes.

The introduction of the pulsed dye laser (PDL) in 1989 revolutionized the treatment of vascular lesions and anomalies and has since been the gold standard. The first-generation PDL emitted laser light at 577 nm, coinciding with the last peak of oxyhemoglobin. Currently available PDLs emit a wavelength of 585 or 595 nm with longer pulse durations. The longer wavelengths and pulse durations allow for greater depth penetration but require higher fluences to compensate for lower absorption beyond 585 nm. Again, the dynamic cooling devices allow for safe-guarding the epidermis under these conditions. Despite being a major advancement, the PDL is still limited in the size of vessels it can coagulate and the depth of penetration of the beam. The therapeutically effective depth of penetration is estimated to be 0.07 mm from the epidermal-dermal junction with poor coagulation beyond 1.16 mm. The vessel size and depth of vessels may be an explanation for the resistance of port-wine stains (PWS, capillary malformations) to treatment and/or incomplete clearance despite multiple PDL procedures. The

same can be said for decreased effectiveness in treating proliferating superficial infantile hemangiomas or the superficial component of compound hemangiomas greater than 3 mm in thickness. Thus it is common for several devices to be used during an extended treatment protocol to address the heterogeneity in vessel size and depth within the vascular lesion. Therapy is first initiated with shorter wavelengths and pulses to target the typical small-diameter (30–50 µm) vessels. Thereafter, longer wavelengths and pulses can be used to target the larger and deeper blood vessels. Laser systems with longer wavelengths currently used for treatment of vascular lesions are the neodymium:yttrium aluminum garnet (Nd:YAG) (1,064 nm) and long-pulsed alexandrite (755 nm). Although not a longer wavelength, the frequency-doubled, potassium titanyl phosphate (KTP) (532 nm) can also be used.

The Nd:YAG, a continuous wave infrared laser (1,064 nm), is not ideal for treating cutaneous vascular lesions due to deep penetration (4–6 mm) and preferential damage to arteries rather than veins. Thermal injury of these deeper vessels may lead to dermal necrosis with increased risk of scarring. This higher risk is thought to be due to partial conversion of oxyhemoglobin to methemoglobin causing a very steep fluence-response curve leading to rapid skin temperature and purpuric changes. The Nd:YAG laser induces shrinkage of vascular lesions by nonspecific thermal damage so it is used primarily for deeper (not cutaneous) lesions such as venous malformations. Delivery of the wavelength transmucosally or interstitially through a bare quartz fiber via a puncture, however, are useful techniques.

The long-pulsed alexandrite has selective absorption of deoxyhemoglobin and 50 to 75% deeper tissue penetration than PDL. The 755-nm wavelength may be used alone or in combination with PDL for improved efficacy of treatment-resistant PWS or hypertrophic lesions without an increase in complications. Permanent hair reduction is a potential side effect of which patients must be warned.

The 532-nm KTP laser emits green light near the 542-nm hemoglobin absorption peak but is absorbed by melanin more than the PDL, which may lead to higher rates of scarring and dyspigmentation. However, at low fluences and longer pulses of 10 to 50 ms, superficial facial vessels respond very well with little morbidity.

12.2 Treatment of Specific Vascular Lesions

12.2.1 Infantile Hemangiomas

Infantile hemangiomas (IHs) are the most common benign tumors of infancy. They have a peculiar, extensively reviewed[2,3] natural history characterized by rapid postnatal proliferation of the tumor followed by variable involution. IHs are classified by degree of involvement of the dermis, with superficial IHs involving the upper layers, deep IHs the lower dermis, and compound IHs (► Fig. 12.1) having both a superficial and deep

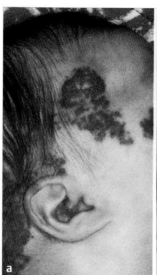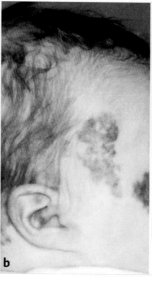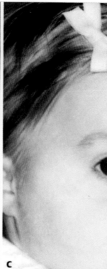

Fig. 12.1 Compound proliferating infantile hemangioma (IH) (**a**) before, (**b**) during, and (**c**) after treatment of the superficial component with the pulsed dye laser (PDL).

component. Multimodality therapy is the norm and involves combinations of observation, laser treatment, medical therapy, and/or surgery. The role of laser therapy can be to effect total resolution of the macular proliferative lesion, retard the proliferation, and/or treat the superficial residuum of involution. Given the excellent safety profile and selectivity of its wavelength, the PDL is the treatment of choice for the superficial component of proliferating and involuting IHs in these children. As discussed, depth of penetration of the 585-nm wavelength is limited; therefore, it is most effective in treating the superficial component that is < 3 mm in thickness. It has been shown to achieve > 95% reduction in proliferating thin lesions after four treatments (7 mm spot size, 1.5–3 ms pulse duration, and up to 10 J/cm^2) spaced 1 month apart versus 85% reduction in color with little change in thickness with the same parameters in those > 3 mm in thickness. So, the PDL has more of a chance of penetrating the entirety of the lesion leading to photocoagulation, cell death, and clearance—the thinner the superficial component. Treatment of thicker lesions leads to reduction in the color but not necessarily in the volume. The PDL, or any interstitial delivery of laser energy, has no proven role in the treatment of the deep component of focal, deep, or compound IHs.[4]

Approximately 10% of proliferating IHs ulcerate, most commonly involving segmental IHs of the perineal area and focal lesions of the lip. The open wounds are painful and, in the diaper area, compounded by soiling and constant need for cleaning. Treatment of ulcerated IHs (▶ Fig. 12.2) involves local wound care, pain management, and laser therapy. The PDL is extremely effective in healing the ulcers in as few as one to two treatments spaced 7 to 10 days apart. A 7 or 10 mm spot size is used with a short pulse duration (1.5 ms–3 ms) and high fluence (10 J/cm^2).[5] Propranolol, a beta-antagonist, has become the first line of medical therapy for IH and is useful in treatment of complicated IHs. The mechanism of action is thought to be by inhibition of vasodilation thus causing vasoconstriction of the IH capillaries, reduction in angiogenesis by downregulation of vascular endothelial factor A, and induction of apoptosis. It is useful in both the proliferative and involution phases of the IH natural course.[6]

Segmental facial IHs (▶ Fig. 12.3) treated concurrently with propranolol and the PDL show more rapid and complete

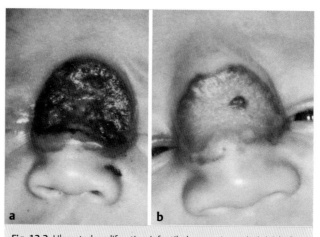

Fig. 12.2 Ulcerated proliferating infantile hemangioma (IH) (**a**) before and (**b**) after two treatments with the pulsed dye laser (PDL). Once the ulceration is healed, the stage is set for more definitive multimodality procedures to achieve a final result.

clearance than those treated with either alone.[7] This approach is more desirable than the use of longer wavelength lasers with deeper penetration due to the risk of epidermal scarring in these young children.

During involution or after it is complete, the PDL is still the laser of choice to reduce the color of the superficial component or treat residual telangiectasias. For the latter, the KTP is also effective. The PDL can also be used to treat residual erythema of scars resulting from surgical approaches used in the management of IH. Very conservative laser resurfacing with the carbon dioxide laser can be used for scar camouflage as well.

12.2.2 Malformations

Malformations, in distinction to IH, are always present at birth, grow commensurate with the patient, and never regress. They are a result of congenital errors in vasculogenesis and are classified by the vessels involved (venous, capillaries, arterial, lymphatic, etc.). These lesions have been extensively reviewed elsewhere as well.[8]

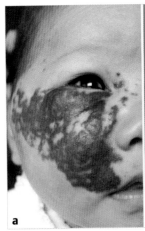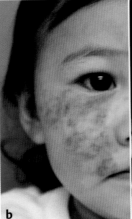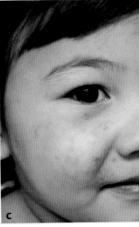

Fig. 12.3 Segmental proliferating infantile hemangioma (IH) (**a**) before, (**b**) during, and (**c**) after concomitant propranolol and pulsed dye laser (PDL) treatments.

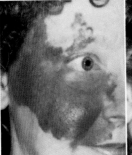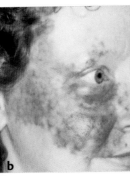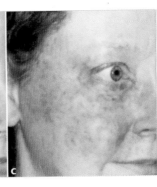

Fig. 12.4 Capillary malformation (port-wine stain [PWS]) (**a**) before, (**b**) during, and (**c**) after 13 pulsed dye laser (PDL) treatments.

Port-Wine Stains

PWS (▶ Fig. 12.4) are a type of vascular malformation, specifically a capillary malformation composed of ectatic vessels in the papillary dermis. Over time, these vessels expand leading to hypertrophy of the involved tissues, nodules, and disfigurement. Avoiding these changes is the impetus for early treatment. PWS most commonly involve the face along the cutaneous distributions of the trigeminal nerve but can be found anywhere on the body. The presence of a PWS in the ophthalmic dermatome merits special attention because 25% of affected children will have an associated ipsilateral vascular malformation of the leptomeninges. This association is known as Sturge-Weber syndrome.

The mainstay of treatment of capillary malformations is laser photocoagulation with the PDL. There is universal improvement in the PWS with laser treatments but only about 20% total clearance. Early treatment leads to better results because the skin of infants is more translucent, the vessels are smaller, and the PWS occupies a smaller surface area.[9,10] The heterogeneity of the vasculature is compounded by variations in optical characteristics of the skin of various parts of the face and among patients, making it difficult to define ideal parameters to achieve maximal clearance. Central face PWS respond less well than those of the lateral face and neck. PWS involving the extremities and lower body respond less well than those of the upper chest. When therapy is first initiated, smaller vessels are targeted with shorter wavelengths and pulse durations. Thereafter, and based on response, longer wavelengths (long-pulsed alexandrite) and pulses are used to target the larger, deeper vessels. The combination of PDL and alexandrite laser therapy produces more rapid results without an increase in complications.[11] The Nd:YAG may be used very judiciously to treat individual hypertrophic nodules.

Venous Malformations

Venous malformations (VMs) (▶ Fig. 12.5) are the most common malformations of the head and neck and the most commonly misdiagnosed as hemangiomas.[12] They are slow-flow lesions that can involve almost any anatomical space and typically present as bluish discolorations of the skin or mucosa with a soft and compressible deep component. They can be small and inconsequential for long periods of time or grow into muscles, viscera, and across multiple spaces leading to marked disfigurement and functional impairment. They are the malformations most commonly associated with coagulopathies. Superficial cutaneous lesions or the mucocutaneous portion of complex lesions may be photocoagulated with the PDL. The Nd:YAG is particularly useful for transmucosal treatment of lip, tongue, and buccal mucosal lesions using a bare fiber in noncontact mode. Power settings of up to 20 W and 0.5 to 1.5 seconds duration pulses are common. Interstitial laser therapy with the same settings is very helpful to induce shrinkage of tongue lesions by thermal injury. There is potential risk to neural structures since the thermal zone of injury is not predictable. To avoid this, the fiber is kept in motion and not allowed to linger in one place. Multiple passes in different directions are used. VMs of the parotid space should not be treated with this modality due to unpredictable risk to the facial nerve. Percutaneous sclerotherapy under image guidance with a variety of agents has become the mainstay of therapy for VMs. It may be

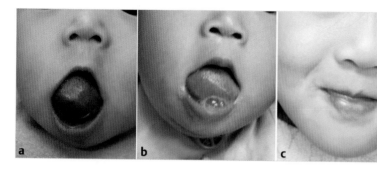

Fig. 12.5 Venous malformation (VM) of the tongue (a) before, (b) during, and (c) after interstitial neodymium:yttrium aluminum garnet (Nd:YAG) laser therapy and concomitant sclerotherapy over a period of 3 years. The child has been decannulated of her tracheotomy.

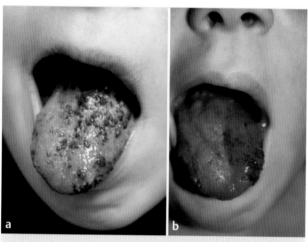

Fig. 12.6 Microcystic lymphatic malformation (LM) of the tongue (a) before, and (b) 1 year after carbon dioxide laser resurfacing. Note early recurrence/persistence of cysts that will be re-treated as they become symptomatic.

used as the primary modality or as an adjunct to laser and surgical therapy.

Lymphatic Malformations

Lymphatic malformations (LMs) (▶ Fig. 12.6) are low-flow, relatively uncommon lesions that are descriptively classified as macrocystic, microcystic, or mixed. The clinical presentation is varied ranging from focal superficial skin lesions to diffuse, infiltrative lesions of multiple anatomical spaces. The clinical course ranges from innocuous to life-threatening lesions. As with other malformations, the overall clinical course is relentless, variable progression with bouts of acute exacerbation due to infection or trauma. Sclerotherapy or surgery for macrocystic lesions and surgery for microcystic lesions is the norm. Laser therapy is confined to resurfacing of mucosal lesions with the carbon dioxide laser in ablative mode.[13] The depth of ablation is determined visually with the goal being to obliterate the spaces and allow remucosalization. The procedures are repeated as the lesions recur and become symptomatic. Relief between treatments is often measured in years.

Facial Telangiectasias

Facial telangiectasias and erythema are among the most common indications for cutaneous laser therapy. They are small-diameter (0.1–1.0 mm) vessels that appear as simple, linear,

superficial blue or red vessels or as a collection of vessels appearing as a field of erythema and commonly located in the midface, cheeks, and chin. Likewise, spider telangiectasias are typically located on the cheeks and consist of radially branching linear vessels emanating from a central arteriole. Telangiectasias are very effectively treated with a variety of laser systems. The PDL, KTP, diode (800, 810, and 930 nm), and long-pulsed alexandrite lasers are all effective. Vessel clearance can be accomplished with stacking pulses of lower fluence and longer duration, obviating the need for posttreatment purpura in cosmetically sensitive patients. Procedures are spaced 4 to 6 weeks apart.[14]

12.3 Conclusion

Advances in laser technology have allowed for more selective photothermolysis and more efficient therapeutic responses with less risk. Currently, lasers play an integral role in the management of vascular anomalies. Clinical trials are ongoing in the use of lasers in addition to topical and systemic medical therapy to modulate the wound-healing response and revascularization of skin. These may open the door for further improvement in results and options for treatment of cutaneous vascular lesions.[15,16]

References

[1] ISSVA Classification. International Society for the Study of Vascular Anomalies. April 2014. Available at: http: issva.org/content.aspx?page_id=22&club_id=298433&module_id=152904. Accessed May 2014

[2] Hochman M, Adams DM, Reeves TD. Current knowledge and management of vascular anomalies: I. hemangiomas. Arch Facial Plast Surg 2011; 13: 145–151

[3] Burns AJ, Navarro JA, Cooner RD. Classification of vascular anomalies and the comprehensive treatment of hemangiomas. Plast Reconstr Surg 2009; 124 Suppl: 69e–81e

[4] Burns AJ, Navarro JA. Role of laser therapy in pediatric patients. Plast Reconstr Surg 2009; 124 Suppl: 82e–92e

[5] Thomas RF, Hornung RL, Manning SC, Perkins JA. Hemangiomas of infancy: treatment of ulceration in the head and neck. Arch Facial Plast Surg 2005; 7: 312–315

[6] Storch CH, Hoeger PH. Propranolol for infantile haemangiomas: insights into the molecular mechanisms of action. Br J Dermatol 2010; 163: 269–274

[7] Reddy KK, Blei F, Brauer JA, et al. Retrospective study of the treatment of infantile hemangiomas using a combination of propranolol and pulsed dye laser. Dermatol Surg 2013; 39: 923–933

[8] Hochman M, Adams DM, Reeves TD. Current knowledge and management of vascular anomalies, II: malformations. Arch Facial Plast Surg 2011; 13: 425–433

[9] Ortiz AE, Nelson JS. Port-wine stain laser treatments and novel approaches. Facial Plast Surg 2012; 28: 611–620

[10] Chapas AM, Eickhorst K, Geronemus RG. Efficacy of early treatment of facial port wine stains in newborns: a review of 49 cases. Lasers Surg Med 2007; 39: 563–568

[11] Izikson L, Nelson JS, Anderson RR. Treatment of hypertrophic and resistant port wine stains with a 755 nm laser: a case series of 20 patients. Lasers Surg Med 2009; 41: 427–432

[12] Hassanein AH, Mulliken JB, Fishman SJ, Greene AK. Evaluation of terminology for vascular anomalies in current literature. Plast Reconstr Surg 2011; 127: 347–351

[13] Glade RS, Buckmiller LM. CO2 laser resurfacing of intraoral lymphatic malformations: a 10-year experience. Int J Pediatr Otorhinolaryngol 2009; 73: 1358–1361

[14] Geronemus RG. Treatment of spider telangiectasias in children using the flashlamp-pumped pulsed dye laser. Pediatr Dermatol 1991; 8: 61–63

[15] Jia W, Sun V, Tran N, et al. Long-term blood vessel removal with combined laser and topical rapamycin antiangiogenic therapy: implications for effective port wine stain treatment. Lasers Surg Med 2010; 42: 105–112

[16] Tremaine AM, Armstrong J, Huang YC, et al. Enhanced port-wine stain lightening achieved with combined treatment of selective photothermolysis and imiquimod. J Am Acad Dermatol 2012; 66: 634–641

13 Treatment of Acne Rosacea

David A. F. Ellis and Tee Sin Lee

13.1 Definition of Acne Rosacea

Acne rosacea is a chronic, inherited cutaneous condition involving persistent erythema of the convexities of the central face (cheeks, chin, nose, and central forehead) lasting for at least 3 months, and is characterized by remissions and exacerbations. It is considered a syndrome encompassing a broad spectrum of clinical signs described as primary and secondary features.[1] Primary features include flushing (transient erythema), nontransient erythema, papules and pustules, and telangiectasia. Secondary features include burning or stinging, plaque, dry appearance, edema, ocular manifestations, peripheral location, and phymatous changes. A typical patient presents with some but not all of the possible manifestations. Understanding the disease is of importance because of its prevalence, as well as significant lifestyle and treatment implications associated with the diagnosis.

13.2 Classification

In 2002, an expert committee assembled by the National Rosacea Society explicitly defined and classified rosacea into four subtypes and one variant.[1] Evolution from one subtype to another may or may not occur.

- *Subtype 1*: Erythematotelangiectatic—flushing and persistent central facial erythema with or without telangiectasia
- *Subtype 2*: Papulopustular—persistent central facial erythema with transient, central facial papules/pustules
- *Subtype 3*: Phymatous—thickened skin, irregular surface nodularities, and enlargement; may occur on the nose, chin, forehead, cheeks, or ears
- *Subtype 4*: Ocular—foreign-body sensation in the eye, burning or stinging, dryness, itching, ocular photosensitivity, blurred vision, telangiectasia of the sclera, periorbital edema
- *Variant*: Granulomatous—noninflammatory; hard; brown, yellow, or red cutaneous papules; or nodules of uniform size

13.3 Pathophysiology, Epidemiology, and Impact

Although rosacea has been described since the 14th century[2] and has been one of the most common skin disorders, its pathogenesis remains unclear and controversial and has also been the subject of prolonged study. However, there are several key components in its development and these include[3]:

- Vasculature
- Climatic exposures (wind and sun)
- Dermal matrix degeneration and endothelial damage
- Molecular biological changes resulting in angiogenesis and vascular leakage
- Neoangiogenesis and vascular endothelial growth factor (VEGF) overexpression
- Chemicals and ingested agents
- Microorganisms (*Demodex* species)
- Reactive oxygen species

There is also a strong hereditary component. In a study in 1996 by the National Rosacea Society, nearly 40% of the respondents indicated they had a family member who also suffered from rosacea.[4] The condition is often called the "curse of the Celts" because it is most common in fair-skinned, fair-haired people of western or northern European descent. However, it can also occur in Asians and African Americans who have darker skin.[1] Rosacea occurs in both men and women, with the onset typically after age 30. Before age 30, people who have extremely red-flushed cheeks through exercise may have rosacea. Unfortunately, there has been no affirmative etiology accounting for this condition.

Rosacea has a major psychosocial impact on patients' quality of life.[5] They are often left with feelings of self-consciousness and isolation. According to the National Rosacea Society, 76% had lowered self-confidence and self-esteem, 65% felt frustrated with the condition, and 41% reported that it had caused them to avoid social gatherings.

13.4 Treatment

There is currently no definitive cure for rosacea. There are only treatment modalities to control the symptoms and to keep them quiescent. The management spans a broad spectrum of therapeutic options due to its complexity. Fluctuations in symptoms, relapses, and the progressive nature of the disease necessitate a detailed understanding of the available treatment options and their corresponding appropriate usage. It is also important to understand that since there is a wide spectrum of disease manifestation, success in treatment may require multiple combined treatment modalities.

Rosacea management can be divided into lifestyle modification, skin care management, pharmacotherapy, laser treatment, and surgery.

13.4.1 Lifestyle Modification

Patients' education is of paramount importance because the disease is likely to wax and wane and accompany them for a long time. They should fully understand the nature of the disease and take control of their management. It is the role of the patient that plays a more vital role than the role of the physician. A more educated and motivated patient is one who will more likely obtain a better result.

Flare-ups and exacerbations of rosacea often appear to be triggered by environmental or lifestyle factors and most are related to flushing. Some of the most common triggers are: sun exposure, emotional stress, hot or cold weather, wind, heavy exercise, alcohol consumption, hot baths, spicy foods, humidity, indoor heat, certain skin care products, heated beverages, certain cosmetics, medications, medical conditions, and certain foods.[6] However, not every trigger affects every patient and the triggers are unique to each individual patient; hence avoidance of every potential factor is unnecessary and impractical. Various studies show that the percentages of patients affected with the various conditions may vary. In a survey by the National Rosacea Society in 2010, alcohol was a trigger for 76% of the patients, with red wine being the most common at 72%, followed by white wine at 49%, and then beer at 42%.[7]

An appropriate management strategy is to take a thorough history to evaluate for the presence of any identifiable triggering agents before initiation of any medical, laser, or surgical therapy. Patients can identify their triggers by keeping a record of the possible rosacea triggers and matching them with their flare-ups of signs and symptoms. In unscientific surveys of patients with rosacea who identified and avoided their personal rosacea triggers, more than 90% reported that their condition had improved in varying degrees.[8]

13.4.2 Skin Care Management

Use of Skin Care and Cosmetic Products

Because rosacea patients have skin that is very sensitive and easily irritated resulting in redness, inflammation, and stinging, everyday skin care to maintain the integrity of the skin barrier while avoiding agents that aggravate or trigger flushing is an important component of rosacea management. It is therefore essential for them to select the mildest and most appropriate skin care products that do not irritate their skin. A useful rule of thumb is to select products that contain no sensory-provoking ingredients, no volatile substances, no minor irritants or allergens, minimal botanical agents, and no unnecessary ingredients. The same principles apply for cosmetic products. They should be advised to avoid any products that cause burning, stinging, itching, or other discomfort. They should also be advised against astringents, toners, menthols, camphor, and waterproof cosmetics that are difficult to remove and require the use of harsh agents that may induce more irritation. New cosmetics should be regularly purchased to minimize microbial contamination and degradation. Brushes are preferred over sponges to avoid abrasion and also brushes can be easily cleaned to decrease bacterial contamination.[9]

Sunscreen

The use of daily broad-spectrum sunscreen is recommended for all patients with rosacea,[10] with protection against both ultraviolet A (UVA) and ultraviolet B (UVB) light. Physical blocking agents such as titanium oxide and zinc oxide can also be used. In addition, the sunscreen should contain protective silicones such as dimethicone or cyclomethicone.

Specialized Skin Care Products

There are two groups of skin care products targeted at patients with rosacea. One is over-the-counter products and the other is a therapeutic line labeled as medical-grade skin care products, which are typically distributed under the care of a treating physician.

Pyratine XR System

This is a moisturizing lotion containing furfuryl tetrahydropyranyladenine as PRK-124 (0.125%, Pyratine XR, Senetek PLC, Napa, California) that is used twice daily for 12 and 48 weeks, and has

been found to be effective for the treatment of mild to moderate rosacea without irritating the skin.[11,12] It is a plant cytokinin shown to have growth modulatory, antioxidative, and antisenescent effects on human skin cells. It reduces redness by inhibiting the enzyme kallikrein, a known and highly significant contributor to a normal inflammatory response. This treatment regimen also decreases skin transepidermal water loss and increases skin moisture content with no evidence of skin irritation, and hence improves the skin barrier function that is compromised in rosacea. It has been shown to significantly reduce erythema by 22% at week 12, with continuous improvement to 45% at week 36. Skin papules and pustules were dramatically reduced by 21% at week 4 with a further 89.5% decrease at week 48. Telangiectasias were decreased by 12% at week 4, with continuous improvement to 27.8% at week 36.

Revaleskin Care Line

The Revaleskin (Revaleskin Products, Inc., Richmond, Virginia) is a medical-grade skin care line marketed for its ability to improve wrinkles, fine lines, and discoloration. The active ingredient is CoffeeBerry whole fruit extract, which is an agent derived from the fruit of the coffee plant, *Coffea arabica*. This extract is rich in polyphenol antioxidants such as chlorogenic acid, condensed proanthocyanidins, quinic acid, and ferulic acid. In general, topical antioxidants exert their effects by downregulating free radical-mediated pathways that damage skin.[13]

Avène Pathology System

Avène (Pierre Fabre Laboratories, France) is a skin care line consisting of four products. First, there is Redness-Relief Dermo-Cleansing Milk for redness-prone sensitive skin. This product contains Ruscus extract that improves microcirculation, dextran sulfate for decongestion and minimizing swelling, hesperidin methyl chalcone (HMC) that protects and strengthens vascular walls, and Avène thermal spring water that is soothing and anti-irritating. The second product is Diroseal, which is an anti-redness night lotion. It contains retinaldehyde that increases epidermal thickness and prevents neoangiogenesis, and also contains dextran sulfate and HMC. The third product is a Redness Relief Soothing Cream with SPF 25 to be used daily. It contains Ruscus extract, HMC, dextran sulfate, Avène thermal spring water, and titanium dioxide. The last product is the Antirougeurs FORT Relief Concentrate, which is to be used daily as an intensive treatment for affected areas following Redness Relief Soothing Cream with SPF 25. It contains saponin-enriched Ruscus extract that acts as a vasoconstrictor that improves cutaneous microcirculation with anti-inflammatory and antiangiogenic properties (reduces VEGF), HMC, and dextran sulfate.

13.4.3 Pharmacotherapy

The goals of pharmacotherapy are to reduce morbidity, minimize irritative symptoms, achieve longevity in disease control, and prevent complications. These can be divided into prescriptive topical and oral medications.

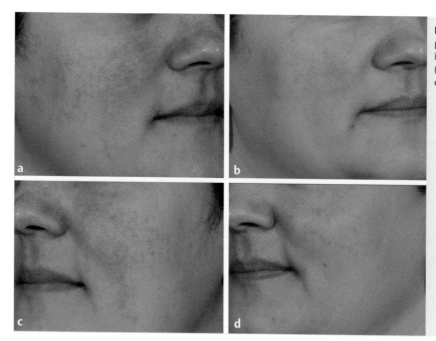

Fig. 13.1 Before (**a, c**) and after (**b, d**) images of a patient with persistent erythema, papules, and intermittent pustules treated with Finacea gel (azelaic acid 15%) (Bayer HealthCare Pharmaceuticals Inc., Whippany, New Jersey).

Topical

Topical medications are mainly used to treat papules, pustules, and early phymatous changes, and include antibiotics, acne agents, immunosuppressants, retinoid agents, and corticosteroids.

The use of antibiotics has been common since the 1950s because microorganisms were thought to be the underlying cause of the disease. However, although treatment philosophy has evolved and bacterial infection is no longer thought to play a major part in the pathogenesis, oral and topical agents continue to be used alone or in combination because of their demonstrated efficacy and also for their anti-inflammatory properties. Topical metronidazole gel 0.75 or 1% is an imidazole, ring-based antibiotic active against various anaerobic bacteria and protozoa and is helpful for mild disease and as an adjuvant to systemic therapy. Erythromycin 2% topical solution is an alternative. Topical clindamycin inhibits bacteria growth by arresting ribonucleic acid (RNA)-dependent protein synthesis; when applied to the skin, it is converted to an active component that inhibits the microorganism, and is effective against mild to moderate papulopustular rosacea.

Agents that have been used to treat acne can be used to treat patients with pustules, papules, and the phymatous type of rosacea. Benzoyl peroxide is converted into benzoic acid when applied to skin and has keratolytic and comedolytic effects. Administration results in free-radical oxygen release that oxidizes bacteria proteins in sebaceous follicles, decreasing the quantity of irritating free fatty acids and anaerobic bacteria. Azelaic acid, which is available in two strengths (15% gel, Finacea [Bayer HealthCare Pharmaceuticals Inc., Whippany, New Jersey]; 20% cream, Azelex [Allergan, Inc., Irvine, California]), has been found to be effective against mild to moderate papulopustular rosacea (▶ Fig. 13.1).[14] It works by reducing the production of reactive oxygen species by neutrophils, decreasing the growth of microorganisms by inhibiting protein synthesis,

and inhibiting follicular keratinization, which may prevent development of comedones. Some patients may report transient burning or stinging. Sodium sulfacetamide and sulfur have also been used topically to treat rosacea. The former has antibacterial properties and the latter is antiseptic with keratolytic action.

The rationale of using an immunosuppressant in rosacea is to inhibit immune reactions resulting from diverse stimuli. Tacrolimus ointment (Protopic) comes in 0.03 and 0.1% and reduces itching and inflammation by suppressing release of cytokines from T cells. It also inhibits transcription of genes encoding IL–3, IL–4, IL–5, and tumor necrosis factor (TNF)-alpha, all of which are involved in early stages of T-cell activation, and inhibits release of preformed mediators from skin mast cells and basophils. It may be of value in treating erythema from active inflammation,[15] but it has been reported to induce a rosacealike eruption.[16] It may not be effective against papules and pustules.

Topical retinoids (tretinoin) have been found to be effective as an adjunct to the management of recalcitrant rosacea.[17] Although effective, recurrence is common; and some patients may experience skin irritation. They inhibit comedones' formation and make keratinocytes in sebaceous follicles less adherent and easier to remove. There is also evidence that they may decrease fibrosis, elastosis, and sebaceous gland hypertrophy.[18]

In certain circumstances, short-term use of a low-strength topical steroid may be considered for rapid resolution of inflammation. However, long-term use often produces rosacealike manifestations (steroid-induced rosacea), and hence should be avoided.

In August 2013, the Food and Drug Administration (FDA) approved brimonidine topical gel for the treatment of erythema associated with rosacea. Brimonidine topical gel users were demonstrated to have significantly greater improvement in facial redness of rosacea than those who used vehicle-controlled gel alone.[19]

Oral

Oral medications include antibiotics targeted at papulopustular rosacea, antiflushing agents aimed at erythematotelangiectatic rosacea, and retinoids targeted at phymatous rosacea.

Oral metronidazole has been shown to be beneficial against papules and pustules, and can be used in combination with the topical form. Erythromycin oral or 2% topical solution inhibits bacterial growth on a molecular level and has proven efficacy in treating ocular rosacea.[20] Tetracyclines and doxycycline are used mainly for their anti-inflammatory properties. The nonantibiotic dosing of doxycycline has become the first-line treatment for many clinicians since 2006. Evidence has suggested that the regimen of 20 to 50 mg of doxycycline every 12 hours is as effective as the older regimen of 100 mg of doxycycline.[21] This could represent a significant cost reduction for many patients. A controlled-release formulation of oral doxycycline is FDA-approved for rosacea with low plasma levels that do not exert antimicrobial effects while retaining anti-inflammatory activity.[22] Topical therapy and/or a controlled-release oral therapy may be used for mild to moderate disease. For severe disease, an oral antibiotic may be used initially with a topical to bring it under control and, once control is achieved, it may be maintained with a topical or controlled-release agent alone for an indefinite period. In some cases, oral tetracycline may be prescribed for patients with ocular involvement; and in some refractory cases, off-label oral trimethoprim-sulfamethoxazole, ampicillin, clindamycin, or dapsone may be used.

There are currently no drugs approved by the FDA to reduce flushing in rosacea; however, certain off-label use may have a moderating effect for moderate to severe flushing. Because there are no broad-spectrum, antiflushing medications, those specific to the cause of flushing should be chosen.[23] Flushing is caused by vasodilation due to an abnormality of cutaneous vascular smooth muscle control that is controlled by circulating vasoactive agents or by autonomic nerves. Antihistamines, aspirin, and other nonsteroidal anti-inflammatory drugs may be used to mediate flushing caused by excessive vasoactive agents. When flushing occurs with sweating, it is usually caused by stimulation of the autonomic system (heat from surroundings, food, or exercise), and can be reduced by cooling of the neck and face with a cold, wet towel or fan, or by avoiding the precipitating factors. In severe cases, alpha-2 agonist clonidine or a beta blocker such as nadolol may be used to reduce neurally mediated flushing. Hormone replacement therapy can be given for women with flushing due to menopause. Oral contraceptives may be helpful in patients who have worsening symptoms with their menstrual cycle. Finally, flushing may have emotional origins and these patients may benefit from psychological counseling or biofeedback.

Isotretinoin, which inhibits sebaceous gland function and keratinization, has been demonstrated to decrease nasal volume in younger patients with less advanced disease, although the volume may increase again after therapy is stopped.[24] During the treatment, numerous large sebaceous glands were reported to be diminished in size and number. Hence it is used in refractory cases of papulopustular rosacea and early stages of phymatous change, when the patulous follicles of incipient rhinophyma are present without contour changes. However, this requires careful monitoring, and long-lasting remission is not common.

13.5 Lasers

Laser therapy has been an effective modality for rosacea patients because of the positive therapeutic effects such as dermal connective tissue remodeling and enhancing the robustness of the epidermal barrier.[25] It is an excellent tool because it can be used to treat the wide spectrum of rosacea manifestations such as flushing, persistent erythema, telangiectasias, and phymatous changes.

13.5.1 Persistent Erythema and Flushing

Intense pulsed light (IPL) is a broad-spectrum polychromatic light-emitting device (515–1,200 nm) that produces high-intensity light during a very short period of time. Its wavelength is controlled by filters, and consequently has multiple targets including melanin and hemoglobin. Adjusting the filters can alter the wavelength to target more of melanin or hemoglobin depending on the objective of the treatment. Traditional IPL filters have a tendency to wear out, whereas the IPL system Limelight by Cutera (Cutera, San Francisco, California) uses real-time calibration to deliver accurate and consistent energy levels. IPL has been shown to be very effective in reducing persistent facial erythema.[26] More recently, the use of Laser Genesis (Cutera), which is a neodymium:yttrium aluminum garnet (Nd:YAG) 1,064-nm wavelength with a patented 300-μs technology, has been combined with the use of IPL. Laser Genesis alone has been shown to reduce erythema and induce new collagen production in the papillary dermis to improve the appearance of wrinkles after three treatment sessions at 1 and 3 months.[27] When combined with IPL, the two lasers have yielded excellent results in reducing facial erythema and flushing in the authors' practice (▶ Fig. 13.2). Laser Genesis is characterized by high-powered 300-μs pulses, high repetition, and the main target is

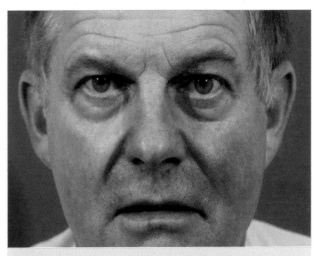

Fig. 13.2 Split-face treatment for facial erythema. Right side of face treated with a combination of intense pulsed light (IPL) system Limelight (Cutera, San Francisco, California) mode A 14 J/cm² and Laser Genesis (Cutera) neodymium:yttrium aluminum garnet (Nd:YAG) 16 J/cm², 5-mm spot size, 0.3 ms at three sessions. Left side of face not treated.

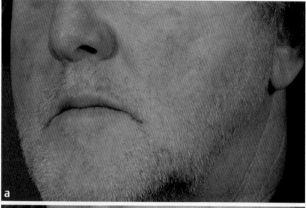

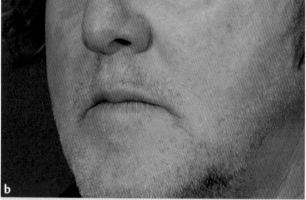

Fig. 13.3 Before (**a**) and after (**b**) images of a patient with erythematotelangiectatic rosacea treated with Limelight (Cutera, San Francisco, California) mode B 18 J/cm2 at five sessions and Excel (Cutera) neodymium:yttrium aluminum garnet (Nd:YAG) 125 to 160 J/cm2 at two sessions.

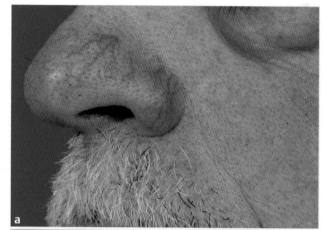

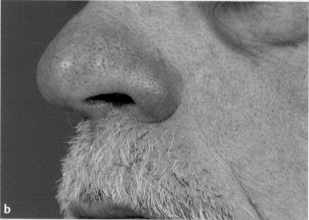

Fig. 13.4 Before (**a**) and after (**b**) images of a patient with nasal telangiectasias treated with Excel (Cutera, San Francisco, California) neodymium:yttrium aluminum garnet (Nd:YAG) 105 to160 J/cm², 5-mm spot size, 10 ms at one session.

the blood vessels in the upper dermis. A spot size of 5 mm allows deep energy absorption to papillary and reticular dermis. Hence, by delivering several thousand micro-pulses, these blood vessels and, in turn, the dermis heat up. Fibroblasts are activated as a result of the heating and new collagen formation is stimulated. This also results in the closure of the tiny blood vessels and improves erythema and flushing associated with rosacea. An average of 8,000 to 10,000 pulses at a fluence of 14 to 17 J/cm² at a 5- to 10-Hz repetitive rate is used for full-face treatment with the end point being erythema or moderate discomfort. A series of five to six treatments are recommended at 2 to 4 weeks apart. With this technology, the epidermis is protected and is safe for dark-skinned patients. There is only minimal discomfort during the process and it involves no downtime, with only mild erythema that lasts for a few hours posttreatment.

13.5.2 Telangiectasias

Telangiectasias are effectively treated with vascular lasers. These include the pulsed dye laser (PDL) (585 or 595 nm), the potassium titanyl phosphate laser (532 nm), the diode-pumped, frequency-doubled laser (532 nm), and IPL. Lasers in these wavelengths selectively target oxyhemoglobin as their chromophore, resulting in vessel reduction with minimal scarring and

collateral damage to surrounding tissues. However, for deeper facial vessels and for bluish vessels (these tend to have slower blood flow, greater depth beneath the skin surface, and greater vessel diameter), longer wavelengths are required, and these include the diode laser (810 nm), the long-pulsed alexandrite laser (755 nm), and the long-pulsed Nd:YAG laser (1,064 nm). We use the Excel Nd:YAG laser (Cutera) that can penetrate 8 mm rather than the 2 mm reached by the PDLs, and it has a longer pulse duration.

Rosacea vessels can be found at the epidermal and dermal layers. Hence we recommend that for the superficial epidermal vessels, the Limelight (IPL) can be used at a fluence of 15 to 18 J/cm² using either mode A (520 nm) or mode B (540 nm) (▶ Fig. 13.3). For the deeper dermal vessels, the Excel Nd:YAG is recommended at a fluence of 140 to 165 J/cm² using 3- to 5-mm spot size and 10- to 15-ms pulse width (▶ Fig. 13.4). A polarized lens can be used to better define the vessels. If the deep vessels appear more reddish, the fluence can be increased when there is inadequate response. If they appear more bluish, the fluence can be decreased and pulse duration increased to achieve better result (fluence of 100 to 150 J/cm² and a pulse duration of 30 ms).

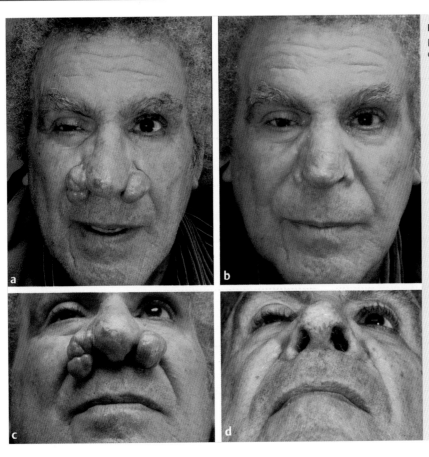

Fig. 13.5 Before (**a, c**) and after (**b, d**) images of a patient with rhinophyma treated with electrocautery recontouring surgery.

13.5.3 Phymatous Changes

Ablative lasers such as the erbium:yttrium scandium gallium garnet (Er:YSGG) and carbon dioxide laser have demonstrated efficacy in the treatment of midfacial thickening and early stages of rhinophyma. They are used as bloodless scalpels to remove excess tissue and recontour the nose. They also have beneficial effects in collagen remodeling, leading to wrinkle improvement.

13.6 Surgery

Rhinophyma describes a large, bulbous, and ruddy nose caused by granulomatous infiltration, commonly as a result of untreated rosacea,[28] with surgery the only treatment option. In the mild form with patulous follicles but no contour changes, topical and oral pharmacotherapy can be used. However, in the moderate to severe forms, when there are contour changes and nodular components, surgical therapy such as cryosurgery, radiofrequency ablation, electrocautery, tangential excision combined with scissors sculpturing, skin grafting, carbon dioxide resurfacing, or dermabrasion may be required. The authors have found excellent results with electrocautery shave excision under conscious sedation (► Fig. 13.5). The patients usually undergo two sessions, approximately 6 months apart. The first session is geared toward major debulking, whereas the second session is usually aimed at achieving symmetry and a more normal nasal contour. Postoperative care involves a regimen of oral analgesia (acetaminophen with codeine), a short course of Vaseline ointment to the treated areas, and cleansing with vinegar soaks every 6 hours. The patients are usually socially acceptable within 3 weeks of the procedure.

13.7 Pearls and Pitfalls

- Understanding rosacea, with effective patient education and compliance constituting part of the treatment paradigm, is of paramount importance in the management of rosacea.
- Treatment is as varied as the clinical presentation spectrum.
- Management often involves multiple treatment modalities including lifestyle modifications, skin care management, pharmacotherapy, laser treatment, and surgery depending on the severity and spectrum of the disease.
- Facial erythema and flushing are treated effectively with a combination of IPL Limelight and Laser Genesis (Nd:YAG).
- Superficial and deep telangiectasias are treated with IPL Limelight and Excel Nd:YAG, respectively.
- A combination of topical (azelaic acid gel) and oral medication (doxycycline 40 mg daily) is best to treat papulopustular rosacea, and oral isotretinoin is added to the combination for the treatment of impending rhinophyma.
- When severe disease results in disfiguring rhinophyma, surgical management is necessary.

References

[1] Wilkin J, Dahl M, Detmar M, et al. Standard classification of rosacea: report of the National Rosacea Society Expert Committee on the classification and staging of rosacea. J Am Acad Dermatol 2002; 46: 584–587

[2] de Bersaques J. Historical notes on rosacea. Eur J Dermatol 1995; 5: 16–22

[3] Chauhan N, Ellis DA. Rosacea: pathophysiology and management principles. Facial Plast Surg Clin North Am 2013; 21: 127–136

[4] Drake L, ed. National Rosacea Society. New evidence shows rosacea may be linked to heredity. Rosacea Review. Fall 1996. Available at: http://www.rosacea.org/rr/1996/fall/article_3.php. Accessed February 15, 2014

[5] Aksoy B, Altaykan-Hapa A, Egemen D, Karagöz F, Atakan N. The impact of rosacea on quality of life: effects of demographic and clinical characteristics and various treatment modalities. Br J Dermatol 2010; 163: 719–725

[6] Drake L, ed. National Rosacea Society. New survey pinpoints leading factors that trigger symptoms. Rosacea Review. Summer 2002. Available at: http://www.rosacea.org/rr/2002/summer/article_3.php. Accessed February 15, 2014

[7] Drake L, ed. National Rosacea Society. Red wine named top alcohol trigger. Rosacea Review. Fall 2010. Available at: http://www.rosacea.org/rr/2010/fall/article_4.php. Accessed February 15, 2014

[8] Drake L, ed. National Rosacea Society. Survey shows lifestyle changes help control rosacea flare-ups. Rosacea Review. Winter 1998. Available at: http://www.rosacea.org/rr/1998/winter/article_3.php. Accessed February 15, 2014

[9] Draelos ZD. Cosmetics in acne and rosacea. Semin Cutan Med Surg 2001; 20: 209–214

[10] Powell FC. Clinical practice. Rosacea. N Engl J Med 2005; 352: 793–803

[11] Ortiz A, Elkeeb L, Truitt A, et al. Topical PRK 124 (0.125%) lotion for improving the signs and symptoms of rosacea. J Drugs Dermatol 2009; 8: 459–462

[12] Tremaine AM, Ortiz A, Elkeeb L, Tran M, Weinstein G. Long-term efficacy and safety of topical PRK 124 (0.125%) lotion (Pyratine-XR) in the treatment of mild-to-moderate rosacea. J Drugs Dermatol 2010; 9: 647–650

[13] Farris P. Idebenone, green tea, and Coffeeberry extract: new and innovative antioxidants. Dermatol Ther 2007; 20: 322–329

[14] Del Rosso JQ, Bhatia N. Azelaic acid gel 15% in the management of papulo-pustular rosacea: a status report on available efficacy data and clinical application. Cutis 2011; 88: 67–72

[15] Bikowski JB. The pharmacologic therapy of rosacea: a paradigm shift in progress. Cutis 2005; 75 Suppl: 27–32, discussion 33–36

[16] Antille C, Saurat JH, Lübbe J. Induction of rosaceiform dermatitis during treatment of facial inflammatory dermatoses with tacrolimus ointment. Arch Dermatol 2004; 140: 457–460

[17] Ceilley RI. Advances in the topical treatment of acne and rosacea. J Drugs Dermatol 2004; 3 Suppl: S12–S22

[18] Yamamoto O, Bhawan J, Solares G, Tsay AW, Gilchrest BA. Ultrastructural effects of topical tretinoin on dermo-epidermal junction and papillary dermis in photodamaged skin. A controlled study. Exp Dermatol 1995; 4: 146–154

[19] Fowler J, Jr, Jackson M, Moore A, et al. Efficacy and safety of once-daily topical brimonidine tartrate gel 0.5% for the treatment of moderate to severe facial erythema of rosacea: results of two randomized, double-blind, and vehicle-controlled pivotal studies. J Drugs Dermatol 2013; 12: 650–656

[20] Hong E, Fischer G. Childhood ocular rosacea: considerations for diagnosis and treatment. Australas J Dermatol 2009; 50: 272–275

[21] van Zuuren EJ, Kramer S, Carter B, Graber MA, Fedorowicz Z. Interventions for rosacea. Cochrane Database Syst Rev 2011: CD003262

[22] Del Rosso JQ, Webster GF, Jackson M, et al. Two randomized phase III clinical trials evaluating anti-inflammatory dose doxycycline (40-mg doxycycline, USP capsules) administered once daily for treatment of rosacea. J Am Acad Dermatol 2007; 56: 791–802

[23] Odom R, Dahl M, Dover J, et al. National Rosacea Society Expert Committee on the Classification and Staging of Rosacea. Standard management options for rosacea, part 2: options according to subtype. Cutis 2009; 84: 97–104

[24] Pelle MT, Crawford GH, James WD. Rosacea: II. Therapy. J Am Acad Dermatol 2004; 51: 499–512, quiz 513–514

[25] Lonne-Rahm S, Nordlind K, Edström DW, Ros AM, Berg M. Laser treatment of rosacea: a pathoetiological study. Arch Dermatol 2004; 140: 1345–1349

[26] Mark KA, Sparacio RM, Voigt A, Marenus K, Sarnoff DS. Objective and quantitative improvement of rosacea-associated erythema after intense pulsed light treatment. Dermatol Surg 2003; 29: 600–604

[27] Schmults CD, Phelps R, Goldberg DJ. Nonablative facial remodeling: erythema reduction and histologic evidence of new collagen formation using a 300-microsecond 1064-nm Nd:YAG laser. Arch Dermatol 2004; 140: 1373–1376

[28] Cohen AF, Tiemstra JD. Diagnosis and treatment of rosacea. J Am Board Fam Pract 2002; 15: 214–217

14 Removal of Tattoos and Permanent Makeup

Louis M. DeJoseph and Danny J. Soares

14.1 History of Tattooing

The history of tattooing dates back to a time as ancient as civilization itself, when this highly symbolic method of expression afforded more than a mere touch of individuality. The iceman *Ötzi*, the 5,200-year-old European Bronze-Age mummy discovered in northern Italy, was covered in punctate tattoos dispersed throughout the skin over his arthritic joints, incurred from multiple ritualistic, therapeutic interventions. In ancient Egypt, dermal tattoos branded criminals, stigmatized prostitutes, and marked social rank. In the 17th century, as European explorers settled into overseas colonies, the practice of tattooing was gradually assimilated into Western culture, with the word *tattoo* itself deriving from *ta-tau,* Tahitian for "the results of tapping." With the Industrial Revolution, the mechanization of conventional tattooing tools allowed for more precise and varied patterns, while the incorporation of multiple pigments provided for multicolored designs. The embrace by popular culture, the military community, and private groups and gangs eventually culminated in the widespread cultural phenomenon that has become evident today.

14.2 Classification of Tattoos

Despite the highly decorative nature of the majority of modern-day tattoos, different types exist (▶ Fig. 14.1), with strong implications for removal technique, clearance, and complications. *Decorative tattoos* constitute the vast majority of those presenting for removal and can be further subdivided into *professional* and *amateur*. Modern professional tattoos reflect a mechanized but refined method of dermal puncturing that incorporates diverse needle-tip sizes and configurations, colorful synthetic pigments, and a standardized sterile technique of dermal ink impregnation. Professional tattoo pigments are purposely introduced into the skin at sufficient depths and volumes that secure long-lasting results. These features promote greater pigment retention and, as a result, render the laser tattoo-removal process significantly more challenging than that seen with amateur tattoos.

Amateur techniques have existed for centuries and represent a more imprecise method of dermal tattooing, often relying upon various carbon-based compounds such as soot, graphite, or India ink for coloration. With their characteristic uniformly black hues, amateur techniques were adopted overseas by American military servicemen, who then subsequently introduced them to growing factions of the U.S. population, such as motorcycle groups and gangs. Amateur tattoo pigments often have more superficial distributions, lower ink volumes, and less-polished designs. As a result, these tattoos, with their traditional dark blue and black pigmentations, often respond well to laser removal.

Cosmetic tattoos have slowly garnered widespread popularity within the realm of permanent makeup, serving to imitate lip or eyeliner, enhance eyebrow definition and shape, and disguise scars or dermal lesions. Permanent makeup has the added benefits of being relatively unchanging, waterproof, and time-saving. They are typically applied by a tattoo artist or a

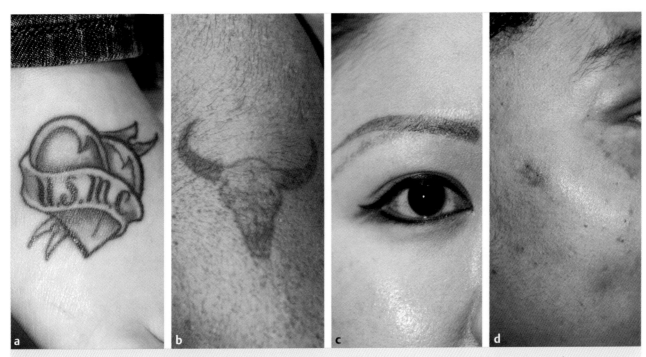

Fig. 14.1 Examples of different tattoo types. (**a**) *Professional* decorative tattoo. (**b**) *Amateur* decorative tattoo. (**c**) *Cosmetic* tattoo (permanent makeup). (**d**) *Traumatic* tattoo.

dermatologist and often employ a variety of red, pink, and flesh color tones containing titanium dioxide and ferric oxide, both of which, incidentally, are known to predispose to paradoxical tattoo darkening upon laser exposure.

Medical tattoos are frequently applied to define radiation ports in patients undergoing radiotherapy or as personal identification and informative medical tags. *Traumatic tattoos* are incurred following superficial dermal trauma resulting from blast exposures, such as firearm or firework explosions and motor vehicle accidents with occupant ejection. As small, high-velocity particles penetrate the injured and exposed dermis, they become permanently lodged within the skin following re-epithelialization. The dermal impregnation of these particles of widely varying caliber yields a permanent tattoo. Often, because these embedded fragments are sulfur-containing, they place the individual at risk for localized reactions, ignition, and even blasts during attempted laser removal.[1]

Regardless of tattoo type, the underlying pathophysiology is characterized by the introduction of pigment-containing particles into the superficial and mid-dermis. This is followed by the gradual but long-lasting incorporation of ink particles into resident fibroblasts and macrophages. Understanding particle properties such as size, absorption spectra, dermal depth, and chemical pigment composition is essential toward achieving maximum tattoo clearance and minimizing complications following laser-tattoo removal. These factors are largely dictated by the tattooing process, and a thorough knowledge of the procedure will assist the cosmetic surgeon in navigating the multiple treatment options and laser settings.

14.3 Technique

The process of dermal tattooing can be defined as the controlled introduction of pigment particles into the dermis through the action of traumatic micro-puncturing of the skin. Modern-day tattoo artists rely heavily on the electric tattoo machine to create elaborate patterns and designs, whereas the variety of pigmented compounds provides for colorful depictions. The electric tattoo machine consists of one or more fine needles (diameter 200–350 μm) contained within a hollow tube. The needle group is soldered onto a bar, which is itself attached to an oscillating unit, allowing for the vertical vibration of the needle tips into and out of the tube. When applied to the skin, each needle produces hundreds of micro-punctures measuring approximately 1 to 2 mm in depth, sufficient to reach the papillary and superficial reticular dermis.[2] When the tip of the needle is immersed into the ink prior to skin application, its action permits the introduction of the pigment into the dermal layer. Tattoo artists use several needle groupings to create different effects. Single needles are used for lining, groups of three or more needles are used for shading, and rows of needles for feathering. Following completion of the work, a healing period over 1 to 2 weeks is allowed to pass before the final appearance is appreciated.

14.4 Histopathology

The sequence of events that follows the placement of a dermal tattoo is similar to any other traumatic injury to the skin

(▶ Fig. 14.2). As the tattoo needle punctures the dermis, cellular injury releases mediators that evoke the early inflammatory response. Despite the introduction of pigment particles, the influx of inflammatory cells is only mild due to the particles' low immunogenicity. Within 24 hours after tattooing, the epidermis begins to peel, akin to that seen with a second-degree burn. In the process, a moderate amount of the deposited tattoo pigment is lost through epidermal shedding and dermal transudation, as well as due to the immediate action of dermal macrophages, which distribute small pigment particles to regional lymph nodes. After 10 to 14 days, the epidermis has fully healed and the majority of the pigment now resides within the superficial and mid-dermis. With passing months and years, due to the chronic phagocytic action of dermal macrophages, the distribution of the remaining pigment particles becomes limited to perivascular fibroblasts and resident phagocytic cells.[3] It is this restricted distribution of pigment particles within long-lived dermal fibroblast and phagocytic cells that gives the tattoo its ultimate long-lasting qualities.

14.5 Ink Particle Properties

With the recent introduction of an entire spectrum of tattoo ink colors, the market for multicolored tattoos has exploded. The treating physician is now often presented with a multitude of synthetic compounds whose properties strongly influence the response to laser-tattoo removal but are otherwise completely unknown. In preparation for tattoo removal, it has become important for the laser surgeon to be cognizant of specific ink particle attributes such as color, size, chemical nature, and laser wavelength absorption peaks, among others.

14.5.1 Color

Tattoo ink color compounds have undergone considerable evolution since the 1980s, with the gradual incorporation of numerous additional colorant groups. Tattoo ink particles can be divided into *pigments* and *dyes*. By definition, a pigment is insoluble and unaffected by the medium in which it is dispersed, resulting in a long-lasting and unchanging color pattern. In contrast, dyes represent water-soluble colorants that tend to chemically react and change with time, resulting in fading attributes. Due to these intrinsic features, the majority of *tattoo inks* incorporate pigments, whereas cosmetic tattoos, also known as *permanent makeup* (PMU), usually consist of organic dyes.[4] The newest types of tattoo inks however, such as the erasable and invisible-fluorescent varieties, also contain organic dyes complexed to beads of polymethylmethacrylate (PMMA) that facilitate the laser-removal process.[5]

Tattoo pigments can be further subdivided into *organic* and *inorganic* compounds. Inorganic pigments, such as metallic oxides, sulfides, and minerals, were widely utilized in tattooing from an early stage. Agents such as cobalt (blue), cadmium sulfide (yellow), mercury sulfide (red), and lead carbonate (white) were commonly employed until their discontinuation due to the occurrence of significant allergic reactions or concerns regarding exposure to toxic heavy metal levels. Metallic pigments in current use today include iron oxide (red, brown), chromium oxide (green), manganese (purple), and titanium

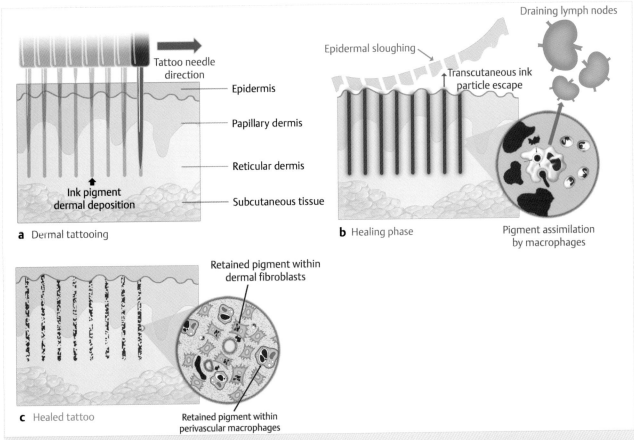

Fig. 14.2 Microscopic features of the tattooing process. (**a**) Dermal tattooing is achieved via the traumatic micro-puncturing of the dermis, depositing ink pigment into the superficial and mid-dermal regions. (**b**) Within 24 hours, an acute inflammatory phase sets in, characterized by epidermal sloughing and mild lymphocytic infiltrates. Early pigment clearance results from transcutaneous ink escape as well as by phagocytic and lymphatic clearance. (**c**) A fully healed tattoo represents dermal impregnation of the dermis with ink pigment, covered by a pigment-free epidermal layer. Following chronic phagocytic and lymphatic clearance, dermal ink particles become restricted to within perivascular resident phagocytic cells and fibroblasts.

dioxide (white). Titanium dioxide and iron oxide deserve special mention because these two pigments are still widely in use and can undergo laser-induced, oxidation-reduction reactions that result in tattoo darkening and a greater likelihood of treatment failure.[6]

Organic tattoo pigments constitute 80% of all modern tattoo ink mixtures and can be chemically categorized into *azo* and *nonazo (polycyclic)* compounds. Azo compounds are often seen in yellow, orange, red, and brown ink mixtures. Azo tattoo pigments have recently received increased scrutiny because some of these compounds have been shown to yield potentially carcinogenic aromatic amines when exposed to the action of quality-switched (Q-switched, QS) lasers.[7] Nonazo compounds, such as dioxazine and phthalocyanine are commonly present in modern violet, blue, and green tattoo inks.

Pigment colors can significantly impact a tattoo's susceptibility to laser removal because they influence laser–particle interactions that strongly depend upon the pigment's intrinsic light-absorption properties. ▶ Fig. 14.3 displays the absorption spectra for several common tattoo colors. Ink pigments, upon being introduced into the dermis, act as external chromophores, and naturally compete with dermal melanin, hemoglobin, and water for absorption of radiant laser energy. The color of a pigment represents the wavelength-specific light reflected off that compound; as such, a red pigment naturally reflects red light and absorbs all other visible wavelengths. In order to maximize laser–chromophore interactions, and therefore pigment clearance, it is often beneficial to utilize a laser wavelength that is closest to the chromophore maximum absorption peaks. For example, the frequency-doubled, QS 532-nm neodymium: yttrium aluminum garnet (Nd:YAG) laser delivers a wavelength that is closest to the maximum absorption peaks for red and orange pigments and has become the preferred laser for removal of those tattoo colors.[8] Black and other dark pigments tend to absorb most wavelengths and therefore respond to most currently available QS lasers. Several additional ink particle and laser properties should be considered when selectively targeting tattoo pigments, such as particle size and thermal relaxation times, as well as particle dermal location and laser depth of penetration, which are discussed next.

14.5.2 Size

The size of a pigment particle has significant consequences on a laser's ability to selectively target the ink while avoiding possible injury to surrounding dermal structures. The length of time that a particle requires to dissipate the heat incurred from laser exposure is termed its *thermal relaxation time* (TRT), and is

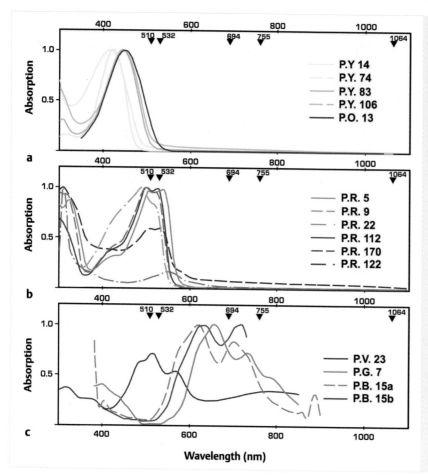

Fig. 14.3 (a–c) Wavelength-dependent absorption of several commonly utilized tattoo pigment colors. Arrowheads indicate the wavelength of common Q-switched (QS) lasers utilized in tattoo removal. P.Y., yellow; P.R., red; P.V., violet; P.G., Green; and P.B., blue. (Adapted with permission from Bäumler W, Eibler ET, Hohenleutner U, Sens B, Sauer J, Landthaler M. Q-switch laser and tattoo pigments: first results of the chemical and photophysical analysis of 41 compounds. Lasers Surg Med 2000; 26(1): 19.)

Table 14.1 Approximate thermal relaxation times of different dermal structures

Structure	Size (μm)	Thermal relaxation time
Tattoo ink particle	0.5–4	10 ns
Melanosome	0.5–1	1 μs
Erythrocyte	7	2 μs
Blood vessel	50	1 ms
Blood vessel	100	5 ms
Blood vessel	200	20 ms
Hair follicle	200	10–100 ms

Data from Bogdan Allemann I, Kaufman J. Laser principles. Curr Probl Dermatol 2011; 42: 7–23.)

directly proportional to the square size of the chromophore. As a result, the smaller the size of a target particle, the shorter is its TRT. The relationship between the TRT and the laser pulse duration can determine the likelihood of collateral thermal injury to surrounding tissues. If the laser pulse duration is greater than the pigment particle's TRT, then thermal damage will be incurred by the particle's immediate surroundings. In contrast, if the pulse duration is shorter than the target particle's TRT, then injury will be avoided.

The thermal relaxation times for common skin structures are listed in ▶ Table 14.1. Because of the size differential between tattoo pigment particles and surrounding dermal structures, adjusting the laser beam's duration to less than the target particle's TRT may help avoid unnecessary collateral skin damage. A frequency-doubled, 532-nm Nd:YAG laser with a pulse duration of 5 nanoseconds (ns) allows for the treatment of a red-colored tattoo without inducing substantial thermal damage to capillaries. The average tattoo pigment particle sizes are diagrammed in ▶ Fig. 14.4, with the majority of compounds existing between 2 to 400 nm. Unfortunately, dermal melanosome sizes significantly overlap with those of tattoo particles, and therefore both have similar thermal relaxation times. To prevent collateral injury to melanocytes, and subsequent dermal dyspigmentation, higher wavelength lasers that minimize melanin competitive absorption, such as the 1,064-nm Nd:YAG, are commonly employed in the treatment of dark blue or black tattoos.[9]

14.6 Tattoo Removal

As the popularity and prevalence of tattoos in the United States have grown, so has the interest in inexpensive and scarless tattoo-removal services. Approximately 24% of the adult American population is estimated to have at least one tattoo, and, when surveyed, 17% of these are actively considering pursuing tattoo removal, with 6% undergoing removal every year.[10] Whereas the motivations for tattoo acquisition often invoke a need for

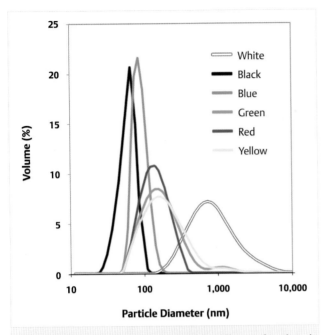

Fig. 14.4 Particle-size profiles obtained by laser diffraction for selected tattoo pigment colors. (Adapted with permission from Høgsberg T, Loeschner K, Löf D, Serup J. Tattoo inks in general usage contain nanoparticles. Br J Dermatol 2011; 165(6): 1215.)

individuality and personal expression, individuals usually seek tattoo removal due to loss of interest or the frequent need for tattoo concealment resulting from previous negative comments, embarrassment, or changes in career.[11] As newer, more rapid techniques of laser-tattoo removal have emerged and the adverse effects and complications have decreased with the development of nonablative modalities, the interest in laser-tattoo removal has seen a very rapid, recent growth. The American Society for Aesthetic Plastic Surgery (ASAPS) estimates that the number of laser tattoo-removal procedures increased by 43% between 2011 and 2012 alone.

14.7 History of Tattoo Removal

A variety of tattoo-removal techniques have been available for as long as tattooing has existed. The oldest method, salabrasion, described by Aetius around 543 AD, induced dermal injury via the application of coarse salt granules to the tattooed skin. Other techniques, such as dermabrasion and caustic (tannic acid and silver nitrate) or thermal (fire, hot coals) means of tissue destruction quickly fell out of favor due to their unacceptably high rates of scarring and dyspigmentation.

The introduction of ablative lasers for dermal resurfacing heralded a new era for tattoo removal and incited a growing interest in the underlying basis of ink particle–laser interactions. In the late 1970s, ablative modalities such as the 10,600-nm carbon dioxide (CO_2) laser resulted in pigment clearance but, due to its indiscriminate targeting of water molecules in the skin, produced dermal fibrosis and scar-tissue formation. Subsequent attempts to selectively target ink particles with the 488/514-nm argon laser also met with challenges, such as

significant dermal scarring, due to excessively long pulse durations (50–200 ms) and resultant nonselective tissue destruction.

In 1983, the principle of *selective photothermolysis* was postulated by Anderson and Parrish. The theory stated that if a particle is exposed to a well-absorbed laser wavelength, thermal tissue injury will be minimized as long as the laser exposure time (pulse duration) is shorter than the particle's *thermal relaxation time*.[12] This new concept revolutionized the approach to laser-tattoo removal and sparked the search for, and development of, ultra short-pulsed lasers, leading to the introduction of *quality-switched technology* into the field of laser dermatology. QS involves the implementation of an electro-optical switch that enables the rapid release of extremely high-energy laser emissions. Modern QS lasers can deliver high-peak power pulses in the range of several nanoseconds (10^{-9} ns) to picoseconds (10^{-12} ps).

14.8 Laser Tattoo Removal

14.8.1 Laser–Pigment Interactions

The dissipation and clearance of tattoo pigment particles following laser exposure is due to several incompletely understood physical interactions. Tattoo-removing lasers have a *photothermal* effect upon pigment particles, in which the radiant energy of the laser is converted into heat, resulting in temperatures in excess of 1,000°C that subsequently produce target vaporization. In addition, the *photoacoustic effect* leads to a rapid, thermally induced ink-particle expansion that incites localized shock waves. This aspect of laser–particle interactions is most significant for tattoo removal because it is thought to result in the fragmentation of ink particles that renders them amenable to phagocytosis and immune clearance. Finally, a laser interaction can also yield a *photochemical effect*, in which permanent cleavage of molecular bonds within the ink pigment induces a shift in its optical properties, leading to a perceived lightening of the tattoo.[13]

14.8.2 Laser Parameters

Different laser parameters should be considered when determining the ideal laser settings in preparation for tattoo removal. Factors such as tattoo type, color, location, and Fitzpatrick skin type should influence the treating physician's choice of laser wavelength, pulse duration, fluence, and spot size. These become important in minimizing adverse reactions and complications.

Wavelength

The wavelength of the chosen laser should ideally match the absorption spectrum of the target tattoo particle. In doing so, thermal injury to the surrounding tissues resulting from competitive absorption by melanin, hemoglobin, and water, is minimized. ▸ Fig. 14.5 shows the range of available lasers along the electromagnetic spectrum and absorption curves for the three primary skin chromophores. Each laser demonstrates intrinsic advantages when applied to different tattoo colors and

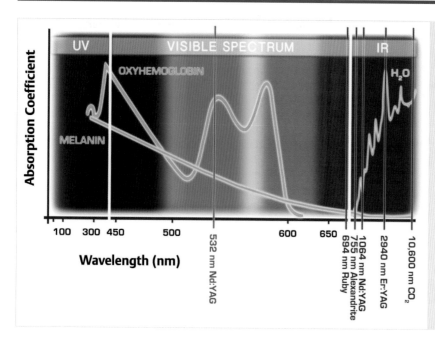

Fig. 14.5 Absorption curves for the intrinsic dermal chromophores: melanin, hemoglobin, and water. Vertical lines mark the wavelengths of commonly used, quality-switched (QS), tattoo removal (532-, 694-, 755-, and 1,064-nm neodymium) and ablative fractional skin resurfacing (2,940-nm erbium and 10,600-nm carbon dioxide [CO_2]) lasers.

Table 14.2 Relative absorption of currently available quality-switched (QS) lasers by tattoo ink color

Ink color	QS laser wavelength-specific relative absorption			
	532 nm	694 nm	755 nm	1064 nm
Black	Very good	Excellent	Excellent	Excellent
Blue	Good	Very good	Excellent	Good
Green	Good	Excellent	Very good	Fair
Brown	Fair	Good	Good	Fair
Red	Excellent	Poor	Poor	Poor
Purple	Good	Fair	Fair	Good
Orange	Good	Fair	Fair	Good
Yellow	Poor	Poor	Poor	Poor
Tan	Good	Poor	Poor	Poor

Reproduced with permission from Parlette EC, Kaminer MS, Arndt KA. The art of tattoo removal. Plastic Surgery Practice. Published January 20, 2008. Available at http://www.plasticsurgerypractice.com/2008/01/the-art-of-tattoo-removal/. Accessed Sept. 13, 2015.

Fitzpatrick skin types. ▶ Table 14.2 lists the different available QS lasers and their color-tattoo applications.[14]

The QS Nd:YAG laser is capable of producing emissions with both 1,064- and 532-nm wavelengths, with the latter due to frequency doubling through a potassium titanyl phosphate (KTP) optical crystal. At 1,064 nm, this laser is well suited to address dark blue or black pigments and, due to its longer wavelength, can afford a deeper level of dermal penetration, which may be useful in the removal of older tattoos. In addition, because melanin absorption is relatively low at 1,064 nm, the Nd:YAG is ideal for the treatment of tattoos in individuals with Fitzpatrick skin types V and VI.[15] The 532-nm pulses, within the green visible spectra, offer a complementary wavelength that is optimal for the treatment of red, orange, and purple pigments. The wavelength output can be modified with the use of special handpieces for conversion to 585- and 650-nm beams that assist in the removal of blue and green pigments, respectively.

The QS ruby laser (QSRL) yields a 694-nm pulse that has demonstrated effectiveness in the treatment of blue, black, and green pigments.[16] Traditional use often results in tattoo clearance without scarring, although temporary hypopigmentation can be encountered.[17] The QS alexandrite laser (QSAL) 755 nm has been similarly applied to blue and black pigments with good results and is currently the laser of choice for the treatment of green tattoos. Rates of 95% pigment removal have been shown with an average of 8.9 treatments with transient hypopigmentation as the most common complication.[18] Whereas black tattoo pigments can theoretically be treated with any of the available QS lasers, the QSRL and QSAL have both been shown to be superior in clearing dark pigments compared to the 1,064-nm Nd:YAG laser, although both carry a greater risk of postprocedure hypopigmentation.[19] In addition, both the QSRL and QSAL are inadequate in the treatment of red pigments.

Pulse Duration

The importance of adequate pulse duration is underscored by the increased thermal damage incurred by surrounding tissues when the pulse duration is greater than the particle's TRT. Most currently available QS lasers with tattoo-removal applications have pulse durations ranging between *5* to *50 ns*. Because the majority of tattoo ink particles measure between 4 to 400 nm, the expected TRTs for carbon particles extend from *19* to *1,000 ps* (0.019–1 ns), which has implied the possibility of improved outcomes with the use of picosecond lasers.[20] Indeed, several studies have demonstrated a more rapid clearance with picosecond lasers than with the conventional nanosecond pulses.[21,22,23]

Fluence

The laser *fluence* represents the energy density delivered upon the target spot size by the laser beam, measured in J/cm^2. The ideal fluence depends upon the target skin depth, tattoo type, color, and target Fitzpatrick skin type, and should be tailored to each specific patient scenario. Higher fluence equates with higher transmitted energy levels and the possibility of greater lightening of the tattoo with fewer treatments, but also the possibility of greater epidermal injury. Often, higher fluences can result in additional collateral thermal injury in patients with darker Fitzpatrick skin types. In the practice of these physicians, individuals with Fitzpatrick skin types I through III are started at a fluence of 3 J/cm^2 that is then increased by 0.4 J/cm^2 up to 5.5 J/cm^2. Those with Fitzpatrick skin types IV through VI are started at 2 J/cm^2 and gradually increased by 0.2 J/cm^2 up to a maximum of 3.0 J/cm^2. In this fashion, superficial pigment levels are addressed initially, with subsequent treatments targeting deeper dermal regions. This practice allows for a stepwise approach that minimizes collateral damage to deeper skin tissues and appendages.[13]

Spot Size

The laser spot size can impact the laser's depth of penetration because a large spot size enhances the depth of penetration by yielding a relative decrease in the amount of scatter that tends to occur at the edges of the laser beam. In this way, a large spot size maximizes the distribution of the laser light while minimizing excess superficial exposure. In contrast, with decreasing spot size, the percentage of scattered waves increases, and more energy is lost on the epidermis. As a result, it is often preferable to keep the spot size as large as possible, as long as the laser fluence is not significantly compromised.[24]

Beam Profile

The laser-beam profile describes how the radiant energy is distributed across the laser spot area. Ideally, the entire spot would have equal maximal energy distribution at both the center and edges of the beam. Instead, most beam profiles follow a Gaussian distribution, where the edges are relatively deprived and the center is energy dense. As a result, spot overlap is usually necessary with most Gaussian-distributed laser beams to achieve a more homogeneous tattoo laser exposure. Newer beam profiles have resulted in improved energy distribution and tattoo clearance.[25]

14.8.3 Laser Tattoo-Removal Technique

Preprocedure

All patients presenting for laser tattoo removal undergo a routine assessment with a full medical history review and physical examination. Patients should be screened for connective tissue and autoimmune disorders that may predispose to abnormal scarring. In addition, patients on chronic immunosuppressants are informed of the possibility of increased clearance time and risk of infection. Preprocedure photography documenting the presenting tattoo is obtained during each visit.

Individuals with dark or tanned skin are instructed to avoid sun exposure and begin topical lightening creams to the tattooed area, respectively, beginning 2 to 3 weeks prior to and during laser-tattoo treatments in order to minimize the chances of scarring and dyspigmentation. All tattoos, especially those with bright- and light-colored inks, should undergo a pre-treatment laser test spot to identify unusual laser reactions such as paradoxical tattoo darkening. If darkening occurs, further counseling should be provided regarding the higher risk of nonclearance, increased number of required sessions, and dermal scarring. Regardless of tattoo type, all patients should be counseled on the need for an average of 6 to 10 or more treatments in order to achieve maximal tattoo eradication.

Tattoo Removal

Protective eye gear of appropriate optical density should be worn at all times by all individuals present during the procedure. The appropriate laser wavelength is chosen depending on the tattoo color, Fitzpatrick skin type, and surgeon preference. These physicians traditionally begin with the QS 1,064-nm Nd:YAG laser for the majority of tattoos because it clears multiple pigments well, especially blue and black, and is safest for use on darker Fitzpatrick skin types. Initially, low-fluence (3 J/cm^2) settings are utilized to target the more superficial pigments and then gradually increased, as previously outlined, using lower fluences for darker Fitzpatrick skin types (2 J/cm^2).

Prior to engaging the laser, the patient's target skin should be cleansed free of any cosmetic products and lotions. Preprocedure topical anesthesia may be instituted with topical anesthetic preparations such as 2.5% lidocaine/2.5% prilocaine cream (EMLA, APP Pharmaceuticals, LLC, Schaumburg, Illinois) or local lidocaine infiltration. If the target area is large, preprocedure oral sedation may be necessary. Additional comfort may be provided by the simultaneous use of refrigerated air (Zimmer Cryo5 Chiller, Zimmer Elektromedizin, Irvine, California) during treatment. Amid laser application, it is important that the user hold the handpiece at a consistent distance from the skin across the entire target tattoo to ensure homogeneous depth of penetration. In addition, overlapping each spot with traditional Gaussian-distributed laser beams is advised. Formation of a mild, white frosting serves as the primary clinical end point during laser administration and equates with adequate pigment particle fragmentation (▶ Fig. 14.6). This immediate but temporary whitening reaction results from the gaseous

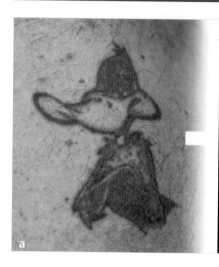
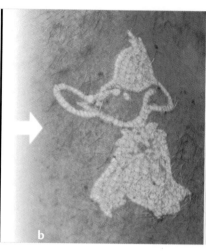

Fig. 14.6 Immediate whitening reaction. **(a)** Black tattoo before and **(b)** immediately after quality-switched (QS) 1,064-nm neodymium:yttrium aluminum garnet (Nd:YAG) laser treatment.

generation and cavitation within dermal tissues that follows exposure to the high-energy beams of QS lasers. If frosting is not witnessed immediately upon laser exposure, laser fluence may be insufficient and it should be increased.

Postprocedure

Immediately following completion of the laser tattoo-removal session, the treated area is covered with an emollient and a nonadherent dressing. The patient is instructed to keep the treated area clean and covered with a protective layer of a topical emollient such as petrolatum (Aquaphor, Beiersdorf Inc., Wilton, Connecticut) at all times to minimize crusting. Sun exposure should be avoided whenever possible following laser treatment. Repeat sessions are performed on a monthly basis until satisfactory clearance has occurred (▶ Fig. 14.7).

14.8.4 Complications

Dyspigmentation

Regional skin dyspigmentation (▶ Fig. 14.8) can occur following laser tattoo removal secondary to collateral melanocyte injury. Specific patient and laser factors predispose to this occurrence—Fitzpatrick skin type and laser wavelength, fluence, and spot size. Individuals with darker Fitzpatrick skin types are at an increased risk for transient hypopigmentation following laser treatments due to the increased levels of epidermal melanin. Lasers with shorter wavelengths are more easily absorbed by the superficial epidermal layers, as well as melanin particles. Due to its longer wavelength, the 1,064-nm QS Nd:YAG laser is capable of delivering higher energy levels to the target chromophore with less melanin absorption than the QS 694-nm ruby and 755-nm alexandrite lasers. As a result, this laser has become the preferred treatment choice for the majority of dark tattoos.

In addition to choosing the most appropriate laser wavelength, both fluence and spot size should be carefully considered. Higher laser fluences beyond those that are necessary for meeting the primary clinical end point only increase the amount of injury delivered to the epidermis and its melanocytes. Smaller spot sizes predispose to increased epidermal injury due to the much greater degree of beam scattering.

All patients with postprocedure dermal hypopigmentation should be counseled on the temporary nature of these pigment changes, typically with resolution within 6 months. Hyperpigmentation, which is often seen with darker Fitzpatrick skin types, may benefit from topical steroid and lightening preparations. Combination agents such as tretinoin, hydroquinone, and fluocinolone (Tri-Luma, Galderma Laboratories, Fort Worth, Texas) may hasten the clearance of postprocedure hyperpigmentation after tattoo removal.[26]

Scarring

The process of laser tattoo removal purposely seeks to produce a targeted dermal injury that can result in ink-particle clearance but also scarring. Dermal scarring is more likely to occur if the treated area is exposed to higher energy levels, melanin content, and increased energy scatter to superficial layers. As previously described, maintaining a large spot size and ensuring pretreatment application of lightening and sunscreen products will assist in minimizing scar formation.

An avoidable but frequent cause of excessive dermal scarring results from an instinctive tendency by treating physicians to increase laser fluence past the clinical plateau phase in refractory cases in the hopes of inducing additional clearance. By default, any increase in laser fluence will also result in a decrease in spot size. The combination of higher energy density and increased dermal scatter will result in the unnecessary transmission of elevated energy to the epidermis and superficial dermis. When faced with a refractory tattoo, the treating physician should consider changing to a different QS laser. This approach often results in maximal clearance with minimal scarring.[27]

Allergic Reactions

Some common tattoo ink pigments are well known to be associated with localized and occasionally systemic allergic responses (▶ Fig. 14.9). Red pigments, in particular, such as those containing *cinnabar* (mercury sulfide) are frequently associated with allergic reactions.[28,29] Recently, allergic reactions to melamine-containing *invisible* tattoos, which are visible only in the dark, have been reported.[30] Patients often present with localized pruritus and an erythematous nodular rash with

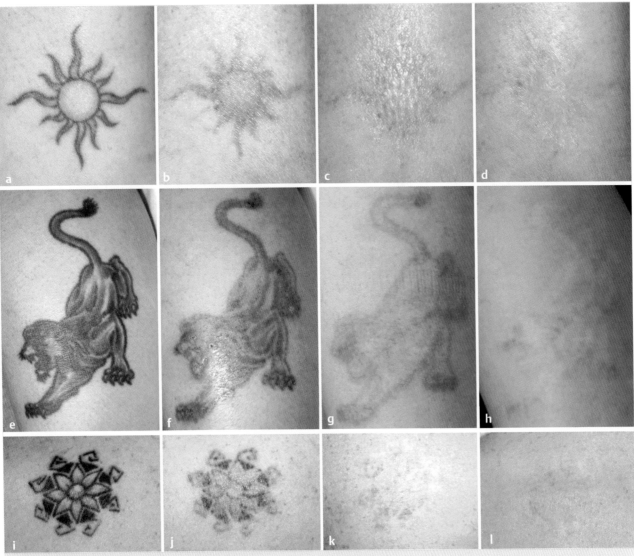

Fig. 14.7 Multicolored tattoo clearance following quality-switched (QS) laser tattoo removal. (**a–d**) Appearance of a black, red, and yellow multicolored tattoo after four treatment sessions with the 1,064- and 532-nm QS neodymium:yttrium aluminum garnet (Nd:YAG) lasers. Notice the initial clearance of the black pigment with the 1,064-nm wavelength, followed by the subsequent lightening of the red and yellow colors with the 532-nm laser output. (**e–h**) Similar multicolored tattoo response to eight treatment sessions utilizing the 1,064- and 532-nm QS Nd:YAG laser wavelengths. (**i–l**) Appearance of a blue, green, and yellow multicolored tattoo with sequential application of the 1,064- and 532-nm QS Nd:YAG, and 755-nm alexandrite lasers, respectively, over six treatment sessions.

dermal scaling. Rarely, patients may also develop signs of an acute systemic reaction, with dyspnea, tachycardia, and hypotension. The use of a test spot prior to proceeding to full tattoo treatment may allow for the identification of at-risk individuals.

Treatment of localized reactions consists of topical or intralesional steroid administration, with systemic steroids reserved for persistent cases. Further and subsequent laser-treatment sessions should be avoided, although some have been successfully treated without complications with the use of simultaneous steroid therapy.[31] These patients should be monitored closely for the development of systemic symptoms that would necessitate immediate intervention, epinephrine administration, and cardiovascular and respiratory support.

Paradoxical Ink Darkening

Ink darkening can occur with specific tattoo colors following exposure to the high-energy beams delivered by traditional QS lasers. The most common culprits include red (ferric oxide) and white (titanium dioxide), but darkening can also be seen with other pigments such as yellow, blue, and green.[32,33] Permanent makeup dyes often incorporate titanium dioxide as a brightening agent and the widely used red and pink colors often contain ferric oxide. When exposed to the laser beam, ferric oxide is converted to its reduced form, *ferrous oxide* (rust colored), whereas titanium (Ti^{4+}) is reduced to Ti^{3+} (blue-black).[34]

Prior to treatment, a test spot should be performed in individuals with tattoo colors at risk for darkening. If a darkening reaction does occur, the patient should be advised that tattoo clearance may require multiple additional sessions, and

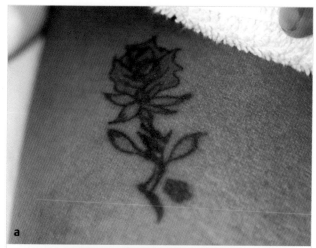

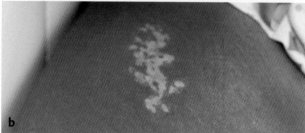

Fig. 14.8 Hypopigmentation following laser tattoo removal. (a) Prior to treatment. (b) Following multisession treatment.

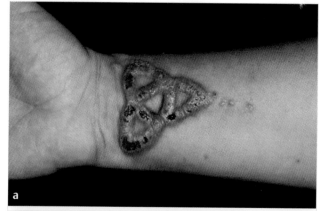

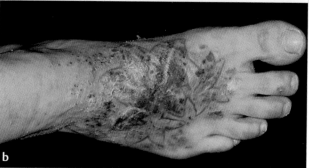

Fig. 14.9 Local and distant allergic reaction following laser treatment of a red pigment-containing tattoo. (a) Appearance of a local allergic reaction to a red, right-ventral wrist tattoo following laser treatment. (b) The patient also developed a distant allergic reaction targeting an untreated right-dorsal foot tattoo. (Reproduced with permission from Harper J, Losch AE, Otto SG, et al. New insight into the pathophysiology of tattoo reactions following laser tattoo removal. Plast Reconstr Surg 2010; 126(6): 314.)

counseled on the possibility of becoming refractory to therapy. Despite this, treatment of darkened tattoos often responds to laser removal just as dark tattoos would, especially for darkened red-containing tattoos, albeit with greater likelihood of a need for additional sessions.[35] Permanent makeup dyes also respond to laser tattoo removal, following ink-darkening reactions, with the 1,064-nm Nd:YAG QS laser.[34]

Darkened tattoos that fail to resolve with conventional QS laser therapy may respond to ablative lasers such as the 10,600-nm CO_2 and 2,940-nm erbium lasers, albeit with an increased risk of dermal scarring. Surgical excision is generally avoided unless specifically requested and is reserved for treatment failures in patients with small tattoos located over favorable regions.

14.8.5 New Developments

Picosecond Lasers

An improved understanding of laser–tattoo particle interactions over the last three decades has promoted the applicability of picosecond lasers in laser tattoo removal. The small dimensions of the average ink particle equate with a short thermal relaxation time, some of which are well into the picosecond range. In theory, the utilization of picosecond beams may induce a more rapid thermal expansion that results in greater ink-particle destruction and subsequent clearance. In addition, the use of picosecond-long pulses would decrease the likelihood of injury to surrounding tissues. Several studies have documented improved results with picosecond lasers compared to traditional nanosecond pulses.[20,21] Picosecond lasers have

also demonstrated the ability to clear tattoos previously refractory to conventional nanosecond lasers.[23]

Accelerated Therapy

Accelerated laser-treatment protocols have recently been introduced to expedite tattoo clearance while avoiding the risk of dermal scarring. Inherent to the adoption of accelerated protocols is the need to await the resolution of the immediate whitening reaction that traditionally follows QS laser tattoo removal—approximately 20 minutes. Kossida et al demonstrated rapid tattoo clearance utilizing a hyperfractionated protocol, termed the *R20 method*, in which four treatment passes were applied 20 minutes apart. Compared to the conventional protocol, the R20 method was much more likely to result in near-complete clearance in a single treatment. Increased epidermal injury, compared to the conventional protocol, was noted but without an elevated risk of permanent dermal scarring.[36] Immediate resolution of the laser-induced whitening reaction can also be achieved with the use of topical perfluorodecaline (PFD), a highly gas-soluble liquid fluorocarbon that clears the frosting within seconds, thereby allowing for immediate subsequent laser passes. Reddy et al demonstrated this technique, labeled the *R0 method*, to be equivalent to the R20 method but with significantly shortened session times.[37]

Combined Q-Switched and Ablative Fractional Laser Therapy

Recent case reports have shown a potential benefit from a combined therapeutic approach employing both QS and fractional CO_2 ablative laser technology for tattoo removal compared to QS laser therapy alone.[38,39] The application of a fractional CO_2 laser over a tattooed region provides additional direct escape routes for transepidermal ink-particle efflux, as well as a potentially more robust inflammatory response for immune-mediated particle clearance.[40] In addition, the dermal micropunctures achieved with the fractional ablative laser modality assist in preventing the formation of postprocedure blisters and may thereby shorten the healing time. Further objective investigations will be required on the use of this dual approach for tattoo removal in order to confirm and establish the significance of such potential benefits.

Erasable Tattoo Inks

The challenging nature of common tattoo pigments that is encountered upon attempted laser removal has highlighted the need for more laser-responsive, reversible tattoos. In an attempt to create an erasable tattoo ink, Freedom-2 has developed *Infinitink* (Freedom-2 Inc., Cherry Hill, New Jersey), a polymethylmethacrylate-complexed bioresorbable dye that can reportedly be cleared with as little as one laser treatment. Laser exposure results in fragmentation of the polymethylmethacrylate beads, leading to dye exposure and subsequent lymphatic clearance. Although already the target of widespread media attention, objective evidence on the suitability and safety of such reversible tattoo ink products is still lacking, and a cautioned approach is still warranted.[5]

14.9 Conclusion

The art of tattooing has represented an ancient, expression-driven, symbolic form of dermal engraving that is strongly defined by permanence but that is frequently challenged by the often-capricious human nature. The resultant growth in the number of tattooed individuals in the United States has been followed by an expected rise in the incidence of requests for tattoo removal. High-powered, QS laser technology has become the gold standard in tattoo removal, often demonstrating the ability to fully clear a tattoo without significant dermal dyspigmentation or scarring. The proper utilization of QS lasers, as applied to tattoo removal, necessitates a thorough understanding of the tattooing process, ink properties, and laser parameters. As the science and technology underlying this therapeutic modality continue to grow, we reach closer to the goal of transforming the permanent nature of the tattoo into an ever-transient one.

References

[1] Taylor CR. Laser ignition of traumatically embedded firework debris. Lasers Surg Med 1998; 22: 157–158

[2] Sperry K. Tattoos and tattooing. Part I: history and methodology. Am J Forensic Med Pathol 1991; 12: 313–319

[3] Sperry K. Tattoos and tattooing. Part II: gross pathology, histopathology, medical complications, and applications. Am J Forensic Med Pathol 1992; 13: 7–17

[4] De Cuyper C, D'Hollander D. Materials used in body art. In: de Cuyper C, Cotapos ML, eds. Dermatologic Complications with Body Art. Berlin Heidelberg, Germany: Springer-Verlag; 2010: 13–28

[5] Bernstein EF. Laser tattoo removal. Semin Plast Surg 2007; 21: 175–192

[6] Timko AL, Miller CH, Johnson FB, Ross E. In vitro quantitative chemical analysis of tattoo pigments. Arch Dermatol 2001; 137: 143–147

[7] Vasold R, Naarmann N, Ulrich H, et al. Tattoo pigments are cleaved by laser light-the chemical analysis in vitro provide evidence for hazardous compounds. Photochem Photobiol 2004; 80: 185–190

[8] Choudhary S, Elsaie ML, Leiva A, Nouri K. Lasers for tattoo removal: a review. Lasers Med Sci 2010; 25: 619–627

[9] Jones A, Roddey P, Orengo I, Rosen T. The Q-switched ND:YAG laser effectively treats tattoos in darkly pigmented skin. Dermatol Surg 1996; 22: 999–1001

[10] Laumann AE, Derick AJ. Tattoos and body piercings in the United States: a national data set. J Am Acad Dermatol 2006; 55: 413–421

[11] Armstrong ML, Roberts AE, Koch JR, Saunders JC, Owen DC, Anderson RR. Motivation for contemporary tattoo removal: a shift in identity. Arch Dermatol 2008; 144: 879–884

[12] Anderson RR, Parrish JA. Selective photothermolysis: precise microsurgery by selective absorption of pulsed radiation. Science 1983; 220: 524–527

[13] Ho DD, London R, Zimmerman GB, Young DA. Laser-tattoo removal—a study of the mechanism and the optimal treatment strategy via computer simulations. Lasers Surg Med 2002; 30: 389–397

[14] Mao JC, DeJoseph LM. Latest innovations for tattoo and permanent makeup removal. Facial Plast Surg Clin North Am 2012; 20: 125–134, v

[15] Lapidoth M, Aharonowitz G. Tattoo removal among Ethiopian Jews in Israel: tradition faces technology. J Am Acad Dermatol 2004; 51: 906–909

[16] Kilmer SL, Anderson RR. Clinical use of the Q-switched ruby and the Q-switched Nd:YAG (1064 nm and 532 nm) lasers for treatment of tattoos. J Dermatol Surg Oncol 1993; 19: 330–338

[17] Scheibner A, Kenny G, White W, Wheeland RG. A superior method of tattoo removal using the Q-switched ruby laser. J Dermatol Surg Oncol 1990; 16: 1091–1098

[18] Fitzpatrick RE, Goldman MP. Tattoo removal using the alexandrite laser. Arch Dermatol 1994; 130: 1508–1514

[19] Leuenberger ML, Mulas MW, Hata TR, Goldman MP, Fitzpatrick RE, Grevelink JM. Comparison of the Q-switched alexandrite, Nd:YAG, and ruby lasers in treating blue-black tattoos. Dermatol Surg 1999; 25: 10–14

[20] Izikson L, Farinelli W, Sakamoto F, Tannous Z, Anderson RR. Safety and effectiveness of black tattoo clearance in a pig model after a single treatment with a novel 758 nm 500 picosecond laser: a pilot study. Lasers Surg Med 2010; 42: 640–646

[21] Ross V, Naseef G, Lin G, et al. Comparison of responses of tattoos to picosecond and nanosecond Q-switched neodymium: YAG lasers. Arch Dermatol 1998; 134: 167–171

[22] Saedi N, Metelitsa A, Petrell K, Arndt KA, Dover JS. Treatment of tattoos with a picosecond alexandrite laser: a prospective trial. Arch Dermatol 2012; 148: 1360–1363

[23] Brauer JA, Reddy KK, Anolik R, et al. Successful and rapid treatment of blue and green tattoo pigment with a novel picosecond laser. Arch Dermatol 2012; 148: 820–823

[24] Bogdan Allemann I, Kaufman J. Laser principles. Curr Probl Dermatol 2011; 42: 7–23

[25] Karsai S, Pfirrmann G, Hammes S, Raulin C. Treatment of resistant tattoos using a new generation Q-switched Nd:YAG laser: influence of beam profile and spot size on clearance success. Lasers Surg Med 2008; 40: 139–145

[26] Torok HM, Jones T, Rich P, Smith S, Tschen E. Hydroquinone 4%, tretinoin 0.05%, fluocinolone acetonide 0.01%: a safe and efficacious 12-month treatment for melasma. Cutis 2005; 75: 57–62

[27] Kirby W, Chen CL, Desai A, Desai T. Causes and recommendations for unanticipated ink retention following tattoo removal treatment. J Clin Aesthet Dermatol 2013; 6: 27–31

[28] Bhardwaj SS, Brodell RT, Taylor JS. Red tattoo reactions. Contact Dermatitis 2003; 48: 236–237

[29] Ashinoff R, Levine VJ, Soter NA. Allergic reactions to tattoo pigment after laser treatment. Dermatol Surg 1995; 21: 291–294

[30] Tsang M, Marsch A, Bassett K, High W, Fitzpatrick J, Prok L. A visible response to an invisible tattoo. J Cutan Pathol 2012; 39: 877–880

[31] Antony FC, Harland CC. Red ink tattoo reactions: successful treatment with the Q-switched 532 nm Nd:YAG laser. Br J Dermatol 2003; 149: 94–98

[32] Goldman MP. Cutaneous and Cosmetic Laser Surgery. Philadelphia, PA: Mosby Elsevier; 2006: 127–130

[33] Fitzpatrick RE, Lupton JR. Successful treatment of treatment-resistant laser-induced pigment darkening of a cosmetic tattoo. Lasers Surg Med 2000; 27: 358–361

[34] Lee CN, Bae EY, Park JG, Lim SH. Permanent makeup removal using Q-switched Nd:YAG laser. Clin Exp Dermatol 2009; 34: e594–e596

[35] Peach AH, Thomas K, Kenealy J. Colour shift following tattoo removal with Q-switched Nd-YAG laser (1064/532). Br J Plast Surg 1999; 52: 482–487

[36] Kossida T, Rigopoulos D, Katsambas A, Anderson RR. Optimal tattoo removal in a single laser session based on the method of repeated exposures. J Am Acad Dermatol 2012; 66: 271–277

[37] Reddy KK, Brauer JA, Anolik R, et al. Topical perfluorodecaline resolves immediate whitening reactions and allows rapid effective multiple pass treatment of tattoos. Lasers Surg Med 2013; 45: 76–80

[38] Weiss ET, Geronemus RG. Combining fractional resurfacing and Q-switched ruby laser for tattoo removal. Dermatol Surg 2011; 37: 97–99

[39] Ibrahimi OA, Syed Z, Sakamoto FH, Avram MM, Anderson RR. Treatment of tattoo allergy with ablative fractional resurfacing: a novel paradigm for tattoo removal. J Am Acad Dermatol 2011; 64: 1111–1114

[40] Wang CC, Huang CL, Sue YM, Lee SC, Leu FJ. Treatment of cosmetic tattoos using carbon dioxide ablative fractional resurfacing in an animal model: a novel method confirmed histopathologically. Dermatol Surg 2013; 39: 571–577

15 Laser Hair Removal

Babar Sultan and Theda C. Kontis

15.1 Historical Perspectives

Hair removal is one of the most common cosmetic procedures performed today. In 2009, industry revenue for hair removal, either personally or by a practitioner, totaled approximately $244 million. It has been practiced since prehistoric times with specific modifications due to local cultural, religious, as well as personal aesthetic preferences. Ancient Egyptian men shaved hair from their heads and faces to prevent grasping during battle; women in the Middle Ages plucked and shaved hair on their eyebrows and anterior hairline to conform to contemporary standards of beauty.[1] Contemporary demand ranges from cases of hirsutism and hypertrichosis to normally distributed body hair that is unwanted. Hirsutism is abnormal hair growth in women in androgen-dependent sites, whereas hypertrichosis is excess hair growth in a body site (anywhere on the body) independent of hormones.

Depilation, the removal of the hair shaft, and epilation, the removal of the hair shaft and bulb, are the two primary methods of hair removal. Shaving is an example of depilation, whereas epilation includes methods such as waxing, electrolysis, and laser hair removal. Epilation hair removal provides results that usually last about 8 weeks; depilation results only last for approximately 2 weeks.[2]

Shaving, an extremely cost-efficient and popular method for men's facial hair and women's legs and underarms, does not alter the hair cycle and is a temporary solution to hair growth.[3] Historically, shaving tools have ranged from sharpened animal teeth and flint to modern electric and nonelectric blades.

Waxing, which has existed since ancient times, provides temporary hair removal and can treat large areas efficiently, albeit at a risk of skin irritation and pain.[4] Electrolysis results in potentially permanent hair removal by a probe passing an electrical current to destroy the hair follicle. It is however a slow and operator-dependent method with wide-ranging rates of complications such as scars and pigment changes.[5] Laser hair removal utilizes the existing melanin in hair follicles for specific targeting called selective photothermolysis. It is important to appreciate the evolution of hair removal because it guides providers about needs for future improvements as well as motivation for patient demands.[6]

15.2 Hair Follicle Growth and Anatomy

The hair follicle is a hormonally active structure with specifically programmed growth. It can be divided into three anatomical portions from superficial to deep: infundibulum, isthmus, and inferior segment (▶ Fig. 15.1). The inferior segment is bordered inferiorly by the base of the follicle and extends superiorly to the erector pili muscle. The isthmus extends from the erector pili muscle to the sebaceous gland duct. The infundibulum extends superiorly to the follicular orifice. The dermal papilla supplies proliferating cells at the base of the follicle.

Melanocytes, located near the infundibulum, provide the pigment that determines hair color.

The hair follicle can be in any one of three different metabolic phases: anagen, catagen, and telogen. Anagen is a period of active growth; catagen involves degradation through apoptosis. Telogen is a resting phase and the relative length of each phase is body-site dependent, although at any given time 90% of the body's hair is in the anagen phase. The follicle can produce various types of hair. Lanugo hairs are found on a fetus and lost during the neonatal period. Vellus hairs have a diameter of 30 μm and are the most prevalent hairs in the body, whereas terminal hairs are much thicker at 300 μm and more ideally suited for laser hair removal.

15.3 Mechanism of Laser Hair Removal

Laser light is unique in that it has one specific wavelength (monochromatic), its rays are parallel (collimated), the rays are in phase with each other (coherent), and are of high intensity. Light from lasers is scattered, transmitted, reflected, or absorbed by the skin surface. Chromophores such as melanin absorb light energy that is in the red or infrared range of electromagnetic radiation (600–1,100 nm). Selective photothermolysis is dependent on the heating and subsequent destruction of the chromophore without collateral damage to surrounding tissue. As described earlier, in the hair follicle there is spatial separation between the location of melanin near the infundibulum and the deeper stem cells. As melanin absorbs the light energy and converts it to heat, the deeper stem cells are thermally injured. The amount of heat absorbed at a given wavelength is determined by the energy density (fluence, measured in joules [J/cm^2]) and the length of time at a given temperature (pulse duration). Selectivity occurs when pulse duration approaches the thermal relaxation time, the time necessary for tissue to cool to half its peak temperature. Therefore, long-pulsed lasers work well if they approach the thermal relaxation time of hair follicles, which is between 10 and 100 ms.[7] Spot size is also an important variable. Due to the phenomenon of lateral scattering of light once it penetrates the skin, the spot size has an effect on the effective depth of light penetration. If all other variables are held constant, a larger spot size will result in an overall greater depth of effect, which is desirable for targeting hair follicles.

The hair in melanin competes with epidermal melanin, increasing the risk of collateral damage in darker skinned individuals. With lighter colored hair, not enough energy may reach the hair follicle stem cells to cause thermal damage. Therefore, the ideal candidate for laser hair removal has light skin and dark hair.

15.4 Types of Lasers

The types of lasers commonly used for hair removal include ruby, alexandrite, diode, and the neodymium:yttrium

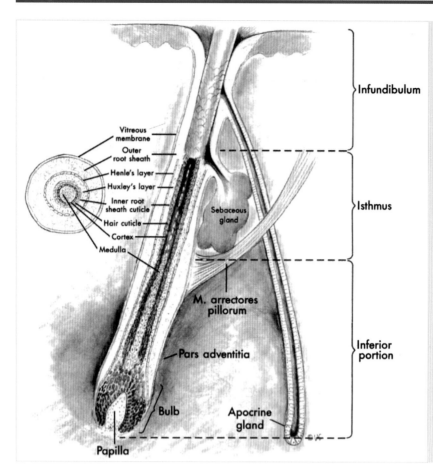

Fig. 15.1 Hair follicle anatomy. The hair follicle can be divided into three anatomical portions from superficial to deep: infundibulum, isthmus, and inferior segment. The inferior segment is bordered inferiorly by the base of the follicle and extends superiorly to the erector pili muscle. The isthmus extends from the erector pili muscle to the sebaceous gland duct. The infundibulum extends superiorly to the follicular orifice. The dermal papilla supplies proliferating cells at the base of the follicle. (Reproduced with permission from Papel I. Facial Plastic and Reconstructive Surgery. 3rd ed. New York, NY: Thieme Medical Publishers; 2009.)

Table 15.1 Hair removal lasers

Laser	Wavelength (nm)	Fitzpatrick skin type
Long-pulsed ruby	694	I and II
Alexandrite	755	I–III
Diode	810	III–V
Neodymium:yttrium aluminum garnet (Nd:YAG)	1,064	IV–VI

aluminum garnet (Nd:YAG) (▶ Table 15.1). Wavelengths of these lasers range from 694 to 1,064 nm. In general, lasers with longer wavelengths are less absorbed by epidermal melanin and have less tissue side effects.[8] Often the intense pulsed light (IPL) device is grouped with laser hair removal instruments but the emission is rather different. Laser light is monochromatic (single wavelength) and has very slight divergence, whereas the IPL device emits light along a range of wavelengths that is non-coherent. The advantages of the IPL mechanism are its low cost and ability to treat large areas; however, more treatments may be required to achieve the same efficacy as compared to the other lasers mentioned. Electro-optical synergy (ELOS) technology combines the benefits of both radiofrequency and IPL technologies for hair removal. The light (optical) component heats the hair follicle, while the radiofrequency modality (electrical) focuses the heat on the hair shaft. This dual treatment system can be used for all skin types since melanin is not targeted.

The long-pulsed ruby laser, which has a wavelength of 694 nm, was approved for hair removal by the Food and Drug Administration (FDA) in 1997 and is effective in treating lighter skinned individuals.[9] The alexandrite laser has a wavelength of 755 nm, and long-term efficacy with long-pulsed alexandrite lasers has been as high as 80.6%. Lloyd and Mirkov[10] studied 11 patients receiving five alexandrite laser treatments to the right groin at 3-week intervals with no evidence of scarring or pigment changes. This procedure is recommended for Fitzpatrick skin types I to III because of reduced competition with epidermal melanin. Lasers with longer wavelengths are less absorbed by epidermal melanin and have less tissue side effects.[8] The diode laser has a wavelength of 810 nm and can be used for slightly darker skin types. The FDA recently approved a diode laser for home use.[11] Such devices offer greater privacy and convenience for the patient and appear to be both safe and effective.[12]

The Nd:YAG laser (1,064 nm) can be used for virtually all skin types. The longer wavelength will penetrate deeper into the skin, while leaving the epidermis undamaged. Although longer wavelength lasers have less side effects in darker skinned individuals, comparisons of efficacy among the different lasers have shown varying results. Chan et al[13] studied 15 Chinese women for mainly axillary hair removal with diode laser on one side and Nd:YAG on the other with 36 weeks of follow-up. Nd:YAG laser treatment was associated with greater immediate post-procedure pain; however, both laser treatments showed similar efficacy with regrowth rates approximately 20% at 6 weeks. Li et al[14] also studied axillary hair removal comparing the efficacy of the diode and Nd:YAG lasers. In their study, 29 Chinese women received three treatments at 4-week intervals. At 8 weeks, there was a higher rate of hair reduction and less postprocedure pain associated with the diode laser side as compared to the Nd:YAG laser-treated side.

Cooling devices are also important to consider during laser hair removal because treatment can be quite painful. Cooling the epidermis not only diminishes pain and side effects at the treatment site, but also allows for the ability to use increased fluence at the procedure site. Cooling can be accomplished by circulating cold water or coolant in the laser handpiece, or applying external forced-air cooling.

15.5 Pretreatment Considerations

As in any treatment offered by a trained provider, a thorough medical history is necessary. Any history of endocrine or menstrual abnormalities, such as polycystic ovary syndrome, could signal a systemic cause for unwanted hair that can be treated medically. Active infection with the herpes simplex virus (HSV) in the area of desired treatment is a contraindication to treatment. If there is a history of HSV infection, prophylactic treatment with valacyclovir a day before treatment is recommended.[15] Although rare now, gold-salt intake is a contraindication because it can cause cutaneous hyperpigmentation (chrysiasis).[16] Active use of isotretinoin is also a contraindication due to impaired tissue healing and skin fragility.

Thorough patient counseling and consent are also important before laser hair removal treatment is initiated. A detailed consent that includes the complications associated with laser hair removal should be obtained (▶ Fig. 15.2). Patients with light-colored hair should be advised that they are poor candidates for laser hair removal. Because hair grows in cycles, laser hair reduction must be performed in a series of procedures, generally, approximately six to eight treatment sessions about 3 to 8 weeks apart. Patients will notice fewer hairs regrow after each successive treatment session. Patients can expect a 10 to 25% hair reduction after each process. Once treatment end point has been reached, patients should understand that periodic touch-up procedures may be required; they will obtain hair reduction but not necessarily permanent hair removal.

Pretreatment tanning increases the competition between epidermal and hair melanin, increasing the risk of collateral injury. Any epilation maneuver that removes the entire hair shaft, such as waxing, electrolysis, threading, or plucking, should be avoided at least 6 weeks prior to treatment. It is recommended that subjects shave 2 to 3 days prior to the procedure, so that fine stubble is present ensuring the presence of the hair shaft but reducing the risk of damage to the skin.

15.5.1 Treatment

Laser-treatment protocols must be strictly followed, including placing laser-use signage on the treatment room door and providing eye protection for all those in the treatment area, since the retina contains a high concentration of melanin. An anesthetic cream or gel may be applied to reduce discomfort associated with the procedure. The cream should be used at an appropriate interval beforehand to allow for complete effect. Local field blocks can also be considered for exquisitely sensitive areas such as the upper lip. If the laser handpiece does not have a cooling mechanism, it is necessary to protect the outer layers of the skin with a cold gel or special cooling device. Treatment causes hair-shaft carbonation and it is important to clean the handpiece and have a mechanism to avoid smoke-plume inhalation.

During the treatment, some hair follicles will be expressed from the skin. A few minutes after the procedure, the treated area will become erythematous and perifollicular edema will develop. Given the experience of the provider, the settings should be adjusted to account for color, thickness, and location of the hair as well as skin color. The practitioner must continually assess the skin during treatment to avoid epidermal injury (▶ Fig. 15.3, Video 15.1).

15.6 Posttreatment Instructions

Perifollicular erythema and edema are the desired end points and the sensation of being sunburned may last several hours. Posttreatment discomfort is generally mild and can last 1 to 3 days. Immediately after the procedure, ice packs may be used and, if needed, mild analgesics such as acetaminophen or ibuprofen can be taken. Patients are advised to avoid sun exposure to the treated area. Should scabbing or blistering occur, they are advised not to pick or abrade the area. Subjects will also notice shedding of additional hair follicles in the posttreatment period. Antiviral medications are prescribed if there is a history of HSV in those who have had the upper lip lasered. Should an epidermal injury occur, topical antibiotic ointments are prescribed and the patient is seen more frequently in follow-up to better assess healing. Treating the hair while in the anagen phase results in most effective long-term treatment; therefore, another procedure session is typically scheduled in 6 to 8 weeks and four to six treatments are generally necessary.

15.7 Complications

In general, laser hair removal is a safe procedure with transient, mild posttreatment complaints of tenderness, erythema, perifollicular edema, and skin irritation. However, first- or second-degree burns, hyperpigmentation or hypopigmentation, and scarring have been described as complications of hair-removal laser treatment.[17] The risk of complications can increase based on patient-specific characteristics such as skin type, body location, and recent sun exposure. Transient hypopigmentation occurs in 10 to 17% of patients and may last several months.[18] Immediate hyperpigmentation occurs in 14 to 25% of patients and transiently lasts several weeks. There is a risk of permanent dyschromia in dark-skinned or heavily tanned individuals. Burns to the skin are the most worrisome complication of laser hair-removal treatments. The likelihood of this complication increases with darker pigmented or tanned skin. The risk of scarring increases with overaggressive treatment, inadequate cooling, or postprocedure infection. For severely injured skin, a topical steroid may be prescribed. Postprocedure infections should be recognized and treated expediently.

<u>Consent for all Laser Procedures</u>

Name: _____

Females only. When was your last menstrual cycle? _____

All laser patients:

- When was the last time you spent time outside or in a tanning bed/booth? _____

- Have you had sunburn in the past two weeks?   ( ) YES ( ) NO

- Do you currently have a self-tanner in the area being treated? ( ) YES ( ) NO

- Do any of your skin care products contain alpha hydroxy   ( ) YES ( ) NO
  acids, glycolic acids, or retinoids (i.e., retinol, Retin-A)?   ( ) YES ( ) NO

- Have you been using a bleaching or lightening product in the
  area being treated?   ( ) YES ( ) NO

- Have you had an injury to the skin in the area to be treated
  since your previous appointment?   ( ) YES ( ) NO

- Have you had an injury to the skin in the area to be treated
  since your previous appointment?   ( ) YES ( ) NO

By signing this form, I acknowledge that blistering, burning, scarring, hyperpigmentation (darkening of the skin), and hypopigmentation (lightening of the skin) are possible risks of laser and light-based procedures. I know that these risks increase with sun exposure and changes in medication.

_____   Evaluator's comments: _____
Client signature   _____
                                          _____
_____   _____
Date   _____
        Evaluator Initials _____

Fig. 15.2 A sample of an informed consent and preprocedure questionnaire for laser hair removal. (*continued*)

Client:_____ Today's Date:____/____/____

Address:_____ Date of Birth:____/____/____

Phone:_____ Alternative Phone:_____ Email:_____

Occupation:_____ Employer:_____

Emergency contact name & number: _____

How did you hear about us? _____

Reason for consultation: _____

Are you currently under a physician's care? ( ) YES   ( ) NO

Are you currently allergic to any medications? ( ) YES   ( ) NO   If yes, please list below:

_____

List all medications you are currently taking (including prescriptions, over-the-counter meds, vitamins, and herb(s):

_____

_____

Does your medication prohibit exposure to sun or light? ( ) YES ( ) NO

Have you been on Accutane in the past 6 months?   ( ) YES ( ) NO

Have you undergone chemotherapy or radiation?   ( ) YES ( ) NO

Do you experience herpes or cold sore breakouts?   ( ) YES ( ) NO

Do you take aspirin, ibuprofen, vitamin E, or other blood thinning medication? ( ) YES ( ) NO

    If YES, how recently? _____

Do you have now, or have you ever had diseases or conditions of: (Please check YES or NO)

	YES	NO		YES	NO
High Blood Pressure	( )	( )	Peripheral Vascular Disorder	( )	( )
Circulatory problems	( )	( )	Diabetes	( )	( )
Heart murmur/MVP	( )	( )	Thyroid Disorder	( )	( )
Irregular heartbeat	( )	( )	Prostate Disease	( )	( )
Phlebitis	( )	( )	Convulsions, Epilepsy, Seizures	( )	( )
Inflammation of vein	( )	( )	HIV/AIDS	( )	( )
Blood clots	( )	( )	Hormonal Condition	( )	( )
Pacemaker	( )	( )	Hepatitis (any type)	( )	( )

Other Diseases or Conditions:

_____

_____

_____

List all surgical procedures and dates:

_____

_____

_____

Fig. 15.2 (continued)

WOMEN: YES   NO

Polycystic Ovarian Syndrome   ( )   ( )

Tumors/Growths/Cysts   ( )   ( )

If YES, when:_____ and where:_____

Menstrual irregularity?   ( )   ( )

Are you pregnant?   ( )   ( )

Are you nursing?   ( )   ( )

Do you plan on becoming pregnant?   ( )   ( )

If YES, when? _____

SKIN:

Do you have redness/darkness from scars? ( )   ( )

Have you ever had skin cancer?   ( )   ( )

If YES, what type? _____ When? _____

Do you wear sunscreen daily?   ( )   ( )

When outside/on vacation?   ( )   ( ) SPF:_____

When were you most recently in the sun?_____ Activity? _____

Duration of exposure? _____

Do you have a history of any skin diseases? ( )   ( )   Which? _____

Do you have problems with healing?   ( )   ( )

Have you had any blistering sunburns?   ( )   ( )   When? _____

Do you develop keloids (raised, bumpy scars)? ( )   ( )

Do you bleed easily?   ( )   ( )

Do you smoke?   ( )   ( )

Do you have any tattoos or permanent makeup? ( ) ( )   Where? _____

Do you develop skin rashes in reaction to any of the following? :

( ) Medications   ( ) Food   ( ) Topical Neosporin   ( ) Environment

( ) Latex   ( ) Bandages   ( ) Anesthetics (novocaine, xylocaine, lidocaine, etc.)

( ) Other, specify: _____

<u>SKIN CONCERNS (Please circle the conditions that apply to you):</u>

Excessive/unwanted hair   Acne   Flushing/blushing   Rosacea   Enlarged pores   Oily skin

Fine lines   Broken capillaries   Age/sun spots   Oily T-Zone   Dry skin   Scarring

Black or whiteheads   Rough, dull tone & texture   Red spots on body   loose skin on face/neck/body

Other (describe): _____

Fig. 15.2 (continued)

SKIN PROCEDURE HISTORY:

Have you undergone any of the following procedures:

Microdermabrasion	( ) YES	( ) NO	When? _____
Chemical peel	( ) YES	( ) NO	When? _____
Laser resurfacing	( ) YES	( ) NO	When? _____
Laser hair removal	( ) YES	( ) NO	When? _____
Botox®	( ) YES	( ) NO	When? _____
Injectable filler	( ) YES	( ) NO	When? _____

(such as Collagen or Restylane®)

Thermage	( ) YES	( ) NO	When? _____
Fraxel	( ) YES	( ) NO	When? _____
Sclerotherapy	( ) YES	( ) NO	When? _____

(vein injections)

IPL/Fotofacial®/Photofacial	( ) YES	( ) NO	When? _____
Facial	( ) YES	( ) NO	When? _____
Waxing/Threading	( ) YES	( ) NO	When? _____

Please disclose any minimally invasive cosmetic surgical procedures you have had:

What type? _____   When? _____

Please disclose any cosmetic surgical procedures that required general anesthesia:

What type? _____   When? _____

_____   ___/___/___
Patient Signature   Date

Fig. 15.2 (continued)

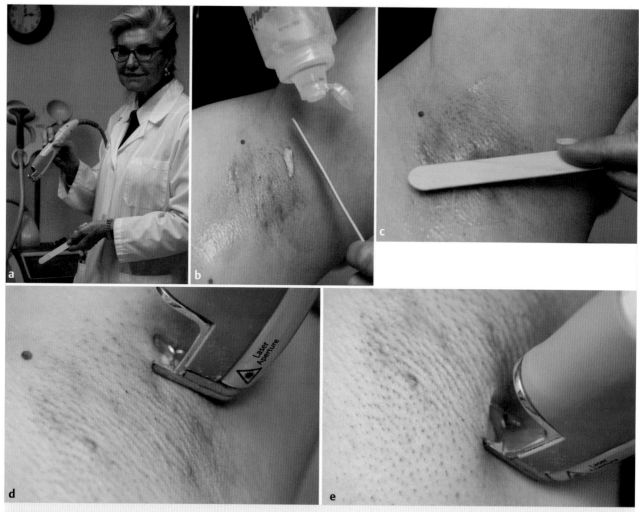

Fig. 15.3 Laser hair removal treatment session. (a) Laser nurse wearing safety glasses, using a neodymium:yttrium aluminum garnet (Nd:YAG) laser to treat axillary hair. (b) Cooling gel applied to axilla after removing deodorant. (c) A thin coating of gel is spread along treatment area. (d) The skin is cooled with the handpiece, lasered, and cooled again. (e) Perifollicular edema is noted at the treatment site.

State laws vary in respect to what level provider may perform laser hair removal. Jalian[19] et al performed an online search of databases involving litigation of laser surgeries performed by nonphysician operators (NPOs). They found that from 2008 to 2011, the number of cases using NPOs increased from 36.3 to 77.8% and that laser hair removal was the most commonly litigated procedure. Physicians should be aware of their state laws and the degree of supervision required when NPOs are performing laser hair-removal treatments.

15.8 Pearls and Pitfalls

- Laser hair removal is not a permanent form of hair removal and often requires multiple sessions for long-term results.
- The ideal candidate for laser hair removal has light-colored skin and dark-colored hair.
- Longer wavelength lasers work better on darker skinned individuals.
- Laser hair removal devices for home use are now FDA-approved.

- Patient counseling is important to optimize expectations and results.
- Settings should be adjusted to account for color, thickness, and location of the hair as well as Fitzpatrick skin type.
- Providers should be aware of potential complications, and early recognition and treatment will decrease the possibility of long-term sequelae.

References

[1] Sherrow V. Hair removal. In: Sherrow V, ed. Encyclopedia of Hair: A Cultural History. Westport, CT: Greenwood Press; 2006: 180–182

[2] Olsen EA. Methods of hair removal. J Am Acad Dermatol 1999; 40: 143–155, quiz 156–157

[3] Ramos-e-Silva M, de Castro MC, Carneiro LV, Jr. Hair removal. Clin Dermatol 2001; 19: 437–444

[4] Liew SH. Unwanted body hair and its removal: a review. Dermatol Surg 1999; 25: 431–439

[5] Wanitphakdeedecha R, Alster TS. Physical means of treating unwanted hair. Dermatol Ther 2008; 21: 392–401

[6] Fernandez AA, França K, Chacon AH, Nouri K. From flint razors to lasers: a timeline of hair removal methods. J Cosmet Dermatol 2013; 12: 153–162

[7] Ross EV, Ladin Z, Kreindel M, Dierickx C. Theoretical considerations in laser hair removal. Dermatol Clin 1999; 17: 333–355, viii

[8] Rao K, Sankar TK. Long-pulsed Nd:YAG laser-assisted hair removal in Fitzpatrick skin types IV-VI. Lasers Med Sci 2011; 26: 623–626

[9] Lask G, Elman M, Slatkine M, Waldman A, Rozenberg Z. Laser-assisted hair removal by selective photothermolysis. Preliminary results. Dermatol Surg 1997; 23: 737–739

[10] Lloyd JR, Mirkov M. Long-term evaluation of the long-pulsed alexandrite laser for the removal of bikini hair at shortened treatment intervals. Dermatol Surg 2000; 26: 633–637

[11] Island TC. TPIA Laser Hair Removal System (TRIA). TRIA Beauty, Inc. Dec. 23, 2009. Available at: http://www.accessdata.fda.gov/cdrh_docs/pdf9/K090820.pdf. Accessed February 13, 2014

[12] Wheeland RG. Permanent hair reduction with a home-use diode laser: safety and effectiveness 1 year after eight treatments. Lasers Surg Med 2012; 44: 550–557

[13] Chan HH, Ying SY, Ho WS, Wong DS, Lam LK. An in vivo study comparing the efficacy and complications of diode laser and long-pulsed Nd:YAG laser in hair removal in Chinese patients. Dermatol Surg 2001; 27: 950–954

[14] Li R, Zhou Z, Gold MH. An efficacy comparison of hair removal utilizing a diode laser and an Nd:YAG laser system in Chinese women. J Cosmet Laser Ther 2010; 12: 213–217

[15] Beeson WH, Rachel JD. Valacyclovir prophylaxis for herpes simplex virus infection or infection recurrence following laser skin resurfacing. Dermatol Surg 2002; 28: 331–336

[16] Almoallim H, Klinkhoff AV, Arthur AB, Rivers JK, Chalmers A. Laser induced chrysiasis: disfiguring hyperpigmentation following Q-switched laser therapy in a woman previously treated with gold. J Rheumatol 2006; 33: 620–621

[17] Weisberg NK, Greenbaum SS. Pigmentary changes after alexandrite laser hair removal. Dermatol Surg 2003; 29: 415–419

[18] Williams R, Havoonjian H, Isagholian K, Menaker G, Moy R. A clinical study of hair removal using the long-pulsed ruby laser. Dermatol Surg 1998; 24: 837–842

[19] Jalian HR, Jalian CA, Avram MM. Increased risk of litigation associated with laser surgery by nonphysician operators. JAMA Dermatol 2014; 150: 407–411

16 Laser Solutions for Scar Management

Jill S. Waibel and Ashley Rudnick

16.1 Introduction

Scars are the result of wounds that affect millions of people in the world and are prevalent in both civilians and wounded warriors injured in military combat. The initial injury may be caused by trauma, surgery, burns, or skin disease (acne, lupus, etc.). Treatment of acute wounds includes systemic stabilization and surgical intervention. Despite the best surgical care, patients continue to have functional impairments and uncomfortable symptoms from scars. Severe cutaneous scars are disfiguring and have many associated symptomatology including pruritus, pain, decreased function, and restricted range of motion. The new goal for scar treatment is that definitive rehabilitation ends with recovery of optimal appearance and function.

Multiple therapeutic options have been used to improve scars.[1] When re-epithelialization and the best surgery have taken their course, there are now new laser options for further scar improvements in function, symptoms, and cosmesis. Lasers are a scientifically precise and effective treatment modality to rehabilitate and improve scars.[2] Lasers have added a powerful tool to improve scar symptoms and deformities.[3]

16.2 Scar Laser Physics

We do not fully understand the biological basis by which scars improve after laser therapy. Scarring is a tissue response, acquired during the second trimester of fetal development at the same time as cellular immunity.[4] Scar tissue has increased vascular and lymphatic channels, as well as changes in collagen structure compared to normal skin. However, in scars the blood vessels, lymphatics, and collagen often are in a chaotic array with resultant decreased physiological function. It is known that in the treatment of healthy skin with a fractional ablative laser, these microscopic thermal injuries are produced in the dermis and stimulate a wound-healing cascade that ultimately leads to tissue remodeling. Normal skin can remodel these microscopic wounds without scarring. Macroscopic thermal burn injury causes the worst scars seen in clinical medicine. It is not understood how macroscopic thermal injury causes scars, and microscopic thermal injury improves scars. The improvements appear to be in the epidermis, dermis, and also have effects in the adnexal skin structures. Many patients report immediate improvement in pruritus, pain, and increased range of motion within hours to weeks after even one treatment session. The skin heals first with improvement of dyschromias followed in time with improvements in texture and topography. Further studies are needed to understand the biological enhancements seen by laser therapy of scars.

16.3 Laser and Surgery Synergy for Treatment of Scars

The treatment of scars is a multispecialty endeavor. A combination approach with medical experts yields optimal scar amelioration. If an injury heals in the presence of tension, hypertrophy often ensues. Understanding the role of tension in the development of a scar is essential to design a successful treatment strategy. If there is significant hypertrophy or contracture present in a scar, surgical intervention is necessary to relieve the tension or there is a high likelihood the scar will reform. After tension relief, hypertrophic and contracture scars are more elastic with new remodeling of collagen; and they are more amenable to laser therapy. However, if a scar has had initial fractional laser therapy, this often makes surgical intervention easier to perform due to thinner collagen bundles.

16.4 Approach to Treatment of Cutaneous Scars

In the initial evaluation of the scar, the physician should determine what characteristics the scar possesses and then choose therapies to address these issues. Some factors to consider before choosing the parameters of a laser device include thickness of the scar (thicker scars need increased depth), age of the scar (younger scars decrease depth and density), body location of the scar (off-face decreases depth and density), skin type of the patient (darker skin types decrease density), and comorbid medical conditions. Next, determine if a scar is hypertrophic, keloid, contracture, or atrophic. Then dyschromia of a scar should be evaluated for erythema, hyperpigmentation, and hypopigmentation. Often, severe scars have many of these characteristics within the same scar. The author's approach is to first use a nonablative laser to treat vascular and pigmented components of a scar and then to utilize fractional ablative tools for ablation of scar tissue, coagulation of microvasculature, and stimulation of subsequent neocollagenesis. The fractional ablative devices are the mainstay of therapy because of their ability to improve all scar types. Repeated laser sessions can occur until achievement of patient and/or physician satisfaction. It is the author's clinical experience, as well as confirmation in published articles, that with each laser session scars continue to improve. In one study for the treatment of an atrophic leishmaniasis scar with a nonablative fractional laser, a 40% improvement resulted after three laser sessions. After ten laser sessions, a 90% improvement was achieved.[5]

16.5 Clinical Indications and Treatment Recommendations

Lasering cutaneous scars requires proper diagnosis of scars as well as an understanding of their histology and biology. The majority of scars result from acne, surgery, trauma, or burns. Techniques and settings for each of these scars are reviewed in the following sections, based on the etiology of the scar.

16.5.1 Acne Scars

Acneiform scars are the result of compromised collagen production during the natural wound-healing process, resulting in

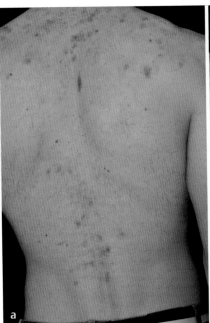
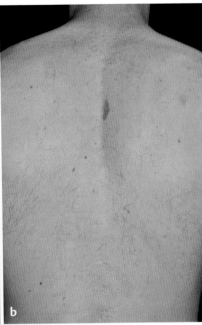

Fig. 16.1 Hypertrophic-/keloidal-type scars on back—fractional laser treatment. (a) Before treatment. (b) After treatment.

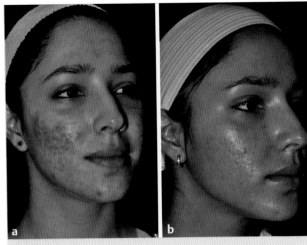

Fig. 16.2 Acne scars—multimodality therapy. (a) Before therapy. (b) After therapy.

cutaneous depressions. Topographical features of acne scarring include perpendicular bundles of collagen that anchor down the skin of the scars. The majority of patients have facial atrophic or *ice-pick* scars. Both result from loss of collagen deposition during the wound-healing process of acneiform lesions. The goals of laser resurfacing are to stimulate collagen and help "plump up" these areas of collagen loss. Given the dermal pathology present with acne scarring, particularly with atrophic scars, therapy modalities should optimally be capable of affecting dermal remodeling at least 1 mm below the skin. Acne scars on the chests and backs of patients are often hypertrophic or keloidal (▶ Fig. 16.1). Treatment of acne scars has traditionally been done with limited success; however, with the advent of deep-reaching, fractional lasers, greater success has been achieved. The acne-scar technique takes a multiprocedural approach (▶ Fig. 16.2). Superficial approaches for skin-surface refinement and pigmentary variation include glycolic acid

chemical peels and topical tretinoin and hydroquinone. Moderate approaches to address deeper scars include punch biopsy and closure, z-plasty transposition flap, fat polysaccharide matrix or collagen, scar subcision, dermabrasion, carbon dioxide (CO_2) laser resurfacing and, most recently, fractional photothermolysis.[6] Advances in laser technology over the last decade have led researchers to study their utilization for the treatment of acne scarring.

Ablative fractional CO_2 lasers have been well studied for acne scarring by Dr. Roy G. Geronemus, MD. In a case series of two to three treatment sessions for moderate to severe acne scarring, there were clinical improvements of 26 to 50% in texture, atrophy, and overall amelioration on topographic analysis. Improvements of 43 to 79.9% in scar depths were obtained; there was a mean depth upturn of 66.8%. A greater degree of improvement was seen with ablative fractional laser technology as opposed to previous studies with nonablative fractional lasers, resulting from deeper dermal penetration of the fractionated CO_2 device. Particularly, it was noted that patients treated for deeper scars on the cheeks with higher energy levels on the second and third treatments received the highest improvement scores.[7] Side effects with the ablative fractional tool were mild to moderate, including posttreatment erythema, edema, and petechiae—all of which resolved within 7 days after each session. Correlating with these clinical data, in vivo studies with this device by Hantash et al have shown tissue ablation and thermal effects as deep as 1 mm into the skin, likely accounting for the effect on moderate to severe acne scarring observed.[8]

In another study with the fractionated CO_2 laser for the treatment of acne scarring, 15 subjects underwent up to three treatments. Patients with a diversity of Fitzpatrick skin types (I–V) were treated, with no complications of short- or long-term hyperpigmentation reported. Of the entire number of subjects, 87% sustained significant improvement in the appearance of acne scarring at 3-month follow-up visits. All patients reported transient erythema that resolved in the first 2 weeks after therapy.[9] Ablative fractional instruments work for all skin types. In

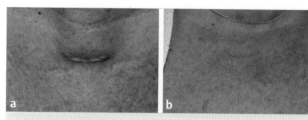

Fig. 16.3 Early thyroidectomy scar—fractional and vascular laser procedure. (**a**) Before procedure. (**b**) After procedure.

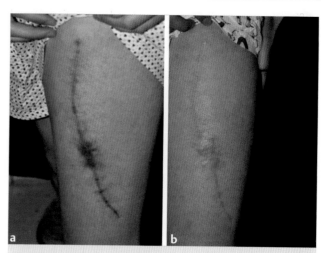

Fig. 16.4 Erythematous, hypertrophic scar—fractional laser treatment. (**a**) Before treatment. (**b**) After treatment.

a prospective study on five Asian patients of skin type IV with moderate to severe atrophic acne scarring, the subjects underwent two, single-pass sessions with an ablative fractional CO_2 laser 6 to 8 weeks apart. Treatment parameters were: fluence, 28 J/cm^2; pulse width, 2.5 ms; spot size, 300 μm; penetration depth, up to 500 μm; and degree of skin coverage, 20%. At 2 months posttreatment, all five patients showed some clinical advancement (four: mild improvement; one: moderate improvement). All patients had erythema that lasted for a mean of 6 days. No other complications, including postinflammatory hyperpigmentation, were observed.[10]

A study was performed on 20 Korean patients with atrophic acne scars treated in a single session with the combined deep and superficial modes of an ablative CO_2 fractional laser. Follow-up results revealed that one patient had clinical improvement of 76 to 100%; nine subjects had enhancements of 51 to 75%; seven patients had moderate advancements of 26 to 50%; and three subjects had minimal to no amelioration. The mean duration of posttherapy crusting or scaling was 6.3 ± 3.0 days, and posttherapy erythema lasted 2.8 ± 4.6 days. A combination of two different treatment modes may provide a new therapy algorithm for acne scars in Asians.[11] Another study treated 13 patients with skin type IV and atrophic scars during three sessions with an ablative fractional CO_2 laser, at an average of 7-week intervals. At 6-month follow-up, 85% of the subjects were rated as having at least a 25 to 50% improvement. At 1 month after three treatments, surface smoothness ($p = 0.03$) and scar volume ($p < 0.001$) significantly improved relative to baseline.[12]

16.5.2 Surgical Scars

All surgical scars improve with fractional ablative laser. First, one must evaluate if the surgical scar is elevated (hypertrophic) or depressed (atrophic). The thicker, hypertrophic scars need deeper treatment depths, whereas more atrophic scars can be dealt with more superficially. Early surgical scars with significant erythema respond to vascular lasers, with or without same-day treatment of fractional lasers (▶ Fig. 16.3).

In a study of 23 Korean women with thyroidectomy scars, a single session was conducted of two passes with a fractional CO_2 laser with a pulse energy of 50 mJ and a density of 100 spots/cm^2. Treatments were performed 2 to 3 weeks after surgery.[13]

Erythematous, hypertrophic scars are seen frequently in the first year after injury. Vascular-specific lasers and light devices, especially the 595-nm pulsed dye laser (PDL), are already well established for such applications, and their use has been highlighted in two recent reviews.[14,15] PDL may be applied alone for small hypertrophic scars, but is often combined with fractional

laser therapy in either concurrent or alternating treatment sessions (▶ Fig. 16.4). Hypertrophic scars develop due to increased proliferation of dermal fibroblasts, resulting in an excess of collagen in the wound that brings about an elevated cutaneous surface.

16.5.3 Burn and Trauma Scars

Hypertrophic burn and traumatic scars are best improved by either ablative or nonablative fractional lasers. Ablative fractional lasers have the capacity to induce a more robust remodeling response than nonablative fractional lasers (▶ Fig. 16.5).[16,17] Ablative lasers have a significantly greater potential depth of thermal injury compared to nonablative lasers, 1.8 mm compared to 4.0 mm, respectively (Lumenis SCAAR FX software). Furthermore, tissue ablation appears to induce a modest immediate photomechanical release of tension in some restrictive scars. An appropriate degree of surrounding thermal coagulation seems to facilitate the subsequent remodeling response. An estimation of scar pliability and thickness through palpation is central to determining appropriate laser pulse energy settings (treatment depth). Treatment depth should not exceed the thickness of the scar. Pigmentary abnormalities (hypopigmentation, hyperpigmentation, dyspigmentation) of scars also improve with fractional therapy (▶ Fig. 16.6).

Flat or atrophic scars from burns and trauma also respond to fractional laser therapy. Atrophic scars are dermal depressions that occur due to collagen destruction during an injury. The goal of laser treatment for atrophic scars is to stimulate collagen production within the atrophic areas (▶ Fig. 16.7 and ▶ Fig. 16.8). Neocollagenesis is stimulated the most from fractional laser therapy, and thus makes it the best choice for flat or thin scars.

16.6 Preoperative and Treatment Considerations

16.6.1 Pretreatment Considerations

As with any procedure, informed consent should include a realistic discussion of therapeutic goals, limitations, and potential complications. A team approach is vital because professional wound care, physical and occupational therapies, and surgical consultation should be available, if possible, throughout the treatment course to optimize outcomes. Pertinent historical information during the initial evaluation includes the time and mechanism of injury, surgical history and schedule of upcoming procedures, previous complications, current limitations and treatment goals, pain and sensory issues, presence of posttraumatic stress disorder (PTSD), and response to current therapy. Physical examination should elicit scar characteristics such as the presence of residual erosions and ulcers, erythema, pliability, textural irregularity, dyspigmentation, and scar thickness and degree of restriction. Associated features that may relate to adjunctive treatments include the presence or absence of residual hair, hyperhidrosis, traumatic tattoos, and related dermatologic conditions such as folliculitis.

Lastly, many patients with severe burn or traumatic scars may have developed PTSD and/or traumatic brain injury (TBI). If patients have either PTSD or TBI other medical paraprofessionals including psychiatrists should be part of the treatment team.

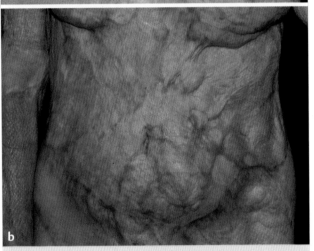

Fig. 16.5 Burn scar—fractional laser procedure. (a) Before procedure. (b) After procedure.

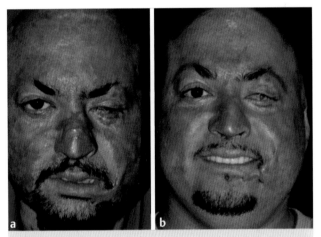

Fig. 16.6 Hypertrophic scar with multiple pigmentary abnormalities—fractional laser therapy. (a) Before therapy. (b) After therapy.

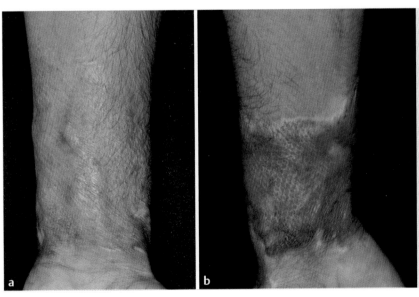

Fig. 16.7 Atrophic scar—fractional laser treatment. (a) Before treatment. (b) After treatment.

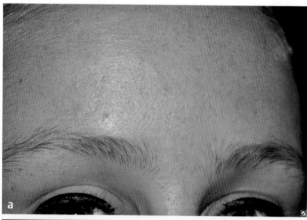
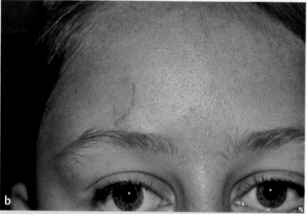

Fig. 16.8 Thin, forehead scar—fractional laser technique. (a) Before technique. (b) After technique.

16.6.2 Fractional Laser Treatment Technique

The majority of treatments are performed in the clinic setting using commercially available topical anesthetic preparations under occlusion for 1 hour or more prior to treatment. Due to large surface areas affected, care must be taken to avoid lidocaine toxicity.[18] Despite an elevated risk for chronic pain issues in this population, pain control during Ablative Fractional Laser (AFL) is frequently not as difficult as it initially appears, given that grafted and scarred sites are often insensate or have reduced sensation. Injectable local anesthetics may be utilized in focal areas, and these measures are often supplemented during treatment with a forced-chilled-air device (Zimmer Cryo, Zimmer Medizin Systems, Irvine, California). Some patients may benefit from systemic preoperative analgesics or anxiolytics. Conscious sedation or even general anesthesia can be employed in instances of large surface area involvement or anticipated poor patient tolerance of the procedure while awake. This is a particularly important consideration in children because multiple treatments are usually required, and children do not tolerate repeated painful interventions well.

With previous discussion in mind, fractional laser treatment technique, parameters, and adjunctive procedures should be applied thoughtfully to minimize the degree of cumulative thermal injury to the tissue. Each treatment is customized at every session according to individual scar characteristics and interval changes. Selected pulse energies are proportional to the scar thickness as estimated by palpation and desired treatment depth without extending beyond the depth of the scar. Aggressive pulse energy settings require a concomitant reduction in procedure density to decrease the potential for bulk heating. Low-density fractional treatment is favored to reduce the risk of complications when treating scars. The treatment area includes the entire scar sheet and a 1 to 2-mm rim of normal skin. Any part of the body may potentially be treated with fractional laser therapy. Procedure parameters should be lowered when treating off-face scars.

16.6.3 When to Treat a Scar

The optimal time to begin fractional laser treatment has yet to be determined. As a general rule, there should be a healed and intact epidermis prior to laser treatment. Treatment of freshly healing wounds with unstable epidermal coverage in the first 1 to 3 months after injury may lead to unpredictable and potentially harmful outcomes. Younger, less mature scars are less tolerant of aggressive processes and should be treated more judiciously in terms of laser settings and combination procedures than more mature scars (years after injury). Mature scars, whether 1 year old or 60 years old, all respond well to laser therapy. A minimum treatment interval of 1 to 3 months between fractional laser treatments is recommended to give scar tissue that is compromised time to heal. Even after just one therapy session, a patient may continue to have improvement for many months up to 1 year.

16.6.4 Postoperative Considerations

Immediately after ablative fractional treatments, petrolatum or a petrolatum-based ointment is applied and continued several times daily until the site is fully epithelialized, usually within 3 or 4 days. Cold compresses are helpful in the first 40 hours to decrease excessive edema and for patient comfort. Patients may resume showering the following day and begin gentle, daily cleansing of the area with mild soap at least twice a day. Dilute vinegar compresses may be initiated, according to the preferences of the treating surgeon and patient. Vinegar may help pH (measurement of acidity) of the skin return to a more normal level and promote healing, as well as discourage bacterial or fungal colonization during this healing period. Patients are allowed to resume essentially normal activity after treatment. Sun avoidance is recommended for 12 weeks after laser therapy. In cases of scar contracture, participation in physical and occupational therapies is highly recommended to take full advantage of the laser effects. Full immersion, such as in a pool or the ocean, is not recommended until the therapy area is fully epithelialized to avoid infections. As with any cutaneous surgical procedure, basic contact and hygiene precautions should be emphasized. Oral antibiotics and antivirals are commonly used for prophylaxis starting 1 day prior to the treatment and continuing up to 1 week after the therapy. Antifungals may be entertained on a case-by-case basis or if the patient develops localized pain or pruritus after laser treatment. When treating facial areas, viral prophylaxis should be considered. Photoprotection should be advocated, including avoidance in the early posttreatment period and application of bland sunblocks once epithelial integrity is restored. Physical sunblocks of zinc or titanium dioxide are less irritating to newly lasered skin. Compression therapy with either silicone gel sheets, tight athletic wear, or medical-compression garments is encouraged, while healing from laser therapy.

16.6.5 Complications

Overall, fractional ablative lasers have a favorable adverse-event rate.[19,20] Safe treatment is based on the avoidance of excessive thermal injury and good laser practices in clinic. General principles applicable to laser selection and therapy technique include applying fractional treatments at low densities, with a relatively narrow beam diameter and pulse width, and minimizing the number of passes. Higher pulse energy settings are typically deeper treatments and necessarily require a concomitant decrease in treatment density; and treatments are frequently performed at the lowest density settings. It is recommended, if possible, to see a patient 1 week after therapy to ensure skin has re-epithelialization and no infections. Patients are advised to call if they experience excessive pain or pruritus.

16.7 Future Directions

Fractional laser technology has revolutionized laser therapy. In the next few years, the fractional ablative tunnels can be utilized for laser-assisted delivery systems (LADS) of a variety of drugs, topical agents, and other living tissue.[21,22,23] Laser-assisted drug delivery may allow for greater precise depth of penetration by existing topical medications, more efficient transcutaneous delivery of large drug molecules, and even systemic drug administration via a transcutaneous route. These zones may be used immediately postoperatively to deliver drugs and other substances to synergistically create an enhanced therapeutic response.

16.8 Summary

Since their introduction, fractional lasers have helped many adults and children with scar deformity. It is very rewarding to be a physician who is part of improving a scar on an infant or an adult. Patients and families are grateful for these medical devices. The medical success of fractional lasers has added greatly to our ability to help heal our patients.

References

[1] Asilian A, Darougheh A, Shariati F. New combination of triamcinolone, 5-Fluorouracil, and pulsed-dye laser for treatment of keloid and hypertrophic scars. Dermatol Surg 2006; 32: 907–915

[2] Kwan JM, Wyatt M, Uebelhoer NS, Pyo J, Shumaker PR. Functional improvement after ablative fractional laser treatment of a scar contracture. PM&R 2011; 3: 986–987

[3] Waibel J, Wulkan AJ, Lupo M, Beer K, Anderson RR. Treatment of burn scars with the 1,550 nm nonablative fractional erbium laser. Lasers Surg Med 2012; 44: 441–446

[4] Larson BJ, Longaker MT, Lorenz HP. Scarless fetal wound healing: a basic science review. Plast Reconstr Surg 2010; 126: 1172–1180

[5] Jung JY, Lee JH, Ryu DJ, Lee SJ, Bang D, Cho SB. Lower-fluence, higher density versus higher-fluence, lower density treatment with a 10,600 nm carbon dioxide fractional laser system: a split-face, evaluator-blinded study. Dermatol Surg 2010; 36: 2022–2029

[6] Leclère FM, Mordon SR. Twenty-five years of active laser prevention of scars: what have we learned? J Cosmet Laser Ther 2010; 12: 227–234

[7] Chapas AM, Brightman L, Sukal S, et al. Successful treatment of acneiform scarring with CO2 ablative fractional resurfacing. Lasers Surg Med 2008; 40: 381–386

[8] Hantash BM, Bedi VP, Kapadia B, et al. In vivo histological evaluation of a novel ablative fractional resurfacing device. Lasers Surg Med 2007; 39: 96–107

[9] Ortiz A, Elkeeb L, Truitt A, Tournas J, Zachary C. Evaluation of a novel fractional resurfacing device for the treatment of acne scarring. Abstract presented at: American Society for Laser Medicine and Surgery Conference; April 2008; Kissimmee, FL

[10] Wang YS, Tay YK, Kwok C. Fractional ablative carbon dioxide laser in the treatment of atrophic acne scarring in Asian patients: a pilot study. J Cosmet Laser Ther 2010; 12: 61–64

[11] Cho SB, Lee SJ, Kang JM, Kim YK, Chung WS, Oh SH. The efficacy and safety of 10,600-nm carbon dioxide fractional laser for acne scars in Asian patients. Dermatol Surg 2009; 35: 1955–1961

[12] Manuskiatti W, Triwongwaranat D, Varothai S, Eimpunth S, Wanitphakdeedecha R. Efficacy and safety of a carbon-dioxide ablative fractional resurfacing device for treatment of atrophic acne scars in Asians. J Am Acad Dermatol 2010; 63: 274–283

[13] Jung JY, Jeong JJ, Roh HJ, et al. Early postoperative treatment of thyroidectomy scars using a fractional carbon dioxide laser. Dermatol Surg 2011; 37: 217–223

[14] Vrijman C, van Drooge AM, Limpens J, et al. Laser and intense pulsed light therapy for the treatment of hypertrophic scars: a systematic review. Br J Dermatol 2011; 165: 934–942

[15] Sobanko JF, Alster TS. Laser treatment for improvement and minimization of facial scars. Facial Plast Surg Clin North Am 2011; 19: 527–542

[16] Oh BH, Hwang YJ, Lee YW, Choe YB, Ahn KJ. Skin characteristics after fractional photothermolysis. Ann Dermatol 2011; 23: 448–454

[17] Anderson R, Donelan M, Hivnor C, et al. Laser Treatment of Traumatic Scar With An Emphasis on Ablative Fractional Laser Resurfacing Consensus Report. JAMA Dermatol 2014;150:187-193

[18] Kim HS, Lee JH, Park YM, Lee JY. Comparison of the effectiveness of nonablative fractional laser versus ablative fractional laser in thyroidectomy scar prevention: a pilot study. J Cosmet Laser Ther 2012; 14: 89–93

[19] Marra DE, Yip D, Fincher EF, Moy RL. Systemic toxicity from topically applied lidocaine in conjunction with fractional photothermolysis. Arch Dermatol 2006; 142: 1024–1026

[20] Graber EM, Tanzi EL, Alster TS. Side effects and complications of fractional laser photothermolysis: experience with 961 treatments. Dermatol Surg 2008; 34: 301–305, discussion 305–307

[21] Waibel J, Wulkan A, Shumaker P. Treatment of hypertrophic scars using laser and laser-assisted corticosteroid delivery. Lasers Surg Med 2013; 45: 135–40

[22] Rkein A, Ozog D, Waibel J. Treatment of atrophic scars with fractionated CO2 laser facilitating delivery of topically applied poly-L-lactic acid. Dermatol Surg 2014; 40: 624–631

[23] Erlendsson AM, Anderson RR, Manstein D, Waibel JS. Developing technology: Ablative fractional lasers enhance topical drug delivery. Dermatol Surg 2014; 40: S142–S146

17 Treatment of Acne Scarring

Cynthia M. Gregg

17.1 Introduction

Acne vulgaris is one of the most common skin conditions in adolescents and adults, and has been reported to affect up to 80% of individuals between the ages of 11 and 30. The causes of acne vulgaris include: hormonal changes, increased sebum production, *propionibacterium acnes* activity, follicular hyperkeratinization, and perifollicular inflammation. The incidence of acne scarring in the general population has been reported between 1 and 30%.[1,2] Acne scarring is a consequence of abnormal wound healing due to damage in the pilosebaceous follicle during inflammation. Recent studies suggest that a patient's risk of scarring correlates with the type and magnitude of the inflammatory response in acne lesions. Cell-mediated immune responses aid in clearance of an antigen but also contribute to the amount of tissue damage. Studies by Holland et al[3] and Holland and Jeremy[4] used immunohistochemical methods to determine the cell-mediated response in developing and resolving inflamed acne lesions. Patients prone to acne scarring have an ineffective early inflammatory response followed by a later increased inflammatory response with greater cellular activation and domination by an influx of macrophages. Acne scars vary in their clinical presentations with a wide range of both pigment and textural alterations in the skin. However, the psychosocial impact of an acne scar cannot be underestimated. Acne scarring can be very distressing to patients and can result in a decreased self-esteem and a diminished quality of life.[5] It is important to note that the degree of an individual's psychosocial distress associated with acne scarring may not correlate with the amount of acne scarring present on examination.

17.2 Acne Scar Classification

Acne scars can be differentiated by color and textural changes in the skin. Postinflammatory erythema may be a resolving acne lesion's initial presentation. Brown shades of postinflammatory hyperpigmentation may lighten and improve with time, whereas hypopigmentation represents the final result of the scarring process. Textural skin changes can be categorized as hypertrophic or atrophic. Hypertrophic scars are confined within the margins of the original injury. They are raised, firm nodular lesions. Keloids resemble hypertrophic scars but are characterized by a disproportionate deposition of collagen with an excess amount outside of the original injury margins. Hypertrophic and keloid scars are a result of excessive collagen deposition at the site of the skin injury where fibrosis has elevated the skin surface focally. In contrast, loss or damage of soft tissue is referred to as an atrophic scar. These acne scars result from collagen destruction in the dermis and soft tissue atrophy. Scar contraction results in the indentation of the skin. Atrophic acne scars are often erythematous initially and can become hypopigmented or hyperpigmented with time. In 2001, Jacob et al proposed a classification of atrophic acne scars into three types: ice-pick, rolling, and boxcar scars. Ice-pick scars are narrow (less than 2 mm), V-shaped epithelial tracts that extend deep into the dermis. Rolling scars are wider (4–5 mm) and are tethered to the subcutaneous tissue, resulting in an undulating appearance. Boxcar scars are sharply delineated round or oval depressions that can be shallow or deep and range in diameters of 1.5–4 mm.[6]

Atrophic acne scarring is by far the most common form of acne scarring, especially on the face.[7] Goodman and Baron proposed a new qualitative grading system for acne scarring with suggested therapies for each scar type (▶ Table 17.1 and ▶ Table 17.2). This grading system has four levels of acne scarring: (1) macular, (2) mild, (3) moderate, and (4) severe. The subdivisions for level 1, macular disease, include erythematous, hypopigmented or hyperpigmented. Grades 2 to 4, mild to severe disease, are classified as being atrophic or hypertrophic. Grade 3, moderate, acne scars can be flattened by manually stretching the skin, and include rolling or shallow boxcar scars. Grade 4 scars are not distensible and include ice-pick, deep boxcar, and significant hypertrophic and keloid acne scars.[8] The lack of a true consensus on a grading scale for acne scarring may limit the ability to clinically standardize the therapeutic approach to acne scars.[9]

17.3 Treatment Options for Acne Scars

Prevention of acne scarring is best achieved through early treatment of active acne. However, once a patient has acne scarring

Table 17.1 Grades of postacne scarring

Grade	Level of disease	Characteristics
1	Macular	Erythematous, hyperpigmented or hypopigmented flat marks visible to patient or observer at any distance
2	Mild	Mild atrophy or hypertrophy that may not be obvious at social distances of 50 cm or more, and may be covered adequately by makeup or the normal shadow of shaved beard hair in men or normal body hair if extrafacial
3	Moderate	Moderate atrophic or hypertrophic scarring that is obvious at social distances of 50 cm or more, and is not covered easily by makeup or the normal shadow of shaved beard hair in men or body hair if extrafacial, but is still able to be flattened by manual stretching of the skin (if atrophic)
4	Severe	Severe atrophic or hypertrophic scarring that is obvious at social distances greater than 50 cm, and is not covered easily by makeup or the normal shadow of shaved beard hair in men or body hair if extrafacial and is not able to be flattened by manual stretching of the skin

(Reproduced with permission from Goodman GJ, Baron JA. The management of postacne scarring. Dermatol Surg 2007; 33: 1175–1188.)

Table 17.2 Global acne-scarring classification: types of scars making up the classification grades

Grade	Level of disease	Examples of scars
1	Macular	Erythematous, hyperpigmented, or hypopigmented flat marks
2	Mild	Mild rolling, small soft papular
3	Moderate	More significant rolling, shallow boxcar, mild to moderate hypertrophic or papular scars
4	Severe	Punched-out atrophic (deep boxcar), ice-pick, bridges and tunnels, marked atrophy, dystrophic significant hypertrophy or keloid

(Reproduced with permission from Goodman GJ, Baron JA. The management of postacne scarring. Dermatol Surg 2007; 33: 1175–1188.)

the treatment should be individualized to meet the needs of the patient. It is important to establish realistic expectations for patients. Patient education regarding the nature of acne scarring and the inability to remove the scar is imperative in the preoperative evaluation and consultation. Treatment for acne scars can be divided into medical, procedural, and surgical options. Typically, a wide variety of acne scars can exist in each individual patient, necessitating knowledge of the range of treatment modalities available.

17.3.1 Medical Options

Topical retinoids are recommended as part of a combination treatment for inflammatory acne disease. Topical retinoids stimulate collagen formation, increase dermal collagen synthesis, and improve elastic fibers.[10,11] Use of a 0.05% topical tretinoin for 4 months was reported to improve the appearance of facial ice-pick scars.[12] Topical treatments including retinoic acid, hydroquinone, azelaic acid, and kojic acid are effective in decreasing postinflammatory hyperpigmentation.[13,14] Tretinoin causes epidermal thickening, compaction of the stratum corneum, increased granular thickness, increased collagen synthesis, and decreased melanin content, which results in a decrease of postinflammatory hyperpigmentation and improved appearance of facial rhytids and scars.

Options for treatment of hypertrophic and keloid scars include the glucocorticoids (triamcinolone, hydrocortisone, methyl prednisone, and dexamethasone). The glucocorticoids have anti-inflammatory properties and inhibit fibroblast growth while degrading collagen. Serial intralesional injections spaced 4 to 6 weeks apart can result in flattening and softening of hypertrophic and keloid scars. Injection of cystic, inflammatory acne lesions with steroids may help prevent scarring by decreasing the inflammatory response.[15] Complications from excessive steroid injections include atrophy, hypopigmentation, and telangectasias.[16] A pyrimidine analogue with antimetabolic activity, 5-fluorouracil (5-FU), has been shown to inhibit wound healing. This compound has an inhibitory effect on human fibroblast by inhibiting proliferation and myofibroblast differentiation. Fluorouracil is usually used at a concentration of 50 mg/mL with a total dose between 50 to 150 mg per session. Fluorouracil can be used alone or mixed at a ratio of 80:20 with a low-strength steroid.[8] In a 2002 study by Gupta and Kalra, more than 50% of patients showed significant flattening of keloids as a result of intralesional injections with 5-FU.[17] Additionally, Bleomycin has been shown to flatten hypertrophic scars by inhibiting collagen synthesis through its cytotoxic effects on dividing fibroblasts.[18]

Silicone gel sheeting is recommended as a safe and effective management option for keloid and hypertrophic scars.[19] Several studies report that silicone gels and silicone sheets are equal in efficacy in improvement of scar redness, elevation, pain, and pruritus. Research suggests that the possible mechanism of action of silicone products is not only a result of occlusion but that the magnitude of the occlusion may be an important component in the mechanism of action of silicone. In addition, the decrease in transepidermal water loss and resulting increase in hydration from the occlusion provided by the silicone product may modulate the signaling cascade initiated by the epidermis that stimulates the collagen production by dermal fibroblasts. The use of silicone gels may be better accepted by patients than the silicone sheets due to the decreased visibility of the applied gel on the scar.[20]

17.3.2 Procedural Options

Dermabrasion can be one of the most effective but operator-dependent therapies for acne scarring. It is most effective for rolling, undulating scars and superficial boxcar scars.[21] Several dermabrasion devices exist using either a high-speed brush or diamond cylinder. Diamond fraises are available in varying degrees of coarseness and different shapes. Superficial dermabrasion eliminates the epidermis and a deeper treatment will cause an injury in the papillary dermis. Re-epithelialization occurs by migration of cells stemming from the adnexal structures including the hair follicles, sebaceous glands, and sweat glands. Active inflammatory acne lesions that are present must be treated first and resolved prior to the dermabrasion procedure. A complete re-epithelialization usually occurs within 7 to 10 days after dermabrasion. Postdermabrasion care may include leaving the area open or managing it with occlusive dressings. Complications from dermabrasion include hypertrophic scarring and keloid formation, dyschromia, and infection. Prophylactic treatment of patients with a known history of herpes simplex virus (HSV) and preoperative treatment with antibiotics are recommended. Eczema dermatitis has been reported in 10% of patients and can be treated with topical, intralesional, or systemic steroids.[22] It is recommended that patients wait a minimum of 6 to 12 months after treatment of isotretinoin therapy before undergoing a dermabrasion treatment.[6,7] Isotretinoin reduces the cellular activity of cutaneous adnexal appendages, which hinders the re-epithelialization after the dermabrasion procedure.

Chemical peels differ in their depth of penetration into the skin. In general, patients are open to the option of chemical peels because they are relatively noninvasive; have little downtime; and can improve skin pigmentation, tone, and texture. Superficial peels include alpha hydroxy acids (glycolic, lactic, citric) or beta hydroxy acid (salicylic), Jessner's Solution, modified Jessner's Solution, resorcinol, and low-strength trichloracetic acid (TCA) (< 20%TCA). Light peels are used to treat the most superficial of acne scars and are beneficial for improving postinflammatory hyperpigmentation. TCA solutions of 30 to 40% are primarily considered medium-depth peels. These peels extend down to the papillary dermis. Following a TCA peel, the skin re-epithelializes during the next several days and dermal collagen remodeling may continue for the next several months. During this process there is an increase in the production of collagen, elastin, and glycosaminocans.[23] Deep chemical peels are phenol or croton oil-based. Deep chemical peels using 50% or more TCA and phenol/croton oil-based peels can extend to the reticular dermis and may be more effective for deep atrophic scars; however, they do carry a higher risk for postprocedure dyschromia, milia, and secondary infection. Phenol peels also have an added risk of possible cardiotoxicity and require cardiopulmonary monitoring and intravenous (IV) hydration during the procedure.[24]

Chemical peels are typically performed to treat an entire face or an aesthetic unit. The use of TCA has been refined to only treat the atrophic acne scars, using the chemical reconstruction of skin scars (CROSS) method.[25] This method is reported to improve clinical results with rapid healing times and lower complication rates.[26] The CROSS technique uses focal application of a high concentration (65–100%) of TCA to produce frosting directly in the acne scars. Treatments are often repeated at 6-week intervals and patients can receive a total of six procedures. Histological examination of the treated acne scars revealed coagulative necrosis in the epidermis and necrosis of collagen in the papillary and reticular dermis. This resulted in increased collagen in the treated scars and increased collagen production and fragmentation of elastin fibers in the papillary dermis.[27]

Tissue augmentation using fillers is effective in treating patients with superficial atrophic scars such as undulating, rolling scars. The previously available injectable collagens have been replaced with products containing hyaluronic acid (HA), calcium hydroxylapatite, and poly-L-lactic acid. HA is a polysaccharide that occurs naturally in the body's connective tissue, dermis, umbilical cord, hyaline cartilage, and synovial joint fluid. After the first HA filler was introduced in 2003, a variety of available HA products have become available that differ in their concentration, degree of cross-linking, particle sizes, and longevity.[28] HA fillers may improve the appearance of atrophic acne scars alone or they can be combined with subcision. Disadvantages of using HA fillers include the need for frequent treatments, and HA fillers may only improve the appearance of mildly atrophic scars.

Calcium hydroxylapatite, Food and Drug Administration (FDA) approved in 2006, is a semipermanent filler composed of synthetic bone with microspheres 25 to 45 µm in diameter in a carboxymethylcellulose gel vehicle. The calcium hydroxylapatite (Radiesse, Merz North America, Inc., Raleigh, North Carolina) is biodegradable and stimulates fibroblastic production of collagen. Calcium hydroxylapatite is often appropriate for improving the appearance of shallow, atrophic acne scars.[29] Injectable poly-L-lactic acid (PLLA) (Galderma Pharma SA/ Galderma SA, Lausanne, Switzerland) is a synthetic, long-lasting dermal filler initially approved in 2004 for the correction of facial lipoatrophy associated with treatment for human immunodeficiency virus (HIV) infections. PLLA is a synthetic polymer similar to absorbable suture material. It comes in a lyophilized form and requires reconstitution with sterile water for injection. PLLA stimulates collagen formation due to a foreign-body reaction. Treatment with PLLA may require several sessions over a 4- to 6-month period with lasting results of 24 months or longer. PLLA is used to restore facial volume and several clinical trials and case reports have documented improvement in atrophic facial acne scars.[30,31]

A recent study in 2013 found that the autologous fibroblast procedure was associated with a significantly greater treatment success than the vehicle control for grade 3 (▶ Table 17.1), atrophic, distensible facial acne scars. Autologous fibroblasts are cultured from postauricular, full-thickness, punch biopsies. The autologous fibroblasts were injected into the papillary dermal plane under the atrophic acne scars in three treatment sessions spaced approximately 2 weeks apart. Whereas the mechanism of action of the procedure is not well understood, the improvement in the scar appearance may be due to new collagen production and remodeling of preexisting extracellular matrix in the scarred tissue.[32]

Deep acne scarring can produce severe facial fat atrophy. During the aging process additional soft tissue loss can increase the appearance of the acne scarring and lipoatrophy. Fat augmentation is able to reproduce the youthful appearance of a fuller face by replacing the soft tissue volume. The success of fat grafting is technique-dependent and the treatment requires a second surgical site for harvesting the fat. Improvements and advancements in fat-grafting techniques are resulting in greater consistency and longevity of the procedures.[33,34]

Microneedling or rolling, also referred to as percutaneous collagen induction, utilizes 30-gauge needles introduced into the skin in multiple directions in a controlled fashion. The epidermal trauma heals with transepidermal migration and the dermal trauma heals with collagen remodeling. Skin needling triggers a cascade of growth factors that stimulate wound healing. Histological studies show an increase in collagen and elastin deposition at 6 months posttreatment and a normal stratum corneum; thickened epidermis and normal rete ridges at 12 months posttreatment are displayed.[35,36]

Microneedling or collagen induction therapy is an in-office procedure performed under local anesthetic. Several studies have suggested that it is best utilized for grades 2 and 3 atrophic rolling or shallow boxcar acne scarring with four to six treatment sessions spaced 4 to 6 weeks apart. An advantage of microneedling is that it can be used on all skin types with little downtime.[37,38,39]

Botulinum toxin type A can decrease the appearance of acne scars that are amplified with facial movement. This treatment option is limited but may be applicable for amelioration in the appearance of acne scars in the upper third of the face and the chin area.[40]

Several laser/light therapy options exist to correct the dyschromia of acne scars and to improve the appearance of atrophic acne scars with stimulation of collagen production and remodeling. These include intense pulsed light (IPL) lasers, Q-switched (QS) lasers, the microsecond pulsed neodymium:

yttrium aluminum garnet (Nd:YAG) laser, erbium:yttrium aluminum garnet (Er:YAG) lasers, and erbium:yttrium scandium gallium garnet (Er:YSGG) lasers. Excimer lasers have a wavelength in the ultraviolet (UV) range (308 nm) and provide concentrated melanin stimulation to white scars. Treatment should be deemed unsuccessful if there is no improvement in the hypopigmentation after five to ten sessions of excimer laser therapy.[41]

IPL devices provide noncoherent light of multiple wavelengths ranging from 500 to 1,200 nm that are confined to narrow ranges by the use of filters. A series of IPL procedures spaced 3 to 4 weeks apart can treat several conditions, including reducing the superficial erythema in early acne scars and decreasing postinflammatory hyperpigmentation. IPL devices are able to treat large surface areas due to the larger spot sizes.

The first report of a nonablative laser being used for erythematous facial acne scars was published in 1996.[42] Average clinical improvement in the acne scars 6 weeks after one session with the 585-nm pulsed dye laser (PDL) was 67.5%. A series of treatments with the vascular-specific 585-nm PDL can significantly improve the appearance of erythematous hypertrophic scars by reducing the redness and by induction of dermal collagen remodeling without epidermal damage. PDLs can be used on all skin types. The most common adverse effect of treatment with a PDL is posttreatment purpura that can persist for several days. Other nonablative lasers used to treat atrophic scars are the 1,320-nm Nd:YAG, 1,450-nm diode, and the 1,064-nm Nd:YAG.[43] A study by Tanzi and Alster demonstrated that the 1,320-nm Nd:YAG and the 1,450-nm diode lasers both offer safe and effective clinical improvement of mild to moderate atrophic facial scars. They reported that the maximum clinical improvement was seen 6 months after a series of nonablative laser treatments. However, a decrease of clinical results in a 12-month follow-up evaluation suggests that maintenance treatments may be warranted or needed to enhance or maintain the clinical improvement.[44]

Carbon dioxide (CO_2) laser resurfacing and the Er:YAG laser are two ablative skin-resurfacing techniques used to treat acne scarring. The CO_2 laser with a wavelength of 10,600 nm has as its target extracellular and intracellular water. CO_2 laser resurfacing is useful for hypertrophic scars, boxcar scars, and rolling, undulating scars (▶ Fig. 17.1, ▶ Fig. 17.2, ▶ Fig. 17.3). The ER:YAG laser is a gentler ablative laser resurfacing as compared to the CO_2 laser. The ER:YAG laser is 12 to 18 times more efficiently absorbed by water, leading to a more superficial penetration and less collateral damage with more rapid healing. The photothermal effect of ablative lasers accounts for the shrinkage of collagen and the neocollagenesis and collagen remodeling that leads to marked enhancement of skin-texture irregularity, skin tightening, and lifting. The goal of ablative laser treatments of atrophic scars is to reduce the depth of scar borders and stimulate neocollagenesis. The depth of ablation correlates with the number of passes performed. Treatment of entire cosmetic units has been recommended in order to avoid obvious lines of demarcation between treated and untreated sites. Isotretinoin use within the preceding 6- to 12-month period or a history of keloids is considered a contraindication to ablative laser treatment.[45] Complications of ablative skin resurfacing include hypertrophic scarring, possible ectropion formation, infection, and dyschromia.[46]

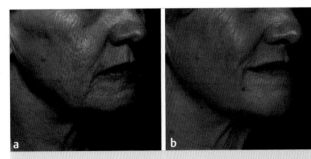

Fig. 17.1 A 60-year-old woman before (**a**) and after (**b**) full ablative carbon dioxide (CO_2) resurfacing of full face for aging skin and moderate acne scars.

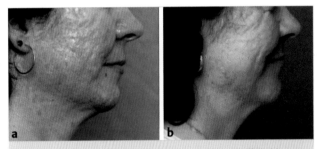

Fig. 17.2 A 42-year-old woman before (**a**) and after (**b**) full ablative carbon dioxide (CO2) resurfacing of full face for marked acne scars.

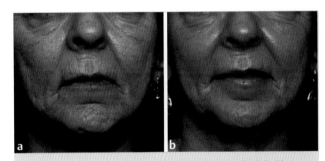

Fig. 17.3 A 58-year-old woman before (**a**) and after (**b**) full ablative carbon dioxide (CO2) resurfacing of full face for aging skin and moderate acne scars. Note cheek and chin areas of scar improvement.

The initial fractional laser was a midinfrared (1,550-nm) wavelength erbium fiber laser used to create microscopic columns of thermal injury in the dermis (microscopic thermal zones [MTZs]) surrounded by zones of viable tissue.[45] Due to the intact residual epidermal/dermal cells surrounding each MTZ, rapid healing occurs. Maintenance of the stratum corneum also ensures continued epidermal barrier function. Several studies have demonstrated a clinical improvement of 50% or more in acne scarring after a series of three consecutive nonablative fractional laser-resurfacing procedures.[45,47,48] In comparison, ablative fractional resurfacing also creates MTZs to stimulate a wound-healing response; however, they also vaporize the stratum corneum. This results in a more immediate postoperative appearance similar to ablative laser resurfacing. Similar to nonablative fractional lasers, clinical refinement of atrophic scarring with ablative fractional lasers results from

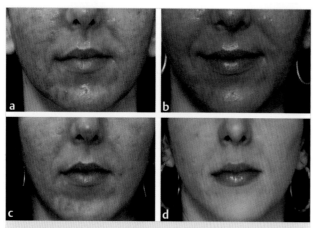

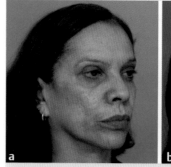

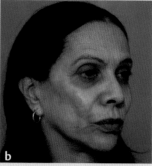

Fig. 17.4 A 38-year-old woman after fractional carbon dioxide (CO_2) resurfacing of full face (Deep FX and Active FX) for moderate acne scars. (**a**) Day 1 posttreatment; (**b**) day 4 posttreatment, immediately after washing face of desquamating epithelium; (**c**) day 5 posttreatment; and (**d**) day 7 posttreatment.

Fig. 17.5 A 55-year-old woman before (**a**) and after (**b**) fractional carbon dioxide (CO_2) resurfacing of full face (Deep FX and Active FX) for moderate acne scars.

both collagen contraction and neocollagenesis (▶ Fig. 17.4 and ▶ Fig. 17.5). Chapas et al first reported success with ablative fractional laser resurfacing with a CO_2 laser in moderate to severe acne scars. Three treatments at monthly intervals resulted in a 26 to 50% enhancement in texture, atrophy, and overall improvement, and topographical analysis revealed the median depths of the scars improved by 66.8%.[49] Hedelund et al presented a randomized, controlled trial evaluating the efficacy and safety of fractional CO_2 laser resurfacing versus no treatment. This clinical blinded study showed an improvement in scar texture with a reduction in the degree of atrophy compared to untreated controlled sites as early as 1 month and up to 6 months after treatment.[50] Ablative fractional lasers may be more effective as compared to nonablative fractional lasers but are associated with higher risks and longer recovery periods. Schweiger and Sundick looked at focally treating acne scars with fractional CO_2 laser resurfacing. The term "focal acne scar treatment" (FAST) is used to describe this double-fractionated approach to the treatment of acne scars in a select patient population. FAST is modeled after the CROSS method of applying a high concentration of TCA to only the acne scar. Based on their case studies, they now include an erbium glass fractional laser treatment 1 month after their FAST treatment in order to reduce any pigmentation abnormalities and localized erythema from the localized CO_2 laser treatment.[51] Radiofrequency devices and plasma energy are two additional options for improving scars through stimulation of collagen remodeling. Radiofrequency instruments and plasma skin resurfacing cause dermal collagen denaturation and stimulate neocollagenesis with minimal side effects. Additional studies evaluating the treatment of acne scarring with these technologies need to be performed.

17.3.3 Surgical Options

Subcision is a technique used to manage atrophic scars by percutaneously releasing scar bands within the dermis and subcutaneous tissue. This strategy was first introduced in 1995 and works best on rolling atrophic scars.[52] Subcision works by releasing the surface from the deeper structures and allowing blood to accumulate under the defect. Successive treatments appear needed to produce further improvement. The procedure involves the insertion of a sharp hypodermic needle (18–26-gauge, depending on scar size and depth), a filter needle, or even a blunt cannula.[53] The bleeding that occurs appears to establish a short-term spacer to keep the tissues from early reattachment. In addition, filler treatments can be used as a spacer after the subcision process. However, it may be the delayed organization of the ecchymosis that results in the new connective tissue under the scar.

A study in 2011 compared subcision versus the 100% TCA (CROSS) technique in the treatment of rolling acne scars. In this study, rolling scars on the left side of the face were treated with the TCA 100% CROSS technique, and subcision was performed on the right side of the face. The research showed that rolling acne scars respond better to subcision than the 100% TCA method, with a statistically greater decrease in scar depth and size.[54]

Surgical scar revision procedures are designed to improve the appearance of a scar by changing its shape and/or direction. Elliptical excision is the most common technique used and is helpful in improving ice-pick, boxcar, hypertrophic, and atrophic acne scars. Elliptical excision of a scar is made parallel to the relaxed skin tension lines (RSTLs), and the length to width ratio should be 3:1. Leaving the dermal aspect of the original scar can help augment the depth of an atrophic acne scar. Scar revision techniques such as Z-plasty, W-plasty, and geometric broken line closure may be helpful to further improve the scar appearance.

Botulinum toxin type A may be a useful adjunct to surgical scar revision. Not only can the decrease in surrounding muscle activity reduce the wound tension but botulinum toxin may have an inhibitory effect on fibroblasts.[55]

In addition to direct excision for acne scarring, a rhytidectomy can be a valuable part of a multimodal approach for the treatment of acne scars. The rhytidectomy procedure can address the effects of facial aging that only magnify the appearance of acne scars. Soft tissue augmentation with fat grafts or injectable PLLA can be performed at the time of the rhytidectomy.[56]

Punch techniques are beneficial for scars with a white atrophic base, sharply punched out ice-pick scars, and some chicken pox and postherpetic scars. Three types of punch methods include punch excision, punch elevation, and punch replacement. Punch excision removes an ice-pick or narrow boxcar scar using a disposable or hair-transplant punch slightly larger than the scar, and the defect is sutured. In performing a punch elevation, the punch is not discarded. The tissue cylinder is incised down to the level of the subcutaneous fat and the scar is allowed to float up until it reaches the level of the surrounding tissue. Punch-replacement grafting is reported to be best when used to treat sharp-walled or deep ice-pick scars with dystrophic or white bases. Punch grafts taken from the postauricular skin can be used to fill the holes left by excising the ice-pick scars. Dermabrasion or laser resurfacing may be performed 4 to 6 weeks later to flatten the grafts for further scar refinement.[57]

17.4 Conclusion

Due to the variety of acne-scar presentations, patients are best served by clinicians who have a thorough knowledge of the medical, procedural, and surgical options that are available. A multimodal approach to improving the appearance of scars may maximize outcomes. In fact, several reports in the medical literature recommend combining several treatment modalities to help patients achieve their goals.[56,58,59,60]

It is essential that clinicians understand a patient's goals and expectations, while also helping the patient comprehend the risks, benefits, and especially the limitations of treating acne scars.

References

[1] Layton AM, Henderson CA, Cunliffe WJ. A clinical evaluation of acne scarring and its incidence. Clin Exp Dermatol 1994; 19: 303–308

[2] Fife D. Practical evaluation and management of atrophic acne scars: tips for the general dermatologist. J Clin Aesthet Dermatol 2011; 4: 50–57

[3] Holland DB, Jeremy AH, Roberts SG, Seukeran DC, Layton AM, Cunliffe WJ. Inflammation in acne scarring: a comparison of the responses in lesions from patients prone and not prone to scar. Br J Dermatol 2004; 150: 72–81

[4] Holland DB, Jeremy AH. The role of inflammation in the pathogenesis of acne and acne scarring. Semin Cutan Med Surg 2005; 24: 79–83

[5] Loney T, Standage M, Lewis S. Not just 'skin deep': psychosocial effects of dermatological-related social anxiety in a sample of acne patients. J Health Psychol 2008; 13: 47–54

[6] Jacob CI, Dover JS, Kaminer MS. Acne scarring: a classification system and review of treatment options. J Am Acad Dermatol 2001; 45: 109–117

[7] Goodman G. Post acne scarring: a review. J Cosmet Laser Ther 2003; 5: 77–95

[8] Goodman GJ, Baron JA. The management of postacne scarring. Dermatol Surg 2007; 33: 1175–1188

[9] Finlay AY, Torres V, Kang S, et al. Global Alliance. Classification of acne scars is difficult even for acne experts. J Eur Acad Dermatol Venereol 2013; 27: 391–393

[10] Schiltz JR, Lanigan J, Nabial W, Petty B, Birnbaum JE. Retinoic acid induces cyclic changes in epidermal thickness and dermal collagen and glycosaminoglycan biosynthesis rates. J Invest Dermatol 1986; 87: 663–667

[11] Varani J, Perone P, Griffiths CE, Inman DR, Fligiel SE, Voorhees JJ. All-trans retinoic acid (RA) stimulates events in organ-cultured human skin that underlie repair. Adult skin from sun-protected and sun-exposed sites responds in an identical manner to RA while neonatal foreskin responds differently. J Clin Invest 1994; 94: 1747–1756

[12] Harris DW, Buckley CC, Ostlere LS, Rustin MH. Topical retinoic acid in the treatment of fine acne scarring. Br J Dermatol 1991; 125: 81–82

[13] Stratigos AJ, Katsambas AD. Optimal management of recalcitrant disorders of hyperpigmentation in dark-skinned patients. Am J Clin Dermatol 2004; 5: 161–168

[14] Goldman MP. The use of hydroquinone with facial laser resurfacing. J Cutan Laser Ther 2000; 2: 73–77

[15] Verbov J. The place of intralesional steroid therapy in dermatology. Br J Dermatol 1976; 94 suppl 12: 51–58

[16] Goette DK, Odom RB. Adverse effects of corticosteroids. Cutis 1979; 23: 477–487

[17] Gupta S, Kalra A. Efficacy and safety of intralesional 5-fluorouracil in the treatment of keloids. Dermatology 2002; 204: 130–132

[18] España A, Solano T, Quintanilla E. Bleomycin in the treatment of keloids and hypertrophic scars by multiple needle punctures. Dermatol Surg 2001; 27: 23–27

[19] Mustoe TA, Cooter RD, Gold MH, et al. International Advisory Panel on Scar Management. International clinical recommendations on scar management. Plast Reconstr Surg 2002; 110: 560–571

[20] Mustoe TA. Evolution of silicone therapy and mechanism of action in scar management. Aesthetic Plast Surg 2008; 32: 82–92

[21] Cooper JS, Lee BT. Treatment of facial scarring: lasers, filler, and nonoperative techniques. Facial Plast Surg 2009; 25: 311–315

[22] Surowitz JB, Shockley WW. Enhancement of facial scars with dermabrasion. Facial Plast Surg Clin North Am 2011; 19: 517–525

[23] Brody HJ. Variations and comparisons in medium-depth chemical peeling. J Dermatol Surg Oncol 1989; 15: 953–963

[24] Bradley DT, Park SS. Scar revision via resurfacing. Facial Plast Surg 2001; 17: 253–262

[25] Lee JB, Chung WG, Kwahck H, Lee KH. Focal treatment of acne scars with trichloroacetic acid: chemical reconstruction of skin scars method. Dermatol Surg 2002; 28: 1017–1021, discussion 1021

[26] Cho SB, Park CO, Chung WG, Lee KH, Lee JB, Chung KY. Histometric and histochemical analysis of the effect of trichloroacetic acid concentration in the chemical reconstruction of skin scars method. Dermatol Surg 2006; 32: 1231–1236, discussion 1236

[27] Yug A, Lane JE, Howard MS, Kent DE. Histologic study of depressed acne scars treated with serial high-concentration (95%) trichloroacetic acid. Dermatol Surg 2006; 32: 985–990, discussion 990

[28] Kontis TC. Contemporary review of injectable facial fillers. JAMA Facial Plast Surg 2013; 15: 58–64

[29] Levy LL, Zeichner JA. Management of acne scarring, part II: a comparative review of non-laser-based, minimally invasive approaches. Am J Clin Dermatol 2012; 13: 331–340

[30] Beer K. A single-center, open-label study on the use of injectable poly-L-lactic acid for the treatment of moderate to severe scarring from acne or varicella. Dermatol Surg 2007; 33 Suppl 2: S159–S167

[31] Sadick NS, Palmisano L. Case study involving use of injectable poly-L-lactic acid (PLLA) for acne scars. J Dermatolog Treat 2009; 20: 302–307

[32] Munavalli GS, Smith S, Maslowski JM, Weiss RA. Successful treatment of depressed, distensible acne scars using autologous fibroblasts: a multi-site, prospective, double blind, placebo-controlled clinical trial. Dermatol Surg 2013; 39: 1226–1236

[33] Coleman SR. Structural fat grafting: more than a permanent filler. Plast Reconstr Surg 2006; 118 Suppl: 108S–120S

[34] Meier JD, Glasgold RA, Glasgold MJ. Autologous fat grafting: long-term evidence of its efficacy in midfacial rejuvenation. Arch Facial Plast Surg 2009; 11: 24–28

[35] Aust MC, Fernandes D, Kolokythas P, Kaplan HM, Vogt PM. Percutaneous collagen induction therapy: an alternative treatment for scars, wrinkles, and skin laxity. Plast Reconstr Surg 2008; 121: 1421–1429

[36] Aust MC, Reimers K, Repenning C, et al. Percutaneous collagen induction: minimally invasive skin rejuvenation without risk of hyperpigmentation-fact or fiction? Plast Reconstr Surg 2008; 122: 1553–1563

[37] Fabbrocini G, De Vita V, Monfrecola A, et al. Percutaneous collagen induction: an effective and safe treatment for post-acne scarring in different skin phototypes. J Dermatolog Treat 2014; 25: 147–152

[38] Fabbrocini G, Fardella N, Monfrecola A, Proietti I, Innocenzi D. Acne scarring treatment using skin needling. Clin Exp Dermatol 2009; 34: 874–879

[39] Majid I. Microneedling therapy in atrophic facial scars: an objective assessment. J Cutan Aesthet Surg 2009; 2: 26–30

[40] Goodman GJ. The use of botulinum toxin as primary or adjunctive treatment for post acne and traumatic scarring. J Cutan Aesthet Surg 2010; 3: 90–92

[41] Rao J. Treatment of acne scarring. Facial Plast Surg Clin North Am 2011; 19: 275–291

[42] Alster TS, McMeekin TO. Improvement of facial acne scars by the 585 nm flashlamp-pumped pulsed dye laser. J Am Acad Dermatol 1996; 35: 79–81

[43] Rivera AE. Acne scarring: a review and current treatment modalities. J Am Acad Dermatol 2008; 59: 659–676

[44] Tanzi EL, Alster TS. Comparison of a 1450-nm diode laser and a 1320-nm Nd:YAG laser in the treatment of atrophic facial scars: a prospective clinical and histologic study. Dermatol Surg 2004; 30: 152–157

[45] Sobanko JF, Alster TS. Laser treatment for improvement and minimization of facial scars. Facial Plast Surg Clin North Am 2011; 19: 527–542

[46] Ward PD, Baker SR. Long-term results of carbon dioxide laser resurfacing of the face. Arch Facial Plast Surg 2008; 10: 238–243, discussion 244–245

[47] Alster TS, Tanzi EL, Lazarus M. The use of fractional laser photothermolysis for the treatment of atrophic scars. Dermatol Surg 2007; 33: 295–299

[48] Cho SB, Lee JH, Choi MJ, Lee KY, Oh SH. Efficacy of the fractional photothermolysis system with dynamic operating mode on acne scars and enlarged facial pores. Dermatol Surg 2009; 35: 108–114

[49] Chapas AM, Brightman L, Sukal S, et al. Successful treatment of acneiform scarring with CO2 ablative fractional resurfacing. Lasers Surg Med 2008; 40: 381–386

[50] Hedelund L, Haak CS, Togsverd-Bo K, Bogh MK, Bjerring P, Haedersdal M. Fractional CO2 laser resurfacing for atrophic acne scars: a randomized controlled trial with blinded response evaluation. Lasers Surg Med 2012; 44: 447–452

[51] Schweiger ES, Sundick L. Focal acne scar treatment (FAST), a new approach to atrophic acne scars: a case series. J Drugs Dermatol 2013; 12: 1163–1167

[52] Orentreich DS, Orentreich N. Subcutaneous incisionless (subcision) surgery for the correction of depressed scars and wrinkles. Dermatol Surg 1995; 21: 543–549

[53] Ayeni O, Carey W, Muhn C. Acne scar treatment with subcision using a 20-G cataract blade. Dermatol Surg 2011; 37: 846–847

[54] Ramadan SAE, El-Komy MHM, Bassiouny DA, El-Tobshy SA. Subcision versus 100% trichloroacetic acid in the treatment of rolling acne scars. Dermatol Surg 2011; 37: 626–633

[55] Zhibo X, Miaobo Z. Botulinum toxin type A affects cell cycle distribution of fibroblasts derived from hypertrophic scar. J Plast Reconstr Aesthet Surg 2008; 61: 1128–1129

[56] O'Daniel TG. Multimodal management of atrophic acne scarring in the aging face. Aesthetic Plast Surg 2011; 35: 1143–1150

[57] Goodman GJ. Treating scars: addressing surface, volume, and movement to expedite optimal results. Part 2: more-severe grades of scarring. Dermatol Surg 2012; 38: 1310–1321

[58] Carniol PJ, Vynatheya J, Carniol E. Evaluation of acne scar treatment with a 1450-nm midinfrared laser and 30% trichloroacetic acid peels. Arch Facial Plast Surg 2005; 7: 251–255

[59] Lee JW, Kim BJ, Kim MN, Mun SK. The efficacy of autologous platelet rich plasma combined with ablative carbon dioxide fractional resurfacing for acne scars: a simultaneous split-face trial. Dermatol Surg 2011; 37: 931–938

[60] Rostan EF. Combining laser therapies for optimal outcomes in treating the aging face and acne scars. Facial Plast Surg Clin North Am 2012; 20: 221–229, vii

18 The Use of Lasers for Skin Pathology

Danielle M. Waymire and Adam A. Ingraffea

18.1 Introduction

The use of lasers for skin pathology has grown dramatically since their initial introduction several decades ago. The quantum theory of radiation, described nearly a century ago, served as the theoretical foundation for the development of lasers. Yet it was not until 1959 that Maiman developed the first laser[1] and later, in 1963, when Dr. Leon Goldman pioneered laser therapy for the field of dermatology by treating various cutaneous conditions with his ruby laser. Laser therapy was further revolutionized when Anderson and Parrish introduced the theory of selective photothermolysis, promoting the selective destruction of targets in the skin without unwanted surrounding thermal damage.[2] Thereafter, advancements in technology, increased ease of operation, and decreased side effects boosted the popularity of laser therapy for cutaneous disease. Although not inclusive of all skin pathologies amenable to laser therapy, this chapter focuses on the laser treatment for hyperpigmented lesions, benign skin lesions, and basal cell carcinomas (BCCs).

18.2 Anatomy

Melanin, hemoglobin, and water are the three chromophores targeted in skin-directed laser therapy. In normal skin, melanin is produced by melanocytes, transferred to keratinocytes, and confined to the epidermis. Hemoglobin is carried within red blood cells that circulate within blood vessels located in the dermis. Water is present in all layers of the skin but is increased in abundance in the dermis and subcutaneous tissue. Melanin, hemoglobin, and water each exhibit characteristic wavelengths of absorption. Exposure to these energy wavelengths induces excitation to a higher energy state. Lasers with corresponding wavelengths selectively target these chromophores to treat cutaneous pathology while limiting surrounding tissue damage.

18.3 Hyperpigmented Lesions

The pathogenesis of skin hyperpigmentation is complex. A single or combination of factor(s) such as photosensitivity, trauma, medication deposition, or neoplasia may result in the clinical observation of skin hyperpigmentation. The classification and treatment of pigmentary disorders is based upon the histological location of the pigment within the epidermis, dermis, or a combination of both the epidermis and dermis. Due to melanin's wide spectrum of absorption, several lasers may be used to target this pigment. Ideal laser therapy targets the abnormal pigment without causing surrounding damage. In general, longer wavelength lasers penetrate deeper in the skin.[3] Thus lasers with a shorter wavelength are commonly utilized for superficial pigmented lesions, whereas the longer wavelength lasers are employed for dermal pigmentation.

Continuous wave and quasicontinuous wave laser systems were the first laser systems implemented to treat pigmentary disorders. However, the pulse duration of these laser systems is longer than the thermal relaxation time of the melanosome, resulting in significant surrounding thermal damage with subsequent scarring and dyspigmentation.[4] More recently, short-pulsed or quality-switched (QS) lasers were developed to selectively target pigment. These laser systems deliver high bursts of energy over a very short period of time and are thus more suitable for treating pigmentary disorders. The main laser systems in use today for pigmentary disorders are the 755-nm QS alexandrite laser, and the 532-nm or 1,064-nm QS neodymium: yttrium aluminum garnet (Nd:YAG) laser.[5] Each laser targets melanin as the chromophore. The type of laser and laser settings are adjusted based upon the skin pathology and location of the pigmentation. Topical, local, and regional anesthesia may be applied for patient comfort. Pigmentary lesions should be treated in a nonoverlapping technique. A "snapping" sound indicates pigment destruction and an ash-gray or white discoloration is produced with treatment. Erythema, hyperpigmentation or hypopigmentation, purpura, and textural changes are possible side effects of each laser. Given the risk for pigmentary alteration, the ideal patient is one with a fair complexion (Fitzpatrick skin types I and II). However, if treatment for a patient with darker skin is indicated, the longer wavelength lasers are associated with less epidermal absorption and thus a decreased risk of posttreatment dyspigmentation.[6] It is essential to perform a test spot on any darker skinned patients before treating large areas of the face. Judicious epidermal cooling and pretreatment and/or posttreatment with bleaching agents, topical steroids, and sun protection may also be of some benefit.

18.3.1 Epidermal Hyperpigmentation

Café-Au-Lait Macules

Café-au-lait macules (CALMs) are well-circumscribed, hyperpigmented macules that present in infancy and may be associated with several underlying genetic syndromes. The hyperpigmentation results from increased pigmentation within the basal layer of the epidermis. Although removal of CALMs with the 532-nm QS Nd:YAG laser has been reported, the results are variable with a high risk of recurrence.[7,8,9,10] Ablative laser therapy using an erbium:yttrium aluminum garnet (Er:YAG) laser system has also been reported.[11] Several treatments may be necessary for resolution.

18.3.2 Combined Epidermal and Dermal Hyperpigmentation

Becker Melanosis

Becker melanosis presents during the second or third decade of life as a unilateral hyperpigmented patch with increased hair growth commonly located on the anterior or posterior chest and shoulder (► Fig. 18.1). Although the exact pathogenesis is unclear, this lesion is regarded as a hamartoma of both ectoderm and mesoderm embryonic tissue with increased pigmentation in the basal layer of the epidermis, a variably increased quantity of melanocytes, hyperplasia of the pilosebaceous units,

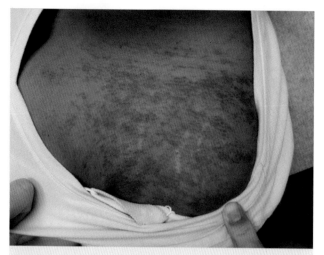

Fig. 18.1 Becker melanosis on the chest of a young woman.

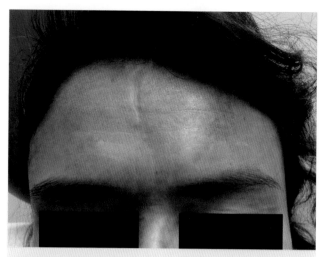

Fig. 18.2 Postinflammatory hyperpigmentation and hydroxychloro-quine-induced pigmentation on the forehead of a woman with dermatomyositis.

and often a smooth-muscle proliferation within the dermis.[12] Ablative, nonablative, QS, and fractional laser systems have been reported to improve the appearance of Becker melanosis.[10,13,14,15,16,17] Terminal hair density may be reduced with long-pulsed 694-nm ruby and 755-nm alexandrite lasers.[14,17] In one comparative trial, a 2,940-nm Er:YAG laser proved to be more efficacious for pigment removal than a 1,064-nm QS Nd:YAG, with fewer treatment sessions required and prolonged results.[16] The QS laser systems, however, are often the preferable method for removal due to their low-side effect profile. However, repeat procedures are often required for recurrent or residual pigmentation. Treatment modality should be based upon the patient's skin type, comorbidities, and preference.

Postinflammatory Hyperpigmentation

Postinflammatory hyperpigmentation results from melanin deposition in the epidermis or the dermis and presents as brown-to-gray macules and patches following trauma to the dermoepidermal junction (▶ Fig. 18.2). Therapy for these lesions has been attempted with 532-nm and 1,064-nm QS Nd:YAG lasers with inconsistent results.[13,18] Since melanin is the chromophore for each laser system, postinflammatory hyperpigmentation is a common and often expected side effect of therapy. Laser therapy for this pigmentary phenomenon should be used with discretion.

18.3.3 Dermal Hyperpigmentation

Drug-Induced Pigmentation

Several systemic medications can cause skin hyperpigmentation. Minocycline and amiodarone are the two more common causative agents. Three clinical and histological categories of minocycline hyperpigmentation exist. A blue-black discoloration in previous sites of inflammation, commonly in acne scars, is characteristic of type I minocycline-associated hyperpigmentation, whereas type II produces blue-gray macules and patches on the surface of the shins, and type III presents with diffuse muddy-brown hyperpigmentation on sun-exposed skin. Histologically, type I and type II minocycline-associated

hyperpigmentation display intracellular and extracellular pigmentation granules within the superficial dermis. To the contrary, type III reveals increased melanin production by melanocytes within the epidermis. Amiodarone-associated hyperpigmentation produces a slate-gray discoloration on photoexposed skin with intracellular yellow-brown pigment granules present histologically.[12] Drug-induced hyperpigmentation may also be caused by chemotherapy agents, antimalarials, heavy metals, psychotropic medications, and other miscellaneous systemic medications (▶ Fig. 18.2). The treatment of choice for drug-induced pigmentation is discontinuation of the inciting agent. Although pigmentation fades over time after discontinuation of the implicated medication, laser therapy may hasten resolution. QS 755-nm alexandrite, QS 1,064-nm Nd:YAG, and fractional 1,550-nm diode laser systems have each been reported to improve minocycline-associated hyperpigmentation.[19,20,21,22,23] Amiodarone-associated hyperpigmentation has been successfully treated with the QS 1,064-nm Nd:YAG.[24] Several treatments are often necessary for complete resolution. Lasers with a higher wavelength may be better suited for individuals with darker skin types to avoid posttreatment dyspigmentation (Fitzpatrick skin types III–VI).

Nevus of Ota

Nevus of Ota is a unilateral bluish-brown patch on the periocular skin (▶ Fig. 18.3) predominantly affecting individuals with a darker skin type (Fitzpatrick skin types III–VI). A proliferation of spindled, pigmented melanocytes within the dermis causes the bluish hyperpigmentation. The term nevus of Ito is used when the hyperpigmentation is localized to the supraclavicular, scapular, or deltoid regions.[12] The QS 755-nm alexandrite and QS 1,064-nm Nd:YAG laser systems, at varying fluences, have successfully lightened the hyperpigmentation.[25,26,27] Postinflammatory hypopigmentation and hyperpigmentation are significant concerns in patients with nevus of Ota, given the propensity for these lesions to affect patients with a darker skin phenotype.[27] Recently, decreased side effects were noted with low-fluence QS 1,064-nm Nd:YAG.[26] Several treatments may be necessary to achieve significant clinical effect.

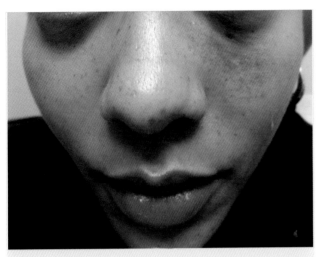

Fig. 18.3 Nevus of Ota on the periorbital skin of a young woman.

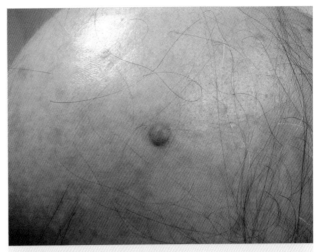

Fig. 18.4 Banal blue nevus on the scalp.

18.4 Benign Skin Lesions

18.4.1 Solar Lentigo and Ephelides

Solar lentigines and ephelides are benign hyperpigmented macules located on photoexposed skin. Solar lentigines result from ultraviolet light exposure. Histologically, an increased number of melanocytes and quantity of melanin is present within the epidermis. Although ephelides may also result from sun exposure, histological examination reveals an increased quantity of melanin within the epidermis without any increase in the number of melanocytes. Both solar lentigines and ephelides are amenable to laser therapy with the QS 755-nm alexandrite laser or the QS 532-nm Nd:YAG laser.[4,10,28] Each lesion turns white after being treated. Typically, two to three treatments repeated every 6 to 8 weeks are necessary for complete resolution. Sun protection and sun avoidance should be emphasized to all patients to prevent recurrence of treated lesions or development of new lesions.

18.4.2 Seborrheic Keratoses

Seborrheic keratoses are benign, pink-to-brown epidermal proliferations with a classic stuck-on appearance commonly affecting adults and older individuals. Both ablative and nonablative laser systems may be utilized for removal.[8,10,29,30,31] However, given the risks of scarring and dyspigmentation with the ablative lasers, QS 532-nm Nd:YAG or long-pulsed 755-nm alexandrite are used more commonly. Repeat treatment may be necessary for complete removal. The advantages of laser treatment versus more economical modalities such as cryotherapy or electrocautery are uncertain.

18.4.3 Melanocytic Nevi

Common acquired melanocytic nevi result from a proliferation of specialized melanocytes or nevoid cells and may be subclassified as junctional, compound, or dermal nevi depending upon the location of the nevus cells within the skin. Blue nevi are blue papules that result from heavily pigmented, spindled melanocytes localized in the dermis (▶ Fig. 18.4). Lastly, congenital melanocytic nevi are proliferations of melanocytes that are present at birth. These lesions may be epidermal, dermal, or both and are clinically classified based upon lesion size into small-, medium-, and giant-sized congenital nevi. Excision with histopathological evaluation is the standard of care for these lesions. The use of lasers for the removal of nevi remains controversial. Although normal-mode ruby, QS, and normal-mode 755-nm alexandrite; QS 532-nm, and 1,064-nm Nd:YAG; 585-nm pulsed dye laser (PDL); and the ablative laser systems may improve the clinical appearance of acquired, blue, or congenital melanocytic nevi, dermal melanocytic nevoid cells often remain after treatment and pose a risk for malignant transformation.[32–44] In general, the longer wavelength lasers are better adapted to reach deeply situated melanocytes to treat blue, congenital, compound, or dermal nevi. The risk of malignant transformation, in addition to the side effects of each type of laser, should be discussed with the patient prior to treatment. Each patient should be monitored for recurrence or malignant transformation after therapy completion. In this author's practice, laser surgery is not recommended to treat melanocytic nevi.

18.5 Basal Cell Carcinoma

BCC is a subtype of nonmelanoma skin cancer that develops from malignant progenitor cells located in the interfollicular epidermis or the upper infundibulum of the hair follicle.[45] In 1994, the estimated lifetime risk for the development of BCC of the skin was between 28 to 33%, with more recent reports suggesting an increasing incidence.[46,47] BCCs may be subdivided into clinical and histological subtypes. The four main clinical subtypes are nodular, superficial, morpheaform, and fibroepithelioma of Pinkus (▶ Fig. 18.5). The histological subtypes are nodular, micronodular, superficial, morpheaform or sclerosing, infiltrating, and fibroepithelioma of Pinkus. Treatment for BCCs depends upon the lesion size, location, depth, histopathological subtype, and patient comorbidities. Treatment options include Mohs micrographic surgery, wide–local excision, curettage, cryotherapy, radiation, imiquimod, photodynamic therapy, ingenol mebutate, and vismodegib.

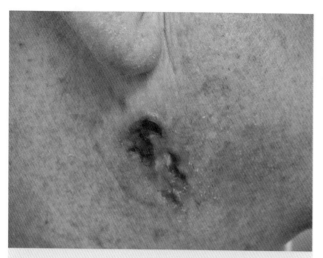

Fig. 18.5 Basal cell carcinoma (BCC) on the lateral neck.

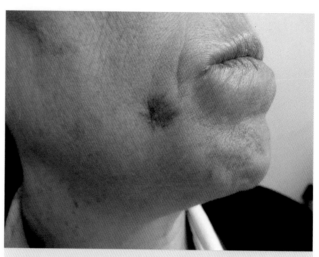

Fig. 18.6 Posttreatment purpura resulting from pulsed dye laser (PDL) therapy.

The use of lasers for the treatment of BCC was introduced by Dr. Leon Goldman in 1968.[48] Compared to traditional surgical management, laser therapy offers a less invasive procedure, often with an improved cosmetic outcome. Furthermore, lasers are useful in anatomical locations where distortion may occur with surgery.[49] These advantages are of increased significance in patients with numerous BCCs. Since its introduction, however, studies have exposed the limitations of lasers in treating larger sized tumors and those with nodular, micronodular, infiltrating, and morpheaform histological subtypes.[50,51,52] Superficial BCCs of a small size were most consistently and successfully treated with laser therapy.

Continuous wave ablative lasers, such as the argon and carbon dioxide (CO_2) lasers, were the first type of laser employed for the treatment of BCCs. However, because continuous wave lasers cause significant nonspecific thermal damage to surrounding tissue with resultant scarring, the high-energy pulsed CO_2 laser (PCO_2) largely replaced the continuous wave CO_2 laser.

Side effects of the PCO_2 laser include erythema, hyperpigmentation or hypopigmentation, acne, milia, contact dermatitis, herpes simplex infection and/or reactivation, local candidiasis, hypertrophic scarring, and ectropion.[53,54] The ideal patient is one with a fair complexion (Fitzpatrick skin type I or II) and a histologically confirmed superficial BCC. Keloidal tendency, herpes simplex virus infection, concurrent isotretinoin use, and ectropion or prior lower blepharoplasty in cases requiring infraorbital treatment are some contraindications to the procedure.[55] Antiviral prophylaxis should be initiated as indicated.

Prior to the procedure, topical, local, or occasionally regional anesthetic is applied. On typical settings, the first pass of the PCO_2 laser will vaporize the epidermis. Studies suggest treating a 1- to 2-mm margin of normal skin in addition to the clinical BCC.[56] Additional passes may be necessary until healthy dermis is identified. After the procedure, a topical emollient is applied to the treated area and kept in place until the skin is re-epithelialized. All patients should be evaluated every 6 to 12 months for at least 3 years thereafter for recurrence.[57]

Recently, the PDL has been employed for the treatment of BCCs. The growth and survival of BCCs has been shown to rely upon their microvasculature.[58] PDL preferentially destroys these ectatic blood vessels within BCCs by targeting hemoglobin within red blood cells. With destruction of the tumor-associated vasculature, BCCs may be eliminated or decreased in size.

Initial use of the 585-nm PDL resulted in poor histological clearance.[50] However, improved success was found using four to five treatments of the 595-nm PDL.[51,59] Complete tumor clearance was more common in smaller tumors less than 1.5 cm and superficial BCCs.[51] Possible side effects of PDL treatment are purpura from red blood cell extravasation of coagulated blood vessels (▶ Fig. 18.6), gray discoloration of the skin, postinflammatory pigmentary alteration, and scarring. The ideal patient is one with a fair complexion (Fitzpatrick skin type I or II) and a histologically confirmed superficial BCC. Cryogen cooling may help to decrease the incidence of pigmentary changes and scarring.

PDL settings should be adjusted as indicated based upon tumor location, size, and depth. Preoperative anesthetics are typically unnecessary. Four to five treatments for each tumor and a narrow margin of normal skin are required to ensure complete tumor removal.[51,56] Close follow-up every 6 to 12 months for at least 3 years after treatment is necessary to evaluate for tumor recurrence.[57]

A few studies have evaluated Nd and Nd:YAG lasers alone or in combination with PDL for the treatment of BCCs.[60,61] These lasers, commonly used for pigmented or vascular lesions and epilation, are speculated to treat BCCs via vascular damage, ablation, necrosis, and hyperthermia.[60,61] A 2.1% recurrence rate was noted with sole treatment of the Nd or Nd:YAG laser therapy.[60] Treatment with both Nd:YAG and PDL showed a 58% tumor clearance with improved resolution in tumors less than 1 cm.[61] Further research is warranted to establish their role in BCC treatment.

References

[1] Maiman T. Stimulated optical radiation in ruby. Nature 1960; 187: 493–494

[2] Anderson RR, Parrish JA. Selective photothermolysis: precise microsurgery by selective absorption of pulsed radiation. Science 1983; 220: 524–527

[3] Sherwood KA, Murray S, Kurban AK, Tan OT. Effect of wavelength on cutaneous pigment using pulsed irradiation. J Invest Dermatol 1989; 92: 717–720

[4] Sobanko JF, Alster TS. Management of acne scarring, part I: a comparative review of laser surgical approaches. Am J Clin Dermatol 2012; 13: 319–330

[5] Stratigos AJ, Dover JS, Arndt KA. Laser treatment of pigmented lesions—2000: how far have we gone? Arch Dermatol 2000; 136: 915–921

[6] Alexis AF. Lasers and light-based therapies in ethnic skin: treatment options and recommendations for Fitzpatrick skin types V and VI. Br J Dermatol 2013; 169 Suppl 3: 91–97

[7] Grekin RC, Shelton RM, Geisse JK, Frieden I. 510-nm pigmented lesion dye laser. Its characteristics and clinical uses. J Dermatol Surg Oncol 1993; 19: 380–387

[8] Fitzpatrick RE, Goldman MP, Ruiz-Esparza J. Laser treatment of benign pigmented epidermal lesions using a 300 nsecond pulse and 510 nm wavelength. J Dermatol Surg Oncol 1993; 19: 341–347

[9] Taylor CR, Anderson RR. Treatment of benign pigmented epidermal lesions by Q-switched ruby laser. Int J Dermatol 1993; 32: 908–912

[10] Kilmer SL, Wheeland RG, Goldberg DJ, Anderson RR. Treatment of epidermal pigmented lesions with the frequency-doubled Q-switched Nd:YAG laser. A controlled, single-impact, dose-response, multicenter trial. Arch Dermatol 1994; 130: 1515–1519

[11] Alora MB, Arndt KA. Treatment of a café-au-lait macule with the erbium:YAG laser. J Am Acad Dermatol 2001; 45: 566–568

[12] Bolognia JL, Jorizzo JL, Schaffer JV, eds. Dermatology. New York, NY: Elsevier Saunders; 2012

[13] Tse Y, Levine VJ, McClain SA, Ashinoff R. The removal of cutaneous pigmented lesions with the Q-switched ruby laser and the Q-switched neodymium: yttrium-aluminum-garnet laser. A comparative study. J Dermatol Surg Oncol 1994; 20: 795–800

[14] Choi JE, Kim JW, Seo SH, Son SW, Ahn HH, Kye YC. Treatment of Becker's nevi with a long-pulse alexandrite laser. Dermatol Surg 2009; 35: 1105–1108

[15] Trelles MA, Allones I, Moreno-Arias GA, Vélez M. Becker's naevus: a comparative study between erbium:YAG and Q-switched neodymium:YAG; clinical and histopathological findings. Br J Dermatol 2005; 152: 308–313

[16] Glaich AS, Goldberg LH, Dai T, Kunishige JH, Friedman PM. Fractional resurfacing: a new therapeutic modality for Becker's nevus. Arch Dermatol 2007; 143: 1488–1490

[17] Nanni CA, Alster TS. Treatment of a Becker's nevus using a 694-nm long-pulsed ruby laser. Dermatol Surg 1998; 24: 1032–1034

[18] Cho SB, Park SJ, Kim JS, Kim MJ, Bu TS. Treatment of post-inflammatory hyperpigmentation using 1064-nm Q-switched Nd:YAG laser with low fluence: report of three cases. J Eur Acad Dermatol Venereol 2009; 23: 1206–1207

[19] Alster TS, Gupta SN. Minocycline-induced hyperpigmentation treated with a 755-nm Q-switched alexandrite laser. Dermatol Surg 2004; 30: 1201–1204

[20] Greve B, Schönermark MP, Raulin C. Minocycline-induced hyperpigmentation: treatment with the Q-switched Nd:YAG laser. Lasers Surg Med 1998; 22: 223–227

[21] Green D, Friedman KJ. Treatment of minocycline-induced cutaneous pigmentation with the Q-switched alexandrite laser and a review of the literature. J Am Acad Dermatol 2001; 44 (2Suppl): 342–347

[22] Nisar MS, Iyer K, Brodell RT, Lloyd JR, Shin TM, Ahmad A. Minocycline-induced hyperpigmentation: comparison of 3 Q-switched lasers to reverse its effects. Clin Cosmet Investig Dermatol 2013; 6: 159–162

[23] Izikson L, Anderson RR. Resolution of blue minocycline pigmentation of the face after fractional photothermolysis. Lasers Surg Med 2008; 40: 399–401

[24] Bernstein EF. Q-switched laser treatment of amiodarone pigmentation. J Drugs Dermatol 2011; 10: 1316–1319

[25] Alster TS, Williams CM. Treatment of nevus of Ota by the Q-switched alexandrite laser. Dermatol Surg 1995; 21: 592–596

[26] Choi CW, Kim HJ, Lee HJ, Kim YH, Kim WS. Treatment of nevus of Ota using low fluence Q-switched Nd:YAG laser. Int J Dermatol 2014; 53: 861–865

[27] Chan HH, Leung RS, Ying SY, et al. A retrospective analysis of complications in the treatment of nevus of Ota with the Q-switched alexandrite and Q-switched Nd:YAG lasers. Dermatol Surg 2000; 26: 1000–1006

[28] Wang CC, Sue YM, Yang CH, Chen CK. A comparison of Q-switched alexandrite laser and intense pulsed light for the treatment of freckles and lentigines in Asian persons: a randomized, physician-blinded, split-face comparative trial. J Am Acad Dermatol 2006; 54: 804–810

[29] Fitzpatrick RE, Goldman MP, Ruiz-Esparza J. Clinical advantage of the CO2 laser superpulsed mode. Treatment of verruca vulgaris, seborrheic keratoses, lentigines, and actinic cheilitis. J Dermatol Surg Oncol 1994; 20: 449–456

[30] Mehrabi D, Brodell RT. Use of the alexandrite laser for treatment of seborrheic keratoses. Dermatol Surg 2002; 28: 437–439

[31] Culbertson GR. 532-nm diode laser treatment of seborrheic keratoses with color enhancement. Dermatol Surg 2008; 34: 525–528, discussion 528

[32] Duke D, Byers HR, Sober AJ, Anderson RR, Grevelink JM. Treatment of benign and atypical nevi with the normal-mode ruby laser and the Q-switched ruby laser: clinical improvement but failure to completely eliminate nevomelanocytes. Arch Dermatol 1999; 135: 290–296

[33] Westerhof W, Gamei M. Treatment of acquired junctional melanocytic naevi by Q-switched and normal mode ruby laser. Br J Dermatol 2003; 148: 80–85

[34] Rosenbach A, Williams CM, Alster TS. Comparison of the Q-switched alexandrite (755 nm) and Q-switched Nd:YAG (1064 nm) lasers in the treatment of benign melanocytic nevi. Dermatol Surg 1997; 23: 239–244, discussion 244–245

[35] Al-Hadithy N, Al-Nakib K, Quaba A. Outcomes of 52 patients with congenital melanocytic naevi treated with ultrapulse carbon dioxide and frequency doubled Q-switched Nd:YAG laser. J Plast Reconstr Aesthet Surg 2012; 65: 1019–1028

[36] Chong SJ, Jeong E, Park HJ, Lee JY, Cho BK. Treatment of congenital nevomelanocytic nevi with the CO2 and Q-switched alexandrite lasers. Dermatol Surg 2005; 31: 518–521

[37] August PJ, Ferguson JE, Madan V. A study of the efficacy of carbon dioxide and pigment-specific lasers in the treatment of medium-sized congenital melanocytic naevi. Br J Dermatol 2011; 164: 1037–1042

[38] Funayama E, Sasaki S, Furukawa H, et al. Effectiveness of combined pulsed dye and Q-switched ruby laser treatment for large to giant congenital melanocytic naevi. Br J Dermatol 2012; 167: 1085–1091

[39] Grevelink JM, van Leeuwen RL, Anderson RR, Byers HR. Clinical and histological responses of congenital melanocytic nevi after single treatment with Q-switched lasers. Arch Dermatol 1997; 133: 349–353

[40] Horner BM, El-Muttardi NS, Mayou BJ. Treatment of congenital melanocytic naevi with CO2 laser. Ann Plast Surg 2005; 55: 276–280

[41] Nelson JS, Kelly KM. Q-switched ruby laser treatment of a congenital melanocytic nevus. Dermatol Surg 1999; 25: 274–276

[42] Ostertag JU, Quaedvlieg PJF, Kerckhoffs FE, et al. Congenital naevi treated with erbium:YAG laser (Derma K) resurfacing in neonates: clinical results and review of the literature. Br J Dermatol 2006; 154: 889–895

[43] Reda AM, Taha IR, Riad HA. Clinical and histological effect of a single treatment of normal mode alexandrite (755 nm) laser on small melanocytic nevi. J Cutan Laser Ther 1999; 1: 209–215

[44] Milgraum SS, Cohen ME, Auletta MJ. Treatment of blue nevi with the Q-switched ruby laser. J Am Acad Dermatol 1995; 32: 307–310

[45] Youssef KK, Van Keymeulen A, Lapouge G, et al. Identification of the cell lineage at the origin of basal cell carcinoma. Nat Cell Biol 2010; 12: 299–305

[46] Miller DL, Weinstock MA. Nonmelanoma skin cancer in the United States: incidence. J Am Acad Dermatol 1994; 30: 774–778

[47] Rogers HW, Weinstock MA, Harris AR, et al. Incidence estimate of nonmelanoma skin cancer in the United States, 2006. Arch Dermatol 2010; 146: 283–287

[48] Goldman L, Rockwell RJ, Jr, Meyer R, Otten R. Investigative studies with the laser in the treatment of basal cell epitheliomas. South Med J 1968; 61: 735–742

[49] Choudhary S, Tang J, Elsaie ML, Nouri K. Lasers in the treatment of nonmelanoma skin cancer. Dermatol Surg 2011; 37: 409–425

[50] Allison KP, Kiernan MN, Waters RA, Clement RM. Pulsed dye laser treatment of superficial basal cell carcinoma: realistic or not? Lasers Med Sci 2003; 18: 125–126

[51] Shah SM, Konnikov N, Duncan LM, Tannous ZS. The effect of 595 nm pulsed dye laser on superficial and nodular basal cell carcinomas. Lasers Surg Med 2009; 41: 417–422

[52] Horlock N, Grobbelaar AO, Gault DT. Can the carbon dioxide laser completely ablate basal cell carcinomas? A histological study. Br J Plast Surg 2000; 53: 286–293

[53] Bernstein LJ, Kauvar ANB, Grossman MC, Geronemus RG. The short- and long-term side effects of carbon dioxide laser resurfacing. Dermatol Surg 1997; 23: 519–525

[54] Nanni CA, Alster TS. Complications of carbon dioxide laser resurfacing. An evaluation of 500 patients. Dermatol Surg 1998; 24: 315–320

[55] Alster TS. Cutaneous resurfacing with CO2 and erbium:YAG lasers: preoperative, intraoperative, and postoperative considerations. Plast Reconstr Surg 1999; 103: 619–632, discussion 633–634

[56] Campolmi P, Brazzini B, Urso C, et al. Superpulsed CO2 laser treatment of basal cell carcinoma with intraoperatory histopathologic and cytologic examination. Dermatol Surg 2002; 28: 909–911, discussion 912

[57] Rowe DE. Comparison of treatment modalities for basal cell carcinoma. Clin Dermatol 1995; 13: 617–620

[58] Chen GS, Yu HS, Lan CC, et al. CXC chemokine receptor CXCR4 expression enhances tumorigenesis and angiogenesis of basal cell carcinoma. Br J Dermatol 2006; 154: 910–918

[59] Campolmi P, Mavilia L, Bonan P, Cannarozzo G, Lotti TM. 595 nm pulsed dye laser for the treatment of superficial basal cell carcinoma. Lasers Med Sci 2005; 20: 147–148

[60] Moskalik K, Kozlov A, Demin E, Boiko E. The efficacy of facial skin cancer treatment with high-energy pulsed neodymium and Nd:YAG lasers. Photomed Laser Surg 2009; 27: 345–349

[61] Jalian HR, Avram MM, Stankiewicz KJ, Shofner JD, Tannous Z. Combined 585 nm pulsed-dye and 1,064 nm Nd:YAG lasers for the treatment of basal cell carcinoma. Lasers Surg Med 2014; 46: 1–7

19 Complications in Laser Resurfacing: Avoidance, Recognition, and Treatment

J. Kevin Duplechain

19.1 Introduction

Laser skin resurfacing is one of the most rewarding procedures performed by this author, who has been fascinated by these technologically advanced devices since the days of the original *Star Trek* and is always amazed by the uniqueness of the treatments they deliver. Having an understanding of skin, the nuances of different lasers, and, of course, preventing and managing complications when they occur are the goals of this chapter. It is the author's hope that the information here helps readers to provide patients with uncomplicated treatments and youthful, beautiful skin.

19.2 Adverse Effects of Laser Treatment

Adverse effects of ablative carbon dioxide (CO_2) lasers include prolonged erythema, pigmentary alterations, infections, scarring, acne flares, milia, contact dermatitis, pruritus, and pain during treatment.[1,2] With both fully ablative and fractional CO_2 resurfacing, procedure parameters must be adjusted to accommodate the different characteristics of each anatomical area. Although risks of complications have been reduced by the advent of fractional tools, there is still significant risk associated with these devices.[3,4] The risk of scarring, for example, is greater in the chest, neck, and extremities when compared to the face because of the reduced number of pilosebaceous units in these nonfacial areas.[5] In addition, the depths of the epidermis and dermis (both papillary and reticular) vary significantly on and off the face. Failure to consider these differences when planning and delivering a laser treatment will likely be the source of serious complications.

Complications of ablative erbium:yttrium aluminum garnet (Er:YAG) lasers are similar to those of the CO_2 laser. Nonablative lasers were designed to further reduce adverse effects of skin rejuvenation. Although nonablative energy promotes dermal collagen remodeling and improves photodamage, efficacy is usually less than that of ablative lasers.[6,7] Complications of nonablative erbium-doped fractional lasers have also been reported.[8,9]

19.3 Why Complications Occur

Complications occur as a result of different factors, some controllable and others unpredictable. To better understand the intrinsic risk of any ablative treatment, laser–tissue interaction and the requirements of efficient tissue ablation should be reviewed.

When skin is treated with a 10,600-nm CO_2 laser beam, water in the skin is heated to 100°C and the heated tissue is vaporized. The heat conducted to adjacent tissue results in a zone of coagulation necrosis at a depth and width dependent on the fluence

and dwell time (time for the pulse to be delivered). Fluences greater than 4 to 5 J/cm^2 applied in ≤ 1 ms, the thermal relaxation time (TRT) of human skin, are necessary to ablate the epidermis.[10] When dwell time exceeds the TRT of skin, the surrounding tissue undergoes prolonged, less efficient heating that may result in unexpected and undesired effects including superheating of tissue and char formation. For the CO_2 laser the accepted dwell time or pulse duration to achieve ablation without superheating the surrounding tissue is approximately 0.7 ms. In order for any ablative device to reach a given depth, the length of exposure is increased in the continuous wave (CW) laser, or the number of pulses is increased in the pulsed laser. When the pulse duration is increased beyond the TRT of skin and the thermal effect of the laser–tissue interaction outpaces the velocity of ablation, the result is wider zones of thermal injury. This unseen effect of prolonged pulse width alters treatment density significantly, as illustrated by ▶ Fig. 19.1.

The effect of multiple pulses and pulse width (single, double, or long) within the TRT of skin also deserves discussion. Current fractional lasers permit users to deliver single or multiple pulses over the same area. In a 15-patient study, Bailey and colleagues[11] showed that the mean penetration depth of single-pulse fractional CO_2 laser energy was greater in abdominal skin (mean 582 μm) than in facial skin (mean 415 μm). Data are

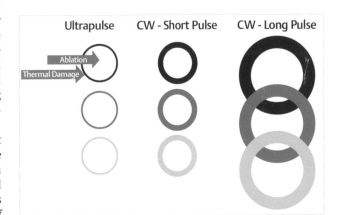

Fig. 19.1 The effect of pulse duration on treatment density in fractional carbon dioxide (CO_2) laser resurfacing. Each circle represents a microthermal wound created by the fractional laser beam. The pulse duration is shortest with the ultrapulse and longest with the long-pulse continuous wave (CW) laser. The circumferential lines represent the areas of thermal damage (i.e., thick lines denote greater thermal damage than thin lines). As the pulse duration increases, the circumferential lines become thicker, the areas of thermal damage increase, and the treatment density increases. At the long pulses the wound areas begin to overlap, resulting in further increases in thermal damage. At this stage the treatment has become fully ablative (i.e., 100% density). This effect is believed to account for the unexpected adverse effects at long pulse durations of fractional resurfacing procedures. (Reproduced with permission from Duplechain JK. Neck rejuvenation: surgical and non-surgical. Facial Plast Surg Clin of North Am. 2014; 22(2): 2003–2016.)

Table 19.1 Dependence of wound width on pulse and energy

Pulse	Energy (mJ)	Mean MTZ depth (µm)		Mean MTZ width (µm)
		Face	Abdomen	Face
Single	15[a]	415[a]	582[a]	312[a]
	30[b]	854[b]	1,345[b]	534[b]
Double	15[b]	881[b]	822[b]	493[b]

MTZ, microthermal zone. Data from:
(a) Bailey SH, Brown SA, Kim Y et al. An intra-individual quantitative assessment of acute laser injury patterns in facial versus abdominal skin. Lasers Surg Med 2011; 43: 99–107
(b) Oni G, Robbins D, Bailey S, Brown SA, Kenkel JM. An in vivo histopathological comparison of single and double pulsed modes of a fractionated CO(2) laser. Lasers Surg Med 2012; 44: 4–10

presented in (► Table 19.1). In a subsequent study using a fractional CO_2 laser, Oni et al[12] compared penetration depths of the same anatomical areas using a single pulse of 30-mJ energy in both areas versus a double pulse of 15-mJ energy in both areas (► Table 19.1). The collective data of the two studies revealed several important relationships. With a single pulse at 15 mJ, depths of injury of facial and abdominal skin (415 and 582 µm, respectively) were similar. With double pulsing at 15 mJ, injury to abdominal skin (822 µm) was more superficial than with a single pulse at 30 mJ (1,345 µm). The difference in depths was 523 µm. A similar comparison for facial skin shows a much smaller difference (881 µm – 854 µm = 27µm), suggesting that laser injury patterns in facial and abdominal skin are not the same. The widths of laser-induced injury in the face and abdomen were also measured. The data showed that for facial skin, the widths of injuries induced by double and single pulses (493 and 312 µm, respectively) at 15 mJ differed by 181 µm, much larger than the 27 µm observed for facial injury depths. When facial injuries induced by single pulses at 30 and 15 mJ were compared, the difference in widths was even larger (534 µm – 312 µm = 222 µm).

This information is presented to demonstrate that lasers operating well within accepted guidelines of efficient skin ablation can still be problematic—especially for different anatomical areas—when higher energy single-pulsed or multipulsed parameters are utilized. A thorough understanding of the effects of varying parameters is key to delivering safe, uncomplicated treatments.

19.4 Patient Selection

The proper selection of patients for laser resurfacing requires input from the patient and the provider. The provider must know the limitations of the instrument being utilized, and whether this tool is capable of delivering the results the patient is seeking. The adage of "under promise and over deliver" is as true in skin rejuvenation as in any procedure performed. Resurfacing can commonly be performed as an adjunct to other procedures such as facelift, blepharoplasty, or other cosmetic processes; however, consideration to which techniques have already been performed is vital to administering safe adjunctive laser resurfacing.

The probability of complications should be carefully evaluated in potential candidates for laser resurfacing. Patients of all skin types are suitable for CO_2 laser resurfacing.[13]Specific risks are often associated with a particular skin type and should be discussed individually. For example, patients with Fitzpatrick skin type IV and above should be counseled more so about the possibility of hyperpigmentation. Patients with a thick epidermis and dermis will see improvement in texture but are unlikely to see as much skin tightening as a patient of northern European ancestry (Fitzpatrick skin type I, with a thin epidermis).

Patients may have conditions or lifestyles for which laser treatment is contraindicated. Such contraindications may be relative or absolute and vary with the practitioner's experience. In general, patients are typically not treated if they cannot avoid sun exposure for at least 1 week. After 1 week, patients may apply a physical sunblock with a titanium or zinc base and resume daily (but reduced) sun exposure. They are advised to minimize sun exposure for about 3 weeks and to avoid extended exposure for 6 weeks. Since this restriction may be problematic, patients who request more aggressive resurfacing are usually treated during the winter period.

Subjects with ongoing acne or active skin infection are not treated. The acne should be stable and in remission for at least 3 months before CO_2 treatment. Resurfacing subjects with an active skin infection could result in severe and serious complications including cellulitis and severe scarring. All patients with or without a history of herpes simplex virus (HSV) are treated prophylactically with an antiviral medication and continued until re-epithelialization has occurred.

Absolute contraindications for ablative skin resurfacing include isotretinoin use within 1 year of the desired procedure, history of keloid formation, immunosuppression (acquired or drug-induced) and neuropsychosis (e.g., facial picking).

19.5 Complications

19.5.1 Erythema

Although cosmetically unacceptable to patients, postoperative erythema is part of healing[14] and is expected after CO_2 laser resurfacing[10] in all patients.[2,15] Diffuse persistent erythema may be associated with allergic or irritant contact dermatitis (► Fig. 19.2)[16,17] and superficial infections[17] including bacterial or fungal.

The residual thermal damage or heating with either a CO_2 or Er:YAG laser treatment is most likely responsible for prolonged erythema. Single-pass ablative treatments alone are unlikely to result in significant erythema unless comorbidities such as infection occur. Ross and coworkers,[18] in their 13-patient study of wrinkle reduction and adverse effects, compared microscopic and clinical injuries resulting from four-pass treatment with an Er:YAG laser and single-pass treatment with a CO_2 laser. Periorbital and perioral areas of the face were treated on one side with the Er:YAG laser and on the other side with the CO_2 laser. Both lasers produced ablation of 60 µm of the epidermis and residual thermal damage of the upper 20 µm of the dermis. These results showed that with the treatment parameters used in the study, a single pass with the CO_2 laser produced injuries similar to those of four passes of the Er:YAG laser.

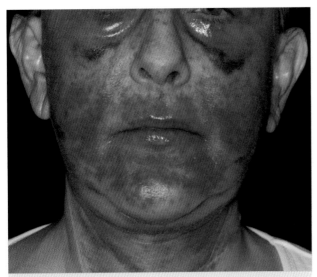

Fig. 19.2 A 61-year-old woman who underwent carbon dioxide (CO_2) resurfacing and was treated with a petrolatum aftercare product. The erythema and pustules are often associated with this type of product.

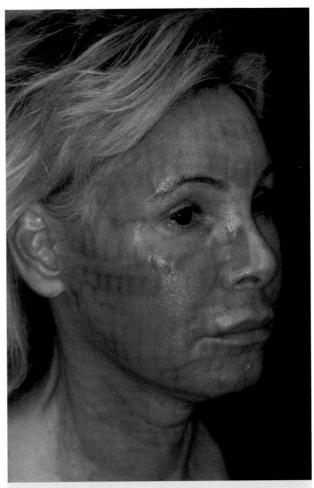

Fig. 19.3 A 55-year-old woman who underwent fractional carbon dioxide (CO_2) resurfacing. Cross marks and stamping effect of the fractional device are significant at 6 days after treatment. Erythema persisted more than 6 weeks due to high density and energy settings.

Erythema was significantly less ($p < 0.04$) after 2 weeks on the CO_2 laser-treated sides than on the Er:YAG-treated sides and the differences resolved 6 weeks after treatment. Tanzi and Alster,[19] in their 100-patient study of subjects who underwent either single-pass CO_2 or multiple-pass Er:YAG resurfacing, reported postoperative erythema persisting for 4.5 and 3.6 weeks, respectively.

The pulse frequency can also contribute to the degree of erythema. High-frequency treatments reduce the treatment time, but when frequency rates approach the TRT of skin, overheating of the skin can occur. For example, at a frequency of 600 Hz, the laser fires every 1.5 ms. Cooling time between pulses is approximately 0.8 ms, assuming the pulse duration is 0.7 ms, the TRT of human skin. At 250 Hz, the cooling time is 3.3 ms, or 412.5% longer than the 0.8 ms cooling time at 600 Hz. This longer cooling time allows for some of the thermal component of the injury to dissipate before the next pulse is delivered. This helps prevent the buildup of heat, classically known as a heat sink. Some devices also provide random patterns of ablation so that no two pulses are adjacent. This may also help prevent excessive erythema.

Transient erythema after treatment with a fractional laser[8,9,20] and all types of nonablative treatments[21] has been reported. Erythema persisting longer than 4 days on the face and longer than 7 days on the neck and chest has been noted in 1.1% of patients after ablative fractionated CO_2 laser treatment.[5] With fractionated resurfacing, erythema is considered prolonged if it persists longer than 4 days with nonablative treatments and longer than 1 month with ablative procedures. The risk of prolonged erythema after fractionated laser resurfacing increases with multiple passes and inadvertent pulse stacking.[20]

▶ Fig. 19.3 shows a patient in whom erythema persisted more than 6 weeks after fractional CO_2 laser resurfacing. The contributing factors were thought to be long pulse width and high density with inefficient ablation.

Treatments of erythema include hydrocortisone 1% cream used sparingly and for a short time[10] and, to reduce inflammation, topical ascorbic acid after re-epithelialization is complete.[15,22] Hydrocortisone 2.5% cream and hydrocortisone valerate 0.2% cream have also been suggested for erythema and pruritus. Many physicians apply steroid creams after re-epithelialization has occurred because healing may be delayed if the steroid is given before re-epithelialization is complete.[23] The use of topical steroid creams during the re-epithelialization following resurfacing has been implicated in increased infection rates.[24] If scarring develops, intralesional triamcinolone 10 mg/mL or 5 fluorouracil along with pulsed dye laser treatment is recommended promptly because delay in treatment may lead to hypertrophic scarring.[10,15] These treatment options may help reset healing by decreasing the production of collagen, reducing the amount of extracellular matrix deposition, and/or modulating certain growth factors implicated in wound healing.[25] Intense pulsed light has been used successfully to remove erythema and hyperpigmentation after CO_2 laser resurfacing of the periorbital area.[26] Persistent erythema following laser resurfacing requires vigilant treatment because patients are often homebound for several months, resulting in significant dissatisfaction toward the physician.

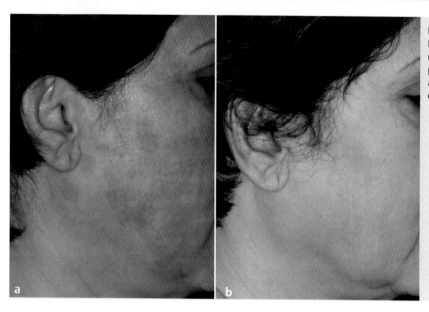

Fig. 19.4 (a) A 32-year-old, Fitzpatrick skin type IV woman who underwent fractional CO_2 laser resurfacing 3 weeks post-treatment. (b) Note persistence of hyperpigmentation at 6 weeks after treatment, believed to be related to excessively long pulse width and high density.

19.5.2 Hyperpigmentation

Hyperpigmentation occurs approximately 4 weeks after CO_2 laser resurfacing in more than 30% of all patients and nearly 100% of dark-skinned patients.[27] It may also occur in skin types I, II, and III, even without sun exposure.[13] Hyperpigmentation is often due to inadvertent sun exposure shortly after laser treatment.[28] The amount of heat deposited into the skin is considered a primary source of hyperpigmentation by many. Frequency, density, and prolonged heating of the skin all contribute to this problem (▶ Fig. 19.4). Since pigmentary changes may be emotionally disturbing, patients should be warned of this possibility before the procedure.[22,28,29] Hyperpigmentation usually resolves within several months without treatment but may persist for 6 to 9 months.[28] Resolution may be expedited with topical glycolic, retinoic, or azelaic acid; hydroquinone; light glycolic acid peels (30–40%); or both; and regular use of broad-spectrum sunscreens.[22] The postoperative use of an anti-hyperpigmentation regimen (4% hydroquinone bleaching agent, kojic acid or mild lactic acid peeling, and sunscreen) has been shown to reduce the incidence of hyperpigmentation from 21 to 6%.[14] Pretreatment with glycolic acid cream or hydroquinone with tretinoin cream appears to provide no reduction in incidence of hyperpigmentation after either CO_2 or Er:YAG laser treatment,[22] although this is controversial.[13,15] However, patients should apply sunscreen with 15 or higher sun protection factor at least 4 weeks before resurfacing and continue regular use after treatment to maintain their clinical improvement.[22]

Hyperpigmentation after treatment with a nonablative 1,500-nm fractional erbium-doped laser has been reported[9] in a small percentage of therapy. In the study of 961 successive treatments, 0.73% of treatments of both facial and nonfacial areas resulted in hyperpigmentation in dark-skinned patients and persisted for a mean of 50.57 days. Techniques to resolve this condition are similar to those of nonfractional lasers. For fractional laser resurfacing, eight studies (most with the 1,500-nm erbium-doped laser) have reported hyperpigmentation in 1 to 32% of patients, depending on the laser system, treatment parameters, and skin types.[20] Procedure is similar to that of nonfractional laser-induced hyperpigmentation.

19.6 Hypopigmentation

Caused by excessive fibrosis and disruption of melanogenesis,[30] hypopigmentation is noticeable skin lightening that may occur 6 to 12 months after CO_2 laser resurfacing,[22] after erythema and hyperpigmentation have resolved. Frequencies after resurfacing range from 1 to 20%.[31] The risk of hypopigmentation is increased with depth of penetration into the reticular dermis[28] and with the amount of thermal injury to the treated areas.[22] It is most pronounced in the presence of melanosis or hyperpigmentation, as in Asian and Hispanic patients.[28] Unlike hyperpigmentation, hypopigmentation may be irreversible and is treated by targeting surrounding depigmented areas with glycolic acid peels or light trichloroacetic acid peels to blend the pigmentary differences between the pale skin and untreated depigmented skin.[22] Hypopigmentation may occur in areas treated aggressively or previously treated by phenol peeling or dermabrasion.[27] Lines of demarcation may be minimized by treating the entire face rather than specific areas (▶ Fig. 19.5).[13,31,32] Melanogenesis may be induced in hypopigmented areas by applying topical Oxsoralen with limited exposure to ultraviolet light to stimulate pigment recovery.[22,31]

Schwartz and colleagues[14] reported an 8% incidence of hypopigmentation in 211 patients undergoing CO_2 facial resurfacing with a 1-year follow-up. These authors emphasized the importance of distinguishing between "pseudohypopigmentation" and true hypopigmentation after facial CO_2 laser resurfacing of sun-damaged skin. Sun-damaged skin is darker than normal, and when a sun-damaged face is treated and the same patient's sun-damaged neck is not treated, one can expect to see a line of demarcation between the treated face (restored to its normal color) and the darker, untreated skin of the neck. The patient should be warned that these lines of demarcation cannot be avoided and, despite treatment with an aggressive skin care regimen, may not be eradicated completely.

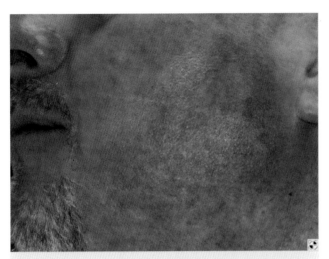

Fig. 19.5 A 55-year-old man treated with fractional carbon dioxide (CO_2) laser resulting in lines of demarcation and permanent hypopigmentation. Areas were re-treated with a superficial ablative CO_2 laser with some improvement.

The risk of hypopigmentation may be lower after Er:YAG laser resurfacing than with the CO_2 laser. As with the CO_2 laser, hypopigmentation may be permanent. Kim et al[33] reported hypopigmentation in 13.7% of 190 patients treated with a short-pulsed, variable-pulsed, or dual-mode Er:YAG laser. Hypopigmentation appeared in 8% of patients treated with the short-pulsed laser, 15.3% of patients treated with the variable-pulsed laser, and in 24.4% of patients treated with the dual-mode laser. The condition became apparent 2 months after treatment and resolved without treatment within 12 months in 85% of cases.

Hypopigmentation is uncommon in fractional laser resurfacing.[20] Avram and colleagues[34] noted hypopigmentation within hypertrophic scars on the neck of a patient for several months after fractional laser resurfacing.

19.6.1 Infection

Viral, bacterial, and fungal infections, if they occur, are observed during the first week after resurfacing, before re-epithelialization is complete.[35] Severe cutaneous infections should be treated promptly to prevent atrophic scarring, delayed wound healing, dissemination of the infection, and invasion of other opportunistic pathogens.[35] HSV, the most common infection associated with cutaneous resurfacing, may occur even in patients with no history of HSV infection and despite antiviral prophylaxis.[27] HSV outbreaks can occur in up to 10% of patients who receive appropriate antiviral prophylaxis.[36]

For bacterial infections the most frequent causative agent is *Staphylococcus aureus*.[37] *Pseudomonas, S. epidermidis,* and *Candida* (yeast) infections have also been observed in moist wound environments.[37,38] Infection should be suspected if the patient is experiencing pain, purulent discharge, increased erythema, crusting, or delayed wound healing.[27,39] In this case a broad-spectrum antibiotic should be given until bacterial culture and sensitivity results are available.[35] *Pseudomonas* infection resulting in hypertrophic scarring and dyspigmentation occurred in a patient subjected to overly aggressive CO_2 laser skin resurfacing, delay in diagnosis of a postoperative infection, and failure

to vary the treatment parameters according to the facial or neck area treated.[39]

Viral

Viral infection is indicated by the presence of small superficial erosions (with or without intact pustules or vesicles[40]) accompanied by burning, tingling, or isolated areas of discharge within the treated skin.[27] Antiviral agents should be prescribed for every patient, with or without a history of HSV outbreak because most patients harbor the virus and may be unaware of previous exposure.[41] The need for antiviral prophylaxis on all patients undergoing fractional CO_2 laser resurfacing has been questioned.[5] In a retrospective study of 373 treatments of 287 patients receiving no antiviral prophylaxis, Campbell and Goldman[5] reported a 1.1% incidence of HSV infection compared to 7% for ablative CO_2 laser resurfacing. In a retrospective study of 961 consecutive treatments with a 1,500-nm erbium-doped fractional laser, Graber and colleagues[9] found an incidence of 1.77% for HSV outbreaks. The authors suggested that antiviral prophylaxis was not necessary in all patients undergoing fractional resurfacing with the 1,500-nm erbium-doped laser.

Shamsaldeen et al,[3] using deep fractional CO_2 laser resurfacing on multiple body sites, reported HSV outbreak in 2.2% (n = 11) of 490 treatments of 374 patients. These authors prescribe antiviral agents prophylactically only in patients with a known history of HSV.

Bacterial

Bacterial infections may occur 2 to 10 days after laser resurfacing.[15] The rate of infection with ablative lasers is 0.5 to 4.5% but only 0.1% of patients who undergo fractionated skin resurfacing develop impetigo.[20] Antibiotic prophylaxis is controversial[42] due to the possibility of developing drug-resistant strains of bacteria[38] and evidence that prophylaxis may predispose patients to more pathogenic infections.[15] In their retrospective study of 133 patients who underwent cutaneous CO_2 laser resurfacing, Walia and Alster[42] found no reduction in the rate of infection when antibiotics were administered intraoperatively and postoperatively. Weinstein et al[13] reported a 0.5% incidence of bacterial infection in 1,925 patients (even in those receiving antibiotic prophylaxis) who underwent skin resurfacing with a CO_2 laser.

Fungal

Postoperative *Candida albicans* infections occur infrequently and are often associated with the use of topical antibiotics, diabetes, immunosuppression, and angular cheilitis.[27] Fulton[29] reported a microscopically confirmed *Candida* flare-up of the perioral area after CO_2 laser resurfacing. The pustules were treated successfully with an antiyeast cream (kotoconazole). Cutaneous candidiasis, although rare with fractional laser resurfacing, should be treated promptly with antifungal agents to prevent scarring.[20] Pretreatment with anticandidal agents may be appropriate in patients with a history of frequent vaginal yeast infection.[15,43] ► Fig. 19.6 shows a patient in whom a yeast infection developed after facelift and laser resurfacing.

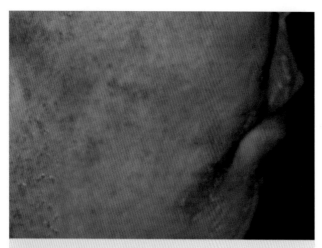

Fig. 19.6 A 58-year-old patient who underwent facelift and laser resurfacing. Note the nonhealing area at the corner of the mouth. Moisture and a history of angular cheilitis were thought to be causative in developing a yeast infection here.

In their study of 1,925 patients undergoing CO_2 laser resurfacing, Weinstein et al[13] observed no fungal or *Candida* infection. They attributed the absence of infection to avoiding the use of occlusive ointments. Shamsaldeen and colleagues,[3] using deep fractional CO_2 laser resurfacing on multiple body sites, reported yeast infection in 1.2% of 490 treatments of 374 patients.

19.6.2 Hypertrophic Scarring

Scars, the most serious complication of ablative laser resurfacing,[13] are observed in up to 2 to 3% of patients.[44] Failure to remove desiccated tissue between laser passes; high-energy treatment densities; overlapped or stacked scans or pulses; poor patient selection; and overly aggressive treatment of the upper lip, neck, periorbital area, or mandible contribute to scar formation.[13,15,31,35,39] The risk of scarring is increased in postoperative wound infection or contact dermatitis, tendency to form keloids, history of radiation treatment, or recent tretinoin use.[15,31,35]

Early indicators of scar formation (abnormal erythema or induration 2 to 4 weeks after treatment[20]) may be treated with potent topical steroids, intralesional steroid injection, occlusive dressing, or pulsed dye laser.[14,15,44] If scarring develops, regression may occur following repeat light fractional resurfacing with ablative or nonablative lasers, injection with 5 fluorouracil, pulsed dye laser, or broadband light therapy. Hypertrophic scars have been observed in fractional CO_2 laser resurfacing particularly in the neck when the reticular dermis was injured (▶ Fig. 19.7).[34,45]

19.6.3 Periocular Laser Complications

Periocular complications include prolonged erythema, hyperpigmentation, hypertrophic scarring, and ectropion. Injuries to the globe are catastrophic and preventable with the use of metal eye shields for all patients undergoing treatment. All health care providers must also be protected from inadvertent

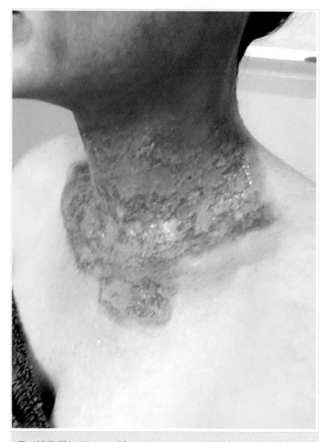

Fig. 19.7 This 46-year-old patient was treated with a carbon dioxide fractional laser in the neck at a density of 35% with a depth of injury at 800 µm. Deep second-degree burns resulted in significant scarring in the neck. Note the loss of skin in the lower neck.

mishaps related to ocular injury. Laser safety glasses with an optical density of + 7 are recommended for CO_2 and erbium lasers. Corneal injuries are most commonly associated with CO_2 and erbium lasers (wavelength > 1,400 nm)

Permanent ectropion has been found in 0.4% of patients after lower lid resurfacing.[46] Risk factors for developing ectropion of the lower lid include previous surgical treatment of the eyelids such as lower lid blepharoplasty, currently planned combined procedures, and laxity of the lower lid. Assessment of the integrity of the lower lid includes preoperative evaluation with a snap test and lid-distraction test. Lower eyelid tightening during the laser resurfacing procedure must be considered if the lid demonstrates poor resting tone.

Tightening of the lower lid can be performed by many techniques; however, this author prefers the following strategy when performing lower lid blepharoplasty and lower eyelid resurfacing as a combined procedure. First, excess fat is resected via a transconjunctival approach when necessary. The lateral retinaculum is then mobilized endoscopically if performing a browlift, and is suspended to the medial component of the superior orbital rim at the level or slightly medial to the lateral canthus. Alternatively it can be mobilized through a small incision at the orbital rim where the suspension suture is to be placed. The orbicularis muscle is then suspended in a similar fashion. Skin excess is removed via a pinch excision technique.

Table 19.2 Comparison of number and percentage of adverse events after carbon dioxide (CO_2) laser resurfacing

Adverse event	No. (%) of adverse events		
	TOE aftercare (n = 99)	Shamsaldeen et al[3] (n = 490, deep fractional ablative)	Nanni and Alster[48] (n = 500, fully ablative)
Milia	5 (5.1)	0 (0)	(11.0)
Acneiform eruption	0 (0)	26 (5.3)	(15.0)
Infection	0 (0)	27 (5.5)	(8.4)
HSV	0 (0)	11 (2.2)	(7.4)
Bacterial	0 (0)	11 (2.2)	(0.0)
Yeast	0 (0)	6 (1.2)	(<1.0)
Hyperpigmentation	2 (2.0)	6 (1.2)	(37.0)
Prolonged erythema	0 (0)	4 (0.8)	(100.0)
Contact dermatitis	0 (0)	4 (0.8)	(11.0)
Scarring	0 (0)	0 (0)	(0.0)
Hypopigmentation	0 (0)	0 (0)	(1.0)
Erythema	–	–	(100.0)
Acne exacerbation	–	–	(15.0)
Total	7 (7.1)	68 (13.9)	–

HSV, herpes simplex virus; TOE, topical oxygen emulsion.
(Reproduced with permission from Duplechain JK, Rubin MG, Kim K. Novel posttreatment care after ablative and fractional CO_2 laser resurfacing. J Cosmet Laser Ther 2014; 16: 77–82.)

Laser resurfacing with the CO_2 laser is then performed. Epidermal ablation at 60 to 80% density is completed. The deeper components of the lid are not treated with the laser because treatment of multiple layers, including the middle lamella, significantly increases the risk of ectropion and is unnecessary when this technique is utilized. Excessive collagen contraction during laser resurfacing may also potentiate eversion of the eyelid.[35]

19.7 Improved Posttreatment Care

The author uses the pulsed ablative CO_2 laser exclusively to rejuvenate skin despite its well-documented adverse effects and the increasing trends in use of less ablative or nonablative fractional lasers. This decision is based on the "gold standard" status of the CO_2 modality and a new aftercare treatment shown in this author's practice to substantially reduce the complications of ablative pulsed CO_2 laser treatment. The details of this posttreatment procedure have been reported[47] and are summarized in the following paragraph.

A 100-patient study evaluated the use of a topical oxygen emulsion (TOE) to reduce adverse effects after treatment with an ablative CO_2 laser alone and in combination with a fractional ablative CO_2 laser. ► Table 19.2 shows the adverse effects observed with TOE as part of aftercare following CO_2 laser resurfacing—fully ablative, fractional ablative, or both in combination. The percentage of patients with adverse effects was limited to 7.1% compared to 0 to 100% reported by Nanni and

Alster[48] after fully ablative CO_2 laser resurfacing and 13.9% reported by Shamsaldeen and colleagues[3] after fractionated ablative CO_2 laser procedures. Infection was not observed in any of the 99 patients who received TOE aftercare.

19.8 Managing the Untoward Event

Dealing with patient dissatisfaction related to resurfacing is as difficult as it is with any other surgical procedure. The visibility of the complication enhances the patient's awareness of the problem, often making the event the center of attention regardless of the many benefits associated with the procedure. Significant attention to the patient with proper skin care, strict guidelines regarding the use of products, and the avoidance of introducing other therapies unless approved by the provider must be clear to the patient. Photographs should be taken at routine intervals to document and provide a means of assessing improvement. Patients will require regular visits that include discussion about improvement and alternative treatment options if initial steps at managing a complication are unsuccessful. Assisting in the management of makeup, skin care, and personal support are paramount to managing the complication.

With proper evaluation, planning, and careful execution of laser resurfacing, superb results can become the "norm" for patients and the health care provider interested in this type of rejuvenation treatment. The results provided when this occurs, the author believes, are still unmatched by other technologies.

19.9 Disclosure

The author is a founder and stockholder of Cutagenesis, Lafayette, Louisiana.

References

[1] Bernstein LJ, Kauvar AN, Grossman MC, Geronemus RG. The short- and long-term side effects of carbon dioxide laser resurfacing. Dermatol Surg 1997; 23: 519–525

[2] Nanni CA, Alster TS. Complications of cutaneous laser surgery. A review. Dermatol Surg 1998; 24: 209–219

[3] Shamsaldeen O, Peterson JD, Goldman MP. The adverse events of deep fractional CO(2): a retrospective study of 490 treatments in 374 patients. Lasers Surg Med 2011; 43: 453–456

[4] Duplechain JK. Fractional CO2 resurfacing: has it replaced ablative resurfacing techniques? Facial Plast Surg Clin North Am 2013; 21: 213–227

[5] Campbell TM, Goldman MP. Adverse events of fractionated carbon dioxide laser: review of 373 treatments. Dermatol Surg 2010; 36: 1645–1650

[6] Khan MH, Sink RK, Manstein D, Eimerl D, Anderson RR. Intradermally focused infrared laser pulses: thermal effects at defined tissue depths. Lasers Surg Med 2005; 36: 270–280

[7] Grema H, Greve B, Raulin C. Facial rhytides—subsurfacing or resurfacing? A review. Lasers Surg Med 2003; 32: 405–412

[8] Fisher GH, Geronemus RG. Short-term side effects of fractional photothermolysis. Dermatol Surg 2005; 31: 1245–1249, discussion 1249

[9] Graber EM, Tanzi EL, Alster TS. Side effects and complications of fractional laser photothermolysis: experience with 961 treatments. Dermatol Surg 2008; 34: 301–305, discussion 305–307

[10] Weinstein C. Carbon dioxide laser resurfacing. Long-term follow-up in 2123 patients. Clin Plast Surg 1998; 25: 109–130

[11] Bailey SH, Brown SA, Kim Y, et al. An intra-individual quantitative assessment of acute laser injury patterns in facial versus abdominal skin. Lasers Surg Med 2011; 43: 99–107

[12] Oni G, Robbins D, Bailey S, Brown SA, Kenkel JM. An in vivo histopathological comparison of single and double pulsed modes of a fractionated CO(2) laser. Lasers Surg Med 2012; 44: 4–10

[13] Weinstein C, Pozner JN, Ramirez OM. Complications of carbon dioxide laser resurfacing and their prevention. Aesthet Surg J 1997; 17: 216–225

[14] Schwartz RJ, Burns AJ, Rohrich RJ, Barton FE, Jr, Byrd HS. Long-term assessment of CO2 facial laser resurfacing: aesthetic results and complications. Plast Reconstr Surg 1999; 103: 592–601

[15] Ratner D, Tse Y, Marchell N, Goldman MP, Fitzpatrick RE, Fader DJ. Cutaneous laser resurfacing. J Am Acad Dermatol 1999; 41: 365–389, quiz 390–392

[16] Papadavid E, Katsambas A. Lasers for facial rejuvenation: a review. Int J Dermatol 2003; 42: 480–487

[17] Blanco G, Clavero A, Soparkar CN, Patrinely JR. Periocular laser complications. Semin Plast Surg 2007; 21: 74–79

[18] Ross EV, Miller C, Meehan K, et al. One-pass CO2 versus multiple-pass Er:YAG laser resurfacing in the treatment of rhytides: a comparison side-by-side study of pulsed CO2 and Er:YAG lasers. Dermatol Surg 2001; 27: 709–715

[19] Tanzi EL, Alster TS. Single-pass carbon dioxide versus multiple-pass Er:YAG laser skin resurfacing: a comparison of postoperative wound healing and side-effect rates. Dermatol Surg 2003; 29: 80–84

[20] Metelitsa AI, Alster TS. Fractionated laser skin resurfacing treatment complications: a review. Dermatol Surg 2010; 36: 299–306

[21] Handley JM. Adverse events associated with nonablative cutaneous visible and infrared laser treatment. J Am Acad Dermatol 2006; 55: 482–489

[22] Alster TS, Lupton JR. Prevention and treatment of side effects and complications of cutaneous laser resurfacing. Plast Reconstr Surg 2002; 109: 308–316, discussion 317–318

[23] Demas PN, Bridenstine JB. Diagnosis and treatment of postoperative complications after skin resurfacing. J Oral Maxillofac Surg 1999; 57: 837–841

[24] Ortiz AE, Tingey C, Yu YE, Ross EV. Topical steroids implicated in postoperative infection following ablative laser resurfacing. Lasers Surg Med 2012; 44: 1–3

[25] Yang Q, Ma Y, Zhu R, et al. The effect of flashlamp pulsed dye laser on the expression of connective tissue growth factor in keloids. Lasers Surg Med 2012; 44: 377–383

[26] Kontoes PP, Vlachos SP. Intense pulsed light is effective in treating pigmentary and vascular complications of CO(2) laser resurfacing. Aesthet Surg J 2002; 22: 489–491

[27] Alster TS, Lupton JR. Treatment of complications of laser skin resurfacing. Arch Facial Plast Surg 2000; 2: 279–284

[28] Apfelberg DB. Side effects, sequelae, and complications of carbon dioxide laser resurfacing. Aesthet Surg J 1997; 17: 365–372

[29] Fulton JE, Jr. Complications of laser resurfacing. Methods of prevention and management. Dermatol Surg 1998; 24: 91–99

[30] Ramsdell WM. Fractional CO2 laser resurfacing complications. Semin Plast Surg 2012; 26: 137–140

[31] McBurney EI. Side effects and complications of laser therapy. Dermatol Clin 2002; 20: 165–176

[32] Ross EV, Grossman MC, Duke D, Grevelink JM. Long-term results after CO2 laser skin resurfacing: a comparison of scanned and pulsed systems. J Am Acad Dermatol 1997; 37: 709–718

[33] Kim YJ, Lee HS, Son SW, Kim SN, Kye YC. Analysis of hyperpigmentation and hypopigmentation after Er:YAG laser skin resurfacing. Lasers Surg Med 2005; 36: 47–51

[34] Avram MM, Tope WD, Yu T, Szachowicz E, Nelson JS. Hypertrophic scarring of the neck following ablative fractional carbon dioxide laser resurfacing. Lasers Surg Med 2009; 41: 185–188

[35] Alster TS, Khoury RR. Treatment of laser complications. Facial Plast Surg 2009; 25: 316–323

[36] Alster TS, Nanni CA. Famciclovir prophylaxis of herpes simplex virus reactivation after laser skin resurfacing. Dermatol Surg 1999; 25: 242–246

[37] Sriprachya-Anunt S, Fitzpatrick RE, Goldman MP, Smith SR. Infections complicating pulsed carbon dioxide laser resurfacing for photoaged facial skin. Dermatol Surg 1997; 23: 527–535, discussion 535–536

[38] Alster TS. Cutaneous resurfacing with CO2 and erbium:YAG lasers: preoperative, intraoperative, and postoperative considerations. Plast Reconstr Surg 1999; 103: 619–632, discussion 633–634

[39] Willey A, Anderson RR, Azpiazu JL, et al. Complications of laser dermatologic surgery. Lasers Surg Med 2006; 38: 1–15

[40] Alster TS, Lupton JR. Erbium:YAG cutaneous laser resurfacing. Dermatol Clin 2001; 19: 453–466

[41] Spruance SL. The natural history of recurrent oral-facial herpes simplex virus infection. Semin Dermatol 1992; 11: 200–206

[42] Walia S, Alster TS. Cutaneous CO2 laser resurfacing infection rate with and without prophylactic antibiotics. Dermatol Surg 1999; 25: 857–861

[43] Fitzpatrick RE, Williams B, Goldman MP. Preoperative anesthesia and postoperative considerations in laser resurfacing. Semin Cutan Med Surg 1996; 15: 170–176

[44] Riggs K, Keller M, Humphreys TR. Ablative laser resurfacing: high-energy pulsed carbon dioxide and erbium:yttrium-aluminum-garnet. Clin Dermatol 2007; 25: 462–473

[45] Fife DJ, Fitzpatrick RE, Zachary CB. Complications of fractional CO2 laser resurfacing: four cases. Lasers Surg Med 2009; 41: 179–184

[46] Apfelberg DB American Society for Aesthetic Plastic Surgery. American Society of Plastic and Reconstructive Surgeons. Summary of the 1997 ASAPS/ASPRS Laser Task Force Survey on laser resurfacing and laser blepharoplasty. Plast Reconstr Surg 1998; 101: 511–518

[47] Duplechain JK, Rubin MG, Kim K. Novel post-treatment care after ablative and fractional CO2 laser resurfacing. J Cosmet Laser Ther 2014; 16: 77–82

[48] Nanni CA, Alster TS. Complications of carbon dioxide laser resurfacing. An evaluation of 500 patients. Dermatol Surg 1998; 24: 315–320

20 Choosing the Right Laser for Your Practice: A Practical Comparison of Available Lasers

Fred G. Fedok, Irina Chaikhoutdinov, and Frank G. Garritano

20.1 Introduction

The modern cosmetic surgery practice provides a network of services to a wide spectrum of patients, addressing multiple patient concerns as well as different age groups, ethnicities, and demographic characteristics. Meeting all of these needs requires the incorporation of both surgical and nonsurgical services. The full-service cosmetic practice is now generally well versed in the use of injectable devices such as botulinum toxin and filler substances. Skin resurfacing with dermabrasion, chemical peeling, and laser technologies has also become a frequent treatment method in many settings to address congenital and acquired skin conditions.

Since lasers first became commercially available in the 1960s, the development and evolution of laser technologies that can be applied to human skin has progressed greatly. Given the broad scope this topic has attained, this review is largely limited to lasers used to treat the face and neck. The goal of this chapter is to provide readers with the information necessary to make an informed assessment about which laser technologies appear to offer a favorable impact to their practices in terms of cost, response to patients' needs, efficacy of technology, and practicality.

20.1.1 Clinical Conditions for Which Patients Seek Treatment and Consultation

A variety of skin conditions are treated with laser therapy within the scope of facial plastic surgery. Photodamage of the skin is characterized by dyschromia, fine rhytids, erythema, telangiectasias, keratosis, and textural changes. Disorganization of collagen fibers and accumulation of ineffective elastin lead to solar elastosis.[1] Variability in skin thickness, with alternating areas of atrophy and hyperplasia, gives skin an overall dry and leathery appearance. Pigmentation irregularity with the presence of lentigines and depigmented areas contributes to an aged appearance.

Laser resurfacing can be used to address skin changes related to aging, including solar damage and rhytids, as well as scarring from acne or trauma. Skin discoloration as part of the aging process is thought by some to be best treated with nonablative therapy or fractionated therapy.[2] Laser therapy can also be used to treat pigmented lesions, vascular malformations, and tattoos.

20.1.2 Patient Demographics

Patient selection and counseling are paramount to achieving optimal outcomes. Realistic expectations should be established and discussed with the patient before treatment. A full medical history should be obtained, with a focus on dermatological history. The physical examination should evaluate pigmented skin lesions for the possible need for biopsy prior to laser therapy.

Any risk factors identified should be discussed with patients as presenting increased risks. Patients with a history of posttraumatic or postinflammatory hyperpigmentation or melasma are at increased risk of hyperpigmentation, as are patients on estrogen therapy. Isotretinoin treatment within the past 6 months is a contraindication to ablative lasers, and these patients should be counseled regarding nonablative lasers. A history of hypertrophic scarring and keloid formation increases scarring risk with deeper laser treatments. Prolonged topical or systemic corticosteroids can delay wound healing and result in areas of atrophic skin healing. Immunocompromised patients, or those who have collagen-vascular disease, can also experience delayed wound healing. A history of perioral or facial herpetic lesions creates a higher risk of recurrence after treatment, and these patients should be started on antiviral prophylaxis. Patients who are currently pregnant or breast-feeding should also avoid laser resurfacing because no studies regarding safety exist.

The Fitzpatrick grading system is a six-level system for designating skin reaction to sun exposure.[3] Laser therapy is ideal for patients with the lightest skin tones, specifically those with Fitzpatrick skin types I through III. Darker skin types carry a risk of postprocedure dyschromia. Additionally, patients with previous postinflammatory hyperpigmentation or melasma, regardless of skin type, are at increased risk of dyschromia.

20.2 Laser Technologies

Lasers are named for the medium that produces the wavelength of laser energy for that specific laser. The laser medium is contained within an optical cavity or resonator and may be a liquid, as in the case of a pulsed dye laser; a solid, as in the case of an erbium:yttrium aluminum garnet (Er:YAG) laser; or a gas, as in the case of the carbon dioxide (CO_2) laser. A general laser design produces photons from an energy source that are made to move parallel to the axis of the optical cavity and are repeatedly reflected between opposing mirrors. The summation of this repetitive interaction causes a stimulated emission to be generated. This laser energy is then transmitted to the operator's handpiece via an articulated tube with mirrors or fiber-optic cable.

Clinically, it is helpful to describe the wavelengths of light associated with particular lasers rather than by using brand names. These designations, such as "1,064-nm neodymium: yttrium aluminum garnet (Nd:YAG)," will guide the clinician to the appropriate use and improve documentation and communication. Critical parameters of the laser emission include the wavelength, pulse characteristics, and fluence. The following sections describe various lasers, along with their general physical characteristics and absorption spectra.[4]

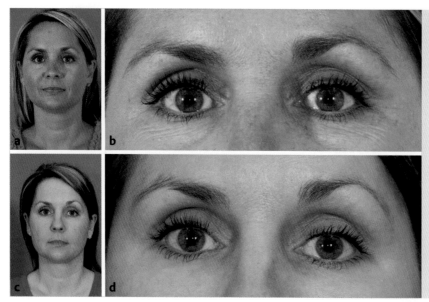

Fig. 20.1 Clinical photographs of patient who underwent 10,600 nm fractional CO_2 laser of face for correction of fine rhytids (patient has undergone previous TCA peeling of acne scars). **(a,b)** Preoperative images; **(c,d)** Postoperative images.

20.3 Lasers for the Treatment of Skin Aging

The rhytids, telangiectasias, laxity, and actinic changes associated with photoaging of the skin can be improved with both ablative and nonablative resurfacing technologies.[5,6,7,8]

20.3.1 The CO_2 10,600-nm Laser

The CO_2 laser became popular for skin resurfacing in the early 1990s and has been the most widely used laser for ablative resurfacing.[9,10,11,12,13] It emits invisible infrared radiation at a 10,600-nm wavelength. This wavelength is primarily absorbed by intracellular and extracellular water, resulting in a number of thermal effects such as tissue necrosis, vaporization, carbonization, and coagulation. In many ways, the dramatic results obtained by the full ablative CO_2 laser still represent the "gold standard" by which other resurfacing modalities are compared. However, its wide application has decreased due to the resulting prolonged healing time, prolonged erythema, and an increased risk of hypopigmentation, infection, and scarring.

Clinically, CO_2 lasers have been applied in the treatment of a variety of cutaneous disorders including age-related photodamage, rhytids, and depressed scars. Since the CO_2 laser penetrates deeper, it is more effective in the remodeling of the deeper layers of the dermis, causing the effacement of coarser rhytids. The more recently introduced fractional CO_2 laser has gained popularity secondary to its improved risk-to-benefit profile, including significantly decreased recovery time.

The use of fractionated CO_2 technologies was reported after 2007.[14,15,16] Similar to the fractionated erbium technologies that preceded them, fractionated CO_2 systems treat cylinders of tissue with laser energy while leaving interspersed areas of untreated tissue. This creates a productive balance between favorable tissue effects, such as correction of epithelial architecture and skin tightening, and any propensity for prolonged healing, erythema, and scarring. Whereas fractional CO_2 lasers

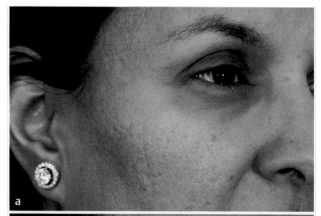

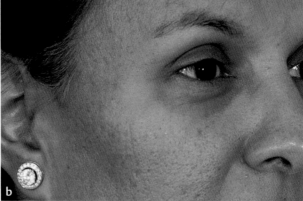

Fig. 20.2 Clinical photographs of patient who underwent single treatment with 10,600 nm fractional CO_2 laser of face for correction of fine rhytids and acne scarring (note absence of postoperative hyperpigmentation in spite of Fitzpatrick IV skin tones). **(a)** Preoperative image; **(b)** Postoperative image.

can be used for fine rhytids, fully ablative treatment is recommended to achieve desired results with deeper rhytids (▶ Fig. 20.1, ▶ Fig. 20.2.)

20.3.2 The Er:YAG 2,940-nm Laser

The erbium laser was introduced for clinical use in the latter part of the 1990s.[17,18,19,20,21,22] This laser has the highest absorption coefficient for water among ablative lasers and given its particular tissue interaction characteristics, it is touted to provide many of the benefits of CO_2 laser treatment with reduced unfavorable sequelae. This may be related to the favorable thermal relaxation times achievable with the Er:YAG platforms compared to the CO_2 platforms.[23,24] The fractionated algorithm further improves its therapeutic margin[25] and provides the ability to adjust for specific patient skin type and degree of photoaging. Although the result is a more measured one, there is a decreased healing time. The Er:YAG laser has also been shown as less effective compared to the ablative CO_2 laser for skin tightening.[26]

The second-generation erbium lasers possess favorable ablative and coagulation properties that make them effective for skin resurfacing. Skin conditions that can be successfully treated with this laser include rhytids, solar elastosis, dyschromias, and actinic photodamage. Additionally, the erbium laser has been described as more effective in the treatment of superficial dyschromias and other actinic changes in the superficial layers of the skin.

20.3.3 Other Superficial Ablative and Nonablative Lasers

The highly successful 1,550-nm fractionated erbium laser expanded the use of erbium lasering for both cosmetic and reconstructive indications.[27,28,29,30,31] At this laser wavelength, patients can be offered a modest but significant improvement in texture, rhytids, and superficial lentigines with markedly reduced downtime. However, because the results can be insufficient for a number of clinical conditions, the popularity of the fractionated CO_2 platforms continues.

Other superficial ablative and nonablative technologies are available for a spectrum of cutaneous applications. These lasers function at 2,790, 1,440, 1,540, 1,550, and 1,064 nm, as well as at other wavelengths.[32,33,34,35,36,37] The clinical effect of these lasers and technologies is frequently not as dramatic as with the ablative and fractionated technologies described earlier; however, the science continues to change, and more effective platforms are being developed.

Nonlaser skin improvement technologies are also available and include plasma, radiofrequency, ultrasound, and light-based technologies. A full discussion of these technologies is beyond the scope of this chapter, and readers are urged to evaluate those reports.

20.4 Lasers for the Treatment of Benign Pigmented Lesions

The Nd:YAG laser produces laser energy at a wavelength of 1,064 nm. It will penetrate up to 2 to 3 mm into the dermis, making it useful in the removal of deeper natural and artificial dermal pigmentations. The 1,064-nm wavelength of the Nd:YAG laser also makes it useful for the removal of blue-black tattoos, but it is relatively poorly absorbed by green pigments.[38,39,]

[40] When the laser beam is passed through a KTP crystal, the laser energy frequency is doubled and the resultant light wavelength is halved to 532 nm. This wavelength is absorbed more superficially in the skin, making it useful for the removal of benign superficial epidermal pigmentations.[41,42]

Lentigines are frequently treated along with rhytids while doing ablative resurfacing. In the patient who does not need general ablative resurfacing, such as the younger patient, the lentigines may be treated more directly. If doubt exists about the diagnosis of a lesion, at least one area of the lesion should be biopsied. When one can be confident that the lesion is indeed benign, the Q-switched (QS), frequency-doubled Nd:YAG laser operating at 532 nm can produce good results.[43,44,45,46,47]

20.5 Lasers for Tattoo Removal

The lightening or removal of traumatic and cosmetic tattoo pigment can be effectively approached with lasers and has similarities to the treatment of naturally occurring pigment lesions. The wavelength of the laser used will depend on the target pigment in the tattoo, and it is advisable that the practitioner (except for the most experienced) use test spots to assess the patient and pigment response before proceeding with treatment of the entire lesion.

The QS alexandrite laser at 755 nm, the QS ruby laser at 694 nm, and the QS Nd:YAG laser at 1,064 nm can be effective in the treatment of lighter skinned individuals with a dark blue or black tattoo pigment. In darker skinned individuals (i.e., Fitzpatrick skin types IV–VI), the QS Nd:YAG laser is preferred because the longer wavelength results in a greater degree of epidermal sparing. For tattoos exhibiting red pigment, the QS Nd:YAG laser operating at 532 nm can be used. Green pigment is frequently difficult to treat and best treated with the QS ruby 694-nm laser.[48,49,50,51,52] Due to the risk of hyperpigmentation and hypopigmentation, treatment is usually limited to light-skinned individuals (▶ Fig. 20.3, ▶ Fig. 20.4.)

20.6 Lasers for the Treatment of Vascular Lesions

Vascular lesions are targeted by a variety of wavelength lasers including the pulsed dye (585–595 nm), the KTP frequency-doubled Nd:YAG (532 nm), and the Nd:YAG (1,064 nm) laser systems.[53,54,55,56,57,58,59] The pulsed dye laser was introduced in 1989, and the first version of these lasers emitted light at 577 nm, which corresponds to the oxyhemoglobin absorption spectrum. Current available pulsed dye lasers emit a wavelength of 585 or 595 nm with longer pulse durations. The 585-nm wavelength gives it excellent specificity to hemoglobin with a minimal risk of hyperpigmentation, hypopigmentation, or skin breakdown. In general, the pulsed dye laser is considered to have a reliable safety margin; and for some authors, it has become the treatment of choice for vascular lesions of various sizes, including port-wine stains, telangiectasias, and hemangiomas.[60,61,62,63,64,65] The KTP frequency-doubled Nd:YAG (532 nm) laser is usually used for smaller lesions such as spider veins and telangiectasias, and the Nd:YAG (1,064 nm) laser has utility in treating reticular veins.[66,67,68]

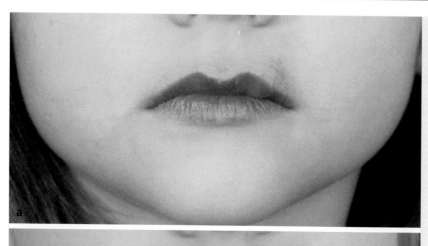

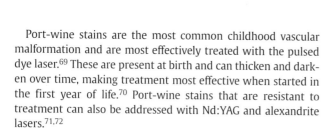

Fig. 20.3 Clinical photographs of patient who underwent single treatment with 1064 nm Nd: YAG laser for treatment of traumatic tattooing of left upper lip. **(a)** Preoperative image. **(b)** Post-operative image.

Port-wine stains are the most common childhood vascular malformation and are most effectively treated with the pulsed dye laser.[69] These are present at birth and can thicken and darken over time, making treatment most effective when started in the first year of life.[70] Port-wine stains that are resistant to treatment can also be addressed with Nd:YAG and alexandrite lasers.[71,72]

Telangiectasias are also most responsive to pulsed dye lasers, usually requiring two to three treatments.[73] The presence of purpura after treatment prognosticates good results. Lasers with longer wavelengths, such as alexandrite and Nd:YAG, can be used for deeper lesions, but they may increase the risk of scarring and ulceration. Certain infantile hemangiomas and pyogenic granulomas have also been treated with laser therapy in an adjunctive fashion, most commonly with pulsed dye lasers. Nd:YAG lasers can be used to assist in treatment of venous malformations when appropriate.

20.7 Lasers for Hair Removal

Prior to the introduction of these laser technologies, modalities such as waxing and electrolysis had been used for hair removal. Laser technology has now become popular for the temporary and semipermanent removal of hair in both women and men for cosmetic purposes, for general grooming, or as part of the treatment or resolution of hirsutism associated with medical conditions such as polycystic ovary disease. Since the targeted chromophore in laser hair removal systems is the melanin

pigment, which is found in the hair shaft and hair follicle epithelium, these lasers are particularly effective.

Although laser hair removal was noted to be available in the 1970s, the first Food and Drug Administration (FDA) approval came with the ruby laser in 1996.[74] This laser has lost popularity due to the development of other technologies that have improved specificity. Alexandrite lasers operating at 755 nm are among the most popular systems, touted to have improved penetration and the ability to treat Fitzpatrick skin types I through IV.[75] The 1,064-nm Nd:YAG laser operating in the long-pulse mode has reported success rates of 70% with five treatments and utility for hair removal even in patients of higher Fitzpatrick skin types.[76]

Diode lasers are popular solid-state lasers that operate at 800 nm and reduce hair density through photothermal destruction of the melanin-containing portions of the hair follicle. These lasers penetrate deeper into the dermis, necessitating epidermal cooling to minimize epidermal and superficial dermal damage, as well as to provide patient comfort. The diode lasers have shown efficacy rates up to 90% and can be used with Fitzpatrick skin types I through IV.[77,78] Patients with dark, coarse hair achieve the most successful outcomes.[79]

Although it does not represent the laser technologies, intense pulsed light (IPL) has become increasingly popular for hair removal. IPL has shown effectiveness comparable to the ruby laser in several studies and statistical equivalence to other devices such as the diode and the alexandrite lasers.[80,81,82]

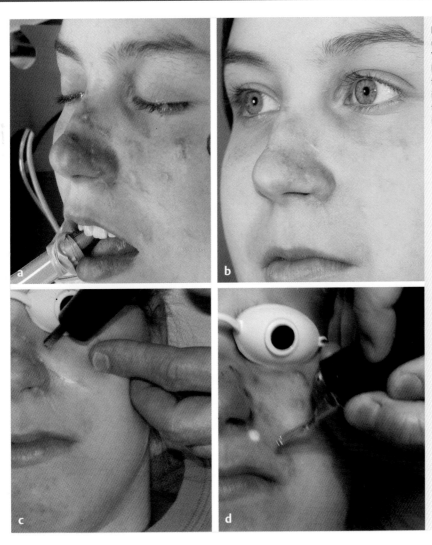

Fig. 20.4 Clinical photographs of patient who underwent single treatment with 1064 nm Nd:YAG laser for treatment of traumatic tattooing of left cheek and nose and 585 nm pulse dye laser treatment of hypertrophic scars. (**a**) Preoperative image. (**b**) Postoperative image. (**c**) Intraoperative image–Nd:YAG laser use. (**d**) Intraoperative image–Pulsed dye laser use.

20.8 Lasers for the Treatment of Scars

Red hypertrophic scars can be effectively treated using the pulsed dye laser with results that are reliable and comparable to the use of intralesional steroid injections.[83] Depressed scars respond quite well to laser resurfacing with both CO_2 and erbium lasers. Acne scars are particularly responsive to a combination of subcision and laser resurfacing ▶ Fig. 20.5.[84,85]

20.9 Available Lasers

There are numerous laser manufacturers offering a variety of laser products that can be used in a facial plastic surgery office (▶ Table 20.1). Some of these products are based on central platforms or main modules that are modified by the addition of different handpieces offering different laser wavelengths and light-based technologies (▶ Fig. 20.6 and ▶ Fig. 20.7). Other laser products have only a single wavelength possible within that one product's system (▶ Fig. 20.8 and ▶ Fig. 20.9). Reasons for this variability are based on the underlying technologies

themselves, the cost of production, and the attainable market prices.

20.10 The Decision to Purchase a Laser for the Office

Before an individual purchases a laser or lasers for the office, a number of questions should be answered.[86] The first question is whether the practitioner has the training and skill level necessary for a given disorder and laser. For instance, if one is contemplating the purchase of a resurfacing laser to manage problems associated with facial aging and sun damage, one should have sufficient knowledge about facial aging with an understanding of why and what rhytids and lentigines to treat. The same questions might be raised related to the purchase of a laser for tattoo removal. Although training is available through several avenues, the fundamental question remains.

Another question to consider is about the prospective patients to be treated. One has to have an idea of the current practice cross-section profile and the likelihood of having sufficient clinical volume to support a particular type of laser practice. For instance, a tattoo-removal laser may be a poor

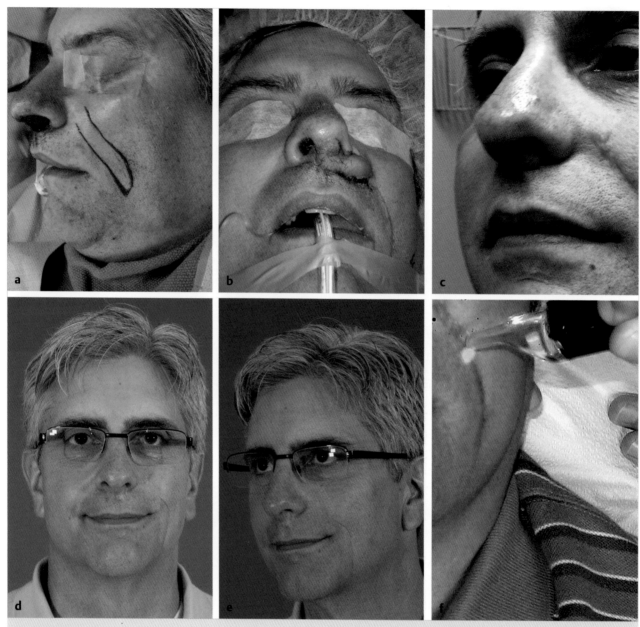

Fig. 20.5 Clinical photographs of patient who underwent treatment with 585 nm pulse dye laser treatment of hypertrophic scars after nasal reconstruction. (**a**) Design of flap prior to surgery. (**b**) Immediately postoperative with the flap turned into the nose. (**c**) Postoperative view demonstrating hypertrophic scar. (**d,e**) Postoperative images. (**f**) Intraoperative image of pulsed dye laser in use.

purchase if the practice does not have patients looking for this service and the surrounding communities do not demonstrate a need.

Finally, one has to assess the local competition and service availability outside of the practice. If so, competitive pricing and other associated factors must be considered. For example, if one lives in a state where nonmedical practitioners can perform laser hair removal—and there are numerous local spas that offer hair removal at prices that would be impractical to perform in of the office—than it would be unrealistic and unwise to purchase a hair-removal laser.

After considering the clinical issues, the technical aspects of the contemplated laser or group of lasers should be examined. Important information includes the possible power settings on

the laser, whether or not it is fractional, and the possible wavelengths within the particular "box." Technical parameters to investigate across multiple machines include the spot size, the settings for duration, and the percentage fractionation. Company representatives, online and brochure information from manufacturers, presentations at meetings, professional publications, and information from colleagues are all useful sources of information. When possible, hands-on experience with the laser through company demonstrations or a visit to a colleague's office can prove invaluable. Evaluation of laser manufacturers and distributors is another critical step. Information about warranties, support and service reliability, and the longevity of the company must be considered.

Table 20.1 Partial listing of various laser manufacturers and products

Manufacturer	Product	Modality	Wavelength (nm)	Applications
Sciton	Joule	Expandable platform		
	BroadBand Light	Broadband Light	420 515 560 590	Acne Pigmented lesions Vascular lesions
	ClearScan ALX	Alexandrite laser	755	Hair reduction, vascular lesions, pigmented lesions, rhytids
	ClearScan YAG	Nd:YAG	1,064	Hair reduction, vascular lesions, vein treatment
	Contour TRL	Er:YAG	2,940	Skin resurfacing
	ProFractional	Er:YAG	2,940	Skin resurfacing
	ProLipo PLUS	Nd:YAG	1,064 1,319	Laser lipolysis
	Pro-V	Nd:YAG	1,319	Endovenous ablative therapy
	ThermaScan	Nd:YAG	1,319	Rhytids, scarring
Ellman	Apex	IPL Er:YAG	Variable 2,940	Acne, sun damage, pigmented/vascular lesions Skin resurfacing
	Cheveux	Diode	810	Hair removal
	Cortex	CO$_2$ Er:YAG	10,600 2,940	Skin resurfacing, pigmented lesions, scars Skin resurfacing
	Medley	Q-switched Nd:YAG/ KTP IPL Er:YAG Diode	1,064/532 Variable 2,940 810	Tattoo removal, pigmented lesions (dark skin) Acne, vascular/pigmented lesions, hair removal Skin resurfacing Hair removal
	Ruby	Q-switched ruby	694	Tattoo removal, pigmented lesions
	Tri-Lase	Q-switched Nd:YAG/ KTP Er:YAG	1,064/532 2,940	Tattoo removal, pigmented lesions (dark skin) Skin resurfacing
Syneron-Candela	Alex TriVantage	Q-switched alexandrite Q-switched Nd:YAG	755 532/1,064	Tattoo removal, pigmented lesions Tattoo removal, pigmented lesions
	Co$_2$re	CO$_2$	10,600	Skin resurfacing
	GentleMax Pro	Alexandrite Nd:YAG	755 1,064	Hair removal Hair removal, vascular/pigmented lesions
	Vbeam Perfecta	Pulsed dye laser	585	Vascular/pigmented lesions
Cutera	Excel V	KTP Nd:YAG	532 1,064	Superficial vascular lesions Vascular lesions, scars, rosacea
	CoolGlide	Nd:YAG	1,064	Hair removal
	Excel	Nd:YAG	1,064	Vascular lesions
	Laser Genesis	Nd:YAG	1,064	Facial rhytids
	Pearl/Pearl Fractional/ Pearl Fusion	YSGG	2,790	Skin resurfacing
	VariLite	Diode	532/940	Vascular/pigmented lesions, cutaneous lesions
Lumenis	Multi-Spot Nd:YAG	Nd:YAG	1,064	Vascular/pigmented lesions, facial rhytids
	ResurFX	Er:Glass	1,565	Skin resurfacing
	IPL with Optimal Pulse Technology	IPL	Variable	Hair removal, vascular/pigmented lesions, skin resurfacing, facial scarring, facial rhytids

Table 20.1 continued

Manufacturer	Product	Modality	Wavelength (nm)	Applications
	LightSheer ET/DUET	Diode	800	Hair removal
	AcuPulse	CO_2	10,600	Skin resurfacing, pigmented lesions
	UltraPulse	CO_2	10,600	Skin resurfacing, facial scarring
	QX MAX	–	532/585/650/1,064	Tattoo removal, hair removal, pigmented/vascular lesions
Alma Harmony series Alma Soprano series Alma Pixel CO_2 series	AFT	Light therapy	300–950	Pigment restoration, acne clearing, vascular lesions, skin rejuvenation, hair removal
	Harmony Alex 755 nm	Alexandrite	755	Hair removal, pigmented lesions
	High Power Laser QS	Q-switched Nd:YAG	532, 1,064	Tattoo removal
	Cooled Laser 1,064 nm	Nd:YAG	1,064	Vascular lesions
	Laser 1,320 nm	Nd:YAG	1,320	Facial rhytids, acne scars
	Pixel Pro 2,940 nm	Er:YAG	2,940	Skin resurfacing
	Soprano ICE	Diode	810	Hair removal
	Pixel CO_2	CO_2	10,600	Skin resurfacing
Cynosure (formerly Palomar)	Acclaim	Nd:YAG	1,064	Hair removal, vascular lesions
	Accolade	Q-switched alexandrite	755	Pigmented lesions, tattoo removal
	Affirm	Nd:YAG	1,320, 1,440	Facial rejuvenation, pigmented lesions
	Apogee	Alexandrite	755	Hair removal, pigmented lesions
	Apogee +	Alexandrite	755	Hair removal, pigmented lesions
	Cynergy	Pulsed dye laser, Nd:YAG	585, 1,064	Vascular lesions
	Elite	Alexandrite, Nd:YAG	755, 1,064	Pigmented lesions, hair removal, vascular lesions
	Elite MPX	Alexandrite, Nd:YAG	755, 1,064	Hair removal, pigmented lesions, vascular lesions, photodamage, facial rhytids
	Elite +	Alexandrite, Nd:YAG	755, 1,064	Hair removal, vascular lesions, pigmented lesions, facial rhytids
	MedLite C6	Q-switched Nd:YAG	532, 1,064	Tattoo removal
	PicoSure	Alexandrite	755	Tattoo removal, pigmented lesions
	Precision Tx	Nd:YAG	1,440	Facial/body sculpting
	RevLite SI	Q-switched Nd:YAG	532, 1,064	Skin resurfacing, tattoo removal, facial rhytids, pigmented lesions
	SmartSkin	CO_2	10,600	Skin resurfacing
	Vectus	Sapphire	800	Hair removal
Fraxel	Fraxel re:pair	CO_2 fractional	10,600	Skin resurfacing, facial rhytids, pigmented lesions, vascular lesions
	Dual 1,550/1,927 nm	Erbium/Thulium	1,550/1,927	Skin resurfacing, facial rhytids, facial scarring, pigmented lesions/dyschromias

Abbreviations: CO_2, carbon dioxide; Er:YAG, erbium:yttrium aluminum garnet; Er:YSGG, erbium:yttrium scandium gallium garnet; IPL, intense pulsed light; KTP, potassium titanyl phosphate; Nd:YAG, neodymium:yttrium aluminum garnet; QS, Q-switched.
Note: This table shows a partial listing of the variety and multitude of laser products. It is not all-inclusive of products or manufacturers.

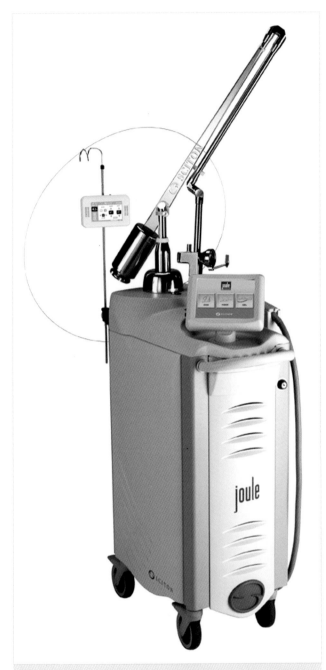

Fig. 20.6 The Sciton Joule. (Courtesy of Sciton, Palo Alto, California.)

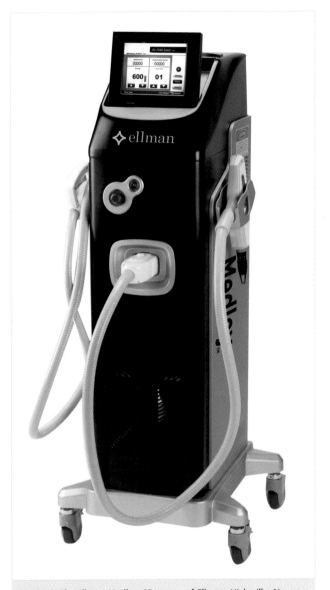

Fig. 20.7 The Ellman Medley. (Courtesy of Ellman, Hicksville, New York.)

If, after these steps, it is decided that one should consider a laser purchase to manage a particular clinical condition or group of clinical conditions, one must then explore the financial issues. The laser-related revenue should be sufficient to offset the laser-related expenses within an acceptable period of time. Although some technology purchases might be acceptable loss leaders to generate traffic into the practice from which other revenue sources might be derived, it is most desirable that the lease or purchase of technologies and equipment produce a positive financial outcome.

The financial burden of the lease or purchase of a laser has several components, some obvious up front, some not. In considering the financial investment or expense of the laser, one has to take into account the laser purchase price, any cost of leasing or servicing a loan, service contracts, maintenance costs, storage and transportation costs, if necessary, and the cost of any disposables necessary for treatment. One also must be aware of associated costs, such as cabinetry for storage of supplies, and any ancillary equipment used with the laser, such as cooling devices. When all of these expenses are weighed, one must create a pro forma based on anticipated charges, procedure volume, and expenses. An important consideration at this point is the physician opportunity cost of doing laser treatments relative to other revenue-generating procedures, as well as the potential increased revenue if one practices in a state that allows nonmedical practitioners to use lasers. Ideally, the break-even point should occur within 2 years of a laser purchase.[87] Beyond this time frame, there is a risk that technology changes might make the equipment obsolete, with more attractive and competitive products in the community. This financial

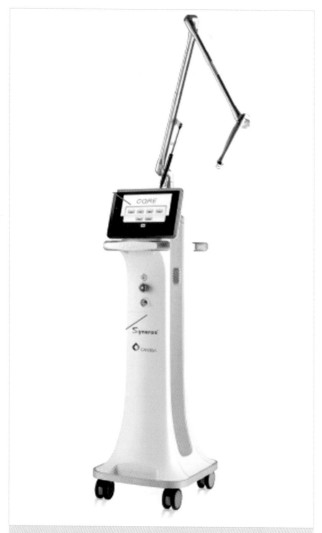

Fig. 20.8 The Syneron Co₂re. (Courtesy of Syneron Medical Ltd., Yokneam, Israel.)

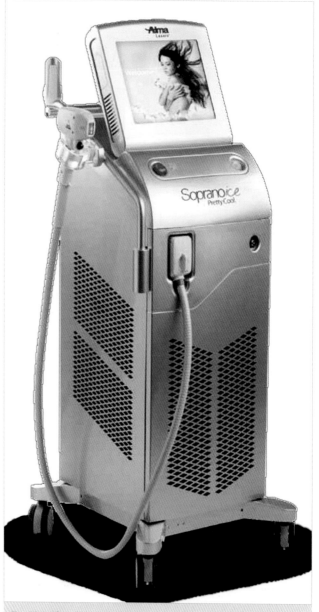

Fig. 20.9 The Alma Soprano. (Courtesy of Alma Lasers, Buffalo Grove, Illinois.)

analysis is something that should be carried out with each equipment purchase or practice-asset acquisition.[88]

20.11 The Survey

To assess the laser technologies that active practices have found useful, a survey was conducted with members of the American Academy of Facial Plastic and Reconstructive Surgery.[89] Members were polled using an online 5-question survey to evaluate preferences regarding laser purchases and uses. The 100 respondents reported that the lasers they purchased most commonly included fractionated CO_2 (46%), ablative CO_2 (31%), Nd:YAG (27%), and Er:YAG (25%). Many members owned more than one laser. The lasers most frequently used via lease agreement were fractionated CO_2 and ablative CO_2 (25 and 21%, respectively). When queried regarding the laser they would like to have access to, 47% responded that they would like access to a fractionated CO_2 laser, with 29% citing a pulsed dye laser. The laser used most commonly was the fractionated CO_2 (31%), followed by the ablative CO_2 (13%). Members advised that physicians starting a new practice acquire a fractionated CO_2 laser (63%), a pulsed dye laser (17%), and an Er:YAG laser (15%) (▶ Fig. 20.10).

20.12 Conclusion

The acquisition of laser technologies for a facial plastic surgery practice is one of the more important decisions to be made in starting and maintaining a practice. Whether or not to purchase a laser is a question that should be based on the practice profile, the demographics of the practice, the practitioner skill-set, and the desire to treat a particular spectrum of clinical issues. The decision-making process should include a well-thought-out

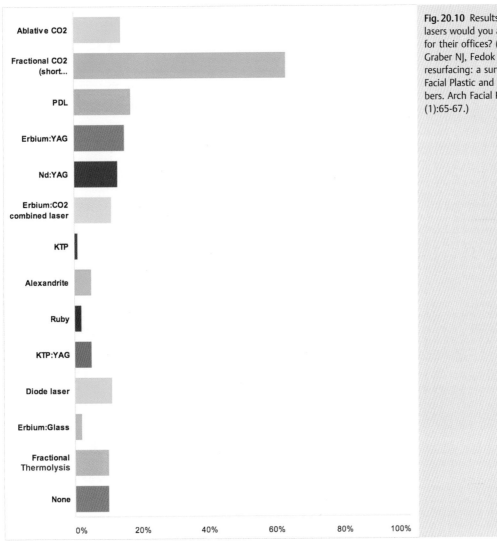

Fig. 20.10 Results of survey question: What lasers would you advise new physicians to obtain for their offices? (Data from Park SS, Khalid AN, Graber NJ, Fedok FG. Current trends in facial resurfacing: a survey of American Academy of Facial Plastic and Reconstructive Surgery members. Arch Facial Plast Surg. 2010 Jan-Feb;12 (1):65-67.)

assessment of the return on investment of acquiring the technology. There is a variety of manufacturers' products available to choose from, and most are credible and sound. Various resurfacing technologies continue to be among the most popular technologies sought after in facial plastic surgery practices.

Among the respondents in current practices, it was found that those products most acquired for practices included fractionated resurfacing technologies, hair-removal lasers, and lasers to treat vascular lesions. Although not a part of the survey because it is not a laser technology, the authors would also remark that IPL technologies are frequently cited by facial plastic surgery practices as attractive technologies for purchase.

References

[1] Kligman LH. Photoaging. Manifestations, prevention, and treatment. Dermatol Clin 1986; 4: 517–528

[2] Tierney EP, Hanke CW. Review of the literature: treatment of dyspigmentation with fractionated resurfacing. Dermatol Surg 2010; 36: 1499–1508

[3] Fitzpatrick TB. The validity and practicality of sun-reactive skin types I through VI. Arch Dermatol 1988; 124: 869–871

[4] Fedok FG, Garritano F, Portela A. Cutaneous lasers. Facial Plast Surg Clin North Am 2013; 21: 95–110

[5] Alster TS, Kauvar AN, Geronemus RG. Histology of high-energy pulsed CO2 laser resurfacing. Semin Cutan Med Surg 1996; 15: 189–193

[6] Alster T, Hirsch R. Single-pass CO2 laser skin resurfacing of light and dark skin: extended experience with 52 patients. J Cosmet Laser Ther 2003; 5: 39–42

[7] Fitzpatrick RE, Goldman MP, Satur NM, Tope WD. Pulsed carbon dioxide laser resurfacing of photo-aged facial skin. Arch Dermatol 1996; 132: 395–402

[8] Goldman MP. CO2 laser resurfacing of the face and neck. Facial Plast Surg Clin North Am 2001; 9: 283–290, ix

[9] Fitzpatrick RE. Laser resurfacing of rhytides. Dermatol Clin 1997; 15: 431–447

[10] Fitzpatrick RE. CO2 laser resurfacing. Dermatol Clin 2001; 19: 443–451, viii

[11] David LM, Sarne AJ, Unger WP. Rapid laser scanning for facial resurfacing. Dermatol Surg 1995; 21: 1031–1033

[12] Lowe NJ, Lask G, Griffin ME, Maxwell A, Lowe P, Quilada F. Skin resurfacing with the UltraPulse carbon dioxide laser. Observations on 100 patients. Dermatol Surg 1995; 21: 1025–1029

[13] Alster TS, West TB. Resurfacing of atrophic facial acne scars with a high-energy, pulsed carbon dioxide laser. Dermatol Surg 1996; 22: 151–154, discussion 154–155

[14] Goldman MP. Observations on the use of fractionated CO2 laser resurfacing. J Drugs Dermatol 2009; 8: 82–86

[15] Hunzeker CM, Weiss ET, Geronemus RG. Fractionated CO2 laser resurfacing: our experience with more than 2000 treatments. Aesthet Surg J 2009; 29: 317–322

[16] Tierney EP, Eisen RF, Hanke CW. Fractionated CO2 laser skin rejuvenation. Dermatol Ther 2011; 24: 41–53

[17] Alster TS, Lupton JR. Erbium:YAG cutaneous laser resurfacing. Dermatol Clin 2001; 19: 453–466

[18] Bass LS. Erbium:YAG laser skin resurfacing: preliminary clinical evaluation. Ann Plast Surg 1998; 40: 328–334

[19] David LM. Erbium vs CO2 in laser resurfacing: the debate continues. J Cutan Laser Ther 1999; 1: 185–189

[20] Goldberg DJ. Erbium:YAG laser resurfacing: what is its role? Aesthet Surg J 1998; 18: 255–260

[21] Goldman MP. Techniques for erbium:YAG laser skin resurfacing: initial pearls from the first 100 patients. Dermatol Surg 1997; 23: 1219–1221

[22] Weiss RA, Harrington AC, Pfau RC, Weiss MA, Marwaha S. Periorbital skin resurfacing using high energy erbium:YAG laser: results in 50 patients. Lasers Surg Med 1999; 24: 81–86

[23] Ross EV, Naseef GS, McKinlay JR, et al. Comparison of carbon dioxide laser, erbium:YAG laser, dermabrasion, and dermatome: a study of thermal damage, wound contraction, and wound healing in a live pig model: implications for skin resurfacing. J Am Acad Dermatol 2000; 42: 92–105

[24] Shori RK, Walston AA, Stafsudd OM, et al. Quantification and modeling of the dynamic changes in the absorption coefficient of water at 2.94 um. IEEE 2001; 7: 959–970

[25] Cohen JL, Babcock MJ. Ablative fractionated erbium:YAG laser for the treatment of ice pick alar scars due to neodymium:YAG laser burns. J Drugs Dermatol 2009; 8: 65–67

[26] Newman JB, Lord JL, Ash K, McDaniel DH. Variable pulse erbium:YAG laser skin resurfacing of perioral rhytides and side-by-side comparison with carbon dioxide laser. Lasers Surg Med 2000; 26: 208–214

[27] Tanzi EL, Wanitphakdeedecha R, Alster TS. Fraxel laser indications and long-term follow-up. Aesthet Surg J 2008; 28: 675–678, discussion 679–680

[28] Collawn SS. Fraxel skin resurfacing. Ann Plast Surg 2007; 58: 237–240

[29] Bass LS. Rejuvenation of the aging face using Fraxel laser treatment. Aesthet Surg J 2005; 25: 307–309

[30] Chiu RJ, Kridel RW. Fractionated photothermolysis: the Fraxel 1550-nm glass fiber laser treatment. Facial Plast Surg Clin North Am 2007; 15: 229–237, vii

[31] Pham AM, Greene RM, Woolery-Lloyd H, Kaufman J, Grunebaum LD. 1550-nm nonablative laser resurfacing for facial surgical scars. Arch Facial Plast Surg 2011; 13: 203–210

[32] Alam M, Dover JS. Nonablative laser and light therapy: an approach to patient and device selection. Skin Therapy Lett 2003; 8: 4–7

[33] Ang P, Barlow RJ. Nonablative laser resurfacing: a systematic review of the literature. Clin Exp Dermatol 2002; 27: 630–635

[34] Carniol PJ, Farley S, Friedman A. Long-pulse 532-nm diode laser for nonablative facial skin rejuvenation. Arch Facial Plast Surg 2003; 5: 511–513

[35] Chua SH, Ang P, Khoo LS, Goh CL. Nonablative 1450-nm diode laser in the treatment of facial atrophic acne scars in type IV to V Asian skin: a prospective clinical study. Dermatol Surg 2004; 30: 1287–1291

[36] Doshi SN, Alster TS. 1,450 nm long-pulsed diode laser for nonablative skin rejuvenation. Dermatol Surg 2005; 31: 1223–1226, discussion 1226

[37] Fulchiero GJ, Jr, Parham-Vetter PC, Obagi S. Subcision and 1320-nm Nd:YAG nonablative laser resurfacing for the treatment of acne scars: a simultaneous split-face single patient trial. Dermatol Surg 2004; 30: 1356–1359, discussion 1360

[38] Bernstein EF. Laser tattoo removal. Semin Plast Surg 2007; 21: 175–192

[39] Wenzel SM. Current concepts in laser tattoo removal. Skin Therapy Lett 2010; 15: 3–5

[40] Kent KM, Graber EM. Laser tattoo removal: a review. Dermatol Surg 2012; 38: 1–13

[41] Anderson RR, Margolis RJ, Watenabe S, Flotte T, Hruza GJ, Dover JS. Selective photothermolysis of cutaneous pigmentation by Q-switched Nd:YAG laser pulses at 1064, 532, and 355 nm. J Invest Dermatol 1989; 93: 28–32

[42] Kim YJ, Whang KU, Choi WB, et al. Efficacy and safety of 1,064 nm Q-switched Nd:YAG laser treatment for removing melanocytic nevi. Ann Dermatol 2012; 24: 162–167

[43] DePadova-Elder SM, Milgraum SS. Q-switched ruby laser treatment of labial lentigines in Peutz-Jeghers syndrome. J Dermatol Surg Oncol 1994; 20: 830–832

[44] Kono T, Chan HH, Groff WF, et al. Long-pulse pulsed dye laser delivered with compression for treatment of facial lentigines. Dermatol Surg 2007; 33: 945–950

[45] Bassichis BA, Swamy R, Dayan SH. Use of the KTP laser in the treatment of rosacea and solar lentigines. Facial Plast Surg 2004; 20: 77–83

[46] Li YT, Yang KC. Comparison of the frequency-doubled Q-switched Nd:YAG laser and 35% trichloroacetic acid for the treatment of face lentigines. Dermatol Surg 1999; 25: 202–204

[47] Fitzpatrick RE, Goldman MP, Ruiz-Esparza J. Clinical advantage of the CO2 laser superpulsed mode. Treatment of verruca vulgaris, seborrheic keratoses, lentigines, and actinic cheilitis. J Dermatol Surg Oncol 1994; 20: 449–456

[48] Pfeiffer N. Q-switched ruby laser brings scarless tattoo removal. J Clin Laser Med Surg 1990; 8: 10–13

[49] Watts MT, Downes RN, Collin JR, Walker NP. The use of Q-switched Nd:Yag laser for removal of permanent eyeliner tattoo. Ophthal Plast Reconstr Surg 1992; 8: 292–294

[50] Wheeland RG. Tattoo removal using the ruby laser. West J Med 1992; 156: 190

[51] Fitzpatrick RE, Goldman MP, Ruiz-Esparza J. Use of the alexandrite laser (755 nm, 100 nsec) for tattoo pigment removal in an animal model. J Am Acad Dermatol 1993; 28: 745–750

[52] Adrian RM, Griffin L. Laser tattoo removal. Clin Plast Surg 2000; 27: 181–192

[53] Barčot Z, Zupančić B. Pulsed dye laser treatment of vascular lesions in childhood. Acta Dermatovenerol Croat 2010; 18: 201–208

[54] Dias Coelho J, Serrão V. Treatment of vascular lesions of the tongue with Nd:YAG laser. Case Rep Med 2009; 1–2

[55] Cole PD, Sonabend ML, Levy ML. Laser treatment of pediatric vascular lesions. Semin Plast Surg 2007; 21: 159–166

[56] Railan D, Parlette EC, Uebelhoer NS, Rohrer TE. Laser treatment of vascular lesions. Clin Dermatol 2006; 24: 8–15

[57] Rothfleisch JE, Kosann MK, Levine VJ, Ashinoff R. Laser treatment of congenital and acquired vascular lesions. A review. Dermatol Clin 2002; 20: 1–18

[58] Goldberg DJ. Laser treatment of vascular lesions. Clin Plast Surg 2000; 27: 173–180, ix

[59] Ross BS, Levine VJ, Ashinoff R. Laser treatment of acquired vascular lesions. Dermatol Clin 1997; 15: 385–396

[60] McKeown A. Pulsed-dye laser treatment of vascular lesions. Dermatol Nurs 1991; 3: 330–334

[61] Bernstein EF, Kligman A. Rosacea treatment using the new-generation, high-energy, 595 nm, long pulse-duration pulsed-dye laser. Lasers Surg Med 2008; 40: 233–239

[62] Bernstein EF, Kornbluth S, Brown DB, Black J. Treatment of spider veins using a 10 millisecond pulse-duration frequency-doubled neodymium YAG laser. Dermatol Surg 1999; 25: 316–320

[63] Bernstein EF, Lee J, Lowery J, et al. Treatment of spider veins with the 595 nm pulsed-dye laser. J Am Acad Dermatol 1998; 39: 746–750

[64] Choi YS, Suh HS, Yoon MY, Min SU, Lee DH, Suh DH. Intense pulsed light vs. pulsed-dye laser in the treatment of facial acne: a randomized split-face trial. J Eur Acad Dermatol Venereol 2010; 24: 773–780

[65] Cordoro KM, Frieden IJ. Pulsed dye laser for port wine stains. J Am Acad Dermatol 2010; 62: 1065–1066

[66] Eremia S, Li CY. Treatment of leg and face veins with a cryogen spray variable pulse width 1064-nm Nd:YAG laser—a prospective study of 47 patients. J Cosmet Laser Ther 2001; 3: 147–153

[67] Rogachefsky AS, Silapunt S, Goldberg DJ. Nd:YAG laser (1064 nm) irradiation for lower extremity telangiectases and small reticular veins: efficacy as measured by vessel color and size. Dermatol Surg 2002; 28: 220–223

[68] Omura NE, Dover JS, Arndt KA, Kauvar AN. Treatment of reticular leg veins with a 1064 nm long-pulsed Nd:YAG laser. J Am Acad Dermatol 2003; 48: 76–81

[69] Craig LM, Alster TS. Vascular skin lesions in children: a review of laser surgical and medical treatments. Dermatol Surg 2013; 39: 1137–1146

[70] Chapas AM, Eickhorst K, Geronemus RG. Efficacy of early treatment of facial port wine stains in newborns: a review of 49 cases. Lasers Surg Med 2007; 39: 563–568

[71] Li L, Kono T, Groff WF, Chan HH, Kitazawa Y, Nozaki M. Comparison study of a long-pulse pulsed dye laser and a long-pulse pulsed alexandrite laser in the treatment of port wine stains. J Cosmet Laser Ther 2008; 10: 12–15

[72] Alster TS, Tanzi EL. Combined 595-nm and 1,064-nm laser irradiation of recalcitrant and hypertrophic port-wine stains in children and adults. Dermatol Surg 2009; 35: 914–918, discussion 918–919

[73] Tanghetti EA. Split-face randomized treatment of facial telangiectasia comparing pulsed dye laser and an intense pulsed light handpiece. Lasers Surg Med 2012; 44: 97–102

[74] Dierickx CC, Grossman MC, Farinelli WA, Anderson RR. Permanent hair removal by normal-mode ruby laser. Arch Dermatol 1998; 134: 837–842

[75] McDaniel DH, Lord J, Ash K, Newman J, Zukowski M. Laser hair removal: a review and report on the use of the long-pulsed alexandrite laser for hair reduction of the upper lip, leg, back, and bikini region. Dermatol Surg 1999; 25: 425–430

[76] Lorenz S, Brunnberg S, Landthaler M, Hohenleutner U. Hair removal with the long pulsed Nd:YAG laser: a prospective study with one year follow-up. Lasers Surg Med 2002; 30: 127–134

[77] Dierickx CC. Hair removal by lasers and intense pulsed light sources. Dermatol Clin 2002; 20: 135–146

[78] Handrick C, Alster TS. Comparison of long-pulsed diode and long-pulsed alexandrite lasers for hair removal: a long-term clinical and histologic study. Dermatol Surg 2001; 27: 622–626

[79] Campos VB, Dierickx CC, Farinelli WA, Lin TY, Manuskiatti W, Anderson RR. Hair removal with an 800-nm pulsed diode laser. J Am Acad Dermatol 2000; 43: 442–447

[80] Ciocon DH, Boker A, Goldberg DJ. Intense pulsed light: what works, what's new, what's next. Facial Plast Surg 2009; 25: 290–300

[81] Babilas P, Schreml S, Szeimies RM, Landthaler M. Intense pulsed light (IPL): a review. Lasers Surg Med 2010; 42: 93–104

[82] Bjerring P, Cramers M, Egekvist H, Christiansen K, Troilius A. Hair reduction using a new intense pulsed light irradiator and a normal mode ruby laser. J Cutan Laser Ther 2000; 2: 63–71

[83] Alster T. Laser scar revision: comparison study of 585-nm pulsed dye laser with and without intralesional corticosteroids. Dermatol Surg 2003; 29: 25–29

[84] Alexiades-Armenakas MR, Dover JS, Arndt KA. The spectrum of laser skin resurfacing: nonablative, fractional, and ablative laser resurfacing. J Am Acad Dermatol 2008; 58: 719–737, quiz 738–740

[85] Alster T, Zaulyanov L. Laser scar revision: a review. Dermatol Surg 2007; 33: 131–140

[86] Goldman MP. One laser for a cosmetic/dermatologic practice. J Clin Aesthet Dermatol 2011; 4: 18–21

[87] Fabi SG, Metelitsa AI. Future directions in cutaneous laser surgery. Dermatol Clin 2014; 32: 61–69

[88] Jutkowitz E, Carniol PJ, Carniol AR. Financial analysis of technology acquisition using fractionated lasers as a model. Facial Plast Surg 2010; 26: 289–295

[89] Park SS, Khalid AN, Graber NJ, Fedok FG. Current trends in facial resurfacing: a survey of American Academy of Facial Plastic and Reconstructive Surgery members. Arch Facial Plast Surg. 2010 Jan-Feb;12(1):65-67

21 Light Therapy for Aging Facial Skin: Intense Pulsed Light and Infrared Broadband Light

Macrene Alexiades

21.1 Introduction

The clinical signs of aging of the facial skin include rhytids, laxity, and the various aspects of photoaging, including dyspigmentation, erythema/telangiectasia (E/T), solar elastosis, keratosis, and poor texture (▶ Table 21.1).[1,2,3] Over the past several decades, lasers and light-based technologies have been specialized to treat the various categories of skin aging.[1]

Technological advancements have increased not only safety and efficacy but also selectivity. Whereas some devices primarily treat photoaging, others specifically target skin laxity. Among the light-based technologies, intense pulsed light (IPL) has become a well-established form of treatment for photoaging, which includes dyspigmentation, vascularity, solar elastosis, poor texture, and to a lesser degree, rhytids (▶ Table 21.1).[1,2,3,4] Conversely, broadband light in the infrared range has proven to

Table 21.1 Quantitative comprehensive grading scale of rhytids, laxity, and photoaging

Grading scale	Descriptive parameters	Categories of skin aging and photodamage						
		Rhytids	Laxity	Elastosis	Dyschromia	Erythema/Telangiectasia (E/T)	Keratoses	Texture
0.00	None	None	None	None	None	None	None	None
1.00	Mild	Wrinkles in motion, few, superficial	Localized to nasolabial folds (NLFs)	Early, minimal yellow hue	Few (1–3) discrete small (<5 mm) lentigines	Pink E or few T, localized to single site	Few	Subtle irregularity
1.50	mild	Wrinkles in motion, multiple, superficial	Localized, NLFs and early melolabial folds (MLFs)	Yellow hue or early, localized periorbital (PO) elastotic beads (EBs)	Several (3–6), discrete small lentigines	Pink E or several T localized two sites	Several	Mild irregularity in few areas
2.00	Moderate	Wrinkles at rest, few, localized, superficial	Localized, NLFs/MLFs, early jowls, early submental/submandibular (SM)	Yellow hue, localized PO EBs	Multiple (7–10), small lentigines	Red E or multiple T localized to two sites	Multiple, small	Rough in few, localized sites
2.50	Moderate	Wrinkles at rest, multiple, localized, superficial	Localized, prominent NLFs/MLFs, jowls, and SM	Yellow hue, PO and malar EBs	Multiple, small and few large lentigines	Red E or multiple T, localized to three sites	Multiple, large	Rough in several, localized areas
3.00	Advanced	Wrinkles at rest, multiple, forehead, PO and perioral sites, superficial	Prominent NLFs/MLFs, jowls and SM, early neck strands	Yellow hue, EBs involving PO, malar and other sites	Many (10–20) small and large lentigines	Violaceous E or many T, multiple sites	Many	Rough in multiple, localized sites
3.50	Advanced	Wrinkles at rest, multiple, generalized, superficial; few, deep	Deep NLFs/MLFs, prominent jowls and SM, prominent neck strands	Deep yellow hue, extensive EBs with little uninvolved skin	Numerous (>20) or multiple large with little uninvolved skin	Violaceous E, numerous T with little uninvolved skin	Little uninvolved skin	Mostly rough, little uninvolved skin
4.00	Severe	Wrinkles throughout, numerous, extensively distributed, deep	Marked NLFs/MLFs, jowls and SM, neck redundancy and strands	Deep yellow hue, EBs throughout, comedones	Numerous, extensive, no uninvolved skin	Deep, violaceous E, numerous T throughout	No uninvolved skin	Rough throughout

Note: This 4-point grading scale, created by the author of this chapter, has been extensively tested and employed for evaluating laser and energy-based cosmetic treatments.[1,2,3,5,6,24,56]

be an effective treatment selectively targeting skin laxity and rhytids.[5,6] Although IPL and broadband infrared (BBIR) light are less effective than standard ablative laser resurfacing and plastic surgery, respectively, their extremely favorable side-effect profile and immediate recovery and acceptable efficacy have generated high clinical demand among patients.

Clinical improvement of facial rhytids following laser treatment was initially observed when treating other aspects of photoaging.[7,8,9,10,11,12] This finding led to histological and clinical confirmation of neocollagenesis and rhytid reduction following treatment with lasers in the visible, near-infrared, and midinfrared spectrums.[7,8,9,10,11,12] Among the early lasers and light sources, the potassium titanyl phosphate (KTP) laser (532 nm), pulsed dye laser (PDL) (585 and 595 nm), IPL (515–1,200 nm), neodymium:yttrium aluminum garnet (Nd:YAG) (1,064-nm Q-switched, 1,064-nm long pulse, 1,319, and 1,320 nm), diode (980 and 1,450 nm), and erbium glass (Er:glass) (1,540 nm) all demonstrated some degree of efficacy for facial nonablative resurfacing. However, midinfrared devices, owing to deeper penetration of longer wavelengths and lower absorption by epidermal melanin, were the most effective for deeper rhytids and acne scarring after a series of treatments.[10,13,14,15,16,17,18,19,20,21,22,23,24] These findings were followed by the development of BBIR devices, which have delivered significant reductions in rhytids and skin laxity of the face and neck, and a histological correlation of both neocollagenesis and neoelastogenesis.[5,25,26,27,28] In contrast, IPL established itself as a mainstay for the treatment of all categories of photoaging, most notably vascularity and dyspigmentation, and to a lesser degree, rhytids.[4,29,30,31,32,33,34] The histological and ultrastructural effects of IPL include neocollagenesis, and effects on dermal fibroblasts, resulting in induction of collagen, matrix metalloproteinases (MMPs), and transforming growth factor (TGF) gene expression.[4,30,32]

21.2 Intense Pulsed Light

21.2.1 Background

The application of IPL (ranging between 500–1,300 nm) for the treatment of skin aging has proven to be a first-line procedure for the reduction of the signs of photoaging and, to a lesser degree, rhytids.[1,2,3,33] The advantage of IPL is its ability to target both melanin and hemoglobin, resulting in global improvement in dyspigmentation and vascularity. The term *photorejuvenation* was coined in describing the global improvement in multiple parameters of photoaging that is observed with the IPL.[29,31,35,36] Filters may be placed to exclude shorter wavelengths, thereby preferentially targeting various chromophores. Its use for wrinkle reduction has been assessed with evidence of multiple histological changes after treatment.[1,4,30,32] The patient perception of improvement is increased likely due to apparent decreases in dyspigmentation and vascularity, which are more easily detectable than mild changes in rhytids, therefore placing this device in the mainstream of nonablative resurfacing.

21.2.2 Patient Selection: Indications and Contraindications

The ideal patient for treatment with IPL is one who exhibits the signs of photoaging, namely dyspigmentation, vascularity, and mild-to-moderate rhytids of the facial skin (▶ Table 21.1). On physical examination, lentigines and telangiectasias should be present. In addition, fine rhytids and, to a lesser degree, coarse rhytids may respond but this varies from patient to patient. IPL is the treatment of choice for light-skinned patients with photoaging who present at any age with pigment, vascularity, and/or concomitant rhytids. This modality is appropriate for younger patients in their third to fourth decade who manifest early signs of photoaging and fine rhytids, and for whom standard ablative resurfacing may be considered too aggressive. Owing to the lack of thermal injury, patients may receive multiple treatments over the course of many years without developing the textural changes that may be a complication of repeated procedures with fractional laser resurfacing. Therefore it may be recommended in a series, followed by yearly maintenance treatment sessions.

Patients less likely to respond to IPL are those lacking the features of photoaging (▶ Table 21.1). Patients lacking dyspigmentation or vascularity will unlikely be able to appreciate the benefits of IPL. Those presenting primarily with advanced-to-severe rhytids and/or laxity (▶ Table 21.1) are not appropriate candidates for IPL because this device has little-to-no efficacy in the treatment of skin laxity, such as jowels or folds, and limited efficacy on rhytids of an advanced severity. Additionally, patients with more advanced grades 3 to 4 rhytids (▶ Table 21.1) are better candidates for standard or fractional ablative laser resurfacing than IPL, and are less likely to attain appreciable improvement in their rhytids through IPL alone. Those whose primary concern is skin laxity are better candidates for BBIR, other skin tightening technologies, or the surgical facelift. The range of procedure options must be presented at time of consultation.

Contraindications for treatment include: pregnancy, breastfeeding, history of isotretinoin use in the preceding 6 months, keloids, connective tissue disease, or a history of adverse events following IPL. Patients with a history of frequent, recurrent *Herpes simplex* and/or *Staphylococcal* infections should be premedicated with antimicrobial antibiotics such as famciclovir or dicloxacillin, respectively. Tanned or dark-skinned (Fitzpatrick skin type IV or V) patients should be treated only by a highly experienced clinician and with very conservative settings. Alternatively, tanned and/or darkly pigmented skin should be considered relative contraindications. Skin type VI patients are contraindicated because the vast majority of IPL technologies do not provide settings to safely treat such darkly pigmented skin.

Pearls and Pitfalls

The ideal IPL patient presents with the findings of photoaging, manifested by lentigines and telangiectasias (▶ Table 21.1). Proper patient selection will ensure high patient satisfaction.

21.3 Advantages and Disadvantages

The advantages of IPL include the nonablative aspect of the treatment, the absence of perioperative discomfort, and the immediacy of posttreatment recovery. No anesthesia is

Table 21.2 Representative parameters for IPL devices

IPL device	Manufacturer	Spectral output (nm; filtered)	Pulse duration (ms)	Fluence (J/cm²)	Spot size (mm)
Harmony	Alma	420–950	3–50	1–30	40 × 16 30 × 10
Skinstation	Radiancy	400–1,200	10	3–7	36 × 12
Aurora	Syneron	580–980	20–200	10–30	12 × 25
BBL	Sciton	560–1,400	Up to 200	1–40	16 × 46
Xeo	Cutera	500–1,100	Automatic	3–35	10 × 30
PhotoLight	Cynosure	400–1,200	5–80	3–30	46 × 10
StarLux	Cynosure (formerly Palomar)	500–1,200	0.5–600	Up to 50	12 × 12

Abbreviations: BBL, broadband light; IPL, intense pulsed light.
Note: The standard photorejuvenation settings for several IPL devices are shown.

necessary because the treatment is typically painless or associated with minimal discomfort. Immediately following the procedure, the skin may appear slightly erythematous; however, this resolves within minutes. No erythema, blistering, wounding, or obvious crusting should be observed posttreatment, obviating any need for wound care. For these reasons, IPL is considered a "no downtime" process, with patients returning to normal activities immediately following treatment. The other key advantages are the visible improvements that are appreciated by the patient within weeks and engender a high degree of patient satisfaction.

The disadvantages of IPL include the need for multiple treatments, the subtlety of reduction to rhytids, the incompleteness of removal of dyspigmentation/vascularity, and the risk of adverse events. In years past, IPL instruments typically required five to six monthly treatments in order to achieve appreciable results. However, recent technological advancements have boosted treatment efficacy, resulting in shorter required treatment cycles of three monthly sessions. Despite a relatively high level of efficacy in the treatment of photoaging (see section 21.4.3), complete clearance of all lentigines and telangiectasias is unlikely. This must be made clear to the patient at the outset. In addition, IPL is less effective on rhytids, with minimal improvement expected. Another important disadvantage of IPL is the unpredictability of adverse events in certain skin types. For example, patients with actinic bronzing, or excessively photoaged skin on sun-exposed areas, may develop crusting throughout the sun-damaged areas of the skin following a session at conservative settings. Similarly, patients who tan between sessions and do not report this to the clinician may crust following treatment despite relatively low settings. Unexpected crusting typically heals with areas of temporarily decreased pigment levels as compared to surrounding bronzed or tanned skin, causing an uneven color complexion to the skin. This adverse event typically resolves over time without scarring; however, it is very disconcerting to the patient and clinician and must be treated promptly. In the event of crusting, topical corticosteroid and/or silver sulfasalazine ointment and close follow-up should be prescribed. In light of such adverse events, IPL—often given to a physician-extender to perform—can be unpredictable and requires a great deal of oversight and experience.

21.3.1 Pearls and Pitfalls

Always review history and technique settings on every patient prior to treating with IPL. If the patient has had sun exposure in the preceding 6 weeks, decrease the power or energy output on the mechanism or defer treatment until the tan has faded to avoid the pitfall of unexpected crusting posttreatment.

21.4 Preoperative Instructions

Instruct patients to avoid sun exposure prior to and between treatment sessions. Sessions should not be scheduled if the patient has had extensive sun exposure or tanning in the preceding 6 weeks. Patients should immediately report to the clinician performing the procedure any incidence of discomfort during the session and any crusting posttreatment. Patients should be instructed that lentigines form superficial crusts and flake off within 4 to 7 days. Therefore, the patient should not schedule any important social events within 1 week to 10 days following a procedure. Anesthesia is unnecessary for IPL. Premedication with antimicrobials is also unnecessary, except in the aforementioned instances (see section 21.2.2).

21.4.1 Treatment Protocol

Each IPL tool will have different cutoff filters for various applications (▶ Table 21.2). Make certain that the photorejuvenation filter is employed. This typically provides a cutoff at or approximately 500 to 560 nm depending upon the technology. The upper wavelength output on IPL instruments is typically around 1,200 nm. Each device provides guidelines for power or energy output and pulse duration for each skin type. The highest starting fluences and the shortest pulse durations are employed on lighter skin types. Darker skin types and tanned skin require lower fluences and longer pulse durations to avoid thermally heating the melanosomes in the epidermis. See ▸ Table 21.2 for the recommended settings on several IPL devices on the market.

Aqueous gel is applied to the skin surface. Initially, a few test pulses should be performed. Ask patients if they feel any discomfort. The pulse may cause a pinching or fleeting smarting, but should not feel hot or burning. Importantly, a patient's skin should not feel a burning sensation after the pulse has concluded. If this is the case, lower the fluence and lengthen the pulse duration. Pulses are administered in rows across the forehead, followed by each cheek. Great care is taken to ensure that ample aqueous gel is applied so that the IPL handpiece tip makes full contact with the gel and skin. Pulses are administered in passes across each anatomical area. Additional care is taken around the nose to provide a great deal of aqueous gel such that full contact of the laser tip is made. Typically, two to three full-face passes are administered per treatment. The author has found it helpful to administer extra pulses to darker lentigines in order to achieve adequate clinical response. Immediately following a procedure, lentigines should appear to have a slightly erythematous ring surrounding them and slight edema; these findings correlate with their eventual crusting and desquamation.

21.4.2 Postoperative Care/Preventing and Managing Adverse Events

Immediately following treatment, minimal transient erythema is present. The patient should be given an instruction sheet detailing what to expect. Although lentigines will form crusts over the ensuing days and peel off, the remaining skin should not blister or scab. Patients should be told to notify the office immediately if blistering or crusting occurs. If there is vesiculation or crusting following the procedure, wound-care management should be implemented as soon as possible. The patient should be prescribed a silver preparation such as silver sulfasalazine and a topical corticosteroid such as fluocinolone acetonide 0.025% ointment to be applied twice daily. In the case of swelling, edema, or hiving, antihistamine should also be prescribed. Immediately upon identifying vesiculation, prolonged erythema, or thermal burns, ice-cold compresses should be applied for approximately 1 to 3 hours. Following this time period, prolongation of the cold compresses is of diminishing returns. At this point, attention should be turned to topical therapy. It is prudent to bring the patient back to the office the following day to monitor progress and to assist in wound care. Typically, if wound-care instructions are followed, the crusts heal with a transient period of relative hypopigmentation as compared to the surrounding photoaged skin; however, they eventually heal with even pigmentation upon further treatment. In darker skin types, postinflammatory hyperpigmentation may be observed; this eventually resolves without treatment over the course of several months. Topical antipigment agents such as glycolic acid or hydroquinone may speed its resolution. Should irregularity of pigment occur posttreatment, additional IPL treatments serve to even out the pigmentation.

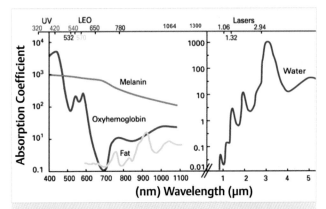

Fig. 21.1 Absorption curves of chromophores in human skin: melanin, hemoglobin, and tissue water. The wavelengths emitted by intense pulsed light (IPL), ranging between 500 and 1,200 nm, are strongly absorbed by melanin and hemoglobin as shown by their absorption curves, resulting in improvements in dyspigmentation and vascularity (left-hand curve). In addition, the near-infrared wavelengths are absorbed by tissue water, which likely accounts for the dermal remodeling that is observed. Broadband infrared (BBIR) light (1,100–1,800 nm) wavelengths, which are more deeply penetrating, are strongly absorbed by tissue water, which accounts for their ability to achieve deep dermal heating and resulting improvements in skin rhytids and laxity (right-hand curve). (Courtesy of Alma Lasers, Caesarea, Israel.)

21.4.3 Clinical, Histological, and Genetic Results

The broad range of wavelengths emitted from IPL devices (ranging from 500–1,300 nm) accounts for the ability of these tools to effectively target both melanin and hemoglobin in the skin (▸ Fig. 21.1).[33] The high absorption of IPL wavelengths by melanin and hemoglobin correlates with the utility of IPL for improving the dyspigmentation and vascularity that characterize photoaged skin (▸ Fig. 21.1).[34,35] As a result, the use of IPL has been consistently demonstrated to result in dramatic improvement in pigment and vascular abnormalities of photodamaged skin.[1,2,4,29,30,31,32,33,34,35,36,37] The author conducted a clinical trial of a combination IPL and radiofrequency technology for the treatment of rhytids, laxity, and photoaging in 28 subjects, employing a quantitative 4-point grading scale of skin aging (▸ Table 21.1).[2,3] In that trial, quantitative analysis demonstrated a mean 10.9% grade reduction per treatment across all categories of skin aging, and a mean 25% grade reduction across all categories of skin aging following an average of 2.4 treatments.[2] Another clinical study calculated high but incomplete clearance rates of lentigines and telangiectasias ranging from 62.5 to 82% following three monthly treatments.[37] Significant descriptive improvements in lentigines have been demonstrated in Caucasian[38] and Asian skin.[39] Additional clinical studies of IPL added to the findings of significant modest-to-moderate reductions in facial telangiectasias.[40,41]

Whereas the efficacy of IPL has been well established in the treatment of dyspigmentation and vascularity, studies conflict on the clinical efficacy of this modality for rhytids. Several split-face randomized trials comparing treatment with IPL alone to IPL in combination with other rejuvenating procedures have documented variable amounts of improvement in fine rhytids after IPL monotherapy.[42,43] In addition, partial improvement after IPL has been detected in several uncontrolled studies.[44,45,46] Other randomized, controlled, split-face trials with IPL showed improvement in dyspigmentation and vascularity, but no change in rhytids.[34,47] For example, one of these was a randomized, split-face trial in which 32 women with mild-to-moderate rhytids received three once-monthly treatments with filtered IPL (530–750 nm, 7.5–8.5 J/cm^2, 2 × 2.5-ms pulses, 10-ms interpulse delay) to one side of the face and no treatment to the other side. Greater improvements in telangiectasias, pigmentation, and skin texture were shown on the IPL side, but there was no significant difference in the effect on rhytids.[34] Variability in the parameters across studies (e.g., fluence, pulse durations, and filtered wavelengths) may account for the inconsistency on the efficacy of IPL for rhytids. Importantly, among the trials that found IPL was ineffective for rhytids, the devices filtered the longer, more deeply penetrating wavelengths of IPL (750–1200 nm), a factor that in the author's opinion likely compromised treatment efficacy.[34,47]

These clinical findings have been accompanied by histological changes indicative of a dermal remodeling effect, but most recently of a more youthful genetic expression program. In a number of studies with histological analysis of skin samples following IPL treatment, increases in extracellular matrix proteins and neocollagenesis have been reported.[4,30,32,48] In contrast, some investigators failed to detect collagen or elastin fiber changes.[49] Recently, the gene expression patterns of IPL-treated skin have been shown to reflect a younger gene expression pattern.[50] In this study, investigators obtained skin samples from younger female volunteers, age < 30, and from site-matched untreated and treated skin of older female volunteers, age > 50—the latter after three monthly IPL treatments. The researchers studied the messenger ribonucleic acid (mRNA) transcript levels of 3,530 genes and identified those genes whose average expression level in older treated skin was closer to younger rather than older untreated skin. Mean gene expression levels in the treated older group were subtracted from mean gene expression levels in the untreated younger group, as well as from the untreated older group. If the difference in gene expression level was less with the untreated younger group compared with the difference with the untreated older group, the gene was operationally defined as "rejuvenated." A total of 1,293 transcripts qualified as "rejuvenated genes." Hierarchical clustering showed that the gene expression pattern of treated older skin more closely resembled that of untreated younger skin than untreated older skin from the same individuals. A twofold to fourfold increase in transcripts among markers typically expressed in younger untreated skin was observed.[49] Thus histological findings are now being accompanied by genetic analysis to identify the proteins involved in youthful skin and support the role of IPL in turning on a more youthful genetic program.

21.4.4 IPL-Mediated Photodynamic Therapy

With the antecedent application of 5-amino levulinic acid (5-ALA) prior to the administration of IPL treatment, greater pigmentary and vascular enhancement is achieved while increasing the degree of improvement of fine wrinkles.[1] The term *photodynamic photorejuvenation* has been applied to the use of IPL in the treatment of actinic keratosis (AK) and photodamage.[50] Among all the light sources, IPL combined with ALA photodynamic therapy (PDT) has been the most extensively studied for use in photorejuvenation, largely stemming from the fact that IPL has independently been shown to rejuvenate skin while spanning wavelengths that activate the downstream photosensitizer of 5-ALA, protoporphyrin IX (PPIX). A randomized, split-face design clinical study comparing ALA IPL to IPL alone demonstrated greater improvement on the ALA side in erythema, dyspigmentation, and fine rhytids following two monthly treatments.[43] Another IPL following a 1- to 2-hour incubation of topical ALA resulted in crusting when fluences above a certain threshold were delivered.[51] ALA IPL varies in both clinical response and side-effect profile, likely due to the variability of different IPL devices in wavelength irradiances (▶ Table 21.2). It should be noted, however, that IPL-mediated PDT typically causes photosensitivity for at least 48 hours posttreatment or longer depending upon the duration of 5-ALA incubation and degree of photodamage and AK. Therefore, proper preoperative and postoperative instructions must be administered to the patient in order to avoid phototoxicity. The author recommends a 1-hour incubation and IPL at photorejuvenation settings with the longest pulse duration, followed by strict bright-light avoidance for 48 hours posttreatment.

21.4.5 Pearls and Pitfalls

In a patient with photoaging and AK, application of 5-ALA followed by IPL should be considered in an effort to optimize clinical outcomes. However, strict bright-light avoidance posttreatment is necessary to avoid phototoxic reactions.

21.5 Broadband Infrared Light

21.5.1 Background

The application of BBIR to the treatment of facial and neck skin rhytids and laxity has contributed greatly to the laser, light, and energy-based technologies designed to treat skin aging.[1] When applied and used properly, BBIR-emitting wavelengths ranging between 800 to 1,600 nm, depending upon the device, yield consistent and reproducible refinements in skin rhytids and laxity to the face and neck without recovery time, side effects, or significant complications.[5,6,52]

Skin laxity on the face and neck is manifested by progressive loss of skin elasticity, loosening of connective tissue framework, deepening and redundancy of skin folds, and progressive prominence of submandibular and submental tissues. A classification scale of skin laxity has been validated that categorizes progressive appearance of hallmark clinical findings into clinical laxity grades (▶ Table 21.1).[2,3] Intrinsic genetic factors and extrinsic factors, such as photoaging, contribute to skin laxity, as evinced by genetic skin disorders with mutations in filaggrin and other elastin genes, and the histopathology findings of solar elastosis of photoaged skin, respectively.[53,54]

Infrared wavelengths were first employed for volumetric heating and treatment of skin laxity with the introduction of the 1,100 to 1,800-nm infrared light device (Titan, Cutera, San Francisco, California), which was Food and Drug Administration

(FDA)-approved for deep dermal heating in 2006.[5,55] Soon after, a variable-depth targeting infrared laser (1,310 nm, Candela Wayland, Massachusetts) was also shown to effectively treat skin laxity.[24] Thus, infrared wavelengths were found to be effective for the treatment of skin laxity, although until now reserved by FDA approval to the treatment of rhytids and/or deep dermal heating.

As BBIR technologies are applied on the skin surface, a major limiting factor in energy delivery to dermal targets is the heating of the epidermis and dermoepidermal junction (DEJ). The risk of thermal injury was particularly prohibitive of fluence delivery when a stationary technique of pulse application was used; this risk has been greatly diminished by the mobile technique developed by the author.[5,56] The mobile protocol was first developed for a radiofrequency technology in an effort to increase the speed and efficiency of radiofrequency energy delivery to dermal structures, while allowing for cooling of epidermal and DEJ structures.[56] Higher fluence delivery was achieved by moving the handpiece on the skin in a continuous motion, which was shown to render the treatment painless and virtually eliminate the risk of burns or complications.[56] In that publication, the author put forth the calculation that the thermal relaxation time of the cutaneous pain sensory nerve fibers was substantially shorter than that of the dermal collagen fibers.[56] Mobile delivery therefore allowed for cooling of these superficial sensory afferents while continuing to deposit energy into the large dermal targets, thereby precluding the firing of pain afferents and rendering the process painless.[56]

The mobile energy delivery approach was subsequently applied to BBIR 1,100 to 1,800 nm (Titan, Cutera) in a successful effort to augment fluence delivery, patient tolerance of high fluences, and to increase safety.[5] As was the case for mobile radiofrequency delivery, the mobile delivery of BBIR precluded the need for topical anesthesia, rendered the treatment painless, and safely allowed for a 30% increase in fluence dosage delivered per pulse, as well as an increase in the pass count to eight passes.[5] This increased energy delivery correlated with higher efficacy and response rates.

21.5.2 Patient Selection: Indications and Contraindications

Careful patient selection is paramount to attaining meaningful improvements and in meeting patient expectations with BBIR. The classification of neck laxity and photoaging into quantitative grades has been previously published and evaluated for clinical trial use by the author (▶ Table 21.1). Treatment with BBIR is indicated for patients with a baseline skin laxity of 2 to 3 on the 4-point quantitative laxity grading scale (▶ Table 21.1). In contrast, patients with severe skin laxity of grades 3.5 to 4 are not proper candidates for BBIR because the degree of improvement is unlikely to yield patient satisfaction. Patients over age 65 are less likely to respond to skin-surface applied nonablative procedures, and should be considered for this treatment approach on a case-by-case basis. Patients with a history of thyroid or parathyroid disease or neoplasia are contraindicated.

The consultation should entail the presentation of all treatment options, including the surgical facelift. Patients should be offered all the treatment options for treating their skin rhytids and laxity, including but not limited to injectables, alternative laser and light-based treatments, surgical options, and no treatment. The rare but real risk of a thermal burn and scar should be discussed during informed consent, in addition to the usual and customary risks and complications of any medical procedure. Premedication and anesthesia are not necessary. BBIR treatments are FDA-approved for deep dermal heating and the application for the treatment of rhytids and skin laxity are off-label.

Pearls and Pitfalls

Proper patient selection is critical to achieving patient satisfaction, with laxity grades 2 to 3 being the ideal candidates and grades 3.5 to 4 being poor candidates for meaningful improvements (▶ Table 21.1). Provide patients with a full understanding of treatment options and level of expected efficacy in order to avoid the pitfall of not meeting patient expectations.

21.5.3 Advantages and Disadvantages

The advantages of BBIR for the treatment of skin rhytids and laxity include the excellent safety profile, lack of downtime, and natural aesthetic outcome. The mobile technique has been associated with no thermal burns to date and no or transient discomfort. Patients report a sense of warmth, but no burning sensation with this treatment approach. As a result, the procedure requires no anesthetic. Whereas transient perioperative and postoperative erythema are desired clinical end points, the erythema resolves within minutes. Therefore, there is no recovery time necessary for the procedure. Adverse events are very rare, particularly with the mobile protocol. Finally, the aesthetic outcomes are exceedingly natural. Because the clinical improvements are due to neocollagenesis and neoelastogenesis without vaporization or coagulation of tissue, the tissue-tightening effect follows the natural vectors to the skin and the texture or color of the skin is not altered as may sometimes be seen with ablative or fractional nonablative technologies.

The disadvantages of this approach include the need for multiple treatments, the need for numerous passes during procedures, the modest efficacy per treatment, and the sometimes-subtle clinical outcomes. For these reasons, the guidelines for the patient consultation and patient selection previously described must be adhered to. Patients should be educated that a range of two to four monthly treatments is necessary for significant improvement. In addition, it is imperative to take baseline digital photographs of all patients so as to track progress with each treatment. It is of paramount importance that the clinician delivers an adequate number of passes in order to attain and maintain target temperature for enough time to induce clinical changes. The number of pulses and/or total energy delivery targets must be followed in order to attain a clinical response. It is advised to review the level of response after the first session with clinical pretreatment and posttreatment photographs. In the author's experience, the patient and clinician should appreciate progress at 1 month following the first procedure, or an alternative treatment course should be considered.

Pearls and Pitfalls

Baseline and follow-up digital photographs are strongly advised at each visit. Progress should be observed at 1 month following the first treatment as a predictor for significant clinical outcome from a treatment series. If the patient does not observe an improvement after the first treatment, a review of baseline and follow-up photographs can serve to prevent the pitfall of patient dissatisfaction.

21.6 Preoperative Instructions

Photography: Baseline and follow-up photography front view, three-quarter views, and from both side views, are necessary. Patients should be advised that clinical results will typically start to manifest at 2 weeks following the first treatment and the results continue to accumulate to approximately 6 months follow-up. It should be explicitly stated that two to four monthly treatment sessions are required for meaningful improvements to be appreciated for patients with baseline laxity grades of 2 to 3. Photographs should be repeated at each treatment and follow-up visit.

Patient preparation: No topical anesthetic is needed for the procedure. A thin 1-mm layer of aqueous ultrasound gel is applied. The typical treatment areas includes the lower face and neck, excluding the thyroid region (▶ Fig. 21.2). Maintain complete contact of the treatment tip with the aqueous gel and skin surface throughout each pulse.

Treatment intervals: Patients with baseline laxity grades 2 to 3 should receive two to four treatments with BBIR at 2- to 4-week intervals.

21.6.1 Treatment Protocols

Broadband Infrared Light—1,100 to 1,800 nm, Titan, Cutera

Early users are advised to start with the 1,100 to 1,800-nm BBIR (Titan, Cutera) using the mobile technique at conservative fluences of 44 to 46 J/cm^2 for the face and 42 to 44 J/cm^2 for the neck. Apply ample aqueous gel to the area to be treated. A series of eight passes to each row as shown in ▶ Fig. 21.2 should be administered, so that the total pulse count for the face and neck should be approximately 800 pulses in total. As one develops experience with the device, the fluence may be titrated up to as high as 50 J/cm^2 for the face and 47 J/cm^2 for the neck, as tolerated by the patient. Special attention should be given to treating the mandibular or bony prominences so that the sapphire tip is in full contact with the gel and parallel with the skin surface. In addition, continual rapid movement of the tip is necessary to prevent discomfort and to virtually eliminate the risk of burns. Total pulse counts for a face and neck treatment will vary depending upon the size of the face and neck, and typically run between 200 and 400 pulses per anatomical site or up to 800 pulses in total. Patients should be followed at a 1-month interval and repeat photography is advised at each visit. Patients should be told at the outset that the final clinical outcome will take 6 months to manifest following the final treatment, paralleling the time course of neocollagenesis and neoelastogenesis. Maintenance treatments are generally advised once every 6 months.

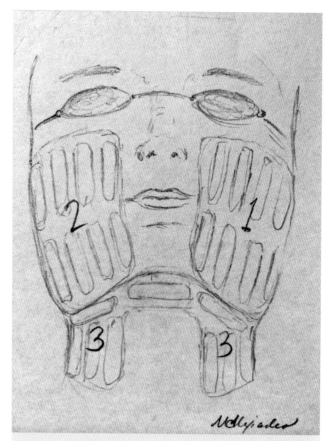

Fig. 21.2 Anatomical treatment areas for application of broadband infrared (BBIR) light. Using the mobile application protocol, procedure should commence on one of the two lower cheek areas. Treatment pulses should be applied sequentially, as described in the treatment protocol, until confluent erythema and heating are attained in a treatment area. The handpiece should be moved to the next procedure area until target temperature and confluence of erythema are achieved. Once all treatment areas are equivalently heated and erythematous, maintenance pulses are administered throughout until total energy delivery, as detailed in the protocols, is reached.

Mobile pulse application: Each light pulse is administered in a mobile, continuous fashion within a localized area measuring approximately 1-handpiece width laterally and vertically. The handpiece is moved with the initiation of each pulse, making oval/circular movements extending approximately one width laterally to the handpiece tip and one length of the handpiece tip vertically. The pulses are delivered in succession along each segment as shown in ▶ Fig. 21.2. A series of 4 to 5 pulses are administered across small grid areas, followed by 6 to 8 passes to each grid area, totaling approximately 200 to 400 pulses per anatomical site per treatment, or up to 800 pulses for lower face and neck. The pulses should be administered in a linear fashion along the jawline, along the upper neck, and in the submental area as shown in ▶ Fig. 21.2. The precise segments or grid areas include: the lower cheek, mid-to-upper cheek, mandible, upper lateral neck, submandibular, and submental areas (▶ Fig. 21.2). The passes are administered in succession to each linear area before commencing in a new area. A minimum of 4, but preferably 7 to 8, passes along each segment each covering an area of approximately 1.5 cm^2 should be administered.

Dose/fluence: Precooling, parallel cooling, and postcooling of the epidermis are applied through continuous contact with a sapphire tip. Each mobile pulse is delivered at a fluence of 46 J/cm^2 to face, 45 J/cm^2 to mandible, and 44 J/cm^2 to neck. The fluence is commenced at 46 J/cm^2 for the mobile protocol to the face; 45 J/cm^2 to the mandible; and 44 J/cm^2 to the neck. If the patient senses momentary transient discomfort, the fluence should be titrated down by 1 J/cm^2 for a final target range on the face of 44 to 50 J/cm^2 and on the neck of 42 to 47 J/cm^2 mobile. For superior periorbital regions, the mobile technique is initiated at fluences ranging from 20 to 24 J/cm^2. The clinician may administer 1 to 2 adjacent pulses to each brow extending to the lateral periorbital region (▶ Fig. 21.2). A total of 4 to 5 passes should be delivered if comfortably tolerated by the patient.

Near-Infrared Broadband Light—800 to 1,600 nm, NIR, Alma Lasers

Following application of aqueous gel to the skin surface, treatment should commence on one lower cheek (▶ Fig. 21.2). A standard setting of 50 W is recommended. Using the mobile technique, the handpiece should be moved across the skin surface in an oval, rotational movement, approximately One-handpiece width in each direction. The clinician should deliver six to eight passes to each treatment area: one cheek, the contralateral cheek, and the submental and lateral neck regions. The sapphire tip is larger on this BBIR device; therefore, treatment is administered to the entire cheek through rapid, rotational motion. Once the patient reports the sensation as "hot," move the handpiece to the next treatment area, either neck or contralateral cheek (▶ Fig. 21.2). Once all three anatomical sites reach the target temperature (i.e., confluent erythema and heating), maintenance passes are administered through rapid motion, successively and continually, until the final energy delivery of 30 kJ is attained. The desired clinical end point is for all treatment areas to be confluently erythematous and for the passes to be continued to all treatment areas in succession until a total of 30 kJ is delivered. Typically, approximately 8 to 9 kJ are delivered per each anatomical site: each cheek and neck/submentum, with subsequent passes throughout to reach 30-kJ total delivered energy.

Perioperative instructions: The patient will report a feeling of warmth; however, the patient should be instructed to alert the clinician immediately should the pulse feel uncomfortable or very hot. If the patient reports discomfort or that the area is very hot, move the handpiece to a new treatment area. Typically, 7 to 8 kJ of energy are delivered to each treatment area in order for confluent erythema and heat sensation to be attained, signaling target temperature has been reached.

Pain evaluations: With any BBIR device, pain should be evaluated while administering each pulse and the fluence titrated up or down to the point of tolerability by the patient. The mobile delivery speed can be increased, in order to allow epidermal cooling and to maximize total energy delivery and safety. Use of the standard stationary technique results in discomfort and requires topical anesthesia at fluences exceeding roughly 30 to 35 J/cm^2 (Titan, Cutera). With the mobile technique, the procedure should be painless at fluences of 44 to 50 J/cm^2 (Titan, Cutera) or 50 W (NIR, Alma Lasers, Buffalo Grove,

Illinois). The clinical study assessing the mobile technique demonstrated perioperative discomfort was rated as a mean of 0.7 ($\pm$ 0.6) on a 0-to-10 visual analog scale (VAS) grading scale.[5,6] In a patient questionnaire asking patients to rate the procedure as painless, mildly painful, moderately painful, or painful, sensation during the treatment was rated as painless by 100% (22 of 22) of patients.[5] In a separate question asking patients whether they sensed rare (< 5) transient moments of heat pain versus frequent (> 5) moments of heat pain versus persistent heat pain during the procedure, 18% (4 of 22) of patients reported only rare transient moments of heat pain during the course of the procedure. None (0%) of the patients reported the procedure as painful, or as sensing frequent or persistent heat pain sensation during the treatment.[5]

Pearls and Pitfalls

Employ the mobile technique to avoid thermal burns and to maximize energy delivery. Apply ample aqueous gel; apply the handpiece in a rapid, oval-circular motion throughout the pulse, and instruct the patient to report any sensation of discomfort. Move to the adjacent treatment area if discomfort is felt in order to avoid any injury to the skin.

21.6.2 Postoperative Care/Preventing and Managing Adverse Events

Safety: Immediately following treatment, minimal erythema and minimal-to-no edema are noted, which resolve within 1 hour. No crusting, dyspigmentation, or scarring should be observed. It is imperative to use adequate gel and maintain full contact of the sapphire tip with the gel and skin surface in order to prevent any epidermal injury. Because the postoperative erythema resolves within minutes, no postoperative care is needed.

The mobile technique has not been associated with thermal burns or other adverse events to date. However, the stationary technique has been associated with rare incidences of thermal burns. To monitor for such an adverse event, the patient should be provided with a postoperative instruction sheet detailing the findings of a burn should this rare complication manifest. The patient should be instructed that any persistent area of redness, blistering, or crusting should be brought to the clinician's attention as soon as possible. This should be treated immediately with cold compresses and topical silver sulfasalazine until the lesion resolves fully. Such burns can be avoided during the stationary technique by applying ample aqueous gel and monitoring carefully along bony prominences to maintain full contact with the gel and skin surface. Lowering the fluence in the periorbital and temporal regions is another precaution to prevent thermal burns to these higher risk areas. Taking great care along the mandible and mental regions is an important precaution, utilizing ample gel and maintaining complete contact during each pulse. Such rare incidences of thermal burns heal completely with exceedingly rare risk of residual scarring.

Clinical evaluations: Clinical results should be evaluated employing the comprehensive 4-point grading scale from photographs at baseline 1-, 3-, and 6-month follow-up visits after the final procedure. Photographs should be evaluated 1 month following the first treatment prior to commencing further therapy to ensure that a desired clinical outcome will be obtained.

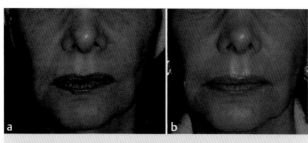

Fig. 21.3 Clinical improvements in lentigines and telangiectasias following intense pulsed light (IPL) treatment. A 70-year-old woman with advanced photoaging is shown at (a) baseline and (b) 1 month following three monthly IPL (Harmony, Alma, Caesarea, Israel) treatments. Significant improvements in lentigines and telangiectasias are observed, resulting in high patient satisfaction and global improvement in skin appearance.

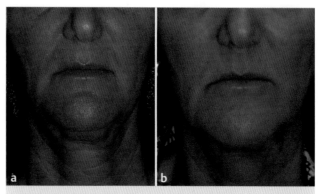

Fig. 21.4 Clinical results from broadband infrared (BBIR) light treatment of skin laxity. (a) A patient prior to and (b) at 2-year follow-up after three monthly treatments with BBIR (Titan, Cutera, San Francisco, California) using the mobile technique at 46 J/cm². The baseline laxity grade (▶ Table 21.1) was rated as 3.75, with a posttreatment laxity grade of 3.00, for a 0.75 grade reduction.

21.6.3 Clinical and Histological Findings

Clinical results in skin laxity and rhytid reduction will typically begin to become evident starting 2 weeks following the first treatment session. Progressive improvements in skin laxity and rhytids are gradually observed over several months, reaching a maximum benefit at 6 to 12 months.[5,24,56] This correlates histologically with the completion of the time course of neocollagenesis.[1,5,57,58,59] Photographic examples of laxity reduction in patients during the follow-up interval from treatment with BBIR using the mobile technique are shown in ▶ Fig. 21.4.

In 2006, the first BBIR (1,100–1,800 nm) light device was introduced and FDA-approved for deep dermal heating. It was soon applied to the treatment of skin laxity on the face and neck in a pilot study of 25 patients treated with a single-treatment infrared 1,100 to 1,800-nm broadband light with the stationary technique at 20 to 40 J/cm² and using topical anesthesia.[57] These findings were reproduced in a subsequent study of 13 patients with facial and neck skin laxity treated with two monthly sessions at 30 to 36 J/cm² and three passes, with 6-month follow-up.[27] A study on Asian skin employed 32 to 40 J/cm², three passes, and three successive monthly treatment sessions, with descriptive improvements in facial skin laxity reported.[58] Of import, among 63 total treatment sessions using the stationary technique, seven incidences of vesiculation and blistering were reported.[58] Another split-face study on Asian skin demonstrated descriptive improvement following two BBIR (1,100–1,800 nm) treatments at 36 to 46 J/cm² on the treated side at 3-month follow-up.[59] One incidence of blistering occurred among the 23 patients treated.[59] In addition, topical anesthesia was required because the stationary application of the device was associated with significant discomfort. Another study of 9 patients demonstrated that application of topical anesthesia followed by infrared broadband light treatment at 30 to 40 J/cm² in one to two sessions yielded descriptive improvements in skin laxity at 1-month follow-up.[60]

Quantitative assessments: The clinical outcomes for the treatment of skin laxity with BBIR using the mobile technique were assessed by quantitative grading employing a tested laxity grading scale, and demonstrated augmented clinical efficacy as compared to the stationary technique.[5] In the clinical study evaluating the mobile technique of BBIR with a 1,100 to 1,800-nm device for the treatment of skin laxity, the mean pretreatment score was 2.9 ± 0.5, the mean posttreatment score was 2.5 ± 0.6, and the mean improvement in prelaxity versus postlaxity grades was 0.4 ± 0.3 (95% confidence interval [CI], 0.2540-0.5415).[5] These represented a statistically significant difference between before and after measurements ($p < .0001$). The mean percentage improvement in laxity grading scores was 14.1 ± 11.3% following a mean of 1.9 serial treatments. The mobile delivery of infrared broadband (1,100–1,800 nm) light yielded consistent clinical improvement in all subjects in the study and afforded a 0.2 laxity grade enhancement per treatment on the 4-point grading scale, while rendering the procedure painless and free of side effects or complications.[5] The mobile delivery allows for cooling of epidermal and DEJ structures, while concurrently allowing for more efficient delivery of 30% higher fluences into the target tissues in the dermis,[5,56] resulting in a more favorable safety profile and higher efficacy.

Histological evaluations of BBIR on skin have demonstrated the induction of collagens and elastin synthesis. In a rat model, greater induction of collagen type I relative to collagen type III was demonstrated by immunostaining in skin sections obtained up to 90 days and 45 days postirradiation, respectively.[61] In postabdominoplasty human skin, irradiation with 30, 45, and 60 J/cm², four passes, demonstrated a difference in the level of collagen fibril alteration among the different fluences. Lower (30 J/cm²) fluences showed less collagen fibril alteration on electron microscopy at the 0- to 1-mm depth as compared to 1- to 2-mm depth, due to the effects of contact cooling at lower fluences. For 45 and 65 J/cm², the entire field demonstrated contracted collagen fibrils.[62] These findings correlate with augmented clinical efficacy in treating rhytids and laxity observed with the mobile technique at high > 46 J/cm² fluences.[5] Finally, BBIR is one of two skin-tightening technologies that have been shown to induce both neocollagenesis and neoelastogenesis.[63] Recently, human-skin biopsies following irradiation at 36 J/cm² using the stationary technique were obtained at 1, 2, and 3 months posttreatment.[63] Immunostains in sun-protected skin demonstrated significant increases in type I collagen until month 1, and in type III collagen and elastin through month 3. In sun-exposed skin, these studies showed increases in type I collagen through month 2, and type III collagen and elastin through month 3.[63] The combined induction of both neocollagenesis and neoelastogenesis likely explain the clinical impact on both rhytids and skin laxity.

21.7 Conclusion

The applications of IPL and BBIR to the treatment of skin aging are two invaluable tools among nonsurgical and nonablative therapeutic modalities. IPL has established itself more than 20 years as a mainstay in the treatment of photoaging, with reproducible improvement in dyspigmentation and vascularity of the facial skin. BBIR has been demonstrated over the past decade as a safe and effective nonsurgical treatment for skin laxity and rhytids. BBIR, when employed with the mobile technique, offers a painless, safe, nonsurgical alternative therapy option for the treatment of skin laxity on the face and neck. The application of the mobile technique allows for 30% higher fluences to be employed, does not require topical anesthesia, renders the treatment painless, and allows for increased pass counts as compared to the stationary approach. Recent advances in genomics and proteomics are identifying the gene expression changes induced by these technologies, supporting their role in inducing a more youthful genetic program in treated skin. The consistency of clinical improvement in photoaging with IPL and skin rhytids and laxity with BBIR supports the continued use of these two approaches in the treatment of skin aging.

References

[1] Alexiades-Armenakas MR, Dover JS, Arndt KA. The spectrum of laser skin resurfacing: nonablative, fractional, and ablative laser resurfacing. J Am Acad Dermatol 2008; 58: 719–737, quiz 738–740

[2] Alexiades-Armenakas M. Rhytids, laxity, and photoaging treated with a combination of radiofrequency, diode laser, and pulsed light and assessed with a comprehensive grading scale. J Drugs Dermatol 2006; Sep;5(8): 731–738

[3] Alexiades-Armenakas M. A quantitative and comprehensive grading scale for rhytids, laxity, and photoaging. J Drugs Dermatol 2006; 5: 808–809

[4] Goldberg DJ. New collagen formation after dermal remodeling with an intense pulsed light source. J Cutan Laser Ther 2000; 2: 59–61

[5] Alexiades-Armenakas M. Assessment of the mobile delivery of infrared light (1100–1800 nm) for the treatment of facial and neck skin laxity. J Drugs Dermatol 2009; 8: 221–226

[6] Alexiades-Armenakas M. Aging facial skin: infrared broad band light technologies. Facial Plast Surg Clin North Am 2011; 19: 361–370

[7] Goldberg DJ, Whitworth J. Laser skin resurfacing with the Q-switched Nd:YAG laser. Dermatol Surg 1997; 23: 903–906, discussion 906–907

[8] Sumian CC, Pitre FB, Gauthier BE, Bouclier M, Mordon SR. Laser skin resurfacing using a frequency doubled Nd:YAG laser after topical application of an exogenous chromophore. Lasers Surg Med 1999; 25: 43–50

[9] Goldberg D, Tan M, Dale Sarradet M, Gordon M. Nonablative dermal remodeling with a 585-nm, 350-microsec, flashlamp pulsed dye laser: clinical and ultrastructural analysis. Dermatol Surg 2003; 29: 161–163, discussion 163–164

[10] Fatemi A, Weiss MA, Weiss RA. Short-term histologic effects of nonablative resurfacing: results with a dynamically cooled millisecond-domain 1320 nm Nd:YAG laser. Dermatol Surg 2002; 28: 172–176

[11] Dayan SH, Vartanian AJ, Menaker G, Mobley SR, Dayan AN. Nonablative laser resurfacing using the long-pulse (1064-nm) Nd:YAG laser. Arch Facial Plast Surg 2003; 5: 310–315

[12] Alam M, Dover JS, Arndt KA. Energy delivery devices for cutaneous remodeling: lasers, lights, and radio waves. Arch Dermatol 2003; 139: 1351–1360

[13] Goldberg DJ. Non-ablative subsurface remodeling: clinical and histologic evaluation of a 1320-nm Nd:YAG laser. J Cutan Laser Ther 1999 Sep;1 (3):153-157

[14] Ross EV, Sajben FP, Hsia J, Barnette D, Miller CH, McKinlay JR. Nonablative skin remodeling: selective dermal heating with a mid-infrared laser and contact cooling combination. Lasers Surg Med 2000; 26: 186–195

[15] Kelly KM, Nelson JS, Lask GP, Geronemus RG, Bernstein LJ. Cryogen spray cooling in combination with nonablative laser treatment of facial rhytids. Arch Dermatol 1999; 135: 691–694

[16] Goldberg DJ. Non-ablative subsurface remodeling: clinical and histologic evaluation of a 1320-nm Nd:YAG laser. J Cutan Laser Ther 1999; 1: 153–157

[17] Goldberg DJ. Full-face nonablative dermal remodeling with a 1320 nm Nd:YAG laser. Dermatol Surg 2000; 26: 915–918

[18] Paithankar DY, Clifford JM, Saleh BA, Ross EV, Hardaway CA, Barnette D. Subsurface skin renewal by treatment with a 1450-nm laser in combination with dynamic cooling. J Biomed Opt 2003; 8: 545–551

[19] Lupton JR, Williams CM, Alster TS. Nonablative laser skin resurfacing using a 1540 nm erbium glass laser: a clinical and histologic analysis. Dermatol Surg 2002; 28: 833–835

[20] Fournier N, Dahan S, Barneon G, et al. Nonablative remodeling: clinical, histologic, ultrasound imaging, and profilometric evaluation of a 1540 nm Er:glass laser. Dermatol Surg 2001; 27: 799–806

[21] Rostan EF, Fitzpatrick RE. Treatment of acne scars with a 1320 Nd:YAG nonablative laser. Lasers Surg Med 2001; 13 Suppl: 31

[22] Tanzi EL, Alster TS. Comparison of a 1450-nm diode laser and a 1320-nm Nd:YAG laser in the treatment of atrophic facial scars: a prospective clinical and histologic study. Dermatol Surg 2004; 30: 152–157

[23] Dahan S, Lagarde JM, Turlier V, Courrech L, Mordon S. Treatment of neck lines and forehead rhytids with a nonablative 1540-nm Er:glass laser: a controlled clinical study combined with the measurement of the thickness and the mechanical properties of the skin. Dermatol Surg 2004; 30: 872–879, discussion 879–880

[24] Alexiades-Armenakas MR. Non-ablative skin tightening with a variable-depth heating 1310 nm wavelength laser in combination with surface cooling. J Drugs Dermatol 2007; 6: 1096–1103

[25] Ruiz-Esparza J. Near painless, nonablative, immediate skin contraction induced by low-fluence irradiation with new infrared device: A report of 25 patients. Dermatol Surg. 2006;32:601-10

[26] Lee M-WC. Comparison of radiofrequency vs. 1100–1800 nm infrared light for skin laxity. Am Soc Derm Surg Abstracts, Atlanta, GA; October 27, 2005

[27] Goldberg DJ, Hussain M, Fazeli A, Berlin AL. Treatment of skin laxity of the lower face and neck in older individuals with a broad-spectrum infrared light device. J Cosmet Laser Ther 2007; 9: 35–40

[28] Kameyama K. Histological and clinical studies on the effects of low to medium level infrared light therapy on human and mouse skin. J Drugs Dermatol 2008; 7: 230–235

[29] Bitter P, Campbell CA, Goldman M. Nonablative skin rejuvenation using intense pulsed light. Lasers Surg Med 2000; 12: 16

[30] Zelickson BD, Kist D. Effect of pulsed dye laser and intense pulsed light source on the dermal extracellular matrix remodeling. Lasers Surg Med 2000; 12: 17

[31] Raulin C, Greve B, Grema H. IPL technology: a review. Lasers Surg Med 2003; 32: 78–87

[32] Huang J, Luo X, Lu J, et al. IPL irradiation rejuvenates skin collagen via the bidirectional regulation of MMP-1 and TGF-β1 mediated by MAPKs in fibroblasts. Lasers Med Sci 2011; 26: 381–387

[33] Babilas P, Schreml S, Szeimies RM, Landthaler M. Intense pulsed light (IPL): a review. Lasers Surg Med 2010; 42: 93–104

[34] Hedelund L, Due E, Bjerring P, Wulf HC, Haedersdal M. Skin rejuvenation using intense pulsed light: a randomized controlled split-face trial with blinded response evaluation. Arch Dermatol 2006; 142: 985–990

[35] Weiss RA, Weiss MA, Beasley KL. Rejuvenation of photoaged skin: 5 years results with intense pulsed light of the face, neck, and chest. Dermatol Surg 2002; 28: 1115–1119

[36] Kulick MI. Photorejuvenation: using intense pulsed light technology in a cosmetic surgery practice. Aesthet Surg J 2001; 21: 255–258

[37] Galeckas KJ, Collins M, Ross EV, Uebelhoer NS. Split-face treatment of facial dyschromia: pulsed dye laser with a compression handpiece versus intense pulsed light. Dermatol Surg 2008; 34: 672–680

[38] Bjerring P, Christiansen K. Intense pulsed light source for treatment of small melanocytic nevi and solar lentigines. J Cutan Laser Ther 2000; 2: 177–181

[39] Negishi K, Tezuka Y, Kushikata N, Wakamatsu S. Photorejuvenation for Asian skin by intense pulsed light. Dermatol Surg 2001; 27: 627–631, discussion 632

[40] Bjerring P, Christiansen K, Troilius A. Intense pulsed light source for treatment of facial telangiectasias. J Cosmet Laser Ther 2001; 3: 169–173

[41] Retamar RA, Chames C, Pellerano G. Treatment of linear and spider telangiectasia with an intense pulsed light source. J Cosmet Dermatol 2004; 3: 187–190

[42] Carruthers J, Carruthers A. The effect of full-face broadband light treatments alone and in combination with bilateral crow's feet Botulinum toxin type A chemodenervation. Dermatol Surg 2004; 30: 355–366, discussion 366

[43] Dover JS, Bhatia AC, Stewart B, Arndt KA. Topical 5-aminolevulinic acid combined with intense pulsed light in the treatment of photoaging. Arch Dermatol 2005; 141: 1247–1252

[44] Goldberg DJ, Cutler KB. Nonablative treatment of rhytids with intense pulsed light. Lasers Surg Med 2000; 26: 196–200

[45] Bitter PH. Noninvasive rejuvenation of photodamaged skin using serial, full-face intense pulsed light treatments. Dermatol Surg 2000; 26: 835–842, discussion 843

[46] Sadick NS, Weiss R, Kilmer S, Bitter P. Photorejuvenation with intense pulsed light: results of a multi-center study. J Drugs Dermatol 2004; 3: 41–49

[47] Jørgensen GF, Hedelund L, Haedersdal M. Long-pulsed dye laser versus intense pulsed light for photodamaged skin: a randomized split-face trial with blinded response evaluation. Lasers Surg Med 2008; 40: 293–299

[48] Prieto VG, Sadick NS, Lloreta J, Nicholson J, Shea CR. Effects of intense pulsed light on sun-damaged human skin, routine, and ultrastructural analysis. Lasers Surg Med 2002; 30: 82–85

[49] Cao Y, Huo R, Feng Y, Li Q, Wang F. Effects of intense pulsed light on the biological properties and ultrastructure of skin dermal fibroblasts: potential roles in photoaging. Photomed Laser Surg 2011; 29: 327–332

[50] Ruiz-Rodriguez R, Sanz-Sánchez T, Córdoba S. Photodynamic photorejuvenation. Dermatol Surg 2002; 28: 742–744, discussion 744

[51] Hall JA, Keller PJ, Keller GS. Dose response of combination photorejuvenation using intense pulsed light-activated photodynamic therapy and radiofrequency energy. Arch Facial Plast Surg 2004; 6: 374–378

[52] Gold MH. Tissue tightening: a hot topic utilizing deep dermal heating. J Drugs Dermatol 2007; 6: 1238–1242

[53] Milewicz DM, Urbán Z, Boyd C. Genetic disorders of the elastic fiber system. Matrix Biol 2000; 19: 471–480

[54] Uitto J. The role of elastin and collagen in cutaneous aging: intrinsic aging versus photoexposure. J Drugs Dermatol 2008; 7 Suppl: s12–s16

[55] Taub AF, Battle EF, Jr, Nikolaidis G. Multicenter clinical perspectives on a broadband infrared light device for skin tightening. J Drugs Dermatol 2006; 5: 771–778

[56] Alexiades-Armenakas M, Dover JS, Arndt KA. Unipolar versus bipolar radiofrequency treatment of rhytids and laxity using a mobile painless delivery method. Lasers Surg Med 2008; 40: 446–453

[57] Ruiz-Esparza J. Near [corrected] painless, nonablative, immediate skin contraction induced by low-fluence irradiation with new infrared device: a report of 25 patients. Dermatol Surg 2006; 32: 601–610

[58] Chua SH, Ang P, Khoo LS, Goh CL. Nonablative infrared skin tightening in type IV to V Asian skin: a prospective clinical study. Dermatol Surg 2007; 33: 146–151

[59] Chan HH, Yu CS, Shek S, Yeung CK, Kono T, Wei WI. A prospective, split face, single-blinded study looking at the use of an infrared device with contact cooling in the treatment of skin laxity in Asians. Lasers Surg Med 2008; 40: 146–152

[60] Ahn JY, Han TY, Lee CK, Seo SJCK, Hong CK. Effect of a new infrared light device (1100–1800 nm) on facial lifting. Photodermatol Photoimmunol Photomed 2008; 24: 49–51

[61] Tanaka Y, Matsuo K, Yuzuriha S, Shinohara H. Differential long-term stimulation of type I versus type III collagen after infrared irradiation. Dermatol Surg 2009; 35: 1099–1104

[62] Zelickson B, Ross V, Kist D, Counters J, Davenport S, Spooner G. Ultrastructural effects of an infrared handpiece on forehead and abdominal skin. Dermatol Surg 2006; 32: 897–901

[63] Tanaka Y, Matsuo K, Yuzuriha S. Long-term evaluation of collagen and elastin following infrared (1100 to 1800 nm) irradiation. J Drugs Dermatol 2009; 8: 708–712

22 Nitrogen Plasma Skin Resurfacing

Stuart H. Bentkover

22.1 Is This Technology Still Relevant?

In 2012, the author reviewed a series of patients who had undergone plasma skin resurfacing (PSR) with the Portrait PSR[3] device,[1] and concluded that plasma skin resurfacing was a relevant and worthwhile procedure for patients with Fitzpatrick skin types I through IV whose major complaints were hyperpigmentation and mild-to-moderate wrinkles everywhere on the face except the upper lip. Since that time, this author continues to use the technology; but its popularity has definitely waned. Fewer patients are willing to accept a week or so of downtime; and with the demise of the original manufacturer (Rhytec, Inc., Waltham, Massachusetts), the procedure has much less Internet presence. Hence, prospective patients are not as familiar with the technology. The new manufacturer of the technology (Energist Medical Group, Swansea, United Kingdom) can supply the necessary parts and service, but it has not reestablished the type of Internet and media presence seen with Rhytec. Downtime, the length of time from the day of the procedure to when a patient may return to relatively normal activity, is comparable to that for nonablative, fractionated carbon dioxide laser resurfacing. In the author's practice, patients with wrinkles or scars deep enough to require a full ablative carbon dioxide laser resurfacing seem more willing to accept the necessary downtime than patients with lesser rhytids and hyperpigmentation. It is important, therefore, to ask if plasma technology is still relevant compared to chemical and laser technologies that have similar effects.

22.2 Historical Perspective

The Portrait PSR[3] device is a class II nonlaser device that was designed to provide a quicker healing alternative to ablative laser treatments for patients with facial rhytids and hyperpigmentation. It was also considerably less expensive than many ablative lasers. Introduced into the U.S. market for cosmetic use by Rhytec in 2005, its launch preceded the launch of a number of fractionated laser devices by 1 or 2 years but was almost simultaneous with others. Its clinical relevance is most commonly compared to that of a fractionated carbon dioxide laser.

The device produces nitrogen plasma in its handpiece. Plasma is an ionized gas that is considered the fourth state of matter. Examples of where plasma is commonly observed in nature include some flat-screen television monitors, electrical storms, and the Aurora Borealis. In this device, an ultrahigh-frequency radio pulse vibrates a tungsten element in the handpiece that excites nitrogen molecules in a stream of nitrogen gas passing through the handpiece. It converts the stable nitrogen gas to unstable ionized nitrogen plasma. Nitrogen plasma is delivered to the skin in one or more passes in a technique similar to that of laser resurfacing (▶ Fig. 22.1).

The original Food and Drug Administration (FDA) approval for the device was for treating facial and nonfacial rhytids, acne scars, and superficial benign skin lesions such as seborrheic keratoses, viral papillomata, and actinic keratoses in Fitzpatrick skin types I through IV. The device is contraindicated in patients prone to keloid formation.

22.3 Comparable Technologies

Ablative and nonablative facial resurfacing techniques are designed primarily to remove wrinkles or scars and rejuvenate skin. *Rejuvenate* is a difficult-to-define term that can include the removal of wrinkles and scars and changes in color and texture of the skin. Some techniques are more efficacious for wrinkles and some are more efficacious for uniformity of skin color. Rejuvenation may also include improvements in overall brightness and luminescence of the skin that may be apparent in photos and in person but are very hard to measure. The various machines and chemical techniques available have varying depths of epidermal and dermal penetration. Virtually all these

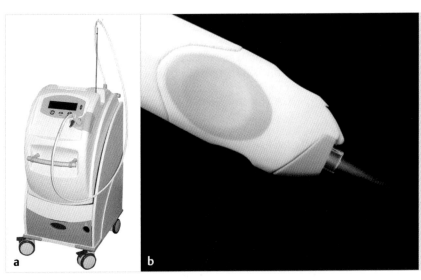

Fig. 22.1 (a) The Portrait plasma skin resurfacing (PSR) device, and (b) a close-up of the delivery end of the handpiece system. (Courtesy of NeoGen by Energist Medical Group, Swansea, United Kingdom; formerly Portrait, Rhytec, Inc., Waltham, Massachusetts.)

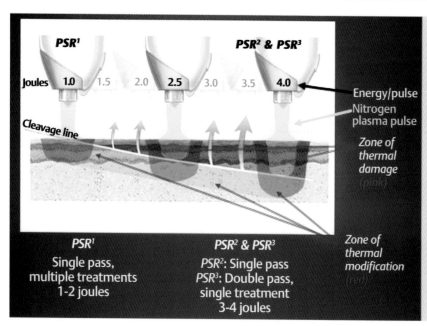

Fig. 22.2 Higher energy delivery leads to more depth of penetration in the zones of thermal damage and thermal modification, lowering the line of cleavage between the two zones deeper into the dermis. (Courtesy of NeoGen by Energist Medical Group, Swansea, United Kingdom; formerly Portrait, Rhytec, Inc., Waltham, Massachusetts.)

technologies claim to stimulate neocollagenesis. With the advent of aesthetic carbon dioxide and erbium laser technology in the mid-1990s, mechanical dermabrasion became less commonly used. Superficial, medium, and deep chemical peels are still common.

The principle by which medical lasers achieve their results is called photothermolysis. Each laser generates a collimated light of a single frequency that can selectively target a specific complimentary color or group of colors, target chromophores. For the carbon dioxide laser (10,600 nm) the primary target of the laser is water.[2] The laser vaporizes skin cells in a very controlled and precise manner.

Lasers commonly used for skin rejuvenation are the 10,600-nm carbon dioxide laser, the 2,940-nm erbium:yttrium aluminum garnet (Er:YAG) laser,[3] and the fractionated erbium 1,550- and 1,410-nm lasers.[4] The depth of penetration for each laser depends on the wavelength of the target chromophore, the number of passes, and the amount of laser energy delivered. Typical depths of penetration for the carbon dioxide laser (10,600 nm) are 450 μm to 1 to 2 mm (although rarely used beyond 1 mm),[2] for the Er:YAG (2,940 nm) laser 3 to 120 μm,[3] and for the erbium fiber, diode (1,550 nm) 250 to 800 μm.[4] By sparing specifically and uniformly spaced areas of untreated skin between targeted skin, fractional technology often provides the ability to treat skin with local or topical anesthesia and shorter postoperative downtime. Fully ablative laser treatments may require a few more days of downtime and may require more intraoperative analgesia or anesthesia. It is important to match the correct technology with the needs and desires of the patient. In skin resurfacing, the patient's very specific goals, the genetic makeup of the patient's skin, the depth and location of the wrinkles or scars, the amount of dyschromia, and tolerance for downtime are important factors in choosing the right technology. The amount of heat delivered to the skin and the depth of that heat penetration are major determinants of the amount of collagen neogenesis. In practice, it seems that around 40 to 44°C is needed for collagen neogenesis. This can also be accomplished to a lesser extent for mild wrinkles and

loss of volume with a bipolar radiofrequency device and no downtime.

22.4 Histological Changes in Plasma Skin Resurfacing

The effect on collagen neogenesis and the mechanisms of healing with plasma skin resurfacing are directly related to the amount of energy delivered to the tissue.[5,6] The histological changes with this device have been most thoroughly studied with delivered energy over 2 joules (J) (the PSR[2], PSR[3], and PSR[2/3] protocols for the device).[5,6,7,8] With energies less than 2 J, slough of the epidermis and treated dermis actually takes longer.

The distribution of heat in the tissue dissipates, according to a predictable Gaussian distribution. Typically, it penetrates to 500 to 600 μm in normally hydrated skin at energies over 3.0 J.[7] This leads to two distinct, histologically visible areas in the skin, a so-called *inner zone of thermal damage* and an *outer zone of thermal modification* (▶ Fig. 22.2). Of particular note is that the epidermis (including the *stratum corneum*) remains largely intact.[5,6] Over time, a line of cleavage forms between these two zones, along which the epidermis and dermis will separate as the skin regenerates. Higher energy leads to a deeper line of cleavage. There is none of the vaporization of tissue seen with a carbon dioxide laser. Protection of this epidermis postoperatively leads to a very predictable slough along the line of cleavage, usually beginning 4 to 5 days after the treatment in energies above 2 J. With energies below 2 J, this process can take 10 days or so.

The preserved epidermis and *stratum corneum* act as a biological dressing. Heat distribution in the *zone of thermal modification* is sufficient to stimulate significant collagen neogenesis. ▶ Fig. 22.3 shows the early histological changes that occur in the epidermis and dermis with plasma energy applied at a typical treatment level of 3.5 J.

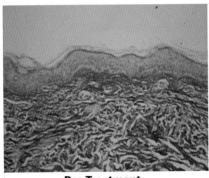
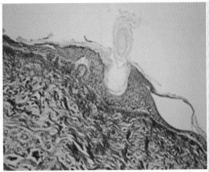

Pre-Treatment **Immediate Post-Treatment: 3.5J**

Fig. 22.3 The immediate effect of application of the nitrogen plasma is heating of the dermis and epidermis, leaving the stratum corneum intact. In clinical practice, the only smoke seen is from heating the hairs. (Courtesy of NeoGen by Energist Medical Group, Swansea, United Kingdom; formerly Portrait, Rhytec, Inc., Waltham, Massachusetts.)

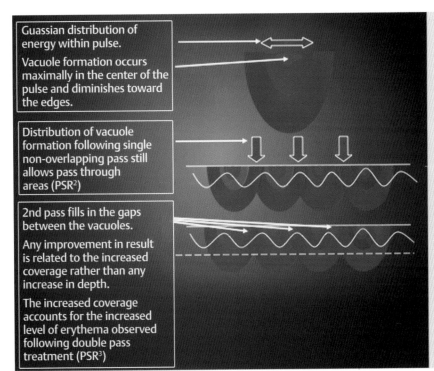

Guassian distribution of energy within pulse.

Vacuole formation occurs maximally in the center of the pulse and diminishes toward the edges.

Distribution of vacuole formation following single non-overlapping pass still allows pass through areas (PSR[2])

2nd pass fills in the gaps between the vacuoles.

Any improvement in result is related to the increased coverage rather than any increase in depth.

The increased coverage accounts for the increased level of erythema observed following double pass treatment (PSR[3])

Fig. 22.4 Effect of a double pass with energies greater than 2 J (PSR[3]). (Courtesy of NeoGen by Energist Medical Group, Swansea, United Kingdom; formerly Portrait, Rhytec, Inc., Waltham, Massachusetts.)

At energies above 2 J, vacuole formation is a prominent feature in the histology.[5,6,7] It is seen in some of the basal epidermal cells at the dermal-epidermal junction. The vacuoles appear to be air-filled spaces that insulate the dermis enough to permit a second pass of plasma without overheating the dermis to the point of irreparable damage. They seem to block deeper penetration of heat with the second pass.[5,6,7] With increasing energy, the depth of the *zones of thermal damage* and *thermal modification* increases, but the second pass at energies over 2 J only fills in the gaps between previously treated spots. It gives a more uniform treatment but not a deeper treatment (▶ Fig. 22.4). A line of skin cleavage forms between a newly regenerated epidermis and old epidermis around day 4 or 5 (▶ Fig. 22.5). The beginning of skin slough on days 4 and 5 is very predictable, and we tell all our patients when to expect this phenomenon. By days 7 to 10 there has been complete remodeling of the epidermis, and collagen neogenesis has begun. There is intense fibroblast activity and neovascularization in the *zone of thermal modification* in the deep dermis that

corresponds with the regeneration of the reticular architecture of the dermis. The *zone of thermal modification* in the upper papillary dermis is reactive. ▶ Fig. 22.6 is a polarized image that shows new collagen in the *zone of thermal modification.* These new collagen fibers assume their normal orientation perpendicular to the skin. Generally, this orientation is not seen with an ablative carbon dioxide laser treatment. By around 90 days, there is a very significant zone of collagen neogenesis at the dermal-epidermal junction (▶ Fig. 22.7).[5,6,7,8] Collagen neogenesis can continue for up to 1 year.

22.5 Plasma Resurfacing Technique

We have used this technology since 2006. Whether in a single treatment over 2 J (so-called *high-energy* treatment) or a multiple treatment approach at energies of or below 2 J (so-called *low-energy* treatment), there is well-documented

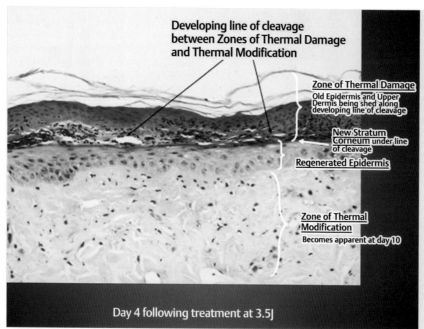

Developing line of cleavage between Zones of Thermal Damage and Thermal Modification

Zone of Thermal Damage
Old Epidermis and Upper Dermis being shed along developing line of cleavage

New Stratum Corneum under line of cleavage

Regenerated Epidermis

Zone of Thermal Modification
Becomes apparent at day 10

Day 4 following treatment at 3.5J

Fig. 22.5 Day 4 after a Portrait nitrogen plasma treatment with 3.5 J. Separation of old epidermis from the new epidermis along the line of cleavage that forms between the zones of thermal damage and thermal modification begins. Usually lasts until day 6 or 7. (Courtesy of NeoGen by Energist Medical Group, Swansea, United Kingdom; formerly Portrait, Rhytec, Inc., Waltham, Massachusetts.)

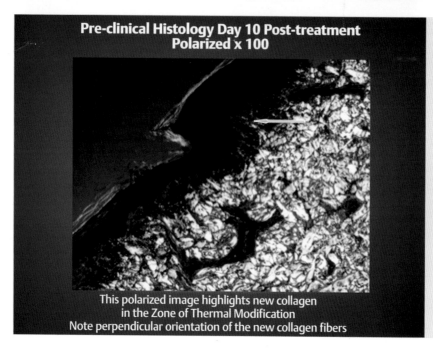

Pre-clinical Histology Day 10 Post-treatment Polarized x 100

This polarized image highlights new collagen in the Zone of Thermal Modification
Note perpendicular orientation of the new collagen fibers

Fig. 22.6 Here a polarized image shows the collagen neogenesis. Much of the new collagen in the dermis is oriented perpendicular to the epidermis. (Courtesy of NeoGen by Energist Medical Group, Swansea, United Kingdom; formerly Portrait, Rhytec, Inc., Waltham, Massachusetts.)

collagen neogenesis; significant decreases in facial rhytids; and overall improvement in the general appearance of facial, neck, chest, and dorsal hand skin.[5,7,8,9,10,11,12,13,14] Although it is claimed that plasma resurfacing can improve some acne scarring by as much as 34%,[10] we have never been able to duplicate this result. We have also not found it useful for deep upper lip wrinkles.

Holcomb et al[13] clearly demonstrated that plasma resurfacing, like carbon dioxide laser resurfacing, can be used simultaneously with facelift and cosmetic eyelid surgery in the properly chosen patient. They had specific recommendations for technique and energy levels.[13] The technique recommendations of Lam and Tzikas[14] published in 2008 are similar to ours.

22.6 Our Current Algorithm for Hyperpigmentation and Facial Rhytids

Whereas our objective is generally long-term efficacy, we also treat rhytids, dyschromia, and minimally depressed scars daily with temporary measures like botulinum toxin, superficial peels, and facial fillers. We treat dyschromia and facial rhytids with long-term measures that may include long-term skin-lightening regimens, Q-switched laser treatments, bipolar radiofrequency procedures, plasma skin resurfacing, fractionated carbon dioxide laser resurfacing, and ablative carbon dioxide laser resurfacing.
► Table 22.1 is our current algorithm for skin rejuvenation.

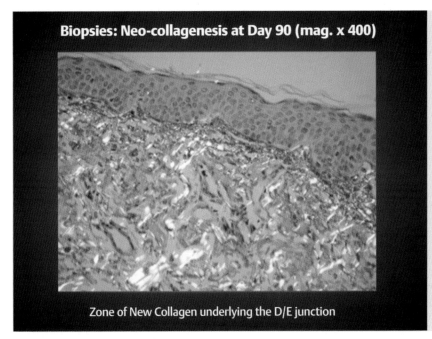

Biopsies: Neo-collagenesis at Day 90 (mag. x 400)

Zone of New Collagen underlying the D/E junction

Fig. 22.7 Plentiful collagen neogenesis at 90 days, much of it perpendicularly oriented. D/E, dermal/epidermal. (Courtesy of NeoGen by Energist Medical Group, Swansea, United Kingdom; formerly Portrait, Rhytec, Inc., Waltham, Massachusetts.)

Table 22.1 The author's current algorithm for skin rejuvenation

Rejuvenation needed	Skin type	Treatment
Hyperpigmentation	Fitzpatrick skin types I–VI	Superficial skin peels (Fitzpatrick skin types I–III only), hydroquinone and tretinoin-based skin care products, Q-switched laser at 532 nm, or plasma skin resurfacing
Mild rhytids around the eyes	Fitzpatrick skin types I–VI, wrinkle severity rating scale (WSRS) 1 and 2[15]	Bipolar radiofrequency
Mild-to-moderate facial rhytids	Fitzpatrick skin types I–IV, WSRS 1 through 3	Plasma skin resurfacing
		Fractionated carbon dioxide laser resurfacing may be recommended for the lower eyelids and crow's-feet in conjunction with a transconjunctival lower eyelid blepharoplasty with fat transposition or as an isolated treatment.
Mild-to-moderate facial rhytids + hyperpigmentation	Fitzpatrick skin types I–IV, WSRS 1 through 3	Plasma skin resurfacing
Moderate-to-severe facial rhytids	Fitzpatrick skin types I–III, WSRS 3 through 5	Carbon dioxide laser resurfacing, fractionated and fully ablative
Moderate-to-severe facial rhytids + hyperpigmentation	Fitzpatrick skin types I–III, WSRS 3 through 5	Carbon dioxide laser resurfacing for deeper rhytids is sometimes combined with plasma skin resurfacing to areas with less deep rhytids for a more even, concomitant treatment of hyperpigmentation.
Long-term follow-up therapy		We recommend long-term follow-up with tretinoin-based products and intermittent use of hydroquinone to maintain uniform skin color. About 50% of the patients adhere to these recommendations.

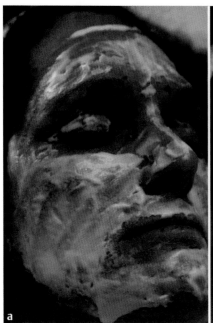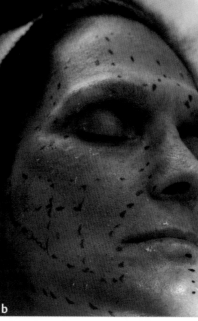

Fig. 22.8 (a) Topical anesthetic cream, and (b) grid to guide the treatment.

22.7 Our Protocol for Plasma Skin Resurfacing

22.7.1 Skin Preparation

In accordance with the original manufacturer's protocols, tretinoin or retinols are discontinued for 4 to 6 weeks before the treatment. We have not verified that this is actually necessary. Before recommending any resurfacing technique, a thorough family history and personal history of how a patient's skin reacts to the sun, injury, and heat are important. Specifically, it is essential to determine the patient's propensity for postinflammatory hyperpigmentation. In New England, we see many patients who appear to have Fitzpatrick skin type III with a significant propensity for hyperpigmentation. Patients of European lineage mixed with Native American ancestry and French Canadian lineage mixed with Native American ancestry are commonplace in New England. Although they may appear to have Fitzpatrick skin type III, we often treat these patients as we would patients with Fitzpatrick skin type IV (see specific treatment protocols in a subsequent section). Whereas we routinely pretreat our carbon dioxide laser resurfacing patients with tretinoin and hydroquinone, we typically treat our plasma resurfacing patients with just hydroquinone. We do not want to thin the *stratum corneum*. Patients are pretreated with 4% hydroquinone for 4 to 6 weeks before the procedure. Hydroquinone is restarted 7 to 10 days after the treatment. We typically restart tretinoin at 3 months postoperative.

22.7.2 Infection Prophylaxis

Viral and bacterial prophylaxis is similar to what we use for the carbon dioxide laser. All patients receiving perioral treatments are started on valacyclovir hydrochloride 1 gm daily for 7 days, starting the day of treatment for *herpes simplex* prophylaxis. All patients are placed on bacterial prophylaxis for 7 days starting the day of treatment. The incidence of methicillin-resistant

Staphylococcus aureus in our community has led to a change from cephalexin prophylaxis to doxycycline or clindamycin in the last 2 years.

22.7.3 Anesthesia

We treat the majority of our patients using topical anesthesia or topical plus subcutaneous local anesthesia in our office procedure room. We also offer the patient 5 to 10 mg of oral diazepam and oxycodone 5 mg, 1 hour prior to the procedure. Our music or the patient's choice of music plays the entire time the patient is in the treatment room. If a patient requests more sedation or general anesthesia, we do the procedure in the same-day surgery unit of our hospital. Our office is located in the same building.

22.7.4 Skin Preparation Day of Surgery

- ▶ Fig. 22.8 illustrates the application of topical anesthetic before the procedure and the grid used to ensure uniform treatment. Consistent with the original investigations, we hydrate the skin for 1 hour before the treatment with a topical anesthetic cream. If the patient is under general anesthesia, an occlusive ointment like Aquaphor (Beiersdorf Inc., Wilton, Connecticut) is just as good. Our current topical anesthetic cream of benzocaine, tetracaine, and lidocaine comes from a local compounding pharmacy and is a ratio of 20:10:10%. If treating without this period of hydration, the energy applied should be decreased about 30%, again consistent with the original Rhytec protocol.

- For treatments of 2 J or less, topical anesthetic alone is usually sufficient.

- For higher energy treatments over 2 J, we use regional blocks and direct infiltration with a total of 15 to 20 mL of 0.5% lidocaine, 1:200,000 epinephrine about 10 minutes before the end of the hydration period. The author blocks all three branches of the trigeminal nerve plus the entire length of the brows, an area of about 4 cm² in front of the tragus, the entire lower eyelid, and about a 1.5-cm wide area along the mandible from the angle of the jaw to the mentum. For the upper lip, an upper dental block is placed, usually after a topical oral anesthetic gel like HurriCaine® (Beutlich Pharmaceuticals, Waukegan, Illinois).

- After removing the topical anesthetic cream with a moist sponge, we draw the grid on the skin with a temporary marker to help ensure that the energy is delivered uniformly. Since this treatment is not chromophore-dependent, the marker can be any color.

22.7.5 Skin Care during Treatment

- We often apply an ice pack to the first side of the face treated, while treating the opposite side. A cooling device that blows cool air also works well.
- The eyes and teeth are protected with moist sponges or by using a slightly bent moist tongue depressor. Plastic scleral shields are safe, but stainless steel scleral shields are contraindicated because of potential heat transmission to the cornea.
- The treatment preserves the *stratum corneum,* and this acts as a biological dressing until the epidermis is regenerated.

22.7.6 Skin Care Posttreatment

- To protect the *stratum corneum,* we apply a petroleum-based ointment (Aquaphor) immediately after the treatment and place a cool gel pack on top of the ointment for 15 to 30 minutes before discharging the patient. The skin is protected from the mask by soft gauze.

22.7.7 Posttreatment Pain Treatment

- This should not be a very painful procedure postoperatively. The pain feels like an intense sunburn and it is usually gone in 1 to 4 hours. The combination of petroleum and ice act as a very effective heat sink, rapidly decreasing the burning sensation. Most patients take oxycodone one time the evening of the procedure and some acetaminophen, 650 to 1,000 mg, or ibuprofen after that. Generally, no pain medication is needed after the first evening. If a patient complains of significant pain the next day, we would become concerned about a possible *herpes simplex* infection. We have never seen such an infection after this procedure, however.

22.7.8 Specific Treatment Protocols

Areas inside the grid marked on the patient's face are treated in rows. Unlike with some lasers, the rows are never laid down in a back and forth manner. According to the original Rhytec protocol, when one row is finished, the next row is started at an adjoining area to the start of the just finished row. This technique is felt necessary to allow for the vacuole formation in already treated areas that protects the dermis from excessive heat delivery. Rhytec also established a specific nomenclature for types of treatments. The choice of treatment protocol depends on the patient's aesthetic goals, the amount of

downtime the patient will tolerate, and the perceived or actual Fitzpatrick skin type:

- PSR[1]—1 to 2 J per pulse in a single pass
- PSR[2]—2 to 4 J per pulse in a single pass
- PSR[3]—2 to 4 J per pulse in a double pass
- PSR[2/3]—PSR[2] and PSR[3] to different parts of the face at the same time

22.7.9 For Fitzpatrick Skin Types I to III

- The *upper eyelids* we treat with a single pass of 2 to 3.3 J (PSR[1] or PSR[2]).
- The *lower eyelids* we treat with two passes at 3.3 to 3.4 J (PSR[3]).
- The *neck, chest, hands,* and *forearms* we treat with a single pass below 2.0 J (PSR[1]) in one to two separate treatment sessions 4 to 6 weeks apart.
- Other areas of the face with thin skin or over bony prominences of the face, like the *superior orbital rim, jawline lateral to the jowl (about a 1.5- to 2-cm wide area anterior to the ear),* and *forehead,* we treat with a single pass (PSR[2]) of usually about 3.3 to 3.5 J.
- The *glabella, nose, upper lip, lower lip/chin,* and the *medial, malar* and *inframalar cheeks,* we generally treat with a double pass (PSR[3]) of 3.3 to 3.8 J. In the PSR[3] protocol the second pass is done at right angles to the first pass. It is done to assure maximum coverage without gaps of untreated skin.

22.7.10 For Fitzpatrick Skin Type IV

Patients with Fitzpatrick skin type IV and some patients with Fitzpatrick skin type III of Native American or mixed Mediterranean lineage, with a significant propensity for hyperpigmentation, usually we treat in a series of lower energy procedures of 1.3 to 2 J in a single pass (PSR[1]) spaced 4 to 6 weeks apart. These patients usually have a primary complaint of diffuse hyperpigmentation. They typically require three to four sessions. We resume hydroquinone 7 to 8 days after peeling. If, after the first two or three low-energy treatments, no evidence of persistent postinflammatory hyperpigmentation is seen and the patient desires more aggressive therapy, another treatment at 2.5 to 3.4 J may be done. The patient must understand and accept the risks of this variation from standard protocol. The patients in ▶ Fig. 22.9 and ▶ Fig. 22.10 are examples of this more aggressive therapy.

22.7.11 Postoperative Period

- As with our laser resurfacing patients, we see all our patients 24 hours after the treatment. We do not allow them to wash their faces for 24 hours.
- Aquaphor should be applied very generously with a vinyl glove. We instruct all our patients in the technique prior to discharge from the procedure but most require repeat instruction at their first postoperative visit.
- After the first 24 hours, we encourage the patient to wash very gently with a mild face wash three times a day and let lukewarm water run over the face in the shower. We are very clear in our instructions for the patient to avoid rubbing and itching. The intact *stratum corneum* is a very important

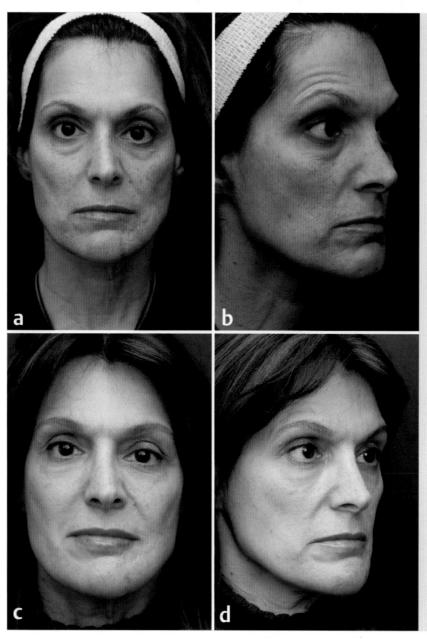

Fig. 22.9 A 53-year-old woman with Fitzpatrick skin type IV (**a, b**) at time of treatment. Treated initially with three treatments 1 month apart at 1.3, 1.6, and 1.9 J. Treated at 3.0 J, 4 months after third procedure. The postoperative photos (**c, d**) are 5 years after the last treatment. (She had a W-plasty of a left chin scar after the last treatment and a transconjunctival lower eyelid blepharoplasty with fat transposition 6 months before the last photo.)

biological dressing, and our patients seem to understand this. Protective Aquaphor is reapplied after each face wash.

- Downtime is always a major issue for patients, so we try to be very realistic about this. With energies above 2 J (PSR[2], PSR[3], or PSR[2/3]), the epidermis very predictably begins to shed in 4 to 5 days and can be completely regenerated in 7 to 8 days. With energies below 2 J (PSR[1]), it can be 2 to 4 days more.
- If there is no significant erythema, we start a mild moisturizer or calming skin care product once the old epidermis has peeled. Sunscreen (sun protection factor [SPF] 50 or above) and a mineral makeup may be used once the patient has stopped peeling.
- If the patient has more significant erythema than is typical, we prescribe desonide ointment or cream twice daily for 10 days. We do not believe that this short course of low-concentration corticosteroid has a negative effect on collagen neogenesis.

- ▶ Fig. 22.11 illustrates a typical postoperative course after a PSR[2/3] treatment, with more than a 4-year follow-up.

22.8 Choosing the Right Patient for Plasma Skin Resurfacing

For maximum wrinkle reduction with rhytids grades 4 and 5 (wrinkle severity rating scale [WSRS][15]), generally we use a fractionated carbon dioxide laser in multiple passes to achieve significant ablation or in the fully ablative mode. Downtime is usually 8 to 10 days. In our experience, the best candidates for plasma resurfacing are patients who desire no more than 1 week of downtime and whose skin can be characterized as follows:

- Grades 1 through 3 wrinkles (WSRS)

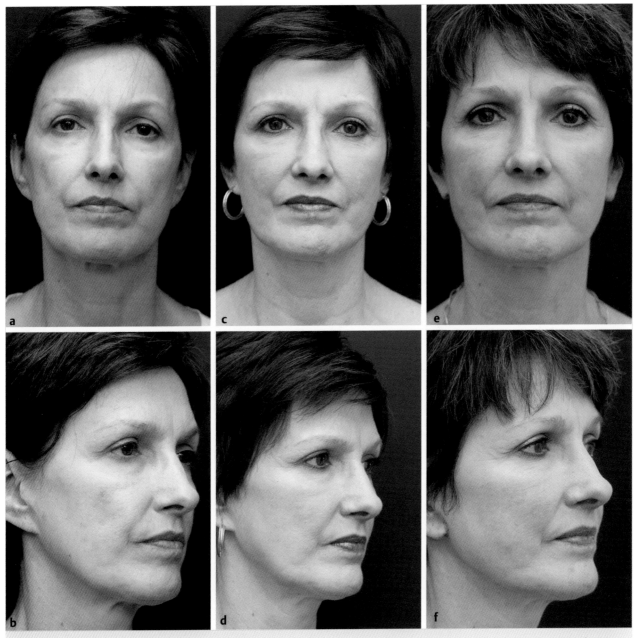

Fig. 22.10 A 56-year-old woman who, at time of treatment, wanted her skin to be clearer and less sallow. She had three treatments 1 month apart at 1.6, 2.0, and 3.3 J, respectively. Also, at the second procedure, the darker spots on her cheeks were treated separately with 3.3 J. Photos are (**a, b**) preoperative, (**c, d**) 4 months postoperative, and (**e, f**) 25 months after the last treatment. There is some pinkness in her skin from recent retinol use and peeling.

- Hyperpigmentation
- Fitzpatrick skin types I through IV

As with any device, it is important not to promise more than the technology can achieve. We learned this early in our experience with this instrument.

22.9 Patient Results

Perhaps the best way to judge the efficacy of this procedure is with a series of photos. In choosing these photos, we made an effort to bring back subjects with as long a follow-up period as possible. Lighting conditions were constant for all photos and automatically white-balanced. Lighter skin color tends to reflect the light more and lighten the photos. Some are the same patients from the author's 2012 publication[1] but with further follow-up. The postoperative protocol for skin care products with this procedure is the same for our laser resurfacing patients and generally includes the long-term, pulsed use of products containing 4% hydroquinone, and tretinoin or retinol in medically therapeutic concentrations.

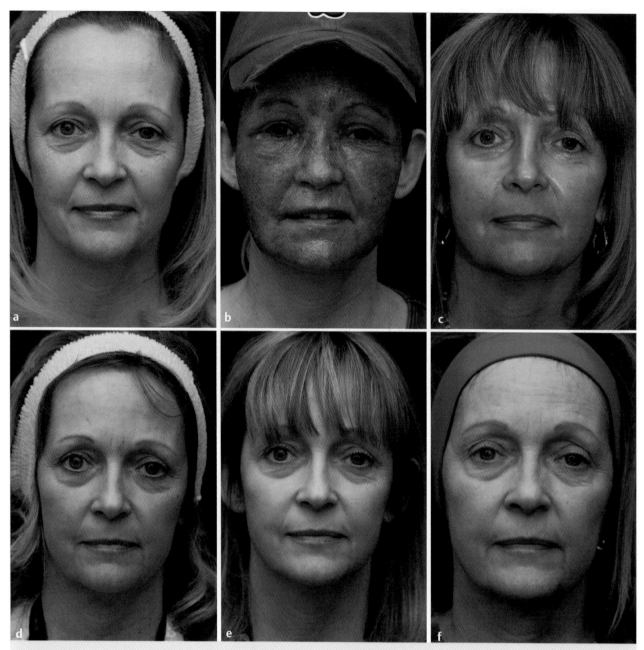

Fig. 22.11 At time of treatment, a 51-year-old woman, Fitzpatrick skin type II, PSR$^{2/3}$ utilized with 3.3 to 3.6 J. Images show a typical healing progression for plasma skin resurfacing. Photos are (**a**) preoperative, (**b**) 1 day postoperative, (**c**) 1 week after treatment, (**d**) 2 weeks postoperative, (**e**) 10 months after, and (**f**) 49 months later.

22.9.1 Who Not to Treat

With shorter downtime, less procedure discomfort, and potentially lower cost, a plasma treatment often appeals to patients in their late 60s or early-to-late 70s. We have found this particularly true if they have done little or nothing to protect or treat their skin previously. Plasma resurfacing is usually not the right choice for these patients. Their rhytids are often too deep and their potential for collagen neogenesis too weak. We have also never been able to equal the degree of improvement in deep upper lip rhytids with plasma resurfacing that we see with the carbon dioxide laser (for smokers, former smokers, and nonsmokers).

22.9.2 Some Reasonable Candidates for Plasma Skin Resurfacing

▶ Fig. 22.9, ▶ Fig. 22.10, ▶ Fig. 22.11, ▶ Fig. 22.12, ▶ Fig. 22.13, ▶ Fig. 22.14 and ▶ Fig. 22.15 show typical results for patients who meet our current criteria for treatment. The only makeup permitted for the photos are lipstick and eyeliner.

The patient in ▶ Fig. 22.11 illustrates a normal progression of early healing for a PSR$^{2/3}$ treatment and a long-term result at more than 4 years. She was treated at 3.3 to 3.6 J.

In ▶ Fig. 22.9 is a patient of Portuguese lineage with Fitzpatrick skin type IV. She was 53 years old at the time of her

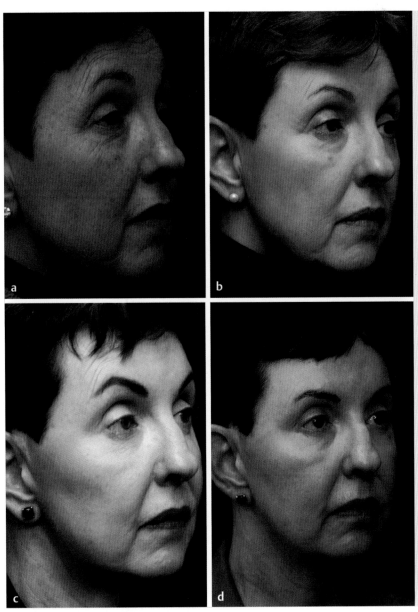

Fig. 22.12 This woman was age 53 at the time of her initial treatment. She was treated with the PSR³ protocol at 3.3 to 3.6 J. At 14 months after the procedure, she had a facelift with a touch-up treatment at 2.3 joules. (**a**) Before treatment. The postoperative photos shown are at (**b**) 1 year, (**c**) 44 months and (**d**) 53 months after the initial treatment.

treatments. Because of her darker skin type, we planned a series of lower energy procedures (PSR¹) 1 month apart. The three sessions were at 1.3, 1.6, and 1.9 J, respectively. Although she saw overall improvement in the quality and texture of her skin along with a modest generalized decrease in hyperpigmentation, she wanted a more profound decrease in the hyperpigmentation after her initial three treatments. The woman wanted her skin to be as close to its color as a teenager and young adult as possible. Therefore, 4 months after the last PSR¹ treatment, we decided to do a fourth treatment at 3.0 J with the PSR²ᐟ³ protocol for further overall lightening of her skin. We discussed the higher risk of postinflammatory hyperpigmentation again before the procedure. She developed some transient postinflammatory hyperpigmentation of her lower eyelids 1 month after this high-energy treatment. This resolved within 30 days by just staying on the same hydroquinone preparation she had been using. The postoperative photos are at 5 years after her last treatment. She underwent a transconjunctival lower lid

blepharoplasty with fat transposition 6 months before the latest photos.

The woman in ▶ Fig. 22.10 had very specific requests. She had experienced multiple skin treatments at other practices prior to plasma. Besides some brown spots on her face, she was bothered by the overall dull and sallow appearance of her skin. By history and lineage she was a Fitzpatrick skin type IV. As with the patient in ▶ Fig. 22.9, we did not adhere to the standard protocol for Fitzpatrick skin type IV. She too wanted maximum clarity in her skin and was willing to risk postinflammatory hyperpigmentation to get there. This treatment, as with the previous patient, "pushed the envelope" so to speak. She started with two low-energy treatments at 1.6 and 2.0 J, 1 month apart. At the second treatment, however, she also had a double pass of 3.3 J (PSR³) to persisting individual brown spots. Her last treatment was a single pass at 3.3 J (PSR²). She experienced no postinflammatory hyperpigmentation. In the set of pictures at 25 months there is some pinkness in her

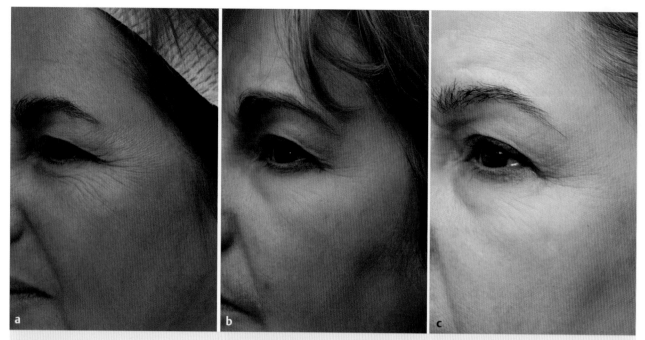

Fig. 22.13 A 52-year-old woman at time of treatment, Fitzpatrick skin type III. PSR$^{2/3}$ technique used with a single pass of 3.2 J to upper eyelids and 3.4 J double pass to lower eyelids and crow's-feet area. (a) Before, (b) 18 months after, and (c) 5 years postoperative.

medial right cheek related to too high a dose of recent retinol use. She was also peeling in that area.

The woman in ▶ Fig. 22.12 was age 53 at the time of her treatment. Her procedure was in accordance with our standard protocols for Fitzpatrick skin type III. She was treated with the PSR^3 protocol at 3.3 to 3.6 J. Like many of our patients, she has been maintained on a hydroquinone or tretinoin regimen since 3 months postoperative. On more than one occasion, strangers have stopped her in stores to comment on the clarity of her skin. At 14 months after her initial plasma treatment she had a superficial muscular aponeurotic system (SMAS) flap facelift and transconjunctival lower lid blepharoplasty with fat transposition. At that time, she also had a touch-up treatment to her temples and peri-oral area (2.3 J). She receives botulinum toxin to the glabella and forehead, calcium hydroxyl apatite to the melolabial creases and midface periodically, and hyaluronic acid to fine lines of her forehead intermittently. The postoperative photos shown are at 1 year, 44 months, and 53 months after the initial treatment. There is significant persistence of overall, uniform improvement in skin color and texture along with a persistent loss of periocular and malar rhytids. At 53 months, there is some return of fine rhytids and some mild dyschromia.

The woman in ▶ Fig. 22.13 was age 52 at the time of her treatment. She has Fitzpatrick skin type III and was treated with the PSR$^{2/3}$ protocol at 3.2 to 3.4 J. She had a single pass on the upper eyelids at 3.2 J and a double pass on the lower eyelids and crow's-feet area at 3.4 J. She does not use any products recommended by us. The postoperative photos are at 18 months and 5 years. The images focus on the results around her eyes. In this case, there was some contracture of the excess skin of her upper eyelids that persists even at 5 years.

The patient in ▶ Fig. 22.14 was age 46 at the time of her treatment. She has Fitzpatrick skin type II and was treated with the PSR$^{2/3}$ protocol at 3.3 to 3.5 J. She was maintained on a vitamin C and hydroquinone system without tretinoin and stopped a few months before the last photos (▶ Fig. 22.14e, f). The postoperative photos are at 2 years and 5.5 years. At 5.5 years there is very good persistence of overall improvement in skin color and texture; however, the patient would probably benefit from a touch-up treatment for the periocular rhytids and a lower lid blepharoplasty with fat transposition.

The patient in ▶ Fig. 22.15 with Fitzpatrick skin type III was treated for large pore size and skin brightening, PSR$^{2/3}$ at 3.3 to 3.5 J. The photos focus on her pore-size improvement. Postoperative photo is at 40 months.

22.10 Conclusion: Plasma Resurfacing Is Still a Relevant and Very Useful Technology

Nitrogen plasma skin regeneration is a skin-resurfacing technique that offers excellent improvement of mild-to-moderate skin rhytids on the wrinkle severity rating scale (WSRS) of 1 to 3, and excellent overall skin rejuvenation in patients with Fitzpatrick skin types I to IV. It is especially efficacious for Fitzpatrick skin types I and II. It also provides excellent improvement in uniformity of skin color and texture in patients with hyperpigmentation and Fitzpatrick skin types I through IV.

22.10.1 Severity of Wrinkles Treated with Plasma

We position this technology between radiofrequency skin tightening for fine lines only (Pelleve, Ellman International, Inc., Hicksville, New York) and fractionated or fully ablative carbon

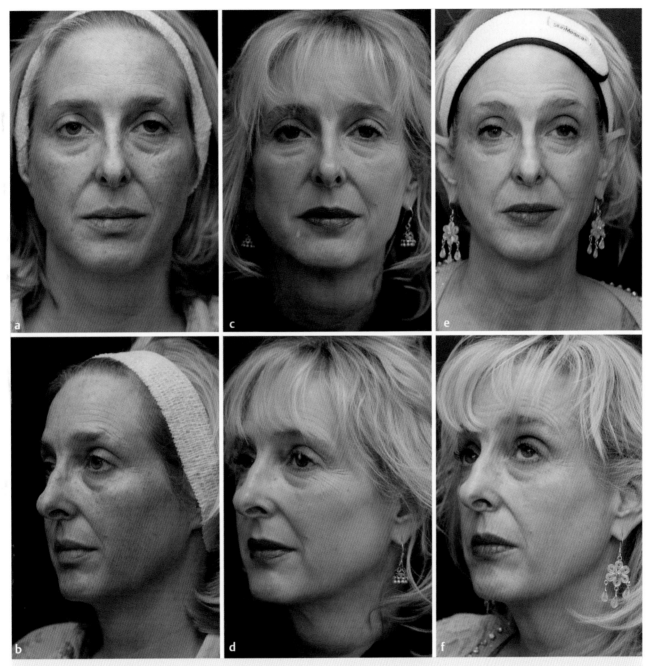

Fig. 22.14 A woman of age 46 at time of treatment. Her primary complaint was hyper-pigmentation and uneven color in her skin. Fitzpatrick skin type II, PSR$^{2/3}$, 3.3 to 3.5 J. (a, b) Before treatment, (c, d) 2 years after, and (e, f) 5.5 years postoperative.

dioxide laser resurfacing for deep wrinkles. We use the radio-frequency treatments for patients of all Fitzpatrick skin types and WSRS grades 1 and 2.

We recommend plasma resurfacing for patients with WSRS grades 1 through 3, and for those with, most commonly, concomitant hyperpigmentation. We also recommend it for pore reduction. We have found plasma resurfacing disappointing for deep upper lip rhytids and not as efficacious as the carbon dioxide laser for acne scars.

We use the fractionated and fully ablative carbon dioxide laser for patients with grades 1 through 5 on the WSRS with or without hyperpigmentation. The laser is also our preferred modality for treating upper lip rhytids and acne scars on Fitzpatrick skin types I through III.

22.10.2 Risk of HypoPigmentation and PostInflammatory HyperPigmentation

We have not seen any hypopigmentation or permanent postinflammatory hyperpigmentation with plasma resurfacing. We are very proactive with hydroquinone in all skin types. Although perhaps not necessary with the Fitzpatrick skin types I and II, this preparation allows us to maximize the energy delivered. Most of the patients we treat with Fitzpatrick skin

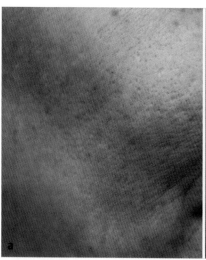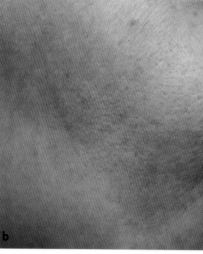

Fig. 22.15 A 54-year old woman at time of treatment, Fitzpatrick III, treated to decrease pore size and for brightening of the skin. PSR[2/3] used at 3.3 to 3.5 J. (**a**) Preoperative and (**b**) 40 months postoperative.

type III come to us, at least partially, because of their hyperpigmentation. In patients with Fitzpatrick skin type IV, the hydroquinone is absolutely necessary. As illustrated with the patient in ▶ Fig. 22.10, Fitzpatrick skin type IV requires a protocol of three to four low-energy treatments ranging usually from 1.3 to 2 J. If a patient with Fitzpatrick skin type IV wants more dramatic wrinkle and hyperpigmentation reduction, we may choose to do another treatment at 3 J or slightly above. The patient must be prepared to risk some postinflammatory hyperpigmentation, but it has never been permanent.

22.10.3 Patient Expectations for Wrinkle Reduction

As with any minimally invasive procedure, setting realistic expectations is very important. If a patient wants maximum wrinkle reduction, the carbon dioxide laser may be a better choice; however, Fitzpatrick skin type IV is an obstacle that usually stops us from treating a patient with the laser. The author still believes that full ablation for severe rhytids with the laser is more comfortable with sedation or general anesthesia, so cost can become a factor in the patient's decision. If the patient is more concerned about skin quality and color than wrinkles, we recommend plasma, and we will treat Fitzpatrick skin type IV in those patients. Patients in their late 60 s and older are not good candidates for plasma resurfacing. Generally, the collagen neogenesis generated by plasma resurfacing in this population is insufficient.

22.10.4 Qualitative Results of Plasma Resurfacing

It is the author's opinion that overall skin radiance, clarity, and uniformity of color with plasma resurfacing is superior to that with the carbon dioxide laser, fractional or fully ablative. We have not presented such comparison photos here; that should be the subject of a separate chapter with blinded observers. We have not seen any of the hypopigmentation with plasma that can be a rare sequela (in our practice) of a deep carbon dioxide laser resurfacing. In plasma-treated patients where the skin has been lightened, it has been purposefully and uniformly

lightened, consistently closer to the color of the patient's facial skin as a teenager (confirmed by patient affirmation and younger photos). Because of what we perceive as better radiance and luminescence with plasma resurfacing, we often use it for cheek and forehead rejuvenation, while using the carbon dioxide laser for deep perioral or periocular rhytids.

References

[1] Bentkover SH. Plasma skin resurfacing: personal experience and long-term results. Facial Plast Surg Clin North Am 2012; 20: 145–162, v–vi

[2] UltraPulse AcuPulse. Specifications of Lumenis UltraPulse® Laser. Lumenis group of companies. 23 Mar 2011. Available at: http://www.aesthetic.lumenis.com/pdf/FINALCO2FamilyBrochure23Mar11.pdf. Accessed November 6, 2011

[3] Lukac M, Perhavec T, Nemes K, Ahcan U. Ablation and thermal depths in VSP Er:YAG laser skin resurfacing. J Laser Health Acad. 2010; 2010(1): 56–71

[4] Rahman Z, Alam M, Dover JS. Fractional laser treatment for pigmentation and texture improvement. Skin Therapy Lett 2006; 11: 7–11

[5] Fitzpatrick R, Bernstein E, Iyer S, Brown D, Andrews P, Penny K. A histopathologic evaluation of the plasma skin regeneration system (PSR) versus a standard carbon dioxide resurfacing laser in an animal model. Lasers Surg Med 2008; 40: 93–99

[6] Tremblay JF, Moy R. Treatment of post-auricular skin using a novel plasma resurfacing system: an in vivo clinical and histologic study[abstract]. Lasers Surg Med 2004; 34 suppl 16: 25

[7] Foster KW, Moy RL, Fincher EF. Advances in plasma skin regeneration. J Cosmet Dermatol 2008; 7: 169–179

[8] Bogle MA, Arndt KA, Dover JS. Evaluation of plasma skin regeneration technology in low-energy full-facial rejuvenation. Arch Dermatol 2007; 143: 168–174

[9] Alster TS, Konda S. Plasma skin resurfacing for regeneration of neck, chest, and hands: investigation of a novel device. Dermatol Surg 2007; 33: 1315–1321

[10] Gonzalez MJ, Sturgill WH, Ross EV, Uebelhoer NS. Treatment of acne scars using the plasma skin regeneration (PSR) system. Lasers Surg Med 2008; 40: 124–127

[11] Elsaie ML, Kammer JN. Evaluation of plasma skin regeneration technology for cutaneous remodeling. J Cosmet Dermatol 2008; 7: 309–311

[12] Groff WF, Fitzpatrick RE, Uebelhoer NS. Fractional carbon dioxide laser and plasmakinetic skin resurfacing. Semin Cutan Med Surg 2008; 27: 239–251

[13] Holcomb JD, Kent KJ, Rousso DE. Nitrogen plasma skin regeneration and aesthetic facial surgery: multicenter evaluation of concurrent treatment. Arch Facial Plast Surg 2009; 11: 184–193

[14] Lam SM, Tzikas TL. Plasma skin resurfacing. In: Shiffman MA, Mirrafati SJ, Lam SM, Cueteaux CG, eds. Simplified Facial Rejuvenation. New York, NY: Springer; 2008: 179–182

[15] Day DJ, Littler CM, Swift RW, Gottlieb S. The wrinkle severity rating scale: a validation study. Am J Clin Dermatol 2004; 5: 49–52

23 Radiofrequency Skin Tightening

Manoj T. Abraham and Neha A. Patel

23.1 Introduction

As modern technologies continue to flourish, there are more and more techniques now available for safer and more effective skin rejuvenation. Traditional methods for nonsurgical skin rejuvenation (such as chemical peels, dermabrasion, and laser resurfacing) are ablative, and involve removing the surface of the skin. However, these more aggressive procedures are associated with complications such as pigmentary changes, scarring, infection, and prolonged recovery. As a result, nonablative methods of skin rejuvenation have gained popularity, both alone and in combination with the other less invasive procedures such as neurotoxins and dermal fillers.[1] Commonly used nonablative skin rejuvenation modalities include radiofrequency (RF), ultrasound, intense pulsed light (IPL), and nonablative lasers. The focus of this chapter is on transcutaneous nonablative radiofrequency (TNRF) skin rejuvenation techniques.

Electromagnetic radiation is released by the flow of charged particles creating an oscillating electrical current. The RF spectrum falls within the 3 kHz to 300 GHz frequency range (► Fig. 23.1), and is assigned for use by medical devices including electrocautery. When the current is applied to tissue, it is transformed into thermal energy (heat) due to tissue resistance to particle movement. The therapeutic benefit of RF treatment is based on this tissue-heating effect. When the RF energy is high intensity and focal, cutting and coagulation are achieved as with electrocautery. Most TNRF skin-rejuvenation devices apply the energy over a broad surface, and concurrently cool the skin surface to protect the epidermis. A reverse thermal gradient is created that allows the heat to be targeted to the dermis and deeper tissues (► Fig. 23.2).[2]

TNRF can be delivered using monopolar, unipolar, bipolar, or newer multipolar devices (► Table 23.1).[3] Monopolar RF instruments require the patient to be grounded and are more deeply penetrating because the current follows the path of least resistance through the skin and deeper tissues and out through the grounding pad. Unipolar RF delivery has one electrode but does not require a separate grounding pad because the grounding plate is within the treatment head. Transcutaneous bipolar devices by their nature penetrate only superficially because the current travels between two surface electrodes (► Fig. 23.3). Variations include needle electrodes that can be inserted into the dermis, which provides for a subdermal as opposed to a truly transcutaneous delivery of energy. The newer multipolar devices combine both unipolar and bipolar energy delivery using multiple electrodes and sophisticated computer algorithms to control the flow of the current; however, the treatment remains more superficial because this energy flow is contained within the treatment tip. The depth of RF penetration can be further modulated by factors such as tissue resistance, and is inversely proportional to the frequency of RF used.

Tissue heating has various effects based on the depth of the tissue targeted. Heating the dermis causes partial denaturation of the skin collagen scaffold with contraction of this framework in the x, y plane as the collagen reanneals, leading to initial skin tightening.[4] This process also stimulates inflammation and a wound-healing response that ultimately results in increased skin collagen production and epidermal thickening (► Fig. 23.4).[5] When monopolar RF is used, energy conduction via collagenous fibrous septa in the deep dermis and tightening of these structures allows for three-dimensional contouring and lifting of the skin (► Fig. 23.5). Additional heating of the fat layer can lead to selective adipose apoptosis, allowing for further contouring.

TNRF was first approved by the U.S. Food and Drug Administration (FDA) in 2002 for the reduction of forehead wrinkles with the Thermage (Solta Medical, Inc., Hayward, California) device (► Fig. 23.6).[6] Since then, many other TNRF tools have been approved for various skin rejuvenation indications

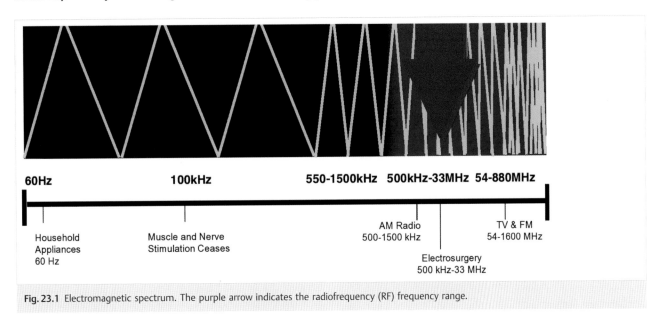

60Hz   **100kHz**   **550-1500kHz**   **500kHz-33MHz**   **54-880MHz**

Household
Appliances
60 Hz

Muscle and Nerve
Stimulation Ceases

AM Radio
500-1500 kHz

TV & FM
54-1600 MHz

Electrosurgery
500 kHz-33 MHz

Fig. 23.1 Electromagnetic spectrum. The purple arrow indicates the radiofrequency (RF) frequency range.

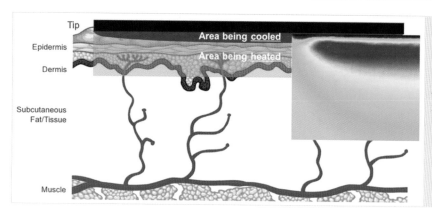

Fig. 23.2 The reverse thermal gradient is depicted in this image. The skin surface is cooled and bypassed, allowing the heat to be delivered only to the deeper levels of the tissue. Inset at right is a thermogram showing the reverse thermal gradient that is created. (Courtesy of Solta Medical, Inc., Hayward, California.)

Table 23.1 Signature radiofrequency skin rejuvenation devices and technologies

MONOPOLAR
Thermage (Solta Medical, Inc., Hayward, California)
Exilis (BTL, Prague, Czech Republic)
truSculpt (Cutera, Brisbane, California)
Pelleve (Ellman International, Inc., Hicksville, New York)
ThermiRF (ThermiAesthetics, Dallas, Texas)

UNIPOLAR
Accent (Alma Lasers, Inc., Ft. Lauderdale, Florida)

BIPOLAR
Elos (Syneron Medical Ltd., Yokneam, Israel)
Aluma (Lumenis Inc., Santa Clara, California)
BodyFX (Invasix, Richmond Hill, Ontario, Canada)

MULTIPOLAR
Regen (Pollogen Ltd., Jerusalem, Israel)
Reaction (Viora, Jersey City, New Jersey)
Freeze (Venus Concepts, Scottsdale, Arizona)
EndyMed (EndyMed Medical Ltd., Caesarea, Israel)

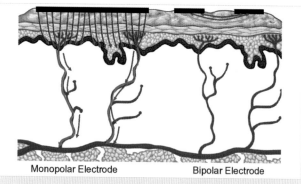

Fig. 23.3 Difference between monopolar and bipolar transcutaneous nonablative radiofrequency (TNRF) treatment. With monopolar treatment, the current (arrows) flows deeper into the skin. With bipolar treatment, the depth of penetration is more bowl-shaped and about one half the distance between the electrodes.

(▶ Table 23.1). In this time span, the Thermage mechanism has evolved over multiple generations and treatment protocols to optimize results, provide more consistency, increase treatment comfort, and decrease the risk of complications.

23.2 Advantages/Disadvantages

A distinct advantage TNRF has over comparable transcutaneous nonablative laser and IPL skin-rejuvenation techniques is that TNRF does not depend on the absorption of light or laser energy by skin chromophores to have a therapeutic effect. Thus, TNRF energy can penetrate more deeply, and can be used with all Fitzpatrick skin types without concern for unsafe levels of energy absorption in patients with tanned or darker skin. Other modalities such as ultrasound and certain nonablative lasers that use energy outside of the visible spectrum, such as infrared, also share this advantage. Conversely, treatments such as TNRF, which target the deeper levels of the skin but bypass and protect the skin surface, do not address superficial skin aging changes including pigment dyschromias, broken capillaries, and skin textural issues—these are better addressed with modalities such as nonablative lasers, IPL, and superficial skin peels and microdermabrasion.

Despite the ability to use TNRF in patients with darker skin types, it is the senior author's experience that patients with thinner skin (often corresponding to a lower Fitzpatrick skin type), see more substantial improvement with TNRF treatment. Patients with thicker skin and higher Fitzpatrick skin types may require repeated TNRF-type treatment or a surgical lift to achieve their aesthetic goals (since ablative skin-resurfacing techniques are also not an option in darker skinned individuals, to avoid skin pigment-related complications).

Because TNRF skin rejuvenation was pioneered by Thermage, their monopolar system has accumulated the most peer-reviewed clinical studies, and remains the gold standard TNRF treatment (▶ Fig. 23.6). Using proprietary capacitive monopolar membrane electrodes, Thermage delivers uniform, volumetric tissue heating, while concurrently cooling and protecting the skin surface with a cryogen spray. The dermis is predictably heated to denature at temperatures of 65 to 75°C,[7] which are up to three or four times higher than other TNRF devices. As a result, a single treatment can be sufficient to provide improvement lasting 2 to 3 years. Pressure and temperature sensors at the treatment tip ensure the electrode membrane is in sufficient contact with the skin prior to energy delivery to prevent localized hot spots. Various disposable treatment tips are available at different sizes and heating profiles to target specific areas of the face and body—since the tips are limited to one-time patient use, there is a disposable cost per procedure.

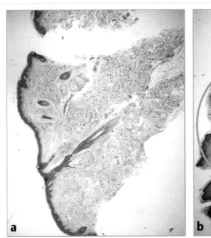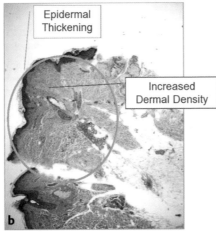

Fig. 23.4 Skin biopsy (**a**) prior to transcutaneous nonablative radiofrequency (TNRF) treatment and (**b**) 4 months after procedure. Note epidermal thickening and increased collagen dermal density. (Courtesy of Julio Barba Gomez, MD and Javier Ruiz-Esparza, MD, Solta Medical, Inc., Hayward, California.)

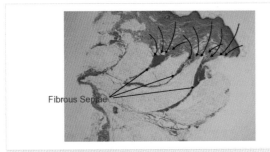

Fig. 23.5 Histology of skin showing the deep dermal fibrous collagen septae, which allow for tightening in the z-axis. (Courtesy of Solta Medical, Inc., Hayward, California.)

Thermage is a monopolar device, and a grounding pad must be placed on the patient. Monopolar energy is more deeply penetrating, and can be more uncomfortable. To address this issue, Thermage rapidly pulses the RF energy many times per second with interwoven cryogen-cooling bursts at each treatment firing; and the latest iteration of the device, the Thermage CPT, incorporates a vibration feature to further distract and minimize discomfort. Deeper penetration of the heat allows the heat to dwell longer, providing greater collagen denaturing. It also allows better three-dimensional lifting and contouring of the skin by tightening the underlying fibrous septa (▶ Fig. 23.5).

There are a few other monopolar TNRF devices available (▶ Table 23.1). The BTL Exilis (BTL, Prague, Czech Republic) device is relatively new and delivers continuous RF energy, as

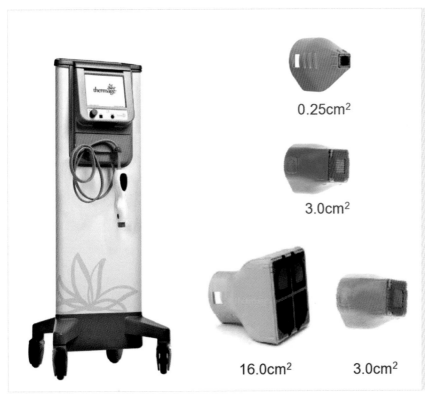

Fig. 23.6 Thermage CPT nonablative radiofrequency (RF) skin rejuvenation system by Solta Medical, Inc. The unit is composed of the computer-controlled RF generator with an integrated cryogen cooling module. The ergonomic handpiece, which incorporates a vibration feature to decrease patient discomfort, is pictured attached to the front of the unit. The various disposable monopolar treatment tips that attach to the handpiece are pictured on the right (not to scale). (Courtesy of Solta Medical, Inc., Hayward, California.)

opposed to individual treatment fires triggered by the operator. The skin surface temperature is monitored continuously to avoid excessive heating. Because the energy is delivered continuously, treatments can be quicker, but more skill is required by the operator.[8] The Ellman (Pelleve, Ellman International, Inc., Hicksville, New York) instrument generator can be used for electrocautery, with add-on aesthetic TNRF treatment handpieces available for skin rejuvenation applications. With the ThermiRF (ThermiAesthetics, Dallas, Texas) tool, cannulas are inserted subcutaneously to deliver RF energy—this therefore cannot truly be considered a TNRF mechanism.

The Accent (Alma Lasers, Inc., Ft. Lauderdale, Florida) system allows the delivery of both unipolar and bipolar TNRF using different handpieces. Unipolar energy delivery is made possible by containing the return grounding plate within the treatment head. Use of 40 MHz RF allows penetration of the heat generated to depths of up to 2 cm, targeting deeper subcutaneous fat.[6] This therapy has been shown to improve the appearance of cellulite.[9] Despite the deeper penetration by the unipolar RF, patients have not found this Accent procedure to be particularly painful. Multiple treatments (from two up to six) may be required to achieve satisfactory improvement.[10] The more superficial bipolar RF handpiece is intended to treat surface wrinkles. Treatment heads on the Accent device are reusable and because there is no separate grounding pad required, there is no consumable cost.

A number of other TNRF devices also employ bipolar energy. The inherent disadvantage of bipolar devices is that the heat does not penetrate as deeply (▶ Fig. 23.3); however, as a result, treatments are in general associated with less pain and studies have shown cosmetic enhancement.[5] Syneron (Elos, Syneron Medical Ltd., Yokneam, Israel) first introduced the concept of combining bipolar RF with other types of energy (IPL, diode laser, infrared) to obtain a synergistic effect. The Aluma system from Lumenis (Lumenis Inc., Santa Clara, California) first used a vacuum device to mechanically suction skin up between bipolar electrodes to maximize dermal penetration,[11] also promoting lymphatic drainage and stimulating circulation. The Aluma device is no longer commercially available, but others including the BodyFX device by Invasix (Invasix, Richmond Hill, Ontario, Canada) have adopted this same treatment mechanism.

Over the past few years, devices that use multipolar TNRF as well as microneedle electrode arrays, fractionated RF delivery, variable RF frequencies, and even combined with magnetic pulses have become available. All of these newer approaches are relatively recent, and although they may hold promise, there currently is a paucity of studies to conclusively support their efficacy.

23.3 Pertinent Anatomy

As skin ages, there is a progressive depletion of the underlying collagen scaffold, resulting in skin that is thinner, more fragile, and prone to wrinkling and sagging. Pores become enlarged and capillaries appear more obvious because there is less collagen surrounding and supporting these structures. Photoaging causes skin damage by solar elastosis where collagen in the dermis becomes disorganized, breaks down and loosens, and elastotic material accumulates in the dermis as the skin's elastic framework degrades.

Ultrastructural studies have shown that TNRF treatment denatures dermal collagen, melting the triple helical configuration of collagen.[4] As the skin cools, the collagen reanneals into tighter, more compact bundles, resulting in initial skin tightening. Longer term, the heat from TNRF treatment is thought to stimulate an inflammatory wound-healing response with activation of dermal fibroblasts. This results in the production of new collagen and elastin.[12] Studies show that there is an increase in newly synthesized type I collagen, as well as total mature type III collagen, at the end of treatment and at 3 months posttreatment compared to baseline.[4,13] Histology of TNRF-treated skin shows a significant rebuilding of the dermal collagen framework as well as epidermal re-thickening (▶ Fig. 23.4). This histological appearance of the skin is more consistent with youthful skin. TNRF may also play a role in treatment of hypertrophic scars by remodeling collagen, and in treating acne due to the heat sterilizing bacteria in the skin.[7]

23.3.1 Indications

TNRF is best for patients requesting subtle, more gradual skin tightening and toning. The ideal patient is in the mid-30s to mid-60s with mild to moderate, but not severe, loosening of the skin.[7] Patients who have had a surgical lift and are looking for some additional touch-up tightening are also good candidates. Patients with more advanced skin sagging may still benefit from the maintenance advantages of TNRF skin rejuvenation—by rebuilding the collagen framework, the pace of additional skin loosening is reversed or slowed.

In the face, TNRF treatment has been shown to tighten the forehead and lift the eyebrows, smooth loose periorbital and eyelid skin, soften the nasolabial folds, and tighten the lower face and anterior neck, thereby softening the marionette folds and better defining the jawline (▶ Fig. 23.7). Body areas targeted include loose skin of the abdomen, flank, buttocks, underarms, and thigh/knee area.

Because dermal layers are affected while the epidermis is spared, TNRF therapy does not treat skin surface issues such as pigment dyschromias and skin texture. However, TNRF can be easily combined with nonablative laser treatments, IPL, superficial skin peels, and microdermabrasion to achieve total skin rejuvenation. Moreover, TNRF therapy can be combined with tissue fillers and neurotoxins in the face to achieve a further cumulative effect (▶ Fig. 23.8). TNRF can also be effectively combined with less invasive surgical procedures such as liposuction and suture suspension, where additional tightening of the skin is required.

23.3.2 Contraindications

The skin surface to be treated must be intact and healthy, without cuts, sores, lesions, blemishes and the like, to allow for safe delivery of the RF energy (▶ Table 23.2). Other absolute contraindications include not treating skin with any metallic tattoos, or other metallic superficial implants. Pregnancy is routinely considered an absolute contraindication for most elective cosmetic procedures. Implanted electronic medical devices such as pacemakers, defibrillators, and pumps are an absolute contraindication for monopolar TNRF procedures that require a grounding pad—unless the implanted device can be safely deactivated

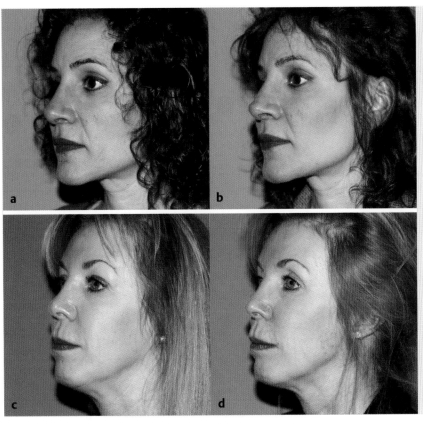

Fig. 23.7 (a–d) Two examples of typical patient results 9 months after transcutaneous nonablative radiofrequency (TNRF) treatment with Thermage. Lifting and stabilization of the brow, tightening of the eyelid skin, and improvement in the midface profile and jawline are evident.

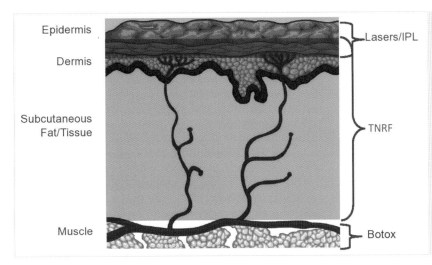

Fig. 23.8 Combining nonablative and less invasive procedures to achieve optimal skin rejuvenation for the face. IPL, intense pulsed light; TNRF, transcutaneous nonablative radiofrequency.

and the patient appropriately monitored during treatment[6] however, this may be only a relative contraindication with bipolar TNRF treatment because the current is locally contained.

Caution is advised in treating patients with active collagen-vascular or autoimmune diseases of the skin, or who have had previous radiation to the area because the ability for the skin to tolerate treatment, heal, and produce new collagen may be impaired. It is also a relative contraindication to treat patients prone to herpetic outbreaks, although this can be addressed effectively by using antiviral prophylaxis prior to treatment. Any implanted metal directly below the skin being treated should be avoided to prevent super-concentration of the heat around the implant, but surrounding areas can be treated

safely. Treatment can be administered safely to areas previously treated with subcutaneous cosmetic fillers and implants, as long as the product is not conductive and does not significantly alter tissue resistance.

23.3.3 Preprocedural

It is critical to correctly set patient expectations prior to TNRF therapy. TNRF treatment does not provide drastic results as do surgical procedures and ablative resurfacing. Appropriate patient selection based on indications and thorough counseling of patients as to the modest, gradual skin tightening that is to be expected will ensure patient satisfaction with the results of treatment.[1]

Table 23.2 Contraindications to transcutaneous nonablative radiofrequency skin rejuvenation

ABSOLUTE CONTRAINDICATIONS
Compromised skin integrity (lacerations, lesions, etc.) Skin with metallic tattoos
Implanted electronic medical devices* (pacemaker, defibrillator, etc.)
Pregnancy
RELATIVE CONTRAINDICATIONS
Systemic disease affecting skin (collagen-vascular, autoimmune, etc.)
Radiated skin Implanted metal in treatment area (plates, screws, joint replacements, etc.)
Skin prone to herpetic or other outbreaks

*Relative contraindication for bipolar devices.

A thorough medical history should be obtained to exclude possible contraindications (▶ Table 23.2), and informed consent should be obtained as per routine. Preprocedural standardized photos should be taken in the same lighting and positioning as postoperative images to best identify and document subtle changes.

Whereas patient discomfort varies from individual to individual and the type of the TNRF device used, most patients will experience a brief hot but tolerable sensation as the RF energy is delivered. It is the senior author's practice to provide oral analgesia and anxiolytic medication to enhance patient comfort during treatment. Antiviral prophylaxis is provided if indicated.

Patients are instructed to not wear makeup (for facial treatment) and to make sure the skin to be treated is clean and free of all skin-care products. Metallic jewelry and accoutrements should not be worn in the areas to be treated. All patients should be aware of the expected, temporary, mild erythema and edema in the areas treated—this is typically self-limited, and resolves within 24 hours.

23.3.4 Periprocedural

Patient comfort is integral to a tolerable TNRF treatment session. This starts with positioning the patient in a private room with a comfortable procedure chair. Oral pain medication and anxiolytics are given sufficiently in advance to provide a therapeutic effect during treatment. Topical anesthetics should not be used with TNRF devices using simultaneous skin surface cooling because this will interfere with patient feedback and sensation of the cooling effect. Patient feedback is important to prevent complications from epidermal overheating. Injected anesthetics have the theoretical disadvantage of altering the depth of RF penetration and are not recommended.

For monopolar TNRF treatment, the patient is grounded appropriately. A temporary ink treatment grid can be used to guide even coverage of the procedure area, especially for multiple-pass regimens. Coupling fluid provided by the manufacturer is applied liberally on the treatment area to allow for maximum conduction of the RF energy from the treatment tip into the skin. If the eyelid skin is being treated directly, plastic eye shields with lubrication are recommended to minimize risk of injury to the globe.

Energy settings must be adjusted based on individual manufacturer recommendations. Areas of thinner skin and areas such as the temple and cheeks, where facial fat pads are more superficial, should be treated with decreased energy settings. Multiple treatment passes using lower energy settings can improve patient comfort and decrease the risk of complications, while providing more consistent clinical outcomes. Because the speed of RF delivery has continued to improve with later generations of TNRF devices, it has facilitated the development of these multiple-pass treatment generations that are not unduly time-consuming to administer. Some devices also feature larger treatment heads to allow for quicker coverage of surface area when treating large areas like the body (▶ Fig. 23.6). In the first set of passes, uniform skin tightening is achieved by covering the entire surface area. The second set of passes provides extra lift by going along superior and lateral vectors. With monopolar TNRF, the final set of passes is used for more precise contouring and skin tightening by targeting the fibrous septa surrounding fat in the subcutaneous layer. Pulses can be stacked to enhance inward contraction; however, time should be given in between pulses to prevent excess heat buildup.[1] The end point of treatment is to achieve appropriate contraction with only mild erythema and edema of the skin.[14]

23.3.5 Postprocedural

Patients should understand that there will be some initial skin tightening seen on the day of treatment as the collagen scaffold denatures and then reanneals. Tightening and toning will continue gradually for several months posttreatment as the skin heals and new collagen is produced. It is recommended that patients desiring additional treatment wait at least 3 months to realize the full effect of the TNRF procedure prior to considering other options. Results can last 2 to 3 years depending on the TNRF device used. Patients with thicker skin typically need more treatments to see improvement. Some TNRF tools that provide more superficial treatment may require multiple and more frequent treatments to achieve the desired outcome.

It is not unusual to have a few small patches of flaky or red skin, possibly due to arcing of the current on the skin surface creating a localized hot spot (most often related to not using sufficient coupling fluid). Patients are advised to use antibiotic ointment on these areas, and they typically resolve without incident in a few days. When treating neck skin, patients may develop focal areas of firmness, most likely due to inflammation of the platysma muscle that is located superficially below the skin surface—this is also a self-limited, transient phenomenon that resolves in a few weeks, and anecdotally is an indication that sufficient energy was utilized to allow for maximum lifting and contouring.[14] Temporary numbness and paresthesias have also been reported, likely due to inflammation of sensory nerves. Patients should be given written postprocedural care instructions to contact the provider concerning any significant or refractory symptoms. Follow-up photos should be scheduled.

23.3.6 Home Care

Aftercare is minimal, but good skin care and sun protection is routinely recommended. Patients are asked to avoid ice and anti-inflammatory medications that may blunt wound healing and collagen formation.[1] Unlike ablative modalities, there is little or no downtime and recovery after TNRF therapy, with patients able to resume their normal social activities immediately after treatment.

23.3.7 Complications

A substantial benefit of TNRF treatment compared to ablative and invasive methods is that complications are much less common and are of lesser magnitude. There was a 0.36% overall incidence of second-degree burns in reports where higher energy levels were used with the original TNRF monopolar devices.[15] With the sophisticated newer instruments currently available that carefully monitor skin surface temperature and modulate RF delivery, skin burns are rarely seen. In addition to superficial burns, blisters, and scars, device complications reported to the FDA include fat loss causing shallow depressions or divots, and incidents of dyschromias, both hyperpigmentation and hypopigmentation. Insufficient use of coupling fluid, tearing or breakdown of the device tip membrane, and high energy settings have been implicated as probable causes. With monopolar TNRF, skin burns have also been reported at the site of the grounding pad, so it is important to ensure the grounding pad is applied correctly. Dry eye or "floaters" may occur—use of lubricating eye ointment and protective plastic corneal shields is recommended when treating around the eyes.

More common side effects include mild-to-moderate pain.[6] As discussed previously, comfort can be enhanced with analgesics and oral anxiolytics. Skin surface depressions related to fat atrophy are usually self-correcting because the skin tightens over time, but fillers can be used if necessary to alleviate uneven contours. In general, complications can be reduced by using lower energy multiple-pass treatment regimens. Avoiding injection anesthesia and general anesthesia to allow for sufficient patient feedback is also helpful to minimize risk of complications.

23.4 Pearls and Pitfalls

- TNRF fits an ideal niche in the aesthetic clinician's practice for patients desiring moderate, gradual, more "natural," subtle, discreet skin tightening, and who have no interest in subjecting themselves to the healing time and risks associated with traditional rejuvenation techniques. By rebuilding the skin's collagen framework, TNRF procedures also provide a theoretical maintenance effect, making the skin less likely to continue to loosen and sag.
- TNRF does not provide the dramatic changes seen with surgical lifting procedures. Patients with considerable skin laxity or those requesting significant changes should be directed to more aggressive skin rejuvenation modalities such as surgical lifts and ablative resurfacing techniques.
- Patient education is critical to ensure realistic expectations and an understanding of the gradual nature of the improvements. If done appropriately, it is the senior author's experience that patients are universally happy with TNRF treatment outcome.
- Because the epidermis is typically cooled and protected with TNRF procedures, skin surface vascular and pigment complexion issues are not addressed. However, because the skin surface is not affected, all Fitzpatrick skin types can be treated safely with TNRF.
- Combining less invasive treatment options like TNRF for skin tightening with neurotoxin to address dynamic lines, fillers to replace volume, IPL treatments for complexion improvement, and superficial peels or microdermabrasion to help texture can often provide a cumulative benefit that each single treatment modality cannot achieve on its own. By addressing each of the individual causes seen with aging skin, the overall improvement achieved can be much more substantial (1 + 1 may actually = 3).
- Newer multiple-pass TNRF treatment protocols are more effective and produce more consistent treatment results with fewer complications compared to the original, high-energy, single-pass treatment regimens. When monopolar TNRF is used, the multiple-pass treatment protocols allow for lifting and contouring the skin in all three dimensions.

References

[1] Abraham M, Rousso J. Capacitive radiofrequency skin rejuvenation. In: Prendergast PM, Shiffman MA, eds. Aesthetic Medicine. Berlin Heidelberg, Germany: Springer; 2012:187–196

[2] Polder KD, Bruce S. Radiofrequency: Thermage. Facial Plast Surg Clin North Am 2011; 19: 347–359

[3] Beasley KL, Weiss RA. Radiofrequency in cosmetic dermatology. Dermatol Clin 2014; 32: 79–90

[4] Zelickson BD, Kist D, Bernstein E, et al. Histological and ultrastructural evaluation of the effects of a radiofrequency-based nonablative dermal remodeling device: a pilot study. Arch Dermatol 2004; 140: 204–209

[5] Ruiz-Esparza J, Gomez JB. The medical face lift: a noninvasive, nonsurgical approach to tissue tightening in facial skin using nonablative radiofrequency. Dermatol Surg 2003; 29: 325–332, discussion 332

[6] Lolis MS, Goldberg DJ. Radiofrequency in cosmetic dermatology: a review. Dermatol Surg 2012; 38: 1765–1776

[7] Sukal SA, Geronemus RG. Thermage: the nonablative radiofrequency for rejuvenation. Clin Dermatol 2008; 26: 602–607

[8] Weiss RA. Noninvasive radio frequency for skin tightening and body contouring. Semin Cutan Med Surg 2013; 32: 9–17

[9] Alexiades-Armenakas M, Dover JS, Arndt KA. Unipolar radiofrequency treatment to improve the appearance of cellulite. J Cosmet Laser Ther 2008; 10: 148–153

[10] Friedman DJ, Gilead LT. The use of hybrid radiofrequency device for the treatment of rhytides and lax skin. Dermatol Surg 2007; 33: 543–551

[11] Gold MH, Goldman MP, Rao J, Carcamo AS, Ehrlich M. Treatment of wrinkles and elastosis using vacuum-assisted bipolar radiofrequency heating of the dermis. Dermatol Surg 2007; 33: 300–309

[12] Hantash BM, Ubeid AA, Chang H, Kafi R, Renton B. Bipolar fractional radiofrequency treatment induces neoelastogenesis and neocollagenesis. Lasers Surg Med 2009; 41: 1–9

[13] el-Domyati M, el-Ammawi TS, Medhat W, et al. Radiofrequency facial rejuvenation: evidence-based effect. J Am Acad Dermatol 2011; 64: 524–535

[14] Abraham MT, Mashkevich G. Monopolar radiofrequency skin tightening. Facial Plast Surg Clin North Am 2007; 15: 169–177, v

[15] Abraham MT, Chiang SK, Keller GS, Rawnsley JD, Blackwell KE, Elashoff DA. Clinical evaluation of non-ablative radiofrequency facial rejuvenation. J Cosmet Laser Ther 2004; 6: 136–144

24 Deep Chemical Peeling

James R. Shire

24.1 Introduction

In the course of this text many types and techniques of facial resurfacing are discussed. My question is: "Why would anyone use a laser when you can get superior, predictable results without a large financial investment by using a peel?" This chapter discusses the deep chemical peel, the true "gold standard" when it comes to resurfacing techniques. Resurfacing is the process of controlled re-epithelialization by creating a wound down to or through the papillary dermis. These resurfacing procedures are used to improve facial surface irregularities including pigmentation disorders, wrinkles, and acne scars, and for treating aged and actinically damaged skin. Various methods of resurfacing have been around for centuries, striving to replace damaged epithelium with new skin. These therapies consist mainly of dermabrasion, lasers, and chemical peels, and their mechanisms of action and guidelines remain constant for whichever technique is used. The goal is to provide smooth skin with even color, tone, and texture without sacrificing the appearance of natural skin. It is critical to understand and avoid the major complications of resurfacing that include pigmentation changes and scarring. The evolution of skin resurfacing has been filled with secret formulas, incorrect scientific dogma, technological advancements, and economic and market pressures. A modern view of the deep chemical facial peel is presented.

24.2 Historic Background

The desire to restore facial skin and improve one's appearance is nothing new. The oldest recorded report of a peel to remove wrinkles is in the Ebers Papyrus written around 1560 BC, which documents a physician using soured milk, oils, and abrasives to resurface and beautify the face and body.[1] In 1892, Edmund Saalfeld published a report that phenol was used to remove freckles, and later, in 1903, New York dermatologist George MacKee reported the use of phenol to treat acne scars.[1,2] Then in 1927, Herbert Otto Bames wrote the first article explaining the use of phenol as the essential element in cosmetic chemical peeling; and Chicago, Illinois, plastic surgeon Joseph Urkov, in 1946, published a 15-year experience treating 2,000 patients using croton oil.[1,2] These were the earliest practitioners experimenting with deep chemical peels in the early 20th century.

But the most colorful and truly innovative techniques in peeling came from the lay peelers of the time. These peelers were cloaked in mystery with French-sounding pseudonyms and "secret ingredients." One of the first lay peelers to gain prominence was Jean DeDesley, whose formula was the absolute standard by which all other peels were judged.[3] Other very well-known peelers in the Hollywood, California, community received their training and formulas from her. These included Arthur Gradé, Venner Kelson, Antoinette LaGassé, Maryanne Coppersmith, and Miriam Maschek during the 1940s to the 1960s.[3] All of their formulas were based on phenol crystals and the presence of croton oil.

The first plastic surgeon to acquire the lay peeler's secret was Adolph Brown, MD. He was an otolaryngology instructor in Chicago, and then moved to southern California. The secret was croton oil. He not only published but, also in 1959, patented the formula that contained water, phenol, croton oil, sesame oil, and cresol.[2] Drs. Litton, Truppman, and Baker were three plastic surgeons in Florida who were in contact with the lay peelers Coopersmith and Maschek.[2,4] They were able to develop peel formulas from them that contained phenol and croton oil as ingredients, but in different concentrations (▶ Table 24.1).

Table 24.1 Comparison of peel formulas in percentages

	Brown (%)	Coopersmith/Litton (%)	Gradé (%)	Kelsen (%)	Maschek (%)	Baker (%)
Water	44.25	50.5	52.42	27.89	51.28	44.02
Phenol 88%	50	48.3	44.79	62.34	47.06	49.25
Croton oil	0.5	0.4	0.2	0.16	0.22	2.08
Sesame oil or olive oil	0.25	–	0.05	6.25	–	–
Cresol or Lysol	5	–	–	3.38	–	–
Glycerin	–	0.8	2.54	–	1.41	–
Septisol[a]	–	–	–	–	–	4.67
Total %	100	100	100	100.02	99.97	100.02

[a]Sandent Co., Murfreesboro, Tennessee.
Data from:
-Hetter GP. An examination of the phenol-croton oil peel: part III. The plastic surgeons' role. Plast Reconstr Surg 2000; 105: 752–763.
-Hetter GP. An examination of the phenol-croton oil peel: part II. The lay peelers and their croton oil formulas. Plast Reconstr Surg 2000; 105: 240–248, discussion 249–251.
-Stone PA. The use of modified phenol for chemical face peeling. Clin Plast Surg 1998; 25: 21–44.

In 1961, Thomas Baker published the first article that provided a simple recipe to make the formula and described the peel regime that he received from the lay peelers. This included a tape mask, removal of the mask, and the use of thymol iodine powder.[5] Then in 1962 Dr. Baker changed the formula by decreasing the volume from 9 to 5 mL, therefore almost doubling the concentration of the croton oil from 1.2 to 2.1%, which created the classic Baker-Gordon formula we all recognize.[1,2,5,6]

The belief during this time was that it was the phenol that was the active agent creating the burn, and that the croton oil was only a mild irritant and might not even be necessary to the peel. This thinking persisted until 1998 when Phillip Stone showed the critical importance of patient selection, skin preparation, vigor and length of rubbing, volume of the peel solution, concentration of croton oil, and that the method and type of occlusion are all responsible for the depth of peel.[4,7] Then in 2000, Gregory Hetter published a four-part series in the journal *Plastic and Reconstructive Surgery* examining the roles of phenol and croton oil and their concentrations in deep chemical peeling.[2,3,6,8] Hetter presented proof that augmenting the concentrations of croton oil increased the depth of peel, and that the phenol was used mainly as a vehicle to deliver the croton oil. With the work of Hetter, all the previous ideas and dogmas of the past 50 to 60 years surrounding the roles and actions of phenol and croton oil have been proven either inaccurate and/or obsolete.

24.3 The Classic Baker-Gordon Peel

When the phrase "deep chemical peel" is discussed or the use of phenol and croton oil are mentioned, the Baker-Gordon peel comes to mind. It is still referred to as the gold standard in peeling and resurfacing techniques. The peel is based on a formula with ingredients that were easy for the surgeon to obtain and create. The classic (1962) formula consists of:
- 3 mL United States Pharmacopeia (USP) liquid phenol (88%)
- 2 mL tap water
- 8 drops liquid soap (Septisol, Sandent Co., Murfreesboro, Tennessee)
- 3 drops croton oil

Note that in the original article, Baker states that if the croton oil is unavailable, it can be eliminated.[1,5] The croton oil was considered an "enhancement" to the formula's keratolytic and penetrating action.

The indications stressed the importance of patient selection due to the bleaching effect of the phenol.[1,5] It was recommended that fair complexions are better suited to the peel and that darker and olive skin will produce a distinct demarcation line. Baker also stated that red-haired, freckled patients, men, and persons of Asian or African descent were all poor candidates for phenol peels. The major indications were the treatment of facial wrinkles, dyschromias, pigmentation irregularities, and actinic and precancerous lesions.

The original articles all recommended that the peel be done under anesthesia, and that the patient needed to be monitored for 1 to 2 days by experienced personnel.[1,5] The patient was degreased of all oils and makeup with ether or acetone. The peeling mixture was painted evenly to cover the entire face and obtain an immediate grayish-white frost. It was applied slowly to minimize the burning sensation and avoid rapid phenol absorption that could result in toxic reactions. The toxicity was most likely due to the large amount of solution that was used and the immediate occlusive dressing that increased absorption. The peel was applied to one region at a time. After each region of the face had been covered with the peeling solution, an occlusive dressing was applied. The dressing of choice was waterproof adhesive tape or a Vaseline occlusive dressing. This was to increase the depth of peel, and produce a longer lasting result. The disadvantages of taping were increased patient discomfort, painful removal process, and the inability of the surgeon to evaluate the peel wound. Application was completed over a 1- to 2-hour period. An assistant watched the eyes for tearing, and carefully blotted any forming tear before it dripped. The tears were thought to deepen the penetration of the burn. The tape was usually removed about 48 hours following the peel. After the tape mask was removed, the peeled area of skin was dusted with thymol iodide. This was to dry the area and forms an eschar. Re-epithelialization usually begins to occur at around 7 to 10 days following the peel, at which point the patient is instructed to use Crisco or cocoa butter. Depending on the individual patient's rate of healing, makeup and sunscreen can be used at about 10 to 15 days. Erythema may persist for up to 3 to 6 months.[1]

Serious complications with the Baker-Gordon peel were described as rare, adding, "However some undesirable results are to be expected." These included hypopigmentation (bleaching effect), which was described as "unavoidable," prolonged erythema, sensitivity to sunlight, scarring, ectropion of the lower eyelid, postpeel hyperpigmentation, infections (more often than not, herpes virus), and milia.[1,5]

24.4 Dispelling the Myths

Phenol and croton oil have been the basis for deep peels beginning with the lay peelers. Then in1962 when the Baker formula was published, it became *the* formula used by plastic surgeons and dermatologists. During this period no one questioned the classic formula or the roles of phenol concentrations or of croton oil in chemical peeling. A set of absolute dogmas developed that persisted for more than 40 years.[6,8] These unchallenged beliefs or "truths" were:
- Phenol is the active ingredient, and there is an "all-or-none" effect.
- Phenol peels deeper in lower concentrations. Highly concentrated phenol prevents deeper penetration of the dermis by denaturing keratin, whereas lower concentrations would penetrate deeper.
- Lower concentrations of phenol are more dangerous.
- The loss of pigmentation or the "porcelain mask" is the result of phenol.

- Phenol has an uncontrollable toxicity.
- Addition of soap lowers the surface tension, thus increasing penetration of the phenol.
- Croton oil is only an irritant.
- Adding an oil "buffers" the solution.

For years the Baker-Gordon peel has been used with varied results, in large part due to the steep learning curve in the "art" of peeling. Controlling the many variables takes much experience. In the late 1990s Stone[4,7] and Hetter[2,3,6,8] published articles describing the role of croton oil and phenol concentrations in chemical peeling. By doing actual studies, the old ideas and dogmas of the past changed, dispelling previous beliefs. In his comprehensive and elegant four-part article in *Plastic and Reconstructive Surgery*, Hetter showed:

- Phenol greater than 50% peels deeper with increasing concentration to a maximum with 88% USP phenol.
- Unoccluded phenol less than 35% does not peel the skin.
- Unoccluded 88% USP phenol without croton oil produces only a light-to-mild peel.
- Phenol does not have an all-or-none effect.
- Croton oil contains a powerful cytotoxic resin
- Minute amounts of croton resin will cause skin burns.
- Small amounts of croton oil added to phenol will cause peeling or skin burns.
- Peel depth increases with augmented concentrations of croton oil.
- Phenol acts as the carrier for the croton oil.
- The depth of the peel is increased by tape occlusion, petroleum-based ointments, and multiple applications of croton oil in phenol.

With this knowledge about the actions and interactions of phenol and croton oil, we can formulate a protocol for deep peeling. Hetter has described in detail the use of serial dilutions of croton oil in phenol, creating solutions with a range of depth of penetrations that can easily be made from stock solutions. (See Chapter 25.)

24.5 Technique for the Deep Chemical Peel: Croton Oil–Phenol

Using the combined knowledge of Baker and his formula and Hetter's studies of croton oil and phenol, the following chemical peel technique has been developed. In addition, the work done by Stone in 1998 showed the critical importance of patient selection, skin preparation, vigor and length of rubbing, volume of the peel solution, concentration of croton oil—and method and type of occlusion—and that all are responsible for the depth of peel. Since 2001, this author has used this technique[9] with superior results and a lack of complications. The peeling procedure involves the prepeel and postpeel care, as well as the formula preparation and actual peeling itself. The peel is based on the original Baker-Gordon formula, with multiple solutions being made varying the amount of croton oil in each; however, an occlusive dressing is never used, and the peeled skin is kept moist throughout the peeling process.

24.5.1 Prepeel

As in all other surgical procedures, patient selection is critical in obtaining the optimum results.[9] Patients with fair or lighter complexions are usually the best candidates. Those patients with olive or darker complexions, marked solar damage, and those with freckles all require full-facial peeling and are not good candidates for regional peels. They do very well with the full-face peels. Regional peels in these patients will leave obvious lines of demarcation and create a noticeable color disparity. Persons of Asian or African descent are not good candidates due to the increased risk of irregular complexion with areas of hypopigmentation and hyperpigmentation occurring.

The consultation preoperatively includes a frank discussion of the principles of resurfacing and the procedure itself. Before and after photos including pictures of the healing process are reviewed with the patient. The healing process is explained in detail to the patient including swelling, discomfort, weeping of the skin, keeping the skin moist, and postpeel erythema. Risks and complications are reviewed in detail and questions are answered. Prescriptions are given at the preoperative visit for cefadroxil monohydrate 500 mg for 7 to 10 days, methylprednisolone dose pack, hydrocodone bitartrate with acetaminophen 7.5/500 mg, or ketorolac tromethamine (Toradol, Roche Pharmaceuticals, Nutley, New Jersey) as needed for discomfort, and valacyclovir HCL 500 to 1,000 mg every 12 hours beginning 2 days prior to the procedure and ending 10 to 12 days postpeel. The patient is instructed to purchase Eucerin cream (Beiersdorf Inc., Wilton, Connecticut) and Aquaphor. A complete written postpeel manual of care with restrictions, do's, and don'ts is reviewed and given to the patient. We do not recommend the use of any exfoliating agents such as retinoids or hydroquinone for 1 month prior to the peel. Any patient-applied pretreatments can vary from patient to patient, and we do not want to change the epidermal kinetics.[9]

Preoperatively, a complete and thorough history and physical examination are required. Evaluation of cardiac, hepatic, and renal function as well as any disorder that affects healing such as diabetes, collagen-vascular disease, history of radiation treatments, medications such as isotretinoin (Accutane, Roche, Nutley, New Jersey), and a history of herpes outbreaks should be well documented. A current electrocardiogram (EKG), complete blood count (CBC), and basic chemistry profile (including electrolytes, blood urea nitrogen [BUN], and liver function tests) are obtained. Standard photos are taken.

Be aware that deep chemical peels should be limited to the face and not extend down to the neck. Peeling the neck will result in hypertrophic scarring.[9]

24.5.2 Deep Peel Formula

Formula preparation used and recommended by this author is based on the Baker-Gordon formula with varying amounts of croton oil used (▶ Table 24.2). The idea behind this formulation is supported by the work of Hetter,[6,8] who has shown that 33% phenol can produce a medium-light, medium-heavy, heavy, or very heavy peel if the concentration of croton oil is changed from 0.35 to 0.7% to 1.1 to 2.1%, respectively. It is to be noted

Table 24.2 Modified formulas to vary the depth of peel

Baker-Gordon	Modified	Modified
3-drop	2-drop	1-drop
3 mL phenol	3 mL phenol	3 mL phenol
2 mL water distilled	2 mL water distilled	2 mL water distilled
8 drops Septisol[a]	8 drops Septisol	8 drops Septisol
3 drops croton oil	2 drops croton oil	1 drop croton oil

[a]Sandent Co., Murfreesboro, Tennessee.

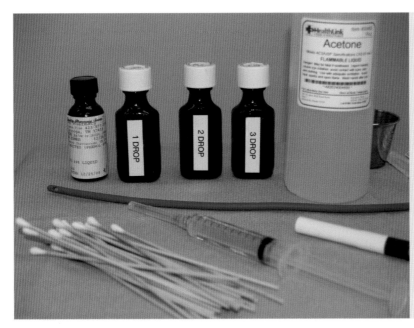

Fig. 24.1 Peel-tray setup contains acetone, freshly mixed peel solution, bupivacaine, and applicators.

that the depth of the peel from 88% phenol has been shown to be less than that produced by 62.5% phenol, which was less than that produced by 48.5% phenol (Baker-Gordon formula).

The formula consists of liquid phenol in a concentration of approximately 88% USP. Croton oil is a powerful cytotoxic resin that increases the depth of peel with boosted concentrations. Distilled water is used as a diluent. Liquid soap Septisol is used as a saponifying agent.

These mixtures are prepared as a fresh batch for each case. It is strongly recommended that each surgeon mixes his own formula and does not entrust this job to a pharmacist, nurse, or other personnel. The formulas are compounded in individual 30-mL, amber glass bottles that are labeled with the patient's name, the date, and the concentration.[9]

24.5.3 The Peeling Procedure

The procedure is performed under conscious sedation anesthesia monitoring with EKG and pulse oximeter. The face is cleansed with Septisol and then degreased with acetone. Removing the oils from the skin allows for even penetration and is a key step in the peeling procedure (▶ Fig. 24.1). Nerve blocks are used to aid in postpeel comfort. Bupivacaine 0.75% is

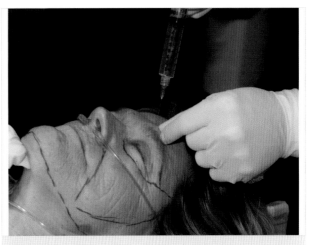

Fig. 24.2 Prepeel nerve block with 0.75% bupivacaine.

used to block the supraorbital, infraorbital, and mental nerves (▶ Fig. 24.2).

The face is divided into treatment zones as described by both Drs. Baker and Hetter.[1,6,9] These zones represent the different skin thicknesses and level of skin appendages. They will

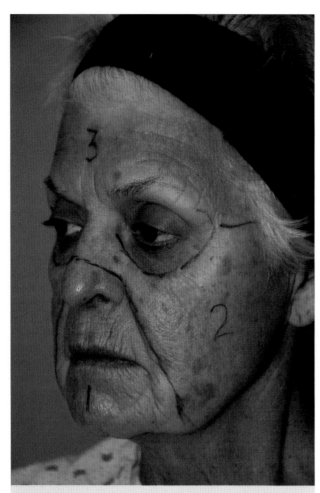

Fig. 24.3 The face is divided into treatment zones.

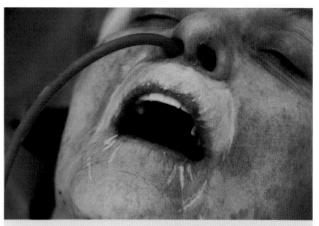

Fig. 24.4 Frosting occurs with the application of the peel solution. Notice that the deep rhytids are pretreated by peeling the base of the rhytid using a fine-tipped applicator stick.

determine the depth of the peel and, in turn, which peel mixture is to be used for each facial zone (▶ Fig. 24.3).

Facial Zones

- Zone 1—Perioral, chin, and lower nose
- Zone 2—Cheeks and upper nose
- Zone 3—Forehead
- Zone 4—Eyelids, periorbital area, temples, and preauricular area

Which formula is to be used where is determined by each individual patient. The 3-drop croton oil mixture is still the formula of choice for deep rhytids. The peel solution is selected and is continuously stirred to keep it in suspension. Cotton-tipped applicators are used to apply the mixture. The deep rhytids are usually pretreated first by applying the solution on a pointed applicator stick to the base of the deep wrinkle line. The areas are then covered by rolling a saturated, cotton-tipped applicator over the area (▶ Fig. 24.4). An entire zone is treated to produce an even, complete coverage. With the application, an

immediate grayish-white frost is observed. We usually complete one zone and allow 10 to 15 minutes between zones. The depth of the peel is determined by how the skin is prepped, the formula used (croton-oil concentration), the amount of solution applied, the amount or vigor of the rubbing that is done, and the number of application layers applied. This is the reason expertise, technique, and the "art" of peeling are critical in obtaining superior results. We do not recommend occlusive dressings—whether tape or a petroleum-based ointment—for the peel area and because an occlusive dressing is not used, thymol iodine powder is also not used or recommended. The depth of peel is increased not by the use of an occlusive dressing, but by the amount of rubbing and the concentration of the solution applied. When an even frost is obtained, a moist dressing of Eucerin cream is heavily applied. The patient is monitored for 1 hour postoperatively and usually has only a minimal-to-mild discomfort level. Toradol or a hydrocodone bitartrate with acetaminophen is used for supplemental relief, if needed.

24.5.4 Postpeel Care

The postoperative care and the healing phase are equally as important to the final result as the peel procedure itself. Detailed instructions are provided to the patient, both in written and verbal form, which answer the patient's questions and allow for the most favorable healing results.

Swelling occurs within the first 24 hours and is usually moderate to severe, especially in the perioral and periorbital areas (▶ Fig. 24.5). The swelling usually peaks around 3 days postpeel and typically begins subsiding on the 5th or 6th day. Initially, the peel area resembles a deep sunburn with the skin darkening and the beginning of a serous exudate. The patient should remain head-elevated as much as possible. The day after surgery, the patient will begin showering the peeled area five to six times a day. This is accomplished by standing in the shower with a fine, wide spray and allowing tepid water to flow over

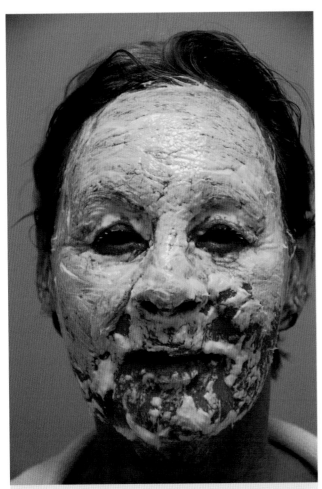

Fig. 24.5 This 72-year-old patient is 1 day postpeel with 3-drop croton oil–phenol peel. Notice there is marked edema and serous exudate with the Eucerin cream (Beiersdorf Inc., Wilton, Connecticut) heavily applied.

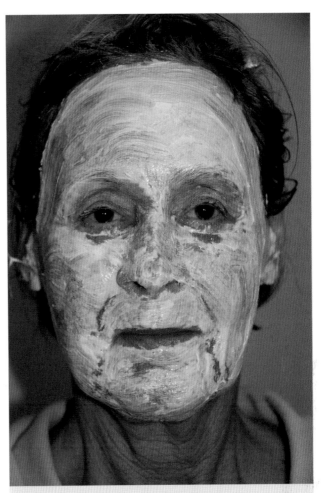

Fig. 24.6 The same patient at 7 days postpeel. The Eucerin cream (Beiersdorf Inc., Wilton, Connecticut) is still present, but the edema and serous exudate have resolved.

the face. The purposes for showering are to provide moisture to the skin and stimulate new skin growth; however, showering is not intended to remove the cream. After the shower, the face is allowed to air-dry and Eucerin cream is then reapplied. The application of the cream should be like frosting a cake. The patient is instructed to keep the face moist at all times, never letting drying or crusting to occur and reapplying the Eucerin cream as needed. The patient is seen daily for the first 4 to 7 days postpeel to monitor the progress of the healing process, the compliance of the patient, and to reassure the patient about the progress of the healing (▶ Fig. 24.6). The peel is usually completed between 9 and 14 days. When re-epithelialization has been completed, the new skin will be an intense pink color (▶ Fig. 24.7). This erythema will slowly fade to a lighter pink and then to a normal skin tone over time. The time line for this varies from individual to individual but the erythema can remain present for up to 3 to 6 months. During this pink phase, it is critical that sunlight be avoided, and the patients protect their new skin with ultraviolet A (UVA)/ultraviolet B (UVB) sunblock (▶ Fig. 24.8 and ▶ Fig. 24.9).

24.6 Complications

Serious complications are rare and mostly avoidable. However, the various complications are discussed with all patients.

Hypopigmentation to some degree is the most commonly reported deep postpeel reaction. It is imperative that the surgeon understand and be able to explain to the patient that although removal of sun-damaged skin, freckles, and solar dyschromias is a lightning of the current skin condition, it is in fact a return to the patient's original skin coloring. The patient is instructed to compare the new skin to an area that has not had previous sun exposure. Severe pigmentation loss and porcelain complexion are due to the use of occlusive dressings (waterproof tape or Vaseline) and are the reasons the Baker-Gordon peel has received an unfair reputation in the past. Pigmentation demarcations are seen in areas of transition between peeled and unpeeled areas. For this reason, patient selection, peeling technique, and the restricted use of regional peeling are crucial.

In the past, *scarring* has been associated with the older techniques of the Baker-Gordon peel. But by using the Baker-Gordon formula, keeping the skin moist with Eucerin cream as opposed to occlusive dressings, and drying the peeled surface

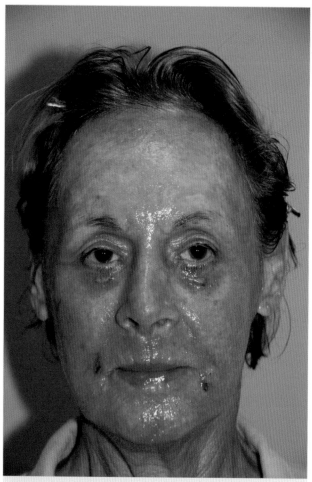

Fig. 24.7 Patient at 13 days postpeel. Re-epithelialization is complete and the patient shows marked erythema.

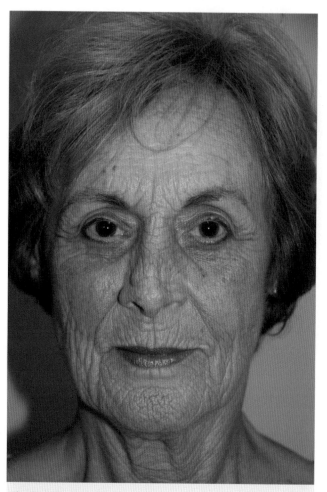

Fig. 24.8 Preoperative view of the same 72-year-old woman with severe deep facial rhytids. Specifically notice the wrinkles in the perioral area and on the nose.

with thymol iodine, scarring has not been an issue. Occasionally, fine, lacy scarring can sometimes be observed immediately postpeel but usually resolves with time and patients are generally unaware of this condition. Scars that do occur are typically minor and can be treated with watchful waiting and/or intralesional steroid injections. The surgeon should also be cautious of patients who have undergone lower lid blepharoplasty in the past, for these patients are at risk of *ectropion*. This can occur in any lid that has been tightened and special care must be taken with these patients.

One of the most common problems that occurs postpeel is *hyperpigmentation*. Patients must be well educated on their sensitivity to the sun and the need to avoid sun exposure during the healing process. Hyperpigmentation occurs more commonly in patients with olive or darker skin and with dark eyes. Exposure to sun, whether it is through a window or reflected light, can easily cause hyperpigmentation during the erythematous period. The use of sunblocks that protect against both UVA and UVB is essential. The sunblock must contain zinc as one of the active ingredients. This sensitivity to sunlight may last for several months until all hints of erythema have resolved. Patients should be advised on the use of sun protection and the avoidance of future tanning. If hyperpigmentation does

develop, begin treatment early with a 2.5%-hydrocortisone cream and a 4- to 8%-hydroquinone cream twice a day topically.

Infections can occur but are extremely rare; nevertheless, all patients are given postoperative antibiotics for 7 days. The most common infection is that of herpes simplex. It is estimated that between 74 and 98% of the population have been exposed to the herpes virus,[10,11] and all patients are therefore treated with valacyclovir 500 to 1,000 mg three times daily beginning 2 days prior to the peel and for 10 days postpeel. Herpetic infections are usually superficial but can result in scarring.

Milia may also occur postpeel as a consequence of the healing process. These are small, inclusion cysts that appear in the first 2 to 6 weeks after the peel and are usually transient in nature. Patients are informed of this and reassured that these will resolve and that they are to be left alone. Patients with fair skin and with a red or flushing complexion may also develop *telangiectasia*. If telangiectasias persist beyond the erythematous phase, they can be treated easily with a vascular laser.

Persistent wrinkles can cause disappointment, both for the patient and for the surgeon. These can usually be avoided with proper patient selection and the use of the proper peeling

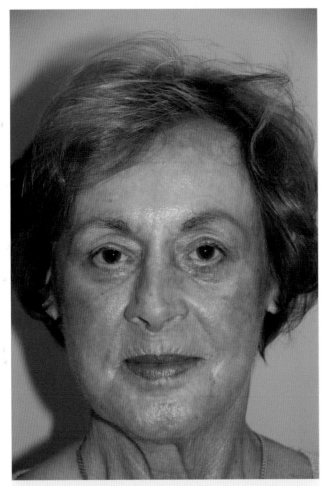

Fig. 24.9 The patient at 3 months postpeel with croton oil–phenol peel. There is still mild erythema, but notice the near-complete removal of the preoperative facial rhytids.

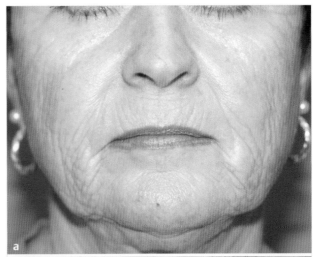

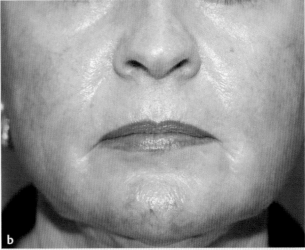

Fig. 24.10 This patient is shown (a) before, and (b) 6 months after 3-drop croton oil–phenol peel.

technique and formula. Repeat touch-up peels can usually be performed after 9 to 12 months and can be handled as an office procedure.

24.7 Conclusion

The Baker-Gordon peel has been referred to as a "phenol" peel because for years that was thought to be the active ingredient. However, as we have now seen, this theory has been found to be completely incorrect. The Baker-Gordon peel is not just the formula; it was the application technique, the use of an occlusive dressing, the process of tape removal and application of thymol iodine, and postpeel treatment that defined the classic peel. All the negativity that existed was a result of this combination of actions and was also based on many scientific falsehoods.

As demonstrated by Hetter, it is the croton oil that is the actual agent that increases the depth of peel through the phenol vehicle, and by varying the croton-oil concentration the depth of peel can be varied. Then Stone showed that the amount of solution, the number of layers applied, and the vigor

of the rubbing of the mixture would impact the depth of peel, therefore allowing the surgeon more control of the peeling process.

For these reasons, the term *Baker-Gordon peel* should only be used as a historical reference and not to describe a deep chemical peel that uses 88% phenol, 3 drops of croton oil, water, and Septisol. We now have a resurfacing spectrum based on this formula by varying the amount of croton oil. To be correct, the deep peel should be referred to as what it really is, a *croton oil–phenol peel*.

Surgeons—by selecting the appropriate patient and formula, and with strict adherence to prepeel preparation, formula blending, postpeel care, and follow-up—will have consistent superior results and some of the happiest and appreciative patients in their practices (▶ Fig. 24.10, ▶ Fig. 24.11, ▶ Fig. 24.12).

Hopefully, we have answered the question of the benefits of peeling versus the laser. One can see that with less than $100 of chemicals, you can obtain predictable results that are far superior to that of the laser, with fewer complications and without the great expense of constantly changing technology.

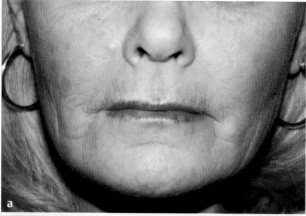
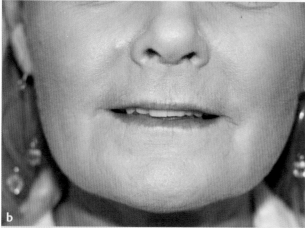

Fig. 24.11 This woman is an example of (a) before procedure, and (b) the 4-year postpeel result of the 3-drop croton oil–phenol peel.

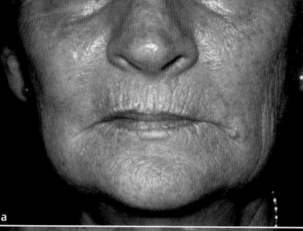
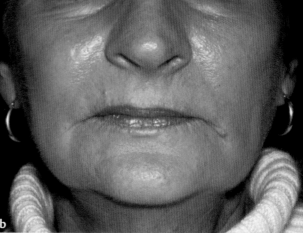

Fig. 24.12 This patient was photographed (a) before, and (b) 6 years after the 3-drop croton oil–phenol peel.

References

[1] Stuzin JM. Phenol peeling and the history of phenol peeling. Clin Plast Surg 1998; 25: 1–19

[2] Hetter GP. An examination of the phenol-croton oil peel: part III. The plastic surgeons' role. Plast Reconstr Surg 2000; 105: 752–763

[3] Hetter GP. An examination of the phenol-croton oil peel: part II. The lay peelers and their croton oil formulas. Plast Reconstr Surg 2000; 105: 240–248, discussion 249–251

[4] Stone PA. The use of modified phenol for chemical face peeling. Clin Plast Surg 1998; 25: 21–44

[5] Baker TJ. Chemical face peeling and rhytidectomy. A combined approach for facial rejuvenation. Plast Reconstr Surg Transplant Bull 1962; 29: 199–207

[6] Hetter GP. An examination of the phenol-croton oil peel: part IV. Face peel results with different concentrations of phenol and croton oil. Plast Reconstr Surg 2000; 105: 1061–1083, discussion 1084–1087

[7] Stone PA, Lefer LG. Modified phenol chemical face peels: recognizing the role of application technique. Facial Plast Surg Clin North Am 2001; 9: 351–376

[8] Hetter GP. An examination of the phenol-croton oil peel: part I. Dissecting the formula. Plast Reconstr Surg 2000; 105: 227–239, discussion 249–251

[9] Shire JR, Cortez EA. Chemical facial resurfacing: the modified phenol-croton oil peel. In: Stucker FJ, deSouza C, Kenyon GS, et al, eds. Rhinology and Facial Plastic Surgery. Berlin Heidelberg, Germany: Springer Verlag; 2009:855–859

[10] Kumar V, Abbas AK, Fausto N, Aster J. Robbins and Cotran Pathologic Basis of Disease. Professional ed. 8th ed. Philadelphia, PA: Saunders Elsevier; 2010

[11] Herpes simplex virus. Univer. Maryland Med Cent. Available at: https://umm.edu/health/medical/altmed/condition/herpes-simplex-virus. Published update 31 May 2013. Accessed 23 June 2015.

25 Multilevel Phenol–Croton Oil Peels

Mark J. Been and Devinder S. Mangat

25.1 Introduction

With medical advancements and an increased life expectancy in modern society there has been heightened interest in optimizing one's quality of life. More than ever, there exists the desire to undo or reverse the facial skin changes that result from sunlight, aging, and genetics. A myriad of technological and medical "breakthroughs" have been produced to meet this demand, yet many are unsubstantiated. Chemical peels remain one of the steadfast and proven tools for facial skin resurfacing. Within this chapter, the advances and techniques associated with the multilevel phenol–croton oil peels are highlighted.

Chemical peels are primarily performed for treatment of rhytids, lentigines, dyschromias, and actinic skin damage. Numerous chemical-peel formulations have been described. Although the art of chemical peeling, or chemexfoliation, has been practiced for centuries, modern-day use was initiated in Hollywood, California, in the 1920s by lay peelers. In the 1950s and 1960s, use of chemical peels moved to the hands of physicians and there was a movement to standardize its practice. Out of this was born the classic Baker-Gordon phenol–croton oil formulation that served as the "gold standard" for deep chemical peels.[1] This peel was utilized by practitioners for decades, yet carried with it the risk of potentially significant complications due to its aggressive nature. In 2000, Hetter eloquently described his findings associated with the phenol–croton oil peel and helped to dispel much of the previously accepted dogma. The publications of Hetter and later Stone serve as the foundation for the advancements that have subsequently occurred in the use of phenol–croton oil peels.

25.2 Patient Selection

Defining the appropriate patient for a chemical peel is of utmost importance. This requires careful attention to both the patient's physical and mental attributes. Physically, one must adhere to appropriate indications, namely rhytids and skin photodamage in the forms of dyschromias and actinic damage (▶ Fig. 25.1). These features must be distinguished from gravitational and other senescent changes including jowling and facial lipoatrophy. Patients who are to undergo phenol–croton oil peels are ideally characterized as those with fair skin, blue eyes, and shallow rhytids. The Fitzpatrick skin type classification is frequently utilized to categorize appropriate patients (▶ Table 5.1).[2] In general, patients with Fitzpatrick skin types I, II, and sometimes III are appropriate patients for the phenol–croton oil peels. Another categorization scheme that is helpful in rating patient skin quality and severity of photodamage is the Glogau skin classification (▶ Table 25.1).[3]

During the initial patient consultation one must develop a sense of the patient's mental preparedness and expectations for a chemical peel. Optimal patient outcomes often necessitate strict adherence to preoperative and postoperative regimens. Lifestyle activities need to be assessed. Patients with habitual sun and smoke exposure should be counseled on the damaging

effects that ultraviolet (UV) radiation and smoke can cause in the first several months following a peel. Those patients who cannot abide by these limitations should be recommended for alternative therapies.

Realistic expectations should be delineated according to the depth of the phenol–croton oil peel to be performed. Erythema is an expected temporary consequence that may last up to 3 months. Patients should ideally be comfortable with the idea of wearing concealing makeup in the intervening time period. To provide the patient with an approximate estimate of the final skin quality following the chemical peel, one may use the patient's axillary skin—provided there has been no history of significant UV exposure. Standardized preoperative photographs should be taken to document the degree of photodamage.

Patients should be screened for other contraindications to performing resurfacing procedures. Relative contraindications include active or frequently recrudescent oral herpes simplex virus (HSV) infections, history of head and neck radiation,

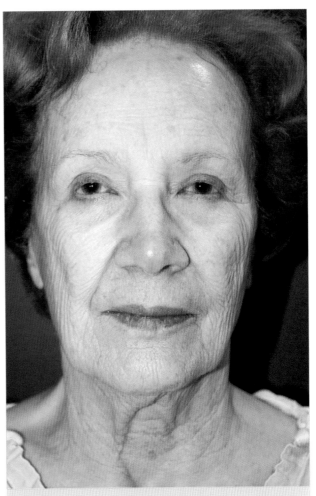

Fig. 25.1 Preoperative photograph of patient demonstrates fair skin, diffuse fine rhytids, and scattered lentigines.

Table 25.1 Glogau photoaging classification

Classification type	Age group	Wrinkling	Typical characteristics
I—Mild	20–30s	No wrinkles	Mild pigmentary changes, minimal wrinkling, no keratoses, little makeup required
II—Moderate	Late 30s or 40s	Wrinkles in motion	Early lentigines, palpable but not visible keratoses, parallel smile lines appear, foundation makeup usually necessary
III—Advanced	50s	Wrinkles at rest	Obvious dyschromias, telangiectasias and keratoses, heavy foundation makeup required
IV—Severe	60–70s	Only wrinkles	Severe photoaging, yellow-gray skin color, history of cutaneous malignancies, no normal skin, cannot wear makeup (cakes and cracks)

Modified with permission from Glogau RG. Aesthetic and anatomic analysis of the aging skin. Semin Cutan Med Surg 1996; 15: 134–138.

diabetes, hypertrophic or keloid scars, and connective tissue disorders. Any patient with elevated estrogen levels is a poor candidate for chemical peels due to the risk of hyperpigmentation. Therefore, those taking oral contraceptives, exogenous hormone replacement, or those planning to become pregnant within 6 months following a peel should be cautioned. Photosensitizing drugs also need to be avoided.

One's ability to re-epithelialize following a chemical peel is dependent upon adnexal structures within the dermis. Any activity that inhibits this process should be considered a contraindication to performing a chemical peel. Isotretinoin use within 6 to 12 months is regarded to be an absolute contraindication due to its inhibition of sebaceous gland activity.

25.3 Choosing Depth of Peel

After selecting appropriately indicated patients, the correct peel depth must be determined. The depth of the chemical peel is based upon the level of skin penetration. Superficial peels are designated as those that induce tissue necrosis limited to the epidermis and will not be included in the discussion of modified phenol–croton oil peels. Medium-depth peels result in destruction of the epidermis with variable necrosis and inflammation of the papillary dermis. Inflammation may extend to the superficial reticular dermis. Deep peels result in epidermis and papillary dermis tissue destruction with inflammation extending to the midreticular dermis. Any deeper tissue destruction would potentially damage the adnexal structures and raise the risk of dyspigmentation and scarring.

Medium-depth chemical peels are often utilized for patients with Glogau level II photodamage. The medium-depth peel can also improve mild and moderate acne scarring. Patients with Glogau levels III and IV are often best treated with deep chemical peels. Specific areas of the face may be treated with different peel depths. Deep rhytids in areas where the skin is thicker, such as the glabella and perioral regions, are better addressed with deep peels, whereas the nasal dorsum and periorbital areas are better suited for medium-depth peels. The Fitzpatrick skin type of a patient should also be a consideration. Greater depth of skin penetration raises the risk of postinflammatory hyperpigmentation (PIH), hypopigmentation, and scarring; therefore, deep peels should be reserved for Fitzpatrick skin types I and II.

25.4 Preprocedural Preparation

A number of prepeel measures may help to optimize healing and final skin outcomes. UV protection in the form of broad-spectrum ultraviolet A (UVA) and ultraviolet B (UVB) sunscreen with at least sun protection factor (SPF) 30 is recommended up to 3 months prior to performing the peel. Doing so stabilizes melanocyte activity and helps prevent prepeel burns or tanning. Sunlight exposure should also be minimized during this time.

Tretinoin is a topical therapy that may be initiated 6 weeks before the peel. There are a number of benefits that can result. Tretinoin aids in re-epithelialization and induces increased melanin distribution.[4] Following tretinoin therapy, the epidermis is thickened and demonstrates decreased corneocyte adhesion, reduced stratum corneum thickness, and neocollagen production. The thickened and uniform epidermis optimizes the execution of the peel, which correlates with improved final results.[5] The recommended dose range is between 0.025 and 0.1% and application is nightly. Possible side effects include erythema, skin irritation, and flaking. For patients sensitive to the effects of tretinoin, treatment should be started with lower concentrations.

Topical hydroquinone (4–8%) and hydrocortisone (1–2.5%) are also effective prepeel medications and can be started 6 weeks prior to the peel. Hydroquinone is particularly effective for patients with lentigines, dyschromias, and patients with higher Fitzpatrick skin types (e.g., types III and IV) because there is an increased risk of PIH in these patients. Hydroquinone inhibits the enzyme tyrosinase within melanocytes, which blocks melanin production. The application of a topical steroid such as hydrocortisone will help to minimize any inflammatory processes prior to undergoing the peel. In treatment of pigmentation, meta-analysis has demonstrated superior improvement with triple combination therapy (tretinoin, hydroquinone, topical steroid) than with monotherapy alone.[6]

All patients undergoing medium and deep peels should be started on antiherpetic prophylaxis. Even if a patient has no prior history of oral HSV outbreaks, the individual should be counseled about that possibility. Latent infections may arise even in the setting of a negative history. Patients with a negative history are regularly started on acyclovir 400 mg three times daily, starting 3 days prior to the peel and continuing 10 to 14 days following the procedure until re-epithelialization is complete. Anyone with a positive history for oral herpetic outbreaks should be provided 1 g of valacyclovir three times daily for the same duration. Herpetic outbreaks following a chemical peel can be devastating to the final results and all precautions should be undertaken to prevent their occurrence.

Because chemical peels intentionally remove the epidermis and portions of the dermis, there is potential for bacterial contamination. Cutaneous flora such as staphylococcal and streptococcal species are the typical causative agents in postpeel cellulitis. Because of its additional utility in treating acne, the authors initiate prophylactic minocycline, 100 mg once daily, starting the day prior to the peel and continuing for 10 days total. Acceptable alternatives include clindamycin, 150 mg three times daily; cephalexin, 250 mg four times daily; or erythromycin, 250 mg four times daily, for the aforementioned duration.

Other precautions should be discussed with the patient to improve uniform depth of penetration during the peel and overall healing. These include avoidance of facial skin waxing, dermabrasion, and electrolysis for 2 to 3 weeks prior to the peel. The chemical peel may be combined with other facial procedures; however, the authors caution against combining the procedure with rhytidectomy procedures as well as transcutaneous lower eyelid blepharoplasty. Decreased blood flow from skin-flap elevation during rhytidectomy may compromise blood flow and impair healing. It is recommended to stagger the peel and rhytidectomy by 6 weeks. Transcutaneous lower eyelid blepharoplasty, combined with the skin-tightening effects of a periorbital chemical peel, places the patient at undue risk for postoperative ectropion.

25.5 Multilevel Phenol–Croton Oil Peels

The multilevel phenol–croton oil peels represent an evolution within medium and deep chemical peels. Aside from the Baker-Gordon phenol-based peel, the only other agent capable of attaining the similar depths was 50% trichloroacetic acid (TCA). Unfortunately, 50% TCA has been shown to significantly increase the risk of postoperative scarring, despite attempts to optimize conditions with various surfactants, emulsifiers, or other additives.[7,8] To achieve depths similar to the 50% TCA peel, but with a more acceptable side-effect profile, multiple combination therapies were developed. Medium-depth peels were described involving application of 35% TCA combined with other agents such as solid carbon dioxide (CO_2), Jessner's Solution, or glycolic acid.[9,10,11] Brody and Hailey[9] and later Brody alone[12] found these three combination peels to have a scarring risk of less than 1%.

Use of the TCA-based peels flourished as a result of the all-or-none qualities of the Baker-Gordon deep peel. For years, there were unsubstantiated assertions made about the nature of the phenol–croton oil peel. These claims were accepted as dogma as early as the 1960s, when this peel was introduced into the plastic surgery arena. The original phenol–croton oil peels were in use by lay peelers in Hollywood, CA, in the 1920s. From this source, as well as Miami, Florida, in the 1950s, physicians were able to extract the lay formulas.[13] Interestingly, most peels contained similar concentrations of croton oil. Litton was the first practitioner to present a phenol–croton oil formula to the American Society of Plastic and Reconstructive Surgery in

Table 25.2 Baker-Gordon formula, 1962

Ingredient	Volume, % total
Phenol USP 88%	3 mL, 49
Distilled water	2 mL, 44
Septisol[a]	8 guttas, 4.5
Croton oil	3 guttas, 2.1

Abbreviation: USP, United States Pharmacopeia.
Note: 27 guttas = 1 mL.
[a]Sandent Co., Murfreesboro, Tennessee.
Modified with permission from Baker TJ. Chemical face peeling and rhytidectomy. A combined approach for facial rejuvenation. Plast Reconstr Surg Transplant Bull 1962; 29: 199–207.

the late 1950s. However, Baker received much attention for his version, which was presented in November 1961 and eventually modified to the classic formulation in 1962 (► Table 25.2).[14]

Intimately linked to the early dogmas of the phenol–croton oil peel were the descriptions presented by Adolph Brown et al.[15] Three primary assertions were outlined: first, that increased concentrations of phenol prevented deeper peels by inducing superficial keratocoagulation that inhibited further penetration deeper into the dermis. Second, Brown claimed that the addition of a saponin lowered surface tension and facilitated augmented depth of penetration by phenol. Finally, he said that croton oil must be included in the solution to act as a "buffer." The literature of the 1960s adopted these premises and then went on to declare further assertions, including that phenol was the only active ingredient within the Baker-Gordon formula and that there was an inverse relationship between the concentration of phenol and the depth of skin penetration. From the time of Brown's initial determinations in the 1960s, there were no well-designed animal or human studies supporting these notions until the 1990s, when Gregory Hetter questioned the role of each of the components in the phenol–croton oil formula.

To begin, a description of croton oil is necessary.[16] This compound is isolated from the seeds of *Croton tiglium*, a small shrub found naturally in India and Sri Lanka. Croton oil is a combination mainly of oleic, linoleic, myristic, and arachidonic acids. Less than 5% of the oil is composed of a resin—this resin has been known for more than a century in the scientific literature to be a skin irritant and possess toxic properties. In 1935, Joseph Spies detailed the toxic properties of the resin as he applied it to the arms of volunteers and observed severe vesiculations of the skin requiring up to 3 weeks to heal.[16] He also noted the resin's poor solubility in a 50:50 phenol to water solution. Hetter elucidated that the real reason to include Septisol (Sandent Co., Murfreesboro, Tennessee), a known surfactant, in the Baker-Gordon formula was to increase the components' solubility.

In Hetter's attempt to disprove the original notions regarding the phenol–croton oil peel, he performed a series of peels at different croton-oil concentrations upon one patient who agreed to undergo the treatments.[16] His findings are the basis for the multilevel phenol–croton oil peels in use today. At the lowest concentration of 18% phenol there was minimal effect. Mild

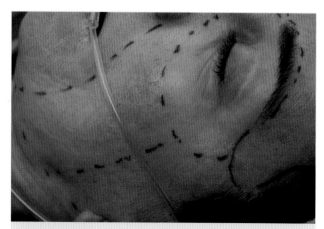

Fig. 25.2 Delineation of facial subunits to customize levels of treatment.

Table 25.3 Hetter phenol–croton oil peel formulas

Croton oil (%)	0.2	0.4	0.8	1.2	1.6
Phenol USP 88% (mL)	3.5	3.0	2.0	1.0	0
Croton oil stock solution* (mL)	0.5	1.0	2.0	3.0	4.0
Septisol[a] (mL)	0.5	0.5	0.5	0.5	0.5
Water (mL)	5.5	5.5	5.5	5.5	5.5

Abbreviation: USP, United States Pharmacopeia.
*Stock solution = 4% croton oil (1 mL croton oil + 24 mL phenol)
[a]Sandent Co., Murfreesboro, Tennessee.

epidermal keratolysis subsequently occurred using 35% phenol, but there was no clear dermal effect. Mild dermal involvement was noted at 50% phenol application. Finally, using 88% phenol, Hetter observed an obvious dermal effect that required 4 to 5 days to heal. The authors use this concentration of phenol alone to achieve a very superficial medium-depth peel.

After discovering the effects of phenol alone, different concentrations of croton oil were added to the peel solution. A croton-oil concentration of 0.7% required 7 days to heal, whereas 2.1% croton oil, equivalent to the concentration in the Baker-Gordon formula, required 11 days to heal.[16]

Based on his observations from these series of treatments, Hetter challenged the previous dogmas regarding phenol–croton oil peels. He deduced that there was a direct correlation between phenol concentration and depth of skin penetration. Furthermore, he showed that the depth of penetration is further enhanced with the addition of increasing concentrations of croton oil. These assertions are consistent with prior investigations by Stegman[17] and subsequent animal model studies.[18]

After completing his treatments on this patient, he used his new-found suppositions in treatment of five additional patients.[19] From these patients he was able to make additional assertions regarding the phenol–croton oil peel. First, he noted that the dilution of croton oil in a constant concentration of phenol shortened patient healing time, suggesting a more shallow depth of penetration. Next, he generalized that phenol concentration has minimal impact on overall depth of tissue injury. He also observed that multiple coats of the peel agent increase the depth of injury, which was later supported in the work of Stone and Lefer.[20]

Johnson et al first described the need for different depths of peeling for individual subunits of the face (▶ Fig. 25.2).[21] Hetter applied this concept by altering the croton-oil concentration in different regions of the face. He found that the nose could tolerate croton-oil concentrations up to 1.2%; however, the cheeks and forehead were limited to 0.8% concentrations and the upper nose, temple, and lateral brow could only tolerate concentrations up to 0.4% croton oil. Overall, Hetter felt that 1% croton oil was the upper threshold before placing the patient at increased risk of scarring and hypopigmentation.[19]

The initial phenol–croton oil formulations were created using droppers, which are inconsistent. Hetter converted drops to mL—25 drops equaled 1 mL. From this conversion, he created a stock solution of 0.04 mL of croton oil per 1 mL of phenol. This allowed him the ability to make varying croton-oil concentrations of 0.4, 0.8, 1.2, and 1.6% in a constant phenol concentration of 35% using phenol, Septisol, and water (▶ Table 25.3). This is in contrast to the Baker-Gordon formula where phenol concentration is approximately 49%.

Stone and Lefer later built upon Hetter's findings by testing three different patients with varying croton-oil concentrations mixed with phenol, the classic Baker-Gordon formula, with and without croton oil, and varying phenol concentrations without croton oil.[20] Their work also demonstrated the importance of technique of application in addition to the concentration and components of the peel solution. In the first patient Stone tested, he showed with repeat biopsies that the classic Baker-Gordon formula with and without croton oil created the same depth of penetration with repeated rubbings and occlusive taping. In the second case, he peeled the patient with alternating concentrations of phenol, 50 and 88%, and alternating concentrations of croton oil, 2.2 and 0.4%, on both thick forehead skin and the thinner nasojugal trough skin. Additionally, he varied the number of rubs using a wrung-out piece of gauze on the nasojugal trough. Biopsies showed that all the formulas created equal histological results and similar fibrosis when applied with 50 rubs. However, by decreasing the amount of rubs, he corroborated Hetter's findings that increasing concentrations of phenol leads to increased depth of skin penetration. Stone's work suggests that an upper threshold of tissue injury can be achieved with varying concentrations of phenol and croton oil when enough applications are undertaken. This finding was confirmed in his third case, when he used lower phenol concentrations with 2.2, 0.4, and 0% croton oil. He found that the aforementioned threshold could be met with all three solutions, but with varying numbers of applications. Stone's conclusion was that croton oil serves to lower the threshold number of applications. In 2009, a porcine animal model study verified the findings that multiple

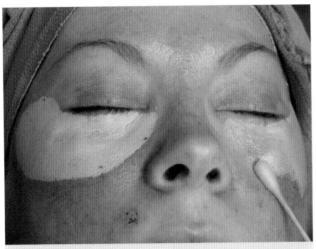

Fig. 25.3 Frosting is evident in the periorbital areas shortly following peel application.

Table 25.4 Chemical peel frosting levels

Level	Frosting characteristics	Approximate depth of penetration
I	Skin erythema with streaks of frosting	Epidermis
II	A light, white frosting with underlying erythema visible	Papillary dermis
III	A solid, white enamel, no erythema present	Reticular dermis

(Modified with permission from Monheit GD. Medium-depth chemical peels. Dermatol Clin 2001; 19: 413–425, vii.)

coatings of the phenol–croton oil peel serve to increase the depth of the peel.[18]

25.6 Peel Technique

Prior to undergoing the chemical peel, the patient's skin must be thoroughly cleaned with acne wash or Septisol the night before or morning of the procedure. Preoperative oral sedation, 10 to 15 mg of diazepam and 100 mg of dimenhydrinate, will help reduce patient anxiety. Antihistamines may also be necessary to decrease oral secretions to further protect the airway.

The patient should be started on intravenous (IV) 0.9% normal saline or lactated ringer before being brought to the operating suite. Prior to supine positioning, the patient's submandibular shadow is marked. This will help demarcate the inferior extent of the chemical peel and avoid unsightly transitions between the treated and untreated skin near the jawline. IV sedation is administered with propofol, and nerve (supraorbital, infraorbital, and mental) blocks with an equal mixture of 2% lidocaine and 0.5% bupivacaine are performed. The authors caution against including epinephrine in the blocks, in order to maximize local blood flow and phenol clearance.

At this time, the entire face is degreased and descaled with an acetone-soaked piece of gauze. Doing so removes any remaining oil and excess stratum corneum and allows for even application of the peel agent. Wrung-out gauze or wide, cotton-tipped applicators may be used for applying the peel. The authors suggest using cotton-tipped applicators for improved control. As previously delineated, the peel depth is dependent upon the amount of solution administered, uniform application of the solution, and the number of strokes applied; hence, control of the peel application is paramount. Advocates of the wrung-out gauze technique favor five to eight strokes for optimal results.[22]

When administering a phenol–croton oil peel, a frost becomes visible within 5 to 20 seconds (▶ Fig. 25.3). This is in contrast to TCA-based peels that may require several minutes for the frost to present. This phenomenon allows the depth of the peel to become quickly apparent and provide a guide to areas in need of reapplication. Medium-depth peels usually elicit levels II and III frosting (▶ Table 25.4).[23] After the frost

presents it will gradually fade over 10 to 15 minutes. There is no need to neutralize the peel because the frost indicates precipitation of keratin by the phenol, the end point of the chemical reaction.

Treatment of subunits of the face can be customized according to inherent levels of photodamage and the thickness of the patient's skin. Thick, sebaceous skin can tolerate higher croton-oil concentrations than thin, dry skin. The authors tend to use 1.2% croton-oil concentrations in areas of thick skin with deep rhytids (Glogau levels III and IV), such as the perioral region. Croton-oil concentrations of 0.8% are commonly used in the forehead, glabella, lateral periorbital region, and cheeks (Glogau levels II and III). Croton-oil peels of 0.4% may be applied to the periorbital region where the skin is thinner. The remainder of the face, including the periphery of treated areas, is handled with the less aggressive 88% phenol solution.

The face is typically divided into three different areas that are treated in 10- to 15-minute intervals. Doing so aids in phenol clearance and lowers risk of adverse events from phenol toxicity, namely cardiac arrhythmias. If a supraventricular arrhythmia occurs, the peel should be halted and the patient must be monitored until there is return to normal sinus rhythm. At that time the peel may resume.

When performing the peel, there are several guidelines that will permit even and uniform application to the entire face. One must be cognizant that a zone of hyperemia will develop on the border of the peeled skin (▶ Fig. 25.4). This represents an unpeeled skin reaction. Ensure adequate application to this region when treating adjacent areas—otherwise a line of untreated skin will be apparent following the peel. One may extend the peel into the hairline as well as across the vermilion border. The peel solution will not affect the hair follicles or lip. For deep rhytids, usually located in the glabella or perioral region, one may use the broken end of a cotton-tipped applicator to individually address the valley of the rhytid.

As with any procedure, great care must be undertaken to prevent iatrogenic injury. When applying the peel around the eyes, one should use a relatively dry cotton tip to avoid inadvertent dripping. The peel may extend 2 to 3 mm below the lower lash line. Should the patient experience any tearing, the tears should be dried immediately to avoid drawing any of the peel solution into the eye. If the peel solution does contact the eye, mineral oil should be applied to neutralize the phenol. Other neutralizing agents include glycerol, propylene glycol, olive oil, castor oil, or cottonseed oil.

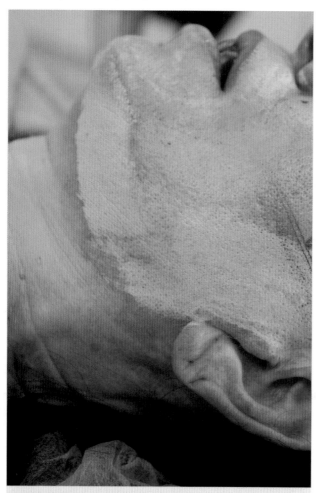

Fig. 25.4 Reactive hyperemia in submandibular area borders the inferior edge of the frosted region.

If incompletely anesthetized, the patient will experience a burning sensation that lasts up to 30 seconds. This burning sensation may return at the end of the procedure and can persist up to 8 hours. The longer lasting bupivacaine will help minimize this discomfort in the immediate postoperative time period.

25.7 Postoperative Care

On awakening from anesthesia, the patient may experience the aforementioned burning discomfort. A fan blown onto the face can provide temporary comfort. As soon as the frost subsides, a bland moisturizing emollient (e.g., Eucerin, Beiersdorf Inc., Wilton, Connecticut) should be applied to the entirety of the peeled area. This does not act as an occlusive dressing; thus, there need not be any worry about increasing the depth of penetration. Patients are directed to continue application of the emollient four to five times daily to ensure adequate coverage. There should be no attempt to vigorously scrub the face and remove all the emollient between applications. The patient should be discharged home with oral narcotic pain medicine. The authors also prescribe temazepam, 30 mg at bedtime, as needed for the first 7 nights.

Healing occurs in four defined stages (▶ Fig. 25.5).[23] The first stage is inflammation, which will increase over the first 12 hours following the procedure. Second, coagulation ensues. The epidermis will become leathery in appearance and separate from the underlying dermis. The dermal injury will manifest in necrotic slough. Use of the emollient will aid clearance of the necrotic tissue from the deep viable dermis. Next, re-epithelialization, which usually begins in 48 to 72 hours, will continue through days 7 to 10 depending on the peel depth. At this point the skin will assume a light shade of pink. The final stage of healing is called fibroplasia. This phase begins at week 1 and continues over 12 to 16 weeks following the peel. During this time there is widespread neoangiogenesis with collagen formation and reorganization.

During the initial 12 weeks following the peel, the patient should avoid UV exposure because uneven pigmentation and hyperpigmentation can result from melanocyte stimulation. In addition, patients' newly formed skin is often too sensitive to tolerate sunscreens for the first 6 weeks. Consequently, patients are educated to strictly avoid direct, prolonged sunlight exposure. To optimize final results, women should avoid becoming pregnant or using exogenous hormones during this time because hyperpigmentation can result.

25.8 Complications

Despite taking all necessary precautions, one may still encounter minor or major postoperative complications. Intraoperatively, the most dreaded complications involve phenol-related cardiotoxicity. Given that the phenol concentration is less in the modified phenol–croton oil peels compared to the Baker-Gordon formula, there is a theoretically reduced likelihood of complications arising. Nevertheless, precautions are taken including preoperative cardiac clearance, IV hydration, oxygen (O_2) administration via nasal cannula, and treatment of facial subunits over intervals of time. A supraventricular arrhythmia can arise 30 minutes following the onset of the peel. In this event, one should discontinue the peel, maintain hydration and oxygenation, and observe for resolution via cardiac monitoring.

Prolonged wound healing occurs when incomplete re-epithelialization lasts longer than 10 days. In this instance, one must assess for infection, contact irritation, or a systemic cause preventing wound healing. Any signs of infection should be treated with appropriate oral antibiotics. Failure to re-epithelialize raises the risk of scarring. When scarring does occur, treatment should be initiated promptly. Triamcinolone acetonide (Kenalog, Bristol-Myers Squibb, Princeton, New Jersey), 20 mg per mL, may be injected intralesionally; nevertheless, too-frequent injection raises the risk of dermal atrophy so caution is urged. Pulsed dye laser administration is another alternative that can be performed every 3 to 4 weeks as needed.

Antiviral prophylaxis must continue until complete re-epithelialization has occurred. Antiherpetic agents inhibit viral replication in the intact epidermal cell. Herpetic outbreaks may occur at any time until re-epithelialization is complete. Posttreatment HSV outbreaks are very uncomfortable for the patient and the wounds increase the risk of scarring. Maximal antiviral therapy should be initiated in the event of an outbreak and continued for 10 to 14 days or until re-epithelialization occurs.

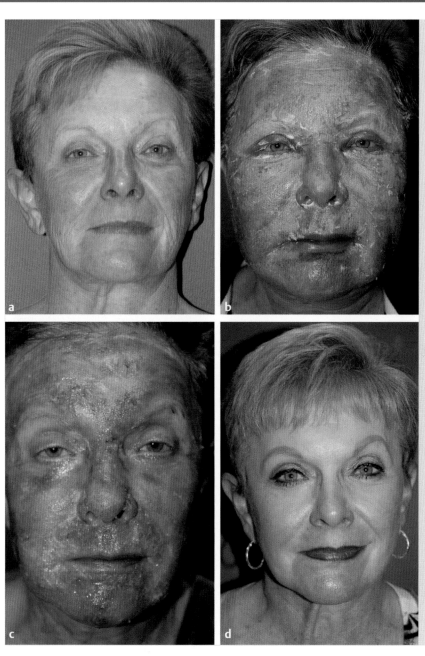

Fig. 25.5 Prior to the procedure and healing over time. (**a**) Preoperative view, (**b**) postoperative day 1, (**c**) postoperative day 6, and (**d**) 7 months after peel.

Patients with sensitive skin or contact dermatitis may experience prolonged erythema. This typically resolves with topical hydrocortisone (2.5%) lotions. For some patients, as the erythema subsides, there will be development of PIH. This is usually seen 3 to 6 weeks after the peel (▶ Fig. 25.6). PIH is most readily observed in darker skinned individuals and areas of the face overlying bony prominences (e.g., malar, zygoma regions). A combination of 0.025% tretinoin, 8% hydroquinone, and 1% hydrocortisone is effective in treating this complication. Alternatively, glycolic and salicylic acid peels have been found effective for treatment of PIH.[24,25,26]

A more problematic dyspigmentation following peels is hypopigmentation. This complication is classically more common when using phenol-based peels. Phenol is believed to eliminate melanocytes' ability to produce melanin. Historically, this occurred much more frequently with the classic Baker-Gordon formula, especially with the use of occlusive taping or thymol iodide masks. Unfortunately, this complication is irreversible. In the event of such an occurrence patients should be counseled on the need to wear concealing makeup.

25.9 Conclusions

In recent decades, laser resurfacing has become popularized and, as a result, the use of chemical peels has become marginalized. The work of Hetter and Stone has overturned outdated dogmas and fallacies involving the phenol–croton oil peels and has reinvigorated their use in medium and deep skin resurfacing. The multilevel phenol–croton oil peels should be considered a safe and effective tool that allows the facial cosmetic surgeon to alter depths of facial resurfacing based on the individual characteristics of the patient, including level of photodamage, skin type, and skin thickness.

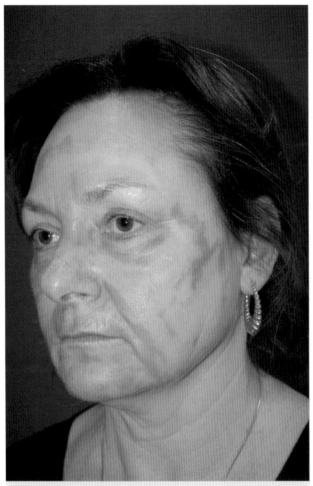

Fig. 25.6 Postinflammatory hyperpigmentation (PIH) 1 month following peel. Most pronounced over left zygoma.

References

[1] Baker TJ. Chemical face peeling and rhytidectomy. A combined approach for facial rejuvenation. Plast Reconstr Surg Transplant Bull 1962; 29: 199–207

[2] Fitzpatrick TB. The validity and practicality of sun-reactive skin types I through VI. Arch Dermatol 1988; 124: 869–871

[3] Glogau RG. Aesthetic and anatomic analysis of the aging skin. Semin Cutan Med Surg 1996; 15: 134–138

[4] Popp C, Kligman AM, Stoudemayer TJ. Pretreatment of photoaged forearm skin with topical tretinoin accelerates healing of full-thickness wounds. Br J Dermatol 1995; 132: 46–53

[5] Hevia O, Nemeth AJ, Taylor JR. Tretinoin accelerates healing after trichloroacetic acid chemical peel. Arch Dermatol 1991; 127: 678–682

[6] Rivas S, Pandya AG. Treatment of melasma with topical agents, peels and lasers: an evidence-based review. Am J Clin Dermatol 2013; 14: 359–376

[7] Brody HJ. Variations and comparisons in medium-depth chemical peeling. J Dermatol Surg Oncol 1989; 15: 953–963

[8] Dinner MI, Artz JS. Chemical peel—what's in the formula? Plast Reconstr Surg 1994; 94: 406–407

[9] Brody HJ, Hailey CW. Medium-depth chemical peeling of the skin: a variation of superficial chemosurgery. J Dermatol Surg Oncol 1986; 12: 1268–1275

[10] Monheit GD. The Jessner's + TCA peel: a medium-depth chemical peel. J Dermatol Surg Oncol 1989; 15: 945–950

[11] Coleman WP, III, Futrell JM. The glycolic acid trichloroacetic acid peel. J Dermatol Surg Oncol 1994; 20: 76–80

[12] Brody HJ. Complications of chemical peeling. J Dermatol Surg Oncol 1989; 15: 1010–1019

[13] Hetter GP. An examination of the phenol-croton oil peel: part II. The lay peelers and their croton oil formulas. Plast Reconstr Surg 2000; 105: 240–248, discussion 249–251

[14] Hetter GP. An examination of the phenol-croton oil peel: part III. The plastic surgeons' role. Plast Reconstr Surg 2000; 105: 752–763

[15] Brown AM, Kaplan LM, Brown ME. Phenol-induced histological skin changes: hazards, technique, and uses. Br J Plast Surg 1960; 13: 158–169

[16] Hetter GP. An examination of the phenol-croton oil peel: part I. Dissecting the formula. Plast Reconstr Surg 2000; 105: 227–239, discussion 249–251

[17] Stegman SJ. A comparative histologic study of the effects of three peeling agents and dermabrasion on normal and sundamaged skin. Aesthetic Plast Surg 1982; 6: 123–135

[18] Larson DL, Karmo F, Hetter GP. Phenol-croton oil peel: establishing an animal model for scientific investigation. Aesthet Surg J 2009; 29: 47–53

[19] Hetter GP. An examination of the phenol-croton oil peel: part IV. Face peel results with different concentrations of phenol and croton oil. Plast Reconstr Surg 2000; 105: 1061–1083, discussion 1084–1087

[20] Stone PA, Lefer LG. Modified phenol chemical face peels: recognizing the role of application technique. Facial Plast Surg Clin North Am 2001; 9: 351–376

[21] Johnson JB, Ichinose H, Obagi ZE, Laub DR. Obagi's modified trichloroacetic acid (TCA)-controlled variable-depth peel: a study of clinical signs correlating with histological findings. Ann Plast Surg 1996; 36: 225–237

[22] Larson DL. Phenol-croton oil peel: an update. Aesthet Surg J 2005; 25: 197–200

[23] Monheit GD. Medium-depth chemical peels. Dermatol Clin 2001; 19: 413–425, vii

[24] Burns RL, Prevost-Blank PL, Lawry MA, Lawry TB, Faria DT, Fivenson DP. Glycolic acid peels for postinflammatory hyperpigmentation in black patients. A comparative study. Dermatol Surg 1997; 23: 171–174, discussion 175

[25] Grimes PE. The safety and efficacy of salicylic acid chemical peels in darker racial-ethnic groups. Dermatol Surg 1999; 25: 18–22

[26] Grimes PE. Management of hyperpigmentation in darker racial ethnic groups. Semin Cutan Med Surg 2009; 28: 77–85

26 Enhanced Medium-Depth Chemical Peels

Phillip R. Langsdon, Dana K. Petersen, and Carol H. Langsdon

26.1 Introduction

Chemexfoliation, whether superficial, medium-depth, or deep, involves controlled destruction of the epidermal and, with sufficient penetration, the dermal tissue. A number of well-characterized chemical agents have been used to improve facial rhytids, scarring, texture and pigmentation irregularities, and general skin imperfections. The type and concentration of the agent, the depth of its penetration, the nature of destruction, and the inflammatory response determine the level of the peel.[1] Medium-depth peeling involves the precise destruction of the skin to the level of the papillary dermis and is effective in stimulating discernible regenerative changes with a relatively quick recovery time.[1]

For centuries, humans have attempted to preserve or restore a youthful appearance of the facial skin. Ancient records indicate that both fruits and wine were used to create topical preparations for such treatments.[2] The acids from these, such as citric and tartaric, have been used for superficial rejuvenation. Lactic acid, an active ingredient of sour milk, was used topically by Egyptian nobility.[3] The exfoliation protocols evolved throughout the generations in many cultures. As science advanced, various natural chemicals were isolated, and more modern agents began to be employed. By the early 20th century, "lay peelers" were using agents that resulted in deeper skin penetration.[4]

Over the following decades, dermatologists and plastic surgeons tried various formulas and protocols; however, there remained little standardization. Although many early 20th-century doctors used peeling to improve superficial scarring and acne, the side effect of wrinkle improvement did not escape notice.[4]

By the mid-1950s, Gillies and Millard began using phenol to treat wrinkled eyelid skin.[5] Then in the early 1960s, Litton began using a phenol–croton oil mixture to treat wrinkled skin not improvable with aging face surgery. In 1966, Baker et al reported the use of phenol with croton oil,[6] expanding awareness in the cosmetic surgery community.

As a more widespread appreciation of wrinkle improvement techniques evolved, so did technology. In the 1990s, lasers became popular tools to resurface the skin. Although some lasers treated more superficially, others, in particular the carbon dioxide (CO_2) laser, possessed the potential to treat deeply. In 1989, David et al[7] demonstrated improvement in the stratum corneum, enhancement in solar elastosis, and the creation of a new subepidermal band of collagen—results similar to those obtained with phenol peeling or dermabrasion. However, the intense thermal tissue insult resulted in longer posttreatment discomfort, persistent erythema, and more intense permanent hypopigmentation than shown with phenol–croton oil formulas.[8] These side effects of deep ablative CO_2 lasers eventually fostered the development of fractionated beam lasers. By design, the fractionated beam is divided into microcolumns of light, sparing the intervening tissue, and thus reducing thermal insult.

Because the chemical peeling components are inexpensive and easy to prepare and apply, there has been a significant resurgence in peeling.[4] Although medium-depth peeling cannot accomplish results comparable to deep-peeling, phenol-based formulas or deep CO_2 laser resurfacing, it has significant potential to ameliorate fine wrinkles and improve skin texture and pigmentation irregularities caused by moderate photodamage and aging.

German dermatologist P. G. Unna first noted the use of trichloroacetic acid (TCA) in chemical peels as early as 1882,[9] and it has been used in peeling for many years since. Previously, TCA peel depth was thought to be related to peel strength, and to a great degree that may be true. Superficial wounding has been quantitated as 10 to 30%, whereas above 50% has the potential to result in deep chemical peeling. TCA at 35 to 50% is considered by some as medium-depth peeling.[10] In any event, there are many variables that impact the various concentrations of TCA upon penetration and thus the level of peeling. Although higher concentrations would certainly peel deeper and in some cases obtain a better result, in some conditions scarring can occur when used above 45%.[11,12] As such, lesser concentrations in combination or as a singular agent are popular options.

TCA is both versatile and chemically stable.[13] It can be utilized in varied concentrations. Further, it does not have the systemic toxicity associated with increasing concentrations, such as seen with phenol peeling.[14]

Combination or multiagent peel therapy has also gained widespread use in medium-depth peeling, not only due to the ability to control frosting (keratin protein denaturation) but also because of the established safety margin.[15] Many of these protocols essentially break down the superficial layers to allow better penetration of TCA.

Common protocols currently employed to enhance medium peeling include 35% TCA alone or in combinations, such as TCA with Jessner's Solution or 70% glycolic acid with TCA. However, there are other options that will allow enhanced penetration of TCA at a lower, safer concentration, thus promoting improved results.

The sequential use of reduced concentrations of TCA (15, 20, and 25%) can provide enhanced results with greater improvement than those typically obtained with lesser concentrations. The technique can reduce fine rhytids, photodamage, and dyschromias, with outcomes approaching those obtained with medium-depth concentrations as well as some fractionated laser treatments. This involves four principles: (1) proper prepeel skin care preparation, (2) good pretreatment skin degreasing, (3) peel application technique that achieves the necessary frosting, and (4) sequential peels over a period of several months.[16]

Proper prepeel daily skin preparation involves the use of an exfoliation cream that results in slight flaking of skin. A 5% or greater glycolic acid product is our preference. Retinoic acid is added in many cases to start the exfoliation process and is continued if necessary to obtain the desired skin preparation. Retinoic acid is discontinued 2 days prior to the peel. This process augments the skin's reparative ability and aids penetration of the peel components.

Just before the peel, the skin is thoroughly washed and then degreased with acetone. Removal of all oils while gently abrading the skin surface also enhances peel penetration.

During the peel application, the skin is carefully observed. The peel is reapplied until proper frosting is obtained; the planned frosting level is dependent upon the skin type and goals. The frosting level is an indication of the peel depth.

The aggressive prepeeling skin care program, immediate prepeel oil removal, and proper frosting level enhance the impact of the weaker TCA concentrations, while avoiding the unpredictability of using higher concentrations. Resuming a daily skin care program once postpeel erythema has subsided in addition to repeated peels can continue to enhance results.

Although higher concentrations of TCA have been used safely, it is the authors' opinion that this protocol using lower concentrations can accomplish equivalent benefits, with a more tolerable peel process, and easier and quicker healing.[16]

26.2 Patient Selection

Fine rhytids, actinic skin changes, mild-to-moderate photoaging, and superficial dyschromias may be improved with medium peeling. The ideal patient is one with fair skin and a Fitzpatrick skin type of I, II, or III. The risk for postprocedural pigmentation abnormalities is higher in individuals with darker skin.

Some patients may present with a history of postinflammatory hyperpigmentation. We exercise caution in peeling these patients and, if peeled, plan to treat any postprocedural pigmentary changes. Patients who are taking hormonal medications have a greater tendency to demonstrate postpeel pigment alterations.[4] We inform these patients that pigment changes may occur, thereby requiring additional treatment after the peeling process.

Superficial acne scarring may occasionally be improved; however, other treatments may be more effective for this condition.

A careful patient history should focus on any skin disorders such as various forms of dermatitis, rosacea, acne, or herpes simplex, so that these conditions may be managed.

A history of radiation exposure, immunosuppression, autoimmune disease, and collagen-vascular disease could potentially compromise the healing process. Isotretinoin (Accutane, Roche, Basel, Switzerland) may also reduce skin-healing capacity. We recommend that patients wait 12 months from the end of isotretinoin therapy before undergoing peeling.

Some patients report that they have sensitive skin. These patients can either undergo a patch test in a small, inconspicuous location before the decision is made to go forward with a full-face, medium-depth peel, or they may be started with a 15% TCA peel.

As with all cosmetic procedures, the physician should understand the patient's desire and communicate realistic expectations. Patients should also comprehend the importance of their roles in the pretreatment and posttreatment skin care regimen. As always, standardized photographic documentation may help record most conditions. However, some photographic details can be difficult to capture due to the limits of lighting, exposure, and camera capabilities.

26.3 Prepeel Preparation

During the initial consultation and after the patient is determined to be an appropriate candidate, the procedure, postprocedural care, alternatives, risks, complications, limitations, and likely further treatment are discussed. No promises of perfection are made. The patient must understand that deeper wrinkles are likely to remain. It is also pointed out that postprocedural erythema, edema, and facial crusting are expected and that multiple peels are often required.

Photographs are obtained with a 100-mm macro-lens. Anteroposterior (AP), oblique, and side full-face views are obtained at 1.5 m. Close-up views are also obtained at 0.6 and/or 0.8 m that include an AP view of the forehead, periorbital, and perioral regions. Oblique right and left cheek views are obtained at 0.8 m. Care must be taken to set exposure and flash settings so that skin irregularities are not obscured in the photograph.

Preprocedural and postprocedural information and instructions are given both orally and in printed form. It is essential that the patient and the patient's family comprehend the expected early discoloration and possible swelling. Patients should also understand their roles in the outcome by properly preparing the skin and adhering to the daily skin care program. They should be realistic and recognize that a series of peels is usually needed to obtain the best result.

We do not normally prescribe antiviral medications unless the patient reports a history of fever blisters. If so, antiviral medication may be started the day prior to the peel and taken for 7 to 14 days after the peel. Valacyclovir or famciclovir may be prescribed at 500 mg/d. If an outbreak occurs, the dose is increased.

The authors' pretreatment program requires a minimum of 2 weeks of aggressive skin preparation with exfoliation, hydration, and protection. Excellent improvements can be seen with this regimen alone (▶ Fig. 26.1 and ▶ Fig. 26.2). Sunscreens and a strong glycolic acid-based exfoliator are used. Glycolic acid is an alpha hydroxy acid derived from sugarcane that initiates keratinocyte dyscohesion and increases type I collagen and hyaluronic acid deposition in the skin.[17] The tightening properties of collagen and the hydrophilic properties of hyaluronic acid give the skin a fuller and less wrinkled appearance.[16] Tretinoin is added in many cases of thick, oily, or resistant skin. Tretinoin (eg., Retin A, Ortho Dermatologics, Los Angeles, California) not only thins the stratum corneum in thick-skinned individuals but also helps prepare the skin for chemical peels by activating dermal fibroblasts and stimulating increased collagen deposition.[16] If the patient cannot tolerate the tretinoin, we use the glycolic cream twice per day as single-modality preparation. The cream application is usually stopped 2 days before the procedure. Hydroquinone is added to the pretreatment regimen, when faced with pigmentation considerations such as spotty hypopigmentation and melasma. Hydroquinone blocks the production of melanin precursors and, consequently, epidermal neopigmentation during the healing phase by inhibiting the enzyme tyrosinase.[18] Hydroquinone 4% cream may be recommended for those patients with Fitzpatrick skin type III or higher, or for those patients with pigmentary dyschromias.[16]

After consent is obtained on the day of the procedure, the patient cleanses the entire face and neck with Septisol (Sandent Co., Murfreesboro, Tennessee) three times and rinses

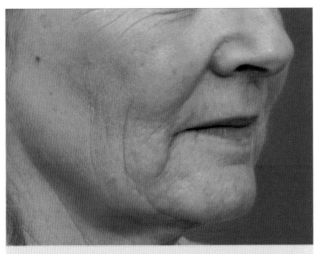

Fig. 26.1 Prior to the initiation of skin care regimen. (Courtesy of The Langsdon Clinic, Germantown, Tennessee.)

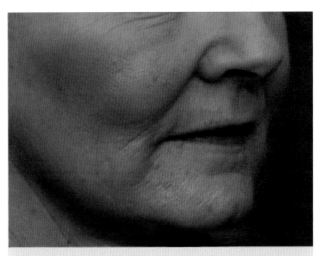

Fig. 26.2 Status after 6 months of dedicated skin care preparation. (Courtesy of The Langsdon Clinic, Germantown, Tennessee.)

thoroughly with tap water. We then degrease the skin with acetone on a cotton ball.

26.4 Trichloracetic Acid Preparation

TCA is naturally found in crystalline form and is mixed weight-by-volume (wt/vol) with distilled water. It is light insensitive, does not require refrigeration, and is stable on the shelf for more than 6 months.[13] The standard concentrations of TCA should be mixed wt/vol to accurately assess the concentration.[1] TCA crystals of 15, 20, and 25 g can be mixed with 100 mL of sterile water to give an accurate concentration of 15, 20, and 25%. We have our solutions prepared by a compounding pharmacy. The pharmacy must double check the concentrate after preparation.

26.4.1 Technique—Enhanced Sequential Trichloracetic Acid Peel

The procedure usually takes approximately 10 minutes. TCA is applied with a saturated (moist, NOT dripping) cotton ball on all facial areas except the eyelids, where a cotton-tipped applicator is used. The periorbital and eyelid areas are typically reserved until the end of the peel, so that we can observe the frosting and reaction of the peel in the thicker regions of the face prior to peeling the thin skin of the eyelids. An even application of the agent is essential to produce a uniform and reliable depth of peel. The time required to obtain the indicated frosting end point varies from patient to patient.[16] It may occur as early as 1 minute after application in thin, dry skin-type patients. It may take longer in thicker, severely aged, or weathered skin. Reapplication of the peel may be required in patients with resistant skin. The level of frosting required is determined by the condition of the skin. Patients with more severe damage may require more advanced frosting. The frosting will be associated with a mild stinging/burning sensation.

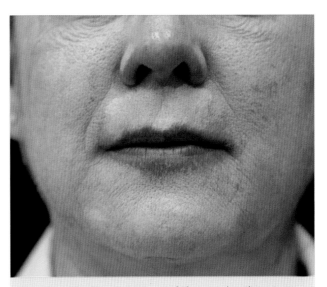

Fig. 26.3 Level 2 frosting. (Courtesy of The Langsdon Clinic, Germantown, Tennessee.)

The peel is performed in aesthetic units. During the procedure, the physician stands at the head of the patient when peeling the forehead, so as to prevent passing the applicator across the patient's body or eyes. The cotton ball is first rolled over the patient's forehead skin and feathered into the hairline and brows.

The perioral region is then peeled, followed by the cheeks. When peeling a cheek region, the peel is feathered onto the earlobe, sideburn, and 1 or 2 cm over the mandibular border. Frosting usually begins within 1 to 2 minutes of application. Both the quality and degree of frost should guide the physician in achieving a uniform peel. Reapplication can help in improving the frosting level. Level 2 frosting (► Fig. 26.3) (white-coated frosting with erythema showing through) is suitable for superficial skin changes, whereas level 3 frosting (solid, white frosting with little or no background of erythema) is used for areas of increased sebaceous glands, thicker skin, and areas of heavy actinic damage.[19]

The epidermal reaction on thicker skin regions helps determine how vigorously to peel the eyelids. If the thicker skin frosts quickly and deeply, then a very superficial eyelid peel can be anticipated. Slow frosting on thicker skin, requiring reapplication, might indicate that more will be required in the eyelid region.

When treatment progresses to the periorbital region, we usually peel the lower eyelids first with the cotton-tipped applicator. In treating the eyelids, special care should be exercised. We stand or sit below the lids, never passing the applicator across the eyes. The patient is asked to look superiorly and the cheek is retracted inferiorly. The skin is usually peeled within 3 mm of the ciliary margin.[20] Any reactive tearing is immediately dried with a clean gauze sponge or cotton-tipped applicator, to prevent any retrograde movement of the peel onto the globe. When treating the upper eyelids, we move to again stand above the patient's head. The patient is asked to close the lids and the brow is retracted superiorly. The peel is carried down to the tarsal groove and is feathered up into the brow. Again, any tearing is immediately dried.

Careful visualization and adequate lighting are imperative during the peeling process. Repeated inspections should be carried out, so as to precisely control the depth of penetration to that determined in the preprocedural plan.

Once the required level of frosting is attained, the solution is washed off with tap water.

26.5 Postpeel Care

Once the discomfort has subsided, erythema and edema will develop and be prominent for the first 48 to 72 hours. Postpeel discomfort is usually limited to the first hour posttreatment. Nonsteroidal, anti-inflammatory medication is typically all that is required.

Beginning the day following the peel, patients are asked to stand in the shower and allow a solid spray of water to wash the face several times a day. Patients should not rub or scrub the peeled areas. After showering, we have the patient gently towel-dry the neck and nonpeeled areas of the head and then allow the water to air-dry. The patient applies Aquaphor cream (Beiersdorf Inc., Wilton, Connecticut) (petrolatum 41%, mineral oil, ceresin, lanolin, alcohol, panthenol, glycerin, and bisabolol) over the entire area that has been peeled. This daily regimen is usually comfortable and eases the sensation of itching. Complete desquamation 4 usually develops as the edema resolves and are typically present from days 4 through 7. Full re-epithelialization is usually complete after 1 week and the face may be gently washed. Continued Aquaphor application is helpful in areas that remain dry. Skin tone is usually normalized by days 10 to 14 but the skin may still be pink for 2 to 4 weeks. Once the pinkness has dissipated, patients can restart their maintenance skin care exfoliation regimen and wear water-based cosmetics.

26.6 Complications

Scarring is a known complication from peels. It is generally accepted that TCA at 35% or less is safe.[11,12] Irregular pigmentation can also occur. Hyperpigmentation is the most common,

which is almost always a transient problem. If it is distressing to the patient, we typically use a skin-bleaching compound such as 4% hydroquinone and 2.5% hydrocortisone cream to improve such areas. Peeling again with either TCA or superficial peeling agents such as 30% salicylic or glycolic acid may be employed to aid in skin tone normalization.

Wound infections are extremely rare after a chemical peel procedure, as long as the patient faithfully follows the postprocedural cleaning instructions. Frequent skin cleansing is usually preventative. If an infection is encountered, oral antibiotics, regular cleansing, and close follow-up should adequately manage the condition.

If a herpetic outbreak occurs, the dose of the antiviral medication is increased. Any ulceration is treated with the addition of a topical antiviral ointment that is applied directly to the ulceration several times a day. Rapid and aggressive treatment of a herpetic outbreak usually resolves without any permanent effect. However, an invasive ulceration can result in scarring at the breakout site. If scarring develops during the healing process, the site can generally later be treated with injectable steroids.[4]

As with any situation, good patient selection, proper preprocedural education, close follow-up, and maintenance of good patient rapport go a long way to help the patient through the resolution of any postpeel sequelae.

26.6.1 Discussion

Although many peel formulas and techniques exist, the enhanced TCA protocol is an effective option for superficial to medium wrinkles, pigmentation abnormalities, and actinically damaged skin. In fact, we feel that the process is at least equal to many fractionated laser treatments. Many patients prefer the treatment since it has little discomfort, is less expensive, and is quick and easy to carry out. The protocol discussed herein allows the skin to achieve an enhanced improvement, with a lower resurfacing morbidity as compared to other modalities, which inflict more heat (as with a laser) or higher and more destructive chemical burns (as with higher concentrations of peeling agents).

We have found that proper pretreatment skin preparation through a daily skin care exfoliation, hydration, and protection program prepares the skin to achieve an enhanced outcome by breaking down the superficial skin layers and stimulating the regenerative capacity to a higher level.

Another factor that enhances the results of the lower concentrations is the proper degreasing along with the technique of achieving the proper frosting level. The degreasing mechanically abrades the surface and removes the oils, thereby improving penetration of the peel. The proper level of frosting is obtained by immediately reapplying the peel to an area of the face that does not frost to the desired level. This technique allows one to frost (penetrate) to a level achieved in other situations by a higher concentration of the peeling agent. The therapy of periodic peeling can sequentially improve the skin until the desired improvement has been obtained (▶ Fig. 26.4, ▶ Fig. 26.5, ▶ Fig. 26.6, ▶ Fig. 26.7). Although, it could be thought that a more aggressive treatment might lessen the time required to improve the skin, it must be remembered that deeper, more aggressive procedures have a higher morbidity

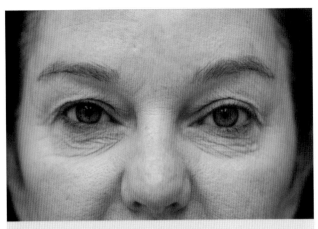

Fig. 26.4 Prior to trichloroacetic acid (TCA) peel (periorbital region). (Courtesy of The Langsdon Clinic, Germantown, Tennessee.)

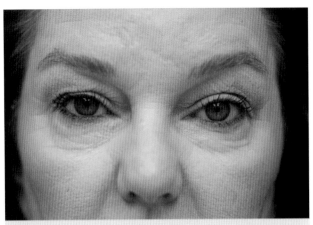

Fig. 26.5 Status after 25% trichloroacetic acid (TCA) peel (periorbital region). (Courtesy of The Langsdon Clinic, Germantown, Tennessee.)

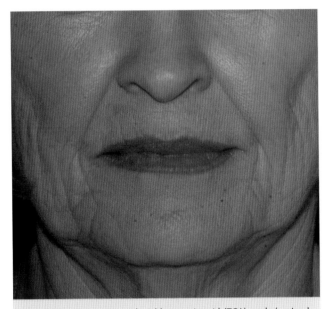

Fig. 26.6 Prior to sequential trichloroacetic acid (TCA) peels (perioral region). Note the fairly deep rhytids. (Courtesy of The Langsdon Clinic, Germantown, Tennessee.)

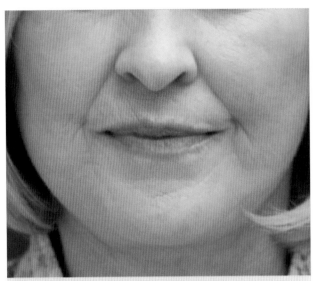

Fig. 26.7 Status after enhanced superficial chemical peeling and facelift. The patient received a total of three peels spaced 6 to 8 weeks apart, with increasing trichloroacetic acid (TCA) concentrations with each peel (15 → 20 → 25%). Note the tremendous improvement in the rhytids. (Courtesy of The Langsdon Clinic, Germantown, Tennessee.)

and risk. In fact, many patients enjoy the less morbid process and consider the periodic peels as an inexpensive yet substantial action in self-improvement. The subsequent tight sensation and smoothing of the tone and texture of the skin provide a strong sense of benefit from this relatively mild process.

Because the peel, as opposed to a laser, does not thermally burn the skin, there is less likelihood of hypopigmentation.

It has been our experience that many patients prefer this peeling technique to more aggressive therapies, unless they possess a level of skin deterioration not improvable with this system. In our involvement in more than 3,000 TCA peels, we have had no scarring and no pigment abnormalities. Posttreatment erythema usually subsides by 2 weeks postprocedure. Discomfort is limited to 1 or 2 minutes during the peel. There is little-to-no postpeel discomfort. We use the enhanced TCA peel protocol in many postfractionated laser patients in order to

continue to refine the patients' results. Many of these patients subsequently tell us that they prefer the peel to the laser.

The enhanced TCA peel alone, however, cannot improve very deep wrinkles. Deep peeling or more ablative-type laser treatments are without question better for deep wrinkles.

26.7 Conclusion

Medium-depth chemical peeling is a safe, effective, and inexpensive tool for facial rejuvenation for conditions such as superficial scarring, wrinkling, photodamage, and pigmentary problems.

The senior author has previously described and regularly employs an enhanced TCA peel technique using a lower concentration of TCA in a manner that achieves the results of medium-depth peeling. This is accomplished via aggressive pre-peel skin exfoliation, sequential peels, pretreatment skin degreasing, and immediate reapplication to the proper frosting level. Enhanced TCA chemical peeling is safe, well tolerated by patients, and offers an exceptional improvement in skin quality.

References

[1] Monheit GD. Chemical peels. Skin Therapy Lett 2004; 9: 6–11

[2] The Incantations and Recipes: Recipe for Transforming an Old Man into a Youth. Breasted, JH, ed. The Edwin Smith Surgical Papyrus Vol 1. Chicago, IL: University of Chicago Press; 1930: 492–498

[3] Brody HJ, Monheit GD, Resnik SS, Alt TH. A history of chemical peeling. Dermatol Surg 2000; 26: 405–409

[4] Langsdon PR, Shires CB. Chemical face peeling. Facial Plast Surg 2012; 28: 116–125

[5] Gillies HD, Millard DR Jr. Principles and Art of Plastic Surgery. Boston, MA: Little Brown; 1957

[6] Baker TJ, Gordon HL, Seckinger DL. A second look at chemical face peeling. Plast Reconstr Surg 1966; 37: 487–493

[7] David LM, Lask GP, Glassberg E, Jacoby R, Abergel RP. Laser abrasion for cosmetic and medical treatment of facial actinic damage. Cutis 1989; 43: 583–587

[8] Langsdon PR, Milburn M, Yarber R. Comparison of the laser and phenol chemical peel in facial skin resurfacing. Arch Otolaryngol Head Neck Surg 2000; 126: 1195–1199

[9] Marmelzat WL. A historical review of chemical rejuvenation of the face. In: Kotler R, ed. Chemical Rejuvenation of the Face. St. Louis, MO: Mosby; 1992: 934–938

[10] Camacho FM. Medium-depth and deep chemical peels. J Cosmet Dermatol 2005; 4: 117–128

[11] Kotler R. Chemical Rejuvenation of the Face. St. Louis, MO: Mosby; 1992

[12] Stegman SJ. Medium-depth chemical peeling: digging beneath the surface. J Dermatol Surg Oncol 1986; 12: 1245–1246

[13] Spinowitz AL, Rumsfield J. Stability-time profile of trichloroacetic acid at various concentrations and storage conditions. J Dermatol Surg Oncol 1989; 15: 974–975

[14] Collins PS. Trichloroacetic acid peels revisited. J Dermatol Surg Oncol 1989; 15: 933–940

[15] Monheit GD. The Jessner's + TCA peel: a medium-depth chemical peel. J Dermatol Surg Oncol 1989; 15: 945–950

[16] Langsdon PR, Rodwell DW, III, Velargo PA, et al. Latest chemical peel innovations. Facial Plast Surg Clin North Am 2012; 20: 119–123

[17] Bernstein EF, Lee J, Brown DB, Yu R, Van Scott E. Glycolic acid treatment increases type I collagen mRNA and hyaluronic acid content of human skin. Dermatol Surg 2001; 27: 429–433

[18] Jimbow K, Obata H, Pathak MA, Fitzpatrick TB. Mechanism of depigmentation by hydroquinone. J Invest Dermatol 1974; 62: 436–449

[19] Brody HJ. Variations and comparisons in medium-depth chemical peeling. J Dermatol Surg Oncol 1989; 15: 953–963

[20] Coleman WP, III, Futrell JM. The glycolic acid trichloroacetic acid peel. J Dermatol Surg Oncol 1994; 20: 76–80

27 Superficial Chemical Peels

Albert J. Fox

27.1 Introduction

Chemical peeling is a popular treatment for rejuvenation of the skin. Superficial chemical peeling used alone or in combination with other treatment modalities can help achieve improvement of aging skin with little downtime and low risk. Chemical peeling agents have been in use for centuries. Women in ancient Rome and Egypt made use of sour milk baths (lactic acid) and rubbed fermented grape skins (tartaric acid) to improve skin texture, taking advantage of the exfoliative effects of the hydroxyl acids present. Today, a variety of peeling agents are available to the clinician to help achieve a desired result.

27.2 Indications for Superficial Peel and Patient Evaluation

The primary clinical indications for superficial chemical peels are for the improvement of mild photoaging (Glogau types I and II), skin texture, acne, actinic keratosis and for improvement of fine rhytids. Superficial peels are ideal for patients whose lifestyles preclude the prolonged recovery required of medium or deep peels. Superficial peels are "patient friendly," allowing patients to return to work the same day, are not painful, and are not associated with hypopigmentation. They are generally safe and rarely are associated with adverse sequelae. Often, superficial peels are performed 1 to 4 weeks apart (▸ Fig. 27.1, ▸ Fig. 27.2, ▸ Fig. 27.3). Maximal results are seen when a series of treatments (six to eight) are performed. Combining a series of peels with a home skin care regimen can result in optimal, long-term changes. Skin care regimens with use of topical vitamin C, retinoids, or low-concentration glycolic acid (GA) promote continued skin improvement and aid collagen production.

A thorough patient history is important prior to any chemical peel regimen. A history of keloid formation, recurrent herpetic outbreaks, medication use such as oral isotretinoin, current use of skin care products, history of silicone injections, prior cosmetic procedures, and overall general health should be obtained. Background on a patient's perceived skin sensitivity is meaningful because it may guide the clinician in choosing more or less aggressive treatments. Evaluations of Fitzpatrick skin type and the skin's overall thickness and oiliness are helpful. Skin that is thicker and more sebaceous may require a pretreatment program with topical retinoids or alpha hydroxy acids (AHAs). Superficial peels can be used to treat all Fitzpatrick skin types (I–VI).

The condition(s) treated by a superficial peel should ideally be limited to the epidermis. Examination of the skin with a Wood lamp will help to identify appropriate candidates (▸ Fig. 27.4). Wood lamp illumination enhances superficial dyschromias, whereas deeper dyschromias demonstrate minimal enhancement under illumination and require more aggressive therapies (medium- or deep-depth resurfacing).[1]

27.3 Basic Chemistry and Histological Changes

AHAs are weak acids that induce their clinical effects by either metabolic or caustic effect.[2] At low concentrations, they reduce corneocyte cohesion, inducing exfoliation of the epidermis.[2] At higher concentrations, their effect is mainly destructive; therefore, AHAs cannot neutralize themselves and need to be neutralized by water or a weak buffer.[2]

Superficial peeling primarily affects the epidermis and uppermost part of the dermis. The stratum corneum becomes thinner, more compact with desquamation.[3] The inflammation stimulates the production of cytokines that in turn stimulate and activate fibroblasts that produce type I and type IV collagen

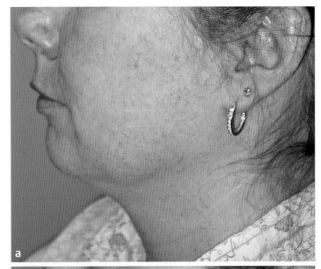
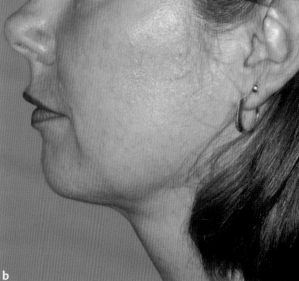

Fig. 27.1 (a) Before a series of glycolic acid (GA) peels. (b) After a series of GA peels.

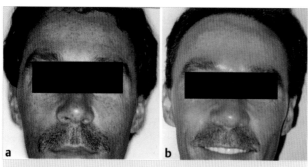

Fig. 27.2 Patient is seen (**a**) prior to a series of glycolic acid (GA) peels, and (**b**) following a series of GA peels.

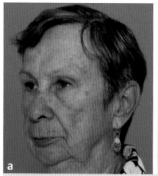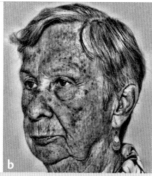

Fig. 27.4 A 70-year-old woman with marked rhytidosis and photo-damage, comparing (**a**) standard photography with a (**b**) computer-generated Wood lamp depiction. (Reproduced with permission from Truswell WH, IV. Aging changes of the periorbita, cheeks, and midface. Facial Plast Surg 2013; 29(1): 3–12.)

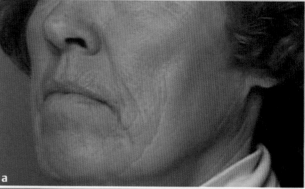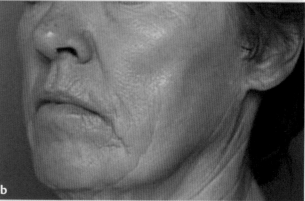

Fig. 27.3 A woman is shown (**a**) before a series of glycolic acid (GA) peels, and (**b**) subsequent to a series of GA peels.

and elastin fibers.[4] Histological studies by Ditre et al[5] showed an increase in collagen and glycosaminoglycans in the papillary and reticular dermis and increased elastic staining in the dermis.[3,5] This increase in collagen and elastin translates into the clinical improvement seen postpeel.

27.4 Classification of Chemical Peels

Chemical peels produce varying clinical effects to the skin depending on their depth of penetration. Chemical agents are classified as very superficial (removing stratum corneum) to deep (extending into reticular dermis) (▶ Table 27.1).[6] Factors such as concentration, duration of contact with the skin, number of coats applied, as well as prepeel skin preparation may impact the depth of a peel and its subsequent clinical effect.

Superficial chemical peels penetrate the level from the stratum granulosum to the upper papillary dermis. Superficial peels are divided into two categories: very light and light. Very light peels exfoliate only the stratum corneum. The agents used include low-concentration GA, Jessner's Solution, salicylic acid, and 10 to 20% trichloroacetic acid (TCA). Light peels injure the entire epidermis and will stimulate collagen deposition and promote epidermal thickening. Light peel agents include 50 to 70% GA, 10 to 35% TCA, and solid carbon dioxide slush (▶ Table 27.1).[6,7]

Table 27.1 Classification of peeling agents

Depth of penetration	Peeling agent
Very superficial (removes stratum corneum)	Microdermabrasion Retinoic acid GA 30–50% (1–2 min) Jessner's Solution (1–3 coats) Resorcinol 20–30% (5–10 min) TCA 10% (1 coat)
Superficial (upper papillary dermis)	GA 50–70% (5–20 min) Jessner's Solution (5–10 coats) Resorcinol 50% (30–60 min) TCA 10–35% (1 coat) Solid CO_2 slush
Medium (papillary dermal)	GA 70% (5–30 min) TCA 35% Modified Baker-Gordon w/2 drops of croton oil
Deep (reticular dermal)	Baker-Gordon phenol formula Hetter Peel

Abbreviations: GA, glycolic acid; TCA, trichloroacetic acid.

27.5 Prepeeling Preparation

Preparation or "priming" of the skin prior to chemical peeling with topical agents may lead to improved and uniform results. This requires good patient compliance with the

Table 27.2 Factors affecting skin reaction and penetration of alpha hydroxy acids

Acid concentration (e.g., 35–70%)
pH and buffering
Contact time with skin
Volume of acid applied
Skin pretreatment and degreasing
Condition of the epidermal barrier

Abbreviation: pH, measurement of acidity in the skin.

pretreatment program for consistent outcomes. Tretinoin applied 4 to 6 weeks in advance of initiating a peel program is commonly utilized. Tretinoin predominantly affects the epidermis with short-term use. Its epidermal effects (thinning and compaction of the stratum corneum and melanocyte suppression) make it an ideal pretreatment agent.[1] Tretinoin enhances penetration of the peeling solutions and accelerates postprocedural epithelialization.[1,7,8] Patients are instructed to apply the tretinoin as uniformly as possible to the face; uneven application can result in uneven or poor uptake of the peeling solution, limiting the effectiveness of the peel.

Reduction in melanogenesis through the use of daily sunscreens is helpful to decrease incidence of postinflammatory hyperpigmentation (PIH). Application of hydroquinone 4% once or twice daily may be helpful to prevent PIH in Fitzpatrick skin types III through VI patients. Hydroquinone causes a reversible depigmentation through inhibition of the enzyme tyrosinase. This inhibits the enzymatic oxidation of 3,4-dihydroxyphenylalanine (dopa) to melanin, effectively suppressing melanin production.[1,4,7]

Although the likelihood of herpes simplex virus (HSV) reactivation with a superficial peel is low, antiviral prophylaxis should be considered because all resurfacing procedures have the potential to stimulate HSV. An active herpes infection is a contraindication to proceeding with a chemical peel. Most commonly used antiviral agents include acyclovir or valacyclovir 500 mg twice daily, started 1 to 3 days prior to procedure and continued for up to 10 to 14 days following the procedure.

27.6 Postpeel Regimen

It is important to avoid scratching or injury to the skin postpeel. Protection from the sun with sunscreen and a hat is recommended. Use of bland moisturizers can soothe newly peeled skin. In cases of prolonged redness or a brisk reaction to a peel, a topical steroid may be helpful. Utilization of a topical steroid may reduce the risk of PIH, especially in Fitzpatrick skin types IV through VI. Initiating or resuming a topical skin care regimen and consideration for maintenance peels will aid in maintaining long-term results of the superficial peels.

27.7 Superficial Chemical Peel Agents

27.7.1 Glycolic Acid

GA is one of the most popular AHAs available over the counter or for physician office use; it is also one of the most common AHAs. GA is obtained from sugarcane, and has the smallest molecular weight of the AHAs and penetrates the skin easily.[2,9] GA is very hydrophilic and the measurement of acidity in the skin (pH) may range from 0.08 to 2.75.[9,10]

It can be purchased in unbuffered concentrations up to 70% in a liquid or gel solution. The unbuffered gel solution provides an ease of application to the skin with 2 × 2 in gauze, sable brush, cotton ball, or cotton-tipped applicator.

Factors affecting the depth of penetration of a glycolic peel include solution concentration, method of application, volume of acid delivered, skin pretreatment, and duration of contact with the skin (▶ Table 27.2).[1] A study by Becker et al[11] demonstrated that varying the pH of the GA will result in varying tissue damage. The study demonstrated that low pH causes greater tissue damage and necrosis than a GA with a higher pH or partially neutralized GA.[11] The range of pH tested in the study varied from 0.6 to 2.75. The duration of application of GA is critical; GA requires neutralization with water or 5% sodium bicarbonate after a brief period (most commonly 2–4 min).[12] Longer periods of application may be required depending upon patient skin response and skin type. However, too long an application period may result in deeper penetration than desired, possibly resulting in injury. Generally, patients with greater photodamaged skin, Glogau classifications III and IV, can tolerate higher concentrations of GA with longer exposure times.[13] Patients with overly sebaceous skin appear to have increased tolerance to GA peels, apparently due either to the amount of surface sebum or to a hyperkeratotic stratum corneum.[13] Virtually all Fitzpatrick skin types (I–VI) can undergo GA peels.

27.7.2 Technique

Proper skin preparation prior to a superficial peel is necessary to obtain maximal results.

A prepeel regimen consisting of tretinoin or low-concentration GA application (e.g., GA pads, 10–15%) is started 2 to 6 weeks before the superficial peel. Prior to application of the peeling agent, the patient's skin is cleansed and degreased. A number of agents can be used: ethanol, acetone, chlorhexidine, ethanol-salicylic acid solution, or Jessner's Solution. These agents can be applied with gauze and help remove debris, sebum, and the stratum corneum.

The peeling agent is applied rapidly with a piece of gauze, large cotton-tipped applicator, cotton ball, or smaller cotton swab (around eyelids, lips). The eyelid skin may be stretched to allow even application. If actinic keratosis, scars, or pigmented macules are present, additional peeling agent can be applied as a second or third coating. The duration of application of the peeling mixture affects penetration and clinical results. When erythema is observed, this indicates epidermal penetration. The

Table 27.3 Jessner's Solution Components

Agent	Amount
Resorcinol	14 g
Salicylic acid	14 g
Lactic acid	14 g
Ethanol	100 mL

peel can be neutralized at this point for a lighter, superficial peel. Dermal penetration may be seen as a white blanch or islands of blanching on the skin; a uniform white frost (as seen with a TCA peel) is not encountered. The patient may experience a mild stinging, heat, or pruritic sensation. Use of a portable cooling fan enhances patient comfort. Neutralization of the peel with water or sodium bicarbonate is performed. If the patient experiences severe erythema, a topical antibiotic ointment, soothing lotion, or mild hydrocortisone cream can be applied 1 to 4 days after the peel. Daily moisturizer and sunscreen are recommended postpeel.

27.7.3 Salicylic Acid

Salicylic acid is a naturally occurring substance found in the bark of the willow tree.[3] Salicylic acid is a beta hydroxy acid, well known for its keratolytic and exfoliative properties of the epidermis. It is also a known comedolytic and is often used in cases of acne and PIH.

Salicylic acid formulations are often 20 or 30% in ethanol or a 50% paste.[2,7] The indications for salicylic acid peels include inflammatory and noninflammatory acne vulgaris, mild dyschromias, and pigmentation.

Like GA peels, the treatment regimen involves a series of four to six peels, 2 to 4 weeks apart. After the skin is prepped and cleansed, the solution is applied for 3 to 5 minutes. A white precipitate of salicylic acid often appears and should not be confused with frosting.[2] This peel is self-limited and neutralization is not required. The face is then gently cleansed. Postpeel care regimen of moisturizers is instituted as needed.

27.7.4 Jessner's Solution

Jessner's Solution was formulated by Dr. Max Jessner in the 1940s. The Jessner's Solution consists of 14 g each of resorcinol, salicylic acid, and lactic acid in ethanol (▶ Table 27.3). Its advantage is the synergistic effects of three keratolytic agents and the benefit of a skin lightening agent (resorcinol) as one of its components.[3,14] Jessner's Solution is applied to prepped skin; typically, mild erythema with white speckling is observed. It is often applied as a single coat; however, two to three coats of the solution can be applied, as indicated by the severity of the patient's skin pathology. The peel will result in 2 to 3 days of light desquamation. Jessner's peels can be used in the treatment of melasma, and are comparable in efficacy to 70% GA with fewer side effects.[15] Jessner's Solution can also be used in combination with other peeling agents such as TCA to achieve more uniform and greater depth of penetration.[6] It has been combined with 5-fluorouracil (5-FU) weekly for 8 weeks for

treatment of actinic keratosis and photoaging.[16] Jessner's Solution needs to be stored in a dark bottle to prevent photooxidation.

27.7.5 Trichloroacetic Acid

TCA is commonly used for superficial peeling. At 10 to 25%, TCA will precipitate superficial epidermal proteins and cause cellular necrosis. TCA is self-neutralizing and does not require water or bicarbonate to terminate the peeling action.[14] Concentrations of 10 to 25% are used for intraepidermal peels. A single coat of 35% TCA is also often classified as a superficial peel (▶ Table 27.1). However, the depth of penetration of 35% TCA will vary with technique, skin preparation, and quality of the epidermal barrier; hence a medium-depth peel can occur.

Once skin has been prepared and degreased with acetone or other agents, TCA may be applied in single or multiple coats using gauze sponges or cotton-tipped applicators. The applicator or gauze is applied with pressure to the skin, taking care that the TCA penetrates to the base of the rhytids.

The depth of the peel is assessed by the skin appearance. Low-concentration TCA (10–20%) often results in mild erythema or erythema with speckled white frosting (level I frosting) corresponding to superficial penetration. This often results in light flaking of the skin 2 to 4 days after the peel. With concentrations of 25% or greater, a white frost with mild background erythema is seen. This corresponds to a full-thickness epidermal peel and may take up to 5 days to heal. If a solid, white frost develops with no erythema showing through, the peel has extended into the papillary dermis and may take 7 days to heal. If the erythema or frosting does not appear uniform, repeat application may be performed. Patients are informed that a stinging or mild burning sensation may be present during and immediately after the peel. Use of a cooling fan during the peel can help alleviate the sensation. Postpeel, cold, wet compresses are applied for patient comfort. A moisturizing cream may then be applied.

27.7.6 Tretinoin

Tretinoin peel is a solution of high-concentration tretinoin (1–5%) in polypylene glycol. The topical tretinoin solution imparts a yellow hue to the skin with application and is painless. A series of five superficial peels with tretinoin 1 to 5% has been reported to improve melasma, ephelides, and acne.[17] The application should be left in place for at least 6 hours. Unlike most peels, the tretinoin peel does not coagulate proteins. It does not require neutralization. Typically, in 2 to 3 days a fine, white desquamation occurs. The peel is very safe and can be used in a layered fashion, over other superficial peeling agents, to potentiate their effects.[18]

27.8 Complications

27.8.1 Infections

Infections are relatively rare with superficial peels, and occur more commonly with medium or deep peels. Common pathogens include *Staphylococci*, *Streptococci*, and *Pseudomonas*. Often these are treated with oral and topical antibiotics.

Herpetic outbreaks can be prevented with acyclovir or valacyclovir prophylaxis. Previous studies have shown a 6.6% HSV infection rate in patients who underwent chemical peels and had no history of infection.[19,20] Prophylactic dosing will need to be increased when active infection occurs. Cutaneous *Candida* infection may also be seen. Perioral pustules develop and may rapidly spread. Patients often will have symptoms of itching or burning. Topical or oral antifungal agents are helpful. Infection often will follow poor wound care. Cultures should be obtained when infection is suspected and acetic acid soaks should be instituted.

27.8.2 Prolonged Erythema

Prolonged erythema may represent a possible contact dermatitis, early impending scarring, or persistent localized inflammation. Treatment includes topical steroids, oral steroid use, rare use of intralesional steroid, avoidance of any irritants, and use of moisturizers. Prolonged erythema can also be treated with pulsed dye laser procedures.

27.8.3 Pigmentation

The most common complication of chemical peeling is pigmentation change. Hyperpigmentation is more typically associated with light peels and hypopigmentation with deep peels. Hyperpigmentation often responds to hydroquinone or kojic acid bleaching agents, retinoic acid, tazarotene cream, and sunscreens.

27.8.4 Milia

Milia or epidermal cysts result from occlusion of the pilosebaceous units. These can be easily treated with a comedonal extractor or use of a fine needle.

27.8.5 Acneiform Dermatitis

Acneic eruptions are not uncommon and may be secondary to reactivation of previously existing acne or occlusion of pores after re-epithelialization. Treatment often involves use of topical or oral antibiotic therapy.

27.8.6 Scarring

Rare with superficial peels, scarring risk escalates with increasing depth of the peel. Early signs of scarring include delayed healing and persistent, indurated, patchy erythema. Therapy options include topical and intralesional steroid, oral steroid, and pulsed dye laser.

27.9 Conclusion

Superficial peels offer many advantages and are useful in the treatment of early signs of aging. Superficial peels have an excellent safety record, can be used on all Fitzpatrick skin types (I–VI), provide for rapid healing with minimal downtime, do not require anesthesia, are affordable, can be combined with other peels or lasers, and can amplify the effects of topical rejuvenating agents. Through their exfoliative properties, many conditions such as melasma, PIH, ephelides, acne vulgaris, fine rhytids, and photoaging changes can be treated successfully. Limitations of superficial peels include the need for multiple peel sessions and minimal effects on deeper rhytids or severe photoaging. To maximize efficacy, a series of chemical peels combined with a topical regimen before and after the peel is recommended. With proper patient selection, patient education, and realistic expectations, the results of superficial peels are often highly satisfactory.

References

[1] Baker TJ, Stuzin JM, Baker TM, eds. Facial Skin Resurfacing. St. Louis, MO: Quality Medical Publishing; 1998
[2] Landau M. Chemical peels. Clin Dermatol 2008; 26: 200–208
[3] Fabbrocini G, De Padova MP, Tosti A. Chemical peels: what's new and what isn't new but still works well. Facial Plast Surg 2009; 25: 329–336
[4] Fischer TC, Perosino E, Poli F, Viera MS, Dreno B Cosmetic Dermatology European Expert Group. Chemical peels in aesthetic dermatology: an update 2009. J Eur Acad Dermatol Venereol 2010; 24: 281–292
[5] Ditre CM, Griffin TD, Murphy GF, et al. Effects of alpha-hydroxy acids on photoaged skin: a pilot clinical, histologic, and ultrastructural study. J Am Acad Dermatol 1996; 34: 187–195
[6] Mendelsohn JE. Update on chemical peels. Otolaryngol Clin North Am 2002; 35: 55–72, vi
[7] Monheit GD, Chastain MA. Chemical peels. Facial Plast Surg Clin North Am 2001; 9: 239–255, viii
[8] Monheit GD. Skin preparation: an essential step before chemical peeling or laser resurfacing. Cosmetic Dermatol. 1996; 9: 13–14
[9] Sharad J. Glycolic acid peel therapy - a current review. Clin Cosmet Investig Dermatol 2013; 6: 281–288
[10] Roberts WE. Chemical peeling in ethnic/dark skin. Dermatol Ther 2004; 17: 196–205
[11] Becker FF, Langford FP, Rubin MG, Speelman P. A histological comparison of 50% and 70% glycolic acid peels using solutions with various pHs. Dermatol Surg 1996; 22: 463–465
[12] Mandy SH, Monheit GD. Dermabrasion and chemical peels. In: Papel ID, ed. Facial Plastic and Reconstructive Surgery. 3rd ed. New York, NY: Thieme Medical Publishers; 2002: 223–240
[13] Murad H, Shamban AT, Premo PS. The use of glycolic acid as a peeling agent. Dermatol Clin 1995; 13: 285–307
[14] Monheit GD. The Jessner's + TCA peel: a medium-depth chemical peel. J Dermatol Surg Oncol 1989; 15: 945–950
[15] Lawrence N, Cox SE, Brody HJ. Treatment of melasma with Jessner's solution versus glycolic acid: a comparison of clinical efficacy and evaluation of the predictive ability of Wood's light examination. J Am Acad Dermatol 1997; 36: 589–593
[16] Katz B. The new fluor-hydroxy pulse peel: a pilot evaluation of a new superficial chemical peel. Cosmet Dermatol 1995; 8: 24–30
[17] Cucé LC, Bertino MC, Scattone L, Birkenhauer MC. Tretinoin peeling. Dermatol Surg 2001; 27: 12–14
[18] Fitzpatrick RE, Goldman MP, Butterwick KJ. Reversal of photoaging in ten weeks: a novel skin peeling system with a uniquely formulated post peel regimen. Int J Cost Surg Aesthet Dermatol. 2001; 3: 199–203
[19] Perkins SW, Balikian R. Treatment of perioral rhytids. Facial Plast Surg Clin North Am 2007; 15: 409–414, v
[20] Perkins SW, Sklarew EC. Prevention of facial herpetic infections after chemical peel and dermabrasion: new treatment strategies in the prophylaxis of patients undergoing procedures of the perioral area. Plast Reconstr Surg 1996; 98: 427–433, discussion 434–435

28 Complications of Chemexfoliation

Phillip R. Langsdon and Dana K. Petersen

28.1 Introduction

Chemexfoliation involves the controlled wounding of the epidermal and dermal tissue, followed by cutaneous regeneration with the goals of improvement of skin texture and tone. Although generally safe, peeling is occasionally associated with adverse cosmetic effects. Aesthetic results as well as unfavorable outcomes are largely related to the depth of wounding.

Peeling has been used for centuries by almost every culture in the world. Ancient records indicate that both fruits and wine were used to create topical preparations for such treatments.[1] These therapies utilized the naturally occurring alpha hydroxy acids (AHAs). AHAs have a marked effect on keratinocytes, by reducing cellular cohesion between terminally differentiated keratinocytes at the lowest levels of the stratum corneum.[2] The more concentrated AHAs have been shown to produce increased amounts of mucopolysaccharides and type I collagen in the dermal layer of skin.[2]

Throughout the last two centuries, chemexfoliation has more rapidly evolved through an increased understanding of many chemical agents. Peel agents include salicylic acid, glycolic acid (GA), pyruvic acid, trichloroacetic acid (TCA), phenol, and croton oil. Although generally safe when used in many of the accepted formulations and concentrations, chemical peeling still carries risks.

Superficial and medium-depth peels induce injury that is limited to the epidermis and papillary dermis.[3] These peels generally help remove the superficial layers and regenerate quickly, usually with few side effects or risks of complications. Deep peels penetrate into the upper layer of the reticular dermis causing a controlled second-degree chemical injury.[4]

Whether a superficial, medium, or deep peel is carried out, once the injury has occurred, the skin goes through an orderly healing process. The intensity of the process will vary with the depth. The phases of this process include inflammation, coagulation, re-epithelialization, and fibroplasia, which generally overlap.[5] Inflammation quickly becomes apparent by the completion of the peel with the appearance of edema and erythema. This phase predominates for the first 12 to 48 hours. The epidermis begins to separate as the coagulation phase begins and a serum exudate appears.

Completion of desquamation usually develops as edema resolves and may take from 4 to 7 days.[6] Deep peeling may take as long as 14 days to heal well enough to accept the application of makeup. Up until about the 10- to 14-day stage in the healing process, skin care maintenance and cleaning are imperative to remove sloughed necrotic epidermis to prevent an infectious process. An infection could convert the peel into a deeper burn and, as a result, potential scarring.

After a week, full re-epithelialization is generally complete in more superficial peels, but may take 10 to 14 days in deeper peels. The skin may still be pink for several weeks postpeel. This may last even longer in fair-skinned individuals.[6]

28.2 Preprocedural and Intraprocedural Considerations of Chemexfoliation

TCA concentrations should be measured weight by volume.[7] TCA is not sensitive to light and is stable on the shelf for more than 6 months.[8] Dates of mixing should be accurately scribed on stored bottles. GA and Jessner's Solution (14% resorcinol, 14% lactic acid, and 14% salicylic acid, in an alcohol base) will lose their potency more rapidly than TCA.[7]

Phenol, an aromatic hydrocarbon, is stable if stored in a dark, glass bottle away from the light. Because it is systemically absorbed through the skin and thought to be potentially toxic to the liver, kidneys, and myocardium, careful handling is critical. For phenol peeling, we use the formula as described in Baker's 1962 publication, with the exception that we use distilled water rather than tap water[9] (phenol United States Pharmacopeia [USP] 88%, 3 mL; distilled water, 2 mL; croton oil, 3 drops; Septisol soap [Sandent Co., Murfreesboro, Tennessee], 8 drops). It is the senior author's practice to mix the solution just prior to the procedure. Phenol in high concentrations will cause precipitation of protein in the keratin layer. This keratocoagulation may slow or prevent additional penetration of the peel affecting the overall outcome.[6]

28.3 Complications and Side Effects of Superficial Chemexfoliation

The popularity of superficial and medium-depth peeling is partly attributed to their safety margins, although they do share a similar general complication profile with deep peeling. Scarring is extremely rare with superficial peels and these lower potency agents typically cause mild and transitory side effects.

Glycolic acid can be utilized at varying concentrations (20–70%). It is capable of causing dermal wounds in higher concentrations (70%) in thin-skinned individuals. Penetration can be variable especially in thicker skin, and reduced concentrations may result in a less uniform outcome.[3] Whereas some patients receive excellent results, others do not; GA peels often require repeated application for optimum improvement.[10] The side effect of intense erythema may occur with high-strength peeling in thin-skinned, fair-complexioned individuals.

Pyruvic acid (40–70%) is an alpha keto acid that may be an effective treatment for mild-to-moderate photoaging or active acne.[11] Although generally safe and effective, it can cause an intense stinging and burning sensation during application. Furthermore, powerful vapors can irritate the respiratory mucosa.[3]

Salicylic acid is a mild beta hydroxy acid used for general skin maintenance as well as controlling acne. In the early 1980s, Shalita demonstrated in a randomized double-blind trial that repeated low concentrations helped resolve inflammatory skin conditions.[11] Salicylic acid can be utilized in various concentrations typically up to 30%. Mild discomfort, burning, irritation, and erythema are quite common but the incidence of major side effects is very low.[12] The predominant risk with this superficial peeling agent is allergic reaction due to salicylate hypersensitivity.[13] Generally, this is a very well-tolerated peel, although the physician should be aware of the rare likelihood of systemic salicylate toxicity.

Jessner's Solution is considered a superficial peeling formula and typically reaches a depth to the upper papillary dermis. The mixture contains lactic acid, salicylic acid, and resorcinol, an alcohol that is structurally similar to phenol.[14] The solution has been in use for more than 100 years as a therapeutic agent to treat hyperkeratotic epidermal lesions. The current formulation was compounded by Dr. Max Jessner to lower the concentration of any one agent and therefore decrease the risk of complications while increasing the keratolytic properties.[10] A modified solution replaces resorcinol with citric acid. Generally, complications are rare with either mixture, and most complaints such as irritation and streaky erythema could be considered side effects rather than true complications. However, both salicylic acid and resorcinol have the potential for systemic toxicity. Salicylism has been reported with repeated Jessner's peels.[10] In addition, persistent erythema is an infrequent side effect and may be treated with topical corticosteroid creams.[10]

Similar to superficial peeling agents, medium-depth TCA peels have a proven safety record. Although TCA in higher concentrations (>45%) may on rare occasion cause scarring,[14] this is much less likely with lower concentrations or TCA combinations (e.g., TCA with Jessner's Solution or TCA with 70% GA) commonly in use.[7] The most frequent side effect, with high concentrations, is irregular pigmentation.[7]

Hyperpigmentation is the most common, which is almost always transient. If it is distressing to the patient, we typically use a skin-bleaching treatment such as 4% hydroquinone and 2.5% hydrocortisone. Alternatively, superficial peels such as 30% salicylic acid, or GA, or repeat medium-depth peeling may normalize pigmentation. Pretreatment and posttreatment of the skin with hydroquinone help prevent pigmentation problems in susceptible individuals.

The risk for postoperative pigmentation abnormalities is higher in individuals with dark skin. Therefore, this is more likely in Fitzpatrick skin types IV through VI. We sometimes consider those patients who present with medium pigmentation and severe deep wrinkles as candidates for medium and deep peeling, if they accept the possibility of postoperative pigment changes and the subsequent need to treat this condition.

Delayed wound healing or persistent erythema may also occur. A superficial peel will typically lose erythema in 3 to 5 days, whereas a medium peel will lose erythema in 15 to 30 days.[7] Erythema, beyond what is expected, may be the result of contact dermatitis (▶ Fig. 28.1) or re-exacerbation of a previous skin disorder. Persistent intense redness may indicate prolonged fibroplasia, which can lead to skin thickening and scarring.[7] If the condition is suspected, topical steroids may help. If scarring occurs, intralesional steroid injection may be of aid.[6]

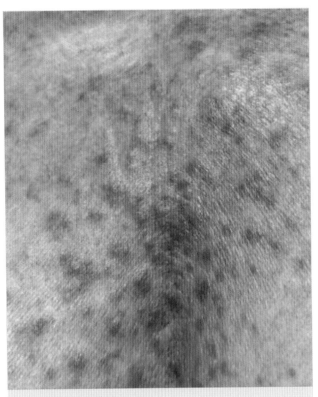

Fig. 28.1 Postoperative dermatitis.

28.4 Complications and Side Effects of Deep Chemexfoliation

With deep phenol/croton oil peeling, hypopigmentation is expected to some degree in the peeled areas. Melanocytes reorganize themselves along the basement membrane and sometimes lose their ability to produce melanin.[4] Contrasts with the nonpeeled areas are sometimes disconcerting. Repeat peeling of the demarcation lines with a feathering technique may be helpful. Loss of pigmentation is a trade-off, not a complication. When one is faced with deeply wrinkled, weather-beaten skin, pigmentary loss can be easily treated with makeup.

Occasionally, an uneven peel may result (▶ Fig. 28.2). It can happen in thick, oily skin or if the areas have not been adequately cleaned with acetone. It may result in spotty pigmentation.[4] If this occurs, hyperpigmented areas can be repeeled when appropriate.

Some degree of erythema can be expected for the first 2 to 3 months following a deep phenol–croton oil peel.[6] Erythema that is particularly intense or persistent can be treated with topical 2.5% hydrocortisone once or twice daily. Most stubborn erythema begins to resolve within 2 to 3 weeks of topical treatment. Rarely, the thickening can progress and, if severe or untreated, result in hypertrophic scarring (▶ Fig. 28.3). The perioral area, specifically the upper lip and the mandibular region, is the most common area for potential scar development.[8]

Phenol is detoxified in the liver, both conjugated and secreted by the kidneys, and has the potential to injure the myocardium. Because of this, patients should be in reasonable health and the peel should be performed with caution and over a period of

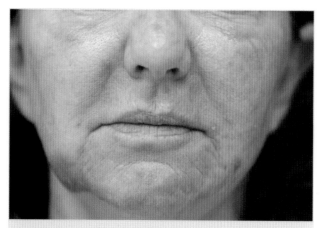

Fig. 28.2 Spotty peeling. This may occur in thick, oily skin.

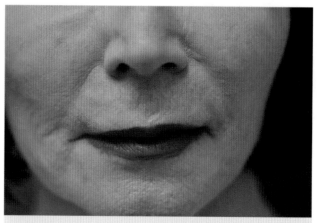

Fig. 28.3 Small lip scar. Kenalog (Bristol-Myers Squibb, Princeton, New Jersey) injections were used to soften the scar.

time to allow the body to manage elevated blood levels of phenol. Patients undergoing a deep phenol peel of more than one third of the face should be closely monitored. Arrhythmias including premature ventricular contractions (PVCs), bigeminy, and premature atrial contractions (PACs) are possible. Patients undergoing simultaneous aesthetic facial surgery have been injected with local anesthetics containing epinephrine and have other medications in circulation that, when combined, could contribute to arrhythmias. Intravenous (IV) hydration and a 15-minute rest period between subunits should protect against any serious problems. If an arrhythmia is noted, procedural pause until the abnormality has resolved with time for IV hydration usually clears the blood levels. The peel can then be resumed as planned with an increase in time spacing between peeling aesthetic units.

Contraction of the lower eyelids can occur with any type of deep peeling. This may result from previous lower eyelid surgery or an age-related weakening of the lower lid. If not severe, the lid position usually recovers as the peel contraction resolves. Injectable triamcinolone may help. In severe cases, if conservative measures do not suffice, a lid-tightening procedure might be indicated.

28.4.1 General Complications of Chemexfoliation

Wound infections are extremely rare after a chemical peel procedure as long as the patient faithfully follows the postoperative cleaning instructions. The best deterrent is frequent skin cleansing. When infection is encountered, an oral antipseudomonal antibiotic, such as ciprofloxacin, and close follow-up with frequent cleansing should adequately manage the situation.

Herpetic outbreaks can occur (▶ Fig. 28.4). A prior history of even a single fever blister makes the likelihood of a herpetic outbreak higher. When patients present with a past history of a fever blister, antiviral medication may help. Patients are started just before the peel and treated for 7 to 14 days postpeel. If a herpetic breakout occurs in spite of the prophylactic dose of antiviral medication, the dose of the antiviral medication is increased. Any skin ulceration is treated with the addition of a topical antiviral ointment several times a day. Rapid and

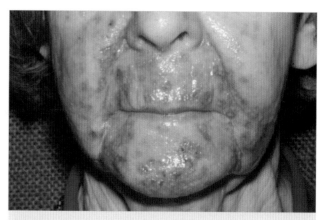

Fig. 28.4 Herpetic outbreak.

aggressive treatment of a herpetic outbreak usually resolves the condition. However, some invasive ulceration can result in scarring at the breakout site. If scarring develops during the healing process, the site can be treated with injectable steroids or scar revision at a later date.

Milia may occur in the early postprocedural period and is a common side effect, not a complication. They are usually self-limiting but may be uncapped with an 18-gauge needle if necessary.

For the first few months after the peel, patients should be mindful of their increased sensitivity to direct sunlight exposure and take appropriate precautions. Sunscreen with a sun protection factor of a least 30 is usually recommended during this time period. Unprotected sun exposure may result in hyperpigmentation.

28.5 Conclusion

Chemexfoliation has gained widespread popularity because, if used properly, and with good patient selection, it is both a safe and reliable tool. Complications such as systemic toxicity, infection, scarring, and abnormal pigmentation may occur. Good patient selection, proper preprocedural education, institution of proper complication treatment, close follow-up, and maintenance of good patient rapport go a long way to help the patient through the resolution of any postpeel sequelae.

References

[1] The Incantations and Recipes: Recipe for Transforming an Old Man into a Youth. Breasted, JH, ed. The Edwin Smith Surgical Papyrus Vol 1. Chicago, IL: University of Chicago Press; 1930: 492–498

[2] Ditre CM, Griffin TD, Murphy GF, et al. Effects of alpha-hydroxy acids on photoaged skin: a pilot clinical, histological and ultrastructural study. J Am Acad Dermatol 1996; 34: 187–195

[3] Pida De Padova M, Tosti A. Complications of superficial and medium chemical peels. In: Tosti A, Beer K, Pida de Padova M, eds. Management of Complications of Cosmetic Procedures. New York, NY: Springer; 2012: 1–7

[4] Mangat DS, Mendelsohn JE. Skin resurfacing-laser or peel. In: Pensak M, ed. Controversies in Otolaryngology. New York, NY: Thieme Medical Publishers; 2001: 164–169

[5] Campbell RM, Monheit CD. Postoperative care and complications. In: Goldberg D, ed. Facial Rejuvenation: A Total Approach. New York, NY: Springer; 2007: 142–146

[6] Langsdon PR, Shires CB. Chemical face peeling. Facial Plast Surg 2012; 28: 116–125

[7] Monheit GD. Chemical peels. Skin Therapy Lett 2004; 9: 6–11

[8] Spinowitz AL, Rumsfield J. Stability-time profile of trichloroacetic acid at various concentrations and storage conditions. J Dermatol Surg Oncol 1989; 15: 974–975

[9] Baker TJ. Chemical face peeling and rhytidectomy. Plast Reconstr Surg 1962; 29: 199–207

[10] Ghersetich I, Brazzini B, Peris K, Cotellessa C, Manunta T, Lotti T. Pyruvic acid peels for the treatment of photoaging. Dermatol Surg 2004; 30: 32–36, discussion 36

[11] Shalita AR. Treatment of mild and moderate acne vulgaris with salicylic acid in an alcohol-detergent vehicle. Cutis 1981; 28: 556–561

[12] Grimes PE. Jessner's solution. In: Tosti A, Grimes PE, Pida De Padova M, eds. Color Atlas of Chemical Peels. New York, NY: Springer; 2006: 57–62

[13] Bari AU, Iqbal Z, Rahman SB. Tolerance and safety of superficial chemical peeling with salicylic acid in various facial dermatoses. Indian J Dermatol Venereol Leprol 2005; 71: 87–90

[14] Stegman SJ. Medium-depth chemical peeling: digging beneath the surface. J Dermatol Surg Oncol 1986; 12: 1245–1246

29 Dermabrasion and Microdermabrasion: Rationale, Application, Safety Concerns, and Complications

Daniel E. Rousso and Sang W. Kim

29.1 Introduction

The history of dermabrasion dates back to 1550 BC when Egyptian physicians used alabaster and pumice to smooth scars and skin blemishes.[1] They recognized that producing partial-thickness abrasion improved the appearance of skin. Modern era dermabrasion was pioneered in 1905 by Kromayer.[2] In 1953, Kurtin refined the dermabrasion technique with modified, powered dental equipment using topical refrigerants and a wire brush.[3]

There are three main modalities for skin resurfacing: chemical peel, laser resurfacing, and mechanical dermabrasion. The contemporary trend favors the use of the laser-resurfacing technique. Many clinicians feel that laser resurfacing allows for more controlled thermal injury and more consistent outcomes with less operator-dependent variability. Whereas the newest laser technology has significantly reduced risk associated with thermal injury to surrounding tissues, in experienced hands, dermabrasion provides great manual control to the depth of destruction without spreading the thermal injury to deeper layers of the skin.

29.2 Mechanism

There are five layers of epidermis: stratum corneum at the surface followed by lucidum, granulosum, spinosum, and basalis. The thickness of epidermis varies depending on age of the patient and location of the skin. Average thickness of facial skin epidermis is approximately 100 µm thick, although at the eyelids it may be only 50 µm thick.[4] Four major cell types are found in the epidermis, including keratinocytes (80%), melanocytes, Langerhans cells, and Merkel cells. In the basalis layer, melanocytes generate skin pigmentation through the actions of the tyrosinase enzyme.[5] The rete ridges are projections of the epidermis into the dermis that help increase the surface area of contact between the two interfaces. In both processes of aging and scar formation, histological changes observed include loss of elastic fiber, atrophy of collagen bundles, and flattening of rete ridges.[6,7]

The dermis consists of papillary and reticular layers. The papillary layer is located below the basement membrane and contains mostly loose collagen and fibrocytes. The reticular layer contains thicker, compact collagen, and the adnexal structures of the skin such as sweat glands, hair follicles, and sebaceous glands. On the hairless part of the face, such as the nose, the sebaceous unit is the predominant adnexal structure. Within the adnexal structures are the epithelial stem cells capable of differentiation and re-epithelialization.[8]

The goal of dermabrasion is to mechanically remove the epidermis while preserving the adnexal structures (▶ Fig. 29.1). This is accomplished with the use of a motorized handpiece and a rotating tip composed of either a wire brush or diamond particle-coated fraise (▶ Fig. 29.2). The depth of injury is controlled by the surgeon carefully abrading the skin to the desired layer (▶ Fig. 29.2). Controlled injury to the epidermis and papillary dermis heals without scarring; however, if the injury penetrates deep into the reticular dermis where the adnexal structures and the epithelial stem cell reservoir are located, then complete re-epithelialization is compromised and scar tissue will develop. Because the skin receives its vascular supply via the arborized papillary plexus and the deep vascular plexus at the dermal-subcutaneous tissue junction, pinpoint bleeding serves as an important landmark to indicate the depth of the papillary dermis.[9]

The healing process is initiated by coagulation of the wound edge and crust formation during the first 24 hours. Locally, activation of coagulation cascade triggers complex signaling pathways including the release of chemotactic and growth factors (i.e., transforming growth factor-beta [TGF-β], fibroblast growth factor [FGF], epidermal growth factor [EGF], transforming growth factor-alpha [TGF-α], and platelet-derived growth factor [PDGF]) involved in endothelial cell and fibroblast proliferation. The proliferative phase begins within the first 24 hours and

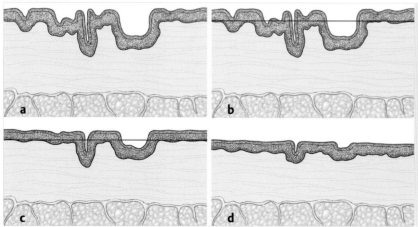

Fig. 29.1 (a) Skin prior to dermabrasion showing multiple imperfections. (b) Dermabrasion is performed to the depth of the papillary dermis. (c) After this has re-epithelialized, a second dermabrasion can be performed (at least 3 months between procedures) in order to achieve further improvement. (d) After this again re-epithelialized, the initial skin imperfections are markedly improved.

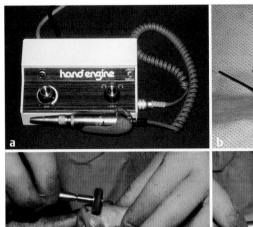
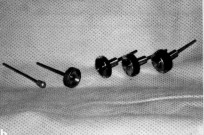
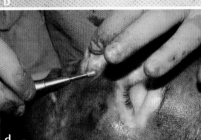

Fig. 29.2 (**a**) Hand engine and handpiece for dermabrasion. (**b**) Diamond fraise (left) and wire brushes (right). (**c**) Wire brush is used to treat broad skin surface. (**d**) Diamond fraise is used to treat nasal alar groove.

continues for up to 3 weeks. During this phase, re-epithelialization happens at the wound margin by migrating epithelial cells from the adnexal structures in the dermis. Epithelial cells fill the defect of the wound margin and proliferate until apposition of advancing epithelial cells inhibits further migration. At the papillary dermal and subcutaneous layers, fibroblast proliferation is initiated and peaks by day 4 after the treatment. With ongoing fibroplasia in the deeper layer, the epidermis begins to thin and retreats to the superficial plane. During this time, fibroblasts produce collagen, elastin, fibronectin, and glycosaminoglycans.[10,11] The maturation phase begins after approximately 3 weeks and continues for up to 18 months after treatment. During this remodeling stage, the collagen is replaced from type III to type I and reorganized from its initial random orientation to a more parallel position relative to the skin surface.[9] The matured collagen fibers contract and coalesce with increased diameter and decreased length. Collagen remodeling also triggers the regression of neovascularization, resulting in improvement of the raised, pink scar from early wound to a flatter, white wound after maturation.

Immunohistochemical studies on facial skin following dermabrasion confirm upregulation of procollagen in papillary dermal fibroblasts.[12] Harmon et al have shown that dermabrasion of evolving scars modulates the expression level of extracellular glycoprotein and the expression pattern from a localized to a more dispersed form.[13] This may promote epithelial cell migration from along the basement membrane and fibroblast movement across the scar boundary to optimize wound healing.

29.3 Indications

Dermabrasion is considered a medium-to-deep skin-resurfacing technique. Whereas numerous indications are described in the literature, the most commonly treated conditions are acne scars, deep facial rhytids, traumatic or iatrogenic scars, actinic damage, and rhinophyma.

29.3.1 Acne Scars

Acne scars that are partial skin thickness respond nicely to dermabrasion treatment. Results may often be improved by a second or third procedure spaced at least 3 months apart. For acne scars that are "ice pick" in nature and extend full thickness, dermabrasion alone is not as effective in improving the appearance of the scar. In these cases, punch grafting is an appropriate therapeutic option. One should perform a punch excision of the deep acne scar, followed by a full-thickness punch graft transferred from a donor site with similar skin color and texture match (▶ Fig. 29.3a, b).[14,15] After 4 to 6 weeks, dermabrasion of the grafted site and surrounding area should be performed (▶ Fig. 29.3c–e). In cases with severe acne scars, one may encounter multiple adjacent acne scars that share subcutaneous tracts. If these areas are deeply dermabraded, it may unroof the tracts resulting in a greater surface deformity.

29.3.2 Deep Facial Rhytids

Many aesthetic surgeons consider dermabrasion to be the treatment of choice for deep, vertical rhytids at the perioral and lip regions. Perkins and Castellano describe combining a full-face deep chemical peel with perioral dermabrasion for optimal deep facial rhytids' rejuvenation.[16] Treatment may need to be repeated for recalcitrant deep rhytids with at least a 12-month interval between sessions.

29.3.3 Scar Revision

For elevated scars with persistent induration and textural change, dermabrasion is a very effective treatment (▶ Fig. 29.4 and ▶ Fig. 29.5).[17] Dermabrasion is not ideal for wide, depressed scars. Because most scars tend to improve over time, conventional wisdom is to observe for at least 6 months prior to planning the revision treatment. However, if the scar is not showing any evidence of improvement, then dermabrasion may be performed within 6 to 8 weeks after the initial wound repair. Yarborough advocated the early use of dermabrasion within 4 to 8

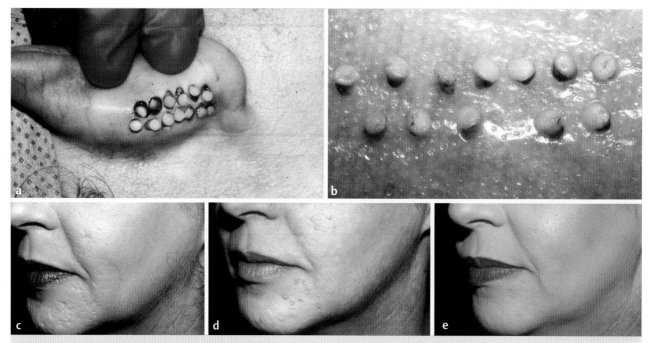

Fig. 29.3 (a) Punch grafts are taken from the postauricular donor site. (b) Full-thickness skin punch grafts. (c) Ice-pick-type acne scars. (d) 3 months after punch grafts were placed. (e) 3 months after dermabrasion performed at the grafted site.

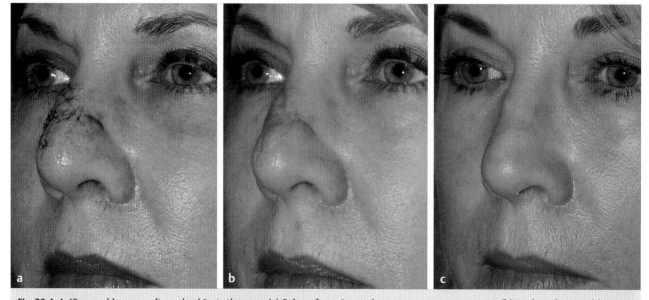

Fig. 29.4 A 48-year-old woman after a dog bite to the nose. (a) 6 days after primary closure at an emergency room. (b) Predermabrasion. (c) 4 years postdermabrasion.

weeks from the initial injury, when high fibroblastic activity is observed. Earlier than 8 weeks, the wound may lack the appropriate tensile strength to achieve optimal results.[8] Brenner and Perro advocated dermabrasion at 6 to 12 weeks after the initial injury, when collagen modeling may be at its peak.[18]

29.3.4 Actinic Damage

The first description of using dermabrasion to treat precancerous skin changes dates back to the 1950s. Numerous studies since then have shown the efficacy of dermabrasion in addressing precancerous lesions.[12,19,20,21] In a series of 23 patients with actinic damages who underwent dermabrasion, 79% were cancer-free at 3 years, 64% at 4 years, and 54% at 5 years. These outcomes were superior to results observed from cryosurgery, 5-fluorouracil, or chemical peel as prophylactic treatment against actinic keratosis.[22]

29.3.5 Rhinophyma

Dermabrasion can be particularly useful in the treatment of rhinophyma (▶ Fig. 29.6 and ▶ Fig. 29.7). Rhinophyma is a

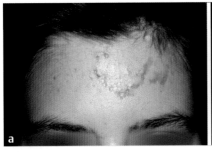
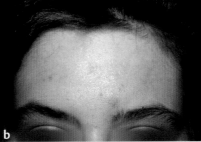

Fig. 29.5 A 27-year-old woman with scar from motor vehicle accident with embedded glass fragments. (a) 2 months from initial injury. (b) 3 months postdermabrasion.

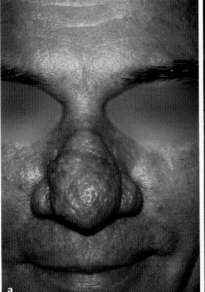
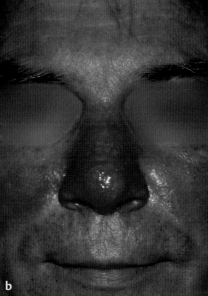
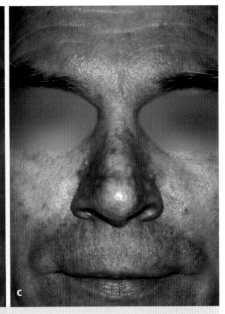

Fig. 29.6 A 54-year-old man with rhinophyma treated with dermabrasion. (a) Predermabrasion. (b) 2 weeks postdermabrasion. (c) 8 months postdermabrasion.

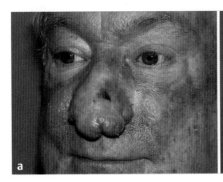
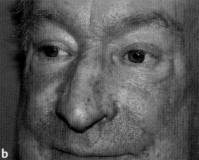

Fig. 29.7 A 57-year-old man with rhinophyma treated with dermabrasion. (a) Predermabrasion. (b) 9 months postdermabrasion.

manifestation of end-stage rosacea and is characterized by sebaceous hypertrophy and inflammation resulting in multiple abscess and skin thickening.[23] This is often a difficult skin condition to manage medically. Surgical treatment is frequently necessary to improve the associated deformity and morbidity. In severe cases, it may be useful to use a scalpel to shave the superficial layers of skin and then complete the process with dermabrasion. When treating a severe case of rhinophyma, controlling the depth of dermabrasion is particularly challenging because one can encounter significant bleeding and sebum exposure. Such an event will obstruct the characteristic features representing the depth of treatment. If dermabrasion is taken

too deep, the treated area will heal with a shiny and unnatural surface lacking any sebaceous pores. When utilized properly, dermabrasion can achieve remarkable results that may be difficult to achieve with any other modality in patients with rhinophyma.

29.4 Contraindications

Dermabrasion is contraindicated for any patients who have decreased adnexal structures of the dermis and therefore may not be able to mount optimal re-epithelialization. Comorbidities associated with poor re-epithelialization include history of radiation treatment to the facial areas, long-term systemic steroid therapy, or history of deep burns.

Patients with active herpetic lesions should delay dermabrasion until any current infection resolves. Active infection may disseminate into newly abraded wounds, and subsequent infection may lead to full-thickness tissue loss.[8] Patients presenting with acne scars may have been or currently may be on systemic isotretinoin (13-cis-retinoic acid). This medication leads to atrophy of the sebaceous glands and may compromise wound healing and re-epithelialization. There are conflicting studies that challenge whether systemic isotretinoin causes atypical scarring after dermabrasion.[24,25] Nevertheless, to minimize any risk of scarring, one should wait at least 6 months and preferably a full year before proceeding with dermabrasion on patients taking systemic isotretinoin.

Medications that contain estrogen or progesterone may lead to pigmentary changes following dermabrasion. Therefore, if possible, it is recommended that patients discontinue such medications for 3 to 6 months posttreatment.

Finally, detailed histories should be obtained to rule out patients with blood-borne pathogens such as human immunodeficiency virus (HIV) or hepatitis B/C virus (HBV/HCV). Dermabrasion treatment can create aerosolization of the blood pathogens. Although blood-borne pathogens may transmit through mucous membrane exposure, there are no known instances of a blood-borne pathogen being transmitted by an aerosol in a clinical setting.[26] Nevertheless, it is good clinical practice for the surgeons and assistants to have appropriate protective shielding against potential aerosol particles (< 10 µm in diameter) and splatter during the procedure.

29.5 Preoperative Preparation

Patients must demonstrate clear understanding of the realistic outcome, posttreatment care, and posttreatment appearance prior to consenting for the treatment. They need to be aware that some pigment changes are expected during the recovery process. Also, they must commit to rigorous posttreatment care in order to achieve the optimal outcome, including protection/avoidance from the sun for at least 3 months posttreatment.

Topical application of tretinoin 0.5% prior to dermabrasion has been shown to improve healing. Patients placed on tretinoin at least several weeks before dermabrasion healed 2 to 3 days faster than those without pretreatment, and had reduced risk of postinflammatory hyperpigmentation.[27]

For patients with a dark skin complexion (Fitzpatrick skin type IV or higher) or history of developing hyperpigmentation after skin resurfacing, hydroquinone 4% topical cream should be initiated several weeks prior to dermabrasion, and resumed soon after posttreatment re-epithelialization. Hydroquinone works by inhibiting the actions of the enzyme tyrosinase, thereby blocking the melanin production involved in skin pigmentation.[5,28]

Oral antiviral prophylaxis against herpes simplex virus (HSV) should be considered for all patients and particularly those with a history of reactivation.

29.6 Technique

The dermabrasion handpiece operates at a range of 1,500 to 50,000 revolutions per minute. The handpiece can accommodate various sizes and types of debrider heads (▶ Fig. 29.2a, b). The two most commonly used debrider heads are the diamond fraise and wire brush. The wire brush abrades skin by creating multiple microscopic lacerations and tends to achieve the required depth more quickly than the diamond fraise (▶ Fig. 29.2c). Nevertheless, this distinction also makes the wire brush more challenging to use for an inexperienced surgeon. A diamond-fraise tip may abrade at a slower rate, but is relatively easier to control and viewed as the safer option. For the areas that are small and hard to reach such as the grooves of the nasal alae or near the eyelids, the diamond fraise should be utilized (▶ Fig. 29.2d). Traditionally, cryogenic agents were applied topically to freeze the skin and create a rigid surface for even treatment. Unfortunately, these agents are no longer available. After the banning of fluorocarbon refrigerants, tumescent anesthesia has been used to induce turgor over the skin with similar effect. The assistant should provide tension and stabilization of the skin being treated, while the surgeon uses the nondominant hand to protect the eyes, nose, and mouth. Gauze should not be used to protect these areas because gauze may actually damage the eyes, nose, or lips when caught with the wire brush. If a deep scar or pitted acne is being treated, one may use gentian violet to stain the epidermis in order to denote these areas after the first pass of dermabrasion.

Typically, the area to be dermabraded is marked in a grid pattern. Most surgeons plan on treating the entire aesthetic facial unit instead of a single spot because the treated and untreated areas of the facial unit tend to blend better and will be easier to camouflage. One should abrade deeper in the area of concern such as the acne scar or deep crease, while feathering lightly in the surrounding area to blend in the texture and color.

Uniform pressure is applied over the treated area, and the movement of the dermabrader is maintained slowly and steadily in a direction perpendicular to the plane of rotation. The depth of treatment is determined through several landmarks. Removal of the epidermal layer is characterized by changes in skin pigmentation (or the ink marking made by the surgeon). The small capillary pinpoint bleeding indicates that the depth of treatment has reached the papillary dermis level. If the superficial reticular dermis is exposed, one will notice the parallel-oriented strand of yellow layer. To optimize the visualization of skin depth and avoid blood pooling, the procedure should be planned to begin in the gravity-dependent areas.

While treating near critical structures of the face such as the lips or the eyes, one should orient the spinning wheel toward these structures. This will prevent the brush from grabbing and retracting the lips or eyelids and causing them to tear or avulse. Bony areas such as the mandible and malar prominence warrant special caution. These areas are naturally more prone to scar formation—likely due to their thin skin and constant tension from facial movements—and should be treated more conservatively.[29]

29.7 Postoperative Care

Application of occlusive dressing or topical ointment such as petroleum jelly has been shown to accelerate the healing process following dermabrasion. The covered wound retains liquid and tends to form less crusting than the wound exposed to the air. The crusting becomes a mechanical barrier for epidermal migration and slows down the re-epithelialization process. The rate of re-epithelialization may increase up to 40%, with complete epithelialization occurring within 24 hours when the wound is appropriately covered.[8] Starting posttreatment day 1, patients are instructed to shower up to six times daily with gentle, lukewarm water to clear crusting at the treated area. Following the rinse, topical ointment should be applied immediately to keep the wound retaining its moisture and prevent crusting formation. Once re-epithelialization has been completed, usually between the 1- and 2-week follow-up visits, topical care can be transitioned from a thick ointment to a gentle skin moisturizer. Ideally, the skin moisturizer should not contain any sunscreen agents because these may irritate the nascent skin. At this point, patients may also begin to wear makeup to camouflage the posttreatment erythema. Water-based makeups are recommended because they are easier to remove. The posttreatment erythema usually subsides after 8 weeks; however, for some patients this may take several months. During the first 3 months patients should avoid any sun exposure. Particularly for recalcitrant ice-pick acne scars and rhinophyma, dermabrasion may be repeated. After the treated area has re-epithelialized, a second dermabrasion may be performed at least 3 months later to remove residual or deep skin defect and achieve further improvement.

29.8 Complications

Approximately 50% of patients will develop milia during 1 month after dermabrasion.[8] Milia are superficial inclusion cysts limited within the epidermis during re-epithelialization (▶ Fig. 29.8a). They are typically self-limiting, but large milia can be opened with an 18-gauge needle for quick resolution. Posttreatment 0.05% topical retinoid has also been shown to be effective in reducing incidence of milia.[27]

Infections at the dermabraded sites include *Staphylococcus aureus* or *Pseudomonas*, *Candida*, or HSV. A bacterial infection may manifest with unusual facial swelling and thick, yellow crusting (*Staphylococcus aureus*) or characteristic odor (*Pseudomonas*) within week 1. A fungal infection may present with persistent irregular patches of erythema and exudates, or reticular white patches (▶ Fig. 29.8b). Herpetic lesions present as disproportionately painful eruptions, often in a dermatome distribution with characteristic vesicles, and may disseminate within the dermabraded site (▶ Fig. 29.8c). Due to the potential for tissue necrosis from the resulting vasculitis, one should address posttreatment herpetic infections aggressively with both oral and topical antiviral medications.

Posttreatment scarring will occur if the depth of dermabrasion penetrates into the reticular dermis. Small fibrotic bands can be managed by instructing patients to massage the area three to four times a day with Mederma cream (Merz Pharmaceuticals, LLC, Frankfort, Germany) or vitamin E oil. More prominent, firm fibrotic bands should be treated with intralesional steroid injection using Kenalog K-10 suspension (Bristol-Myers Squibb, Princeton, New Jersey). The steroid injection should be localized to the fibrotic band because overinjection may lead to atrophy of subcutaneous fat and subsequent unsightly depression. Intralesional steroid should be injected at 3- to 6-week intervals. For a recalcitrant fibrotic scar, higher doses of intralesional steroid injection or serial excision and primary closure may be necessary.

Pigment changes after dermabrasion are a potential risk, especially for patients with Fitzpatrick skin type IV or higher. Posttreatment hyperpigmentation is a common condition, and typically seen starting at 3 to 4 weeks after treatment. Patients

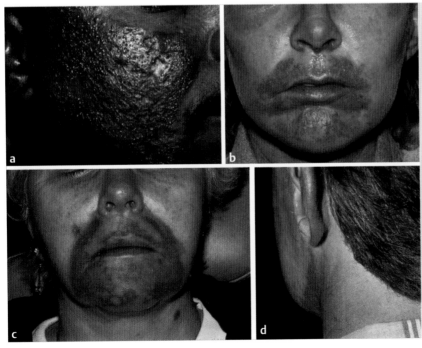

Fig. 29.8 (a) Milia and temporary hyperpigmentation are noted at the treated sites. (b) Tenderness, erythema, and white reticular streaks are signs of candidal infection at the treated site. (c) Postdermabrasion herpetic lesions clinically present as out-of-proportion tenderness with vesicular eruption. (d) Permanent hypopigmentation. Notice the line of demarcation along the angle of mandible.

should be reassured that all hyperpigmentation will resolve over time; however, this may take many weeks and sometimes months. Topical application of 4% hydroquinone and 0.05% tretinoin should be initiated at the earliest sign of hyperpigmentation, and applied diffusely throughout—including the untreated area to help blend. Alternatively, for dark-skinned patients, topical 4% hydroquinone and 0.05% tretinoin may be prescribed 1 month prior to the planned treatment.

Posttreatment hypopigmentation, on the other hand, is a challenging complication (▶ Fig. 29.8d). It may be caused by too-deep treatment resulting in irreversible damage to the melanocytes. Traditionally, the only option was to apply makeup to camouflage the area of hypopigmentation. Recently, Massaki et al described using a fractionated 1,550-nm erbium-doped laser combined with topical bimatoprost and tretinoin or pimecrolimus (Fraxel SR laser; Solta Medical, Hayward, California) to treat for hypopigmentation. After multiple treatments, 11 out of 14 patients demonstrated more than 50% improvement.[30]

29.9 Microdermabrasion

Microdermabrasion is a mechanical-resurfacing technique without the extent of deep-skin penetration achieved using traditional dermabrasion. The typical setup for microdermabrasion includes a handpiece with an outlet and an inlet—a vacuum line that provides the negative pressure and the other line that delivers crystals to generate mechanical abrasion of the skin surface (▶ Fig. 29.9a). The crystals and abraded materials are suctioned out via vacuum to a waste receptacle.

The most commonly used crystal is aluminum oxide. This is an inert ceramic with rough edges and insoluble in water; therefore, it cannot enter the bloodstream. Due to its heavy weight, it does not aerosolize and its size (typically 100 μm) prevents reaching the alveoli if inhaled.[31] Nevertheless, because long-term exposure to aluminum powder has been associated with detrimental cognitive function as observed in miners and factory workers, the U.S. Occupational Safety and Health Administration (OSHA) recommends limiting total exposure to 10 to 15 mg/m³ without respiratory protection.[31,32,33] Another

microdermabrasion modality does not utilize aluminum oxide crystals to abrade the skin. Instead, a specialized handpiece allows the use of attachable tips that are coated with variable grades of fine, diamond particles (▶ Fig. 29.9b). These tips are used to abrade the skin and achieve results that are similar to the use of loose aluminum oxide crystals without some of the less desirable effects of the crystals.

Because the microdermabrasion device was classified by the U.S. Food and Drug Administration (FDA) as a type 1 device (non–life-sustaining), manufacturers do not have to establish performance standards. In addition, the device received an exemption status from the FDA, and thus it can be sold without the FDA clearance letter. As a result, microdermabrasion instruments are not required to establish their efficacy through phase 3 trials, and these tools may be sold to and operated by nonmedical practitioners.[32]

29.10 Indications

In 2011, microdermabrasion was the fourth most widely utilized cosmetic procedure after botulinum toxin, soft-tissue fillers (hyaluronic acid), and laser hair removal.[34] Microdermabrasion is being used to treat a variety of skin conditions including photoaging, dyschromias, scars, acne, enlarged pores, and stretch marks.[35,36] Others have investigated the potential application of utilizing microdermabrasion to enhance transdermal delivery of topical agents by thinning the stratum corneum.[37] Unlike the traditional dermabrasion or other modalities of skin resurfacing, microdermabrasion is not able to penetrate deeply into the epidermis. Therefore, it may be used safely on all skin types with minimal risk for scarring or pigmentation changes.

29.11 Mechanism

Early studies demonstrated some clinical benefits for microdermabrasion with improvement of the skin histological profile. Shim et al examined histological changes of the skin immediately after a single session of 20 passes on abdominal skin ex vivo and after a total of six treatments every 2 weeks to

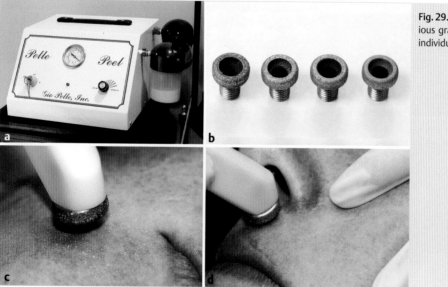

Fig. 29.9 (a) Microdermabrasion device. (b) Various grades of diamond-coated tips. (c, d) Each individual facial subunit is treated one at a time.

the dorsal forearm.[38] Immediately after microdermabrasion, there was thinning and homogenization of the stratum corneum layer of epidermis. However, abrasion did not penetrate through the remaining viable layers of the epidermis. Several studies have noted structural changes in the epidermis and dermis with continuation of regular microdermabrasion treatments, which include regular distribution of melanosomes and less melanization in the epidermis, thickening of the epidermis, mild flattening of the rete ridge pattern, and improvement in hyalinization of the dermis.[39,40,41] None of the histological studies has yet shown that microdermabrasion leads to any significant abrasion of the viable layer of the epidermis; hence, the mechanism behind dermal remodeling remains unclear. Karimipour et al measured significant changes in the expression level of key genes implicated in dermal remodeling after microdermabrasion, despite the minimal epidermal disruption.[42]

Numerous studies have shown improved texture and fine wrinkles of the skin following microdermabrasion treatment.[43,44,45] Whereas several studies have demonstrated objective changes following microdermabrasion including decrease in surface sebum content, flattening of skin wrinkles, and retention of water in the stratum corneum, most of these were transient changes lasting about 1 week posttreatment.[45,46]

29.12 Technique

Depending on the type of microdermabrasion device being utilized, the technique will vary. Microdermabrasion can be performed by a physician, nurse, or licensed aesthetician. After removal of makeup and cleansing, the face is degreased with an isopropyl alcohol pad. A moist pad or equivalent should be used to cover the eyes and ensure complete closure throughout the procedure if a crystal-based device is being used. The extent of abrasion is determined by the rate of the crystal flow or the roughness of the headpiece, the speed of handpiece movement, and the number of passes being performed. If the crystal outflow pressure/suction rate is set too high, one may observe petechiae, especially at the thin-skinned areas. Each pass should be performed in an organized fashion by addressing each aesthetic subunit of the face (▶ Fig. 29.9c,d).

29.13 Posttreatment Care and Complications

There is a minimal downtime associated with microdermabrasion treatment. Slight erythema and petechiae are seen with aggressive microdermabrasion, but are camouflaged with makeup. Treatment is safe for all skin types with minimal risk for any posttreatment pigmentation changes. Potential complication for corneal irritation can be minimized with appropriate precaution when using the crystal-based system near the eyes. Patients are instructed to apply moisturizer and resume use of skin care products including topical tretinoin immediately after the procedure. Prior to treatment, patients should be informed that multiple procedures typically spaced 1 to 2 weeks apart are necessary to achieve the optimal results.

29.14 Conclusion

Dermabrasion and microdermabrasion are two distinct modes of mechanical skin resurfacing. Although the advent of laser technology has led to the diminished use of dermabrasion for skin resurfacing, for certain indications, dermabrasion has clear advantages and utility over other skin-resurfacing techniques. Facial traumatic scars and rhinophyma are two skin conditions that are particularly well suited to treatment with dermabrasion. This approach is unique in the finesse and tactile control of the depth of treatment achieved compared with other resurfacing modalities. The surgeon may use dermabrasion in a manner similar to the way an artist uses a brush to achieve the desired effect. When utilized effectively, dermabrasion can be a powerful tool in the armamentarium of those performing skin-resurfacing surgery. Current studies indicate relatively limited and transient efficacy for microdermabrasion. Nevertheless, given its simplicity and safety, microdermabrasion will continue to play a significant role as a noninvasive method of cosmetic skin rejuvenation.

References

[1] Lawrence N, Mandy S, Yarborough J, Alt T. History of dermabrasion. Dermatol Surg 2000; 26: 95–101

[2] Kromayer E. Rotationsinstrumente: ein neues techisches verfahren in der dermatologischen kleinchirurgic. Dermatol Z. 1905; 12: 26

[3] Kurtin A. Corrective surgical planing of skin; new technique for treatment of acne scars and other skin defects. AMA Arch Derm Syphilol 1953; 68: 389–397

[4] Ha RY, Nojima K, Adams WP, Jr, Brown SA. Analysis of facial skin thickness: defining the relative thickness index. Plast Reconstr Surg 2005; 115: 1769–1773

[5] Gupta AK, Gover MD, Nouri K, Taylor S. The treatment of melasma: a review of clinical trials. J Am Acad Dermatol 2006; 55: 1048–1065

[6] Grunebaum LD, Murdock J, Hoosien GE, Heffelfinger RN, Lee WW. Laser treatment of skin texture and fine line etching. Facial Plast Surg Clin North Am 2011; 19: 293–301

[7] Contet-Audonneau JL, Jeanmaire C, Pauly G. A histological study of human wrinkle structures: comparison between sun-exposed areas of the face, with or without wrinkles, and sun-protected areas. Br J Dermatol 1999; 140: 1038–1047

[8] Yarborough JM, Beeson WH. Aesthetic surgery of the aging face. In: Beeson WH, ed. Aesthetic Surgery of the Aging Face. St. Louis, MO: C.V. Mosby Company; 1986: 142–158

[9] Yarborough JM, Jr. Ablation of facial scars by programmed dermabrasion. J Dermatol Surg Oncol 1988; 14: 292–294

[10] Kanzler MH, Gorsulowsky DC, Swanson NA. Basic mechanisms in the healing cutaneous wound. J Dermatol Surg Oncol 1986; 12: 1156–1164

[11] Goslen JB. Wound healing for the dermatologic surgeon. J Dermatol Surg Oncol 1988; 14: 959–972

[12] Nelson BR, Majmudar G, Griffiths CE, et al. Clinical improvement following dermabrasion of photoaged skin correlates with synthesis of collagen I. Arch Dermatol 1994; 130: 1136–1142

[13] Harmon CB, Zelickson BD, Roenigk RK, et al. Dermabrasive scar revision. Immunohistochemical and ultrastructural evaluation. Dermatol Surg 1995; 21: 503–508

[14] Lowenthal L. Punch biopsy with autograft. Arch Derm Syphilol 1953; 67: 629–631

[15] Arouete J. Correction of depressed scars on the face by a method of elevation. J Dermatol Surg 1976; 2: 337–339

[16] Perkins SW, Castellano R. Use of combined modality for maximal resurfacing. Facial Plast Surg Clin North Am 2004; 12: 323–337, vi

[17] Surowitz JB, Shockley WW. Enhancement of facial scars with dermabrasion. Facial Plast Surg Clin North Am 2011; 19: 517–525

[18] Brenner MJ, Perro CA. Recontouring, resurfacing, and scar revision in skin cancer reconstruction. Facial Plast Surg Clin North Am 2009; 17: 469–487, e3

[19] Epstein E. Planing for precancerous skin. A ten-year evaluation. Calif Med 1966; 105: 26–27

[20] Burks JW, Jr, Brewer JM, Jr, Chernosky ME. Surgical planing for the prevention of cancer of the skin. South Med J 1960; 53: 86–91

[21] Benedetto AV, Griffin TD, Benedetto EA, Humeniuk HM. Dermabrasion: therapy and prophylaxis of the photoaged face. J Am Acad Dermatol 1992; 27: 439–447

[22] Coleman WP, III, Yarborough JM, Mandy SH. Dermabrasion for prophylaxis and treatment of actinic keratoses. Dermatol Surg 1996; 22: 17–21

[23] Tüzün Y, Wolf R, Kutlubay Z, Karakuş O, Engin B. Rosacea and rhinophyma. Clin Dermatol 2014; 32: 35–46

[24] Rubenstein R, Roenigk HH, Jr, Stegman SJ, Hanke CW. Atypical keloids after dermabrasion of patients taking isotretinoin. J Am Acad Dermatol 1986; 15: 280–285

[25] Bagatin E, dos Santos Guadanhim LR, Yarak S, Kamamoto CS, de Almeida FA. Dermabrasion for acne scars during treatment with oral isotretinoin. Dermatol Surg 2010; 36: 483–489

[26] Infection control in dental settings. Centers for Disease Control and Prevention. 6 Dec 2013. Available at: http://www.cdc.gov/. Accessed February 7, 2014

[27] Mandy SH. Tretinoin in the preoperative and postoperative management of dermabrasion. J Am Acad Dermatol 1986; 115: 878

[28] Spencer MC. Topical use of hydroquinone for depigmentation. JAMA 1965; 194: 962–964

[29] McCollough EG, Langsdon PR. Dermabrasion and Chemical Peel: A Guide for Facial Plastic Surgeons. New York, NY: Thieme Medical Publishers; 1988: 30–37

[30] Massaki AB, Fabi SG, Fitzpatrick R. Repigmentation of hypopigmented scars using an erbium-doped 1,550-nm fractionated laser and topical bimatoprost. Dermatol Surg 2012; 38: 995–1001

[31] Sittig M. Aluminum and aluminum oxide. In: Sittig M, ed. Handbook of Toxic and Hazardous Chemicals and Carcinogens. Vol 1. 3rd ed. Park Ridge, NJ: Noyes Publications; 1991: 175–177

[32] Spencer JM. Microdermabrasion. Am J Clin Dermatol 2005; 6: 89–92

[33] Rifat SL, Eastwood MR, McLachlan DR, Corey PN. Effect of exposure of miners to aluminium powder. Lancet 1990; 336: 1162–1165

[34] Statistics on cosmetic surgery ASAPS 2011. American Society for Aesthetic Plastic Surgery. Available at: www.surgery.org. Accessed January 15, 2014

[35] Bhalla M, Thami GP. Microdermabrasion: reappraisal and brief review of literature. Dermatol Surg 2006; 32: 809–814

[36] Karimipour DJ, Karimipour G, Orringer JS. Microdermabrasion: an evidence-based review. Plast Reconstr Surg 2010; 125: 372–377

[37] Lee WR, Tsai RY, Fang CL, Liu CJ, Hu CH, Fang JY. Microdermabrasion as a novel tool to enhance drug delivery via the skin: an animal study. Dermatol Surg 2006; 32: 1013–1022

[38] Shim EK, Barnette D, Hughes K, Greenway HT. Microdermabrasion: a clinical and histopathologic study. Dermatol Surg 2001; 27: 524–530

[39] Shpall R, Beddingfield FC, III, Watson D, Lask GP. Microdermabrasion: a review. Facial Plast Surg 2004; 20: 47–50

[40] Freedman BM, Rueda-Pedraza E, Waddell SP. The epidermal and dermal changes associated with microdermabrasion. Dermatol Surg 2001; 27: 1031–1033, discussion 1033–1034

[41] Rubin MG, Greenbaum SS. Histologic effects of aluminum oxide microdermabrasion on facial skin. J Aesthetic Dermatol. 2000; 1: 237–239

[42] Karimipour DJ, Kang S, Johnson TM, et al. Microdermabrasion: a molecular analysis following a single treatment. J Am Acad Dermatol 2005; 52: 215–223

[43] Coimbra M, Rohrich RJ, Chao J, Brown SA. A prospective controlled assessment of microdermabrasion for damaged skin and fine rhytides. Plast Reconstr Surg 2004; 113: 1438–1443, discussion 1444

[44] Tsai RY, Wang CN, Chan HL. Aluminum oxide crystal microdermabrasion. A new technique for treating facial scarring. Dermatol Surg 1995; 21: 539–542

[45] Tan MH, Spencer JM, Pires LM, Ajmeri J, Skover G. The evaluation of aluminum oxide crystal microdermabrasion for photodamage. Dermatol Surg 2001; 27: 943–949

[46] Rajan P, Grimes PE. Skin barrier changes induced by aluminum oxide and sodium chloride microdermabrasion. Dermatol Surg 2002; 28: 390–393

30 Skin Rejuvenation from the Perspective of the European Facial Plastic Surgeon

Adam P. Stanek

30.1 Introduction

Although the idea of beauty has changed over time within cultures and regions, a human being's longing for it always stays an inveterate part of one's nature.[1] Because our susceptibility to beauty is so strong, it is of huge impact on our lives—whether it be in the choice of our partners or our success at work and in our social lives.[2] In addition, nothing is as fascinating and as expressive as a beautiful human face.[3] And this is the great challenge every facial plastic surgeon in Europe—as well as in other parts of the world—must accept. A stunning growth of public interest in facial rejuvenation confronts a rapidly growing number of physicians from multiple specialities and a plentiful supply from the cosmetic industry providing these services. To meet the demands of this challenging environment appropriately and successfully, facial plastic surgery (FPS) in Europe is in a very constructive process of transitioning from a traditional surgical subspeciality focused on the scalpel—in former times on its use in restricted fields of FPS or limited to the nose exclusively—to a modern, multidisciplinary medical society institutionalized in the European Academy of Facial Plastic Surgery (EAFPS). The academy's members come from all European countries as well as Turkey and Russia, and from different medical fields including dermatology. This variety of specialists has been broadening the European FPS society's horizon and has been expanding its sphere of activity with current scientific insights, progressive development of surgical procedures, modern technology, new clinical applications, and more. Thus dermabrasion, chemical peels, and medical lasers are now part of European FPS.

The first medical use of a laser was for the repair of detached retinas ("spot welding").[4] Further developments made lasers very popular and so they have come to be used today by nearly all medical and surgical specialists for treating a wide range of different conditions. Dermatologists have played a very important role in the evolution and the use of medical lasers to treat a multitude of different cutaneous pathologies and conditions of the entire body—and the face in particular.[5,6] It is very fortunate for the society of FPS to be able to interact with these highly qualified specialists, and it is an enrichment for the EAFPS that dermatologists join to share their knowledge and clinical experience and thereby enhance the high standards of the academy even more.

It is apparent from this that two different developments in European medicine have met: the scalpel and the laser.

30.2 The Scalpel and the European Academy of Facial Plastic Surgery

The history of modern FPS is closely associated with Jacques Joseph (originally, Jakob Lewin Joseph) (▶ Fig. 30.1 and ▶ Fig. 30.2), who is considered to be *the* pioneer of FPS in Europe as well as the rest of the world. It is worthwhile to examine his career and professional transition from a general practitioner to the world's first true facial plastic surgeon. Born September 6, 1865, in Koenigsberg, Prussia (now Poland), the youngest of three children of Rabbi Israel Joseph and his wife, Sara, as a teenager he attended "gymnasium" (high school) in Berlin, Germany. After completing medical school at Friedrich-Wilhelm-University (today Humboldt University) in 1890, he joined a residency program in internal medicine and pediatrics. However, due to his economic situation, he was forced to leave the program and establish a private practice a year later as a general practitioner. Driven by his strong interest in surgery, he was fortunate to again be able to join a residency program at the university's Department for Orthopaedic Surgery in 1892. Here he started a very promising academic career with mentor Prof. Dr. Julius Wolff, a brilliant and highly regarded surgeon at that time. During his surgical training, Joseph appeared more and more to have a penchant for plastic surgery, which would prove to be his temporary undoing. In 1896, the mother of a 10-year-old boy with ear deformity pleaded with him to help her son. Thus—after thorough theoretical preparation and planning—he performed his first otoplasty. The result was beyond any of his expectations and Joseph earned great respect after presenting the case at an academic symposium. Nevertheless, since he had performed this operation without the permission of his superior, Joseph was immediately dismissed and again became a general practitioner. Joseph continued to perform smaller procedures on the face and neck very successfully, and 2 years later he was contacted by a young man for surgical help. The man was suffering from depression due to relentless teasing because of a huge hump on his nose. Again, after thorough preparation, Joseph performed a reduction rhinoplasty on the young man in 1898 with excellent results, earning great respect in the academic world. This finally signaled the start of his career as a plastic surgeon. After 9 years, he had performed more than 200 successful rhinoplasties. Because his first case

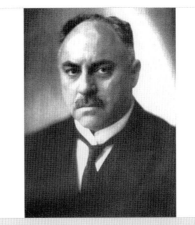

Fig. 30.1 Jacques Joseph, credited with performing the first rhinoplasty.

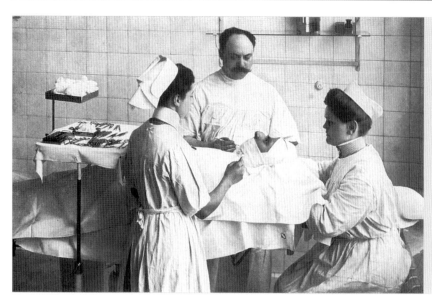

Fig. 30.2 Dr. Joseph in surgery.

was one of the very first rhinoplasties ever performed in the world, Joseph became known as the "father of aesthetic rhinoplasty" or the "father of cosmetic surgery." Meanwhile, he constantly continued extending his surgical work on other areas of the face and neck.

World War I (1914–1918) resulted in an extremely high number of casualties and severe injuries of the face. Those who survived suffered from disfiguring disabilities. As if it were the most natural thing in the world, Joseph decided to help these horribly stigmatized soldiers. He offered his skills and devoted his time and energy to treating as many of them as possible. By doing so, Joseph himself entered a unique field of professional action and personal development. He considered these injured faces to be the "battlefield" ("Schlachtfeld der Gesichtschirurgie") of FPS, and by declaring war on these injuries he became the leading general. During this period, Joseph performed surgery on enormous numbers of wounded soldiers, who quite often presented with overwhelming disfigurements. His infinite patience and endurance, thoroughness and sense of responsibility, and highly developed surgical skills combined with an ingenious and creative pioneering spirit enabled Joseph to revolutionize the surgical techniques and approaches in FPS at that time, helping desperate people get back to (almost) normal lives. Joseph always emphasized the incredible psychological benefit of surgery for his patients. The fact that none of his patients experienced severe or lethal complications owes much to Joseph's demands on safety for his surgical patients.

World War I went on, and to be able to treat the growing number of injured soldiers, a new section at the Department of Otolaryngology at the Charité in Berlin, one of Germany's most reputable academic hospitals, was established: the Department for Facial Plastic Surgery ("Abteilung für Gesichtsplastik"), the first department of this kind in the world. The setting was multidisciplinary and Joseph never grew tired of praising the excellent cooperation of adjoining departments—the Department of Dermatology, in particular, which mutually cared for Joseph's patients. After the section for FPS was closed in 1922, Joseph

established a private clinic for FPS in Berlin, focusing mainly on aesthetic surgery, and continued to work there until he died after a heart attack on February 12, 1934.[7]

His pioneering contributions to FPS had a revolutionary impact on this speciality in Europe—and not only on that continent. Joseph conducted courses in FPS for participants from all over the world. Students Joseph Safim and Gustave Aufricht became leading plastic surgeons in the United States.

Further developments in the European field of FPS plus the ideas of enhancing knowledge, sharing clinical and surgical experience, and education and training in FPS in a multidisciplinary manner—similar to what Joseph had experienced during his work at the section for FPS—led to the establishment of the EAFPS in 1977. In honor of its most important pioneer, it was originally named The Joseph Society.

Closely following the American Academy of Facial Plastic and Reconstructive Surgery (AAFPRS), the EAFPS has the second-highest number of members.

At the turn of the 20th century, while Jacques Joseph explored a large and very fertile field for FPS under compelling time constraints, a German contemporary developed a revolutionary physical theory that laid the essential theoretical foundations for modern laser technology.

30.3 The Laser and Modern Facial Plastic Surgery

In 1916, Albert Einstein published his quantum theory of radiation. Influenced by Niels Bohr's theory of quantum mechanics, published in 1913, here Einstein for the first time described his idea of amplification of stimulated radiation. This concept of stimulated emission of radiation was to become the basis for the development of lasers. However, this work required tremendous effort, intense research, and major contributions by many other scientists over the following four decades. In 1954, U.S. scientists Charles H. Townes and James P. Gordon and their

Russian colleagues Nikolay Basov and Alexander Prokhorov constructed a "maser," a device that created coherent microwave energy.[4] This "forerunner of a laser" laid the groundwork for the first true laser, a ruby laser emitting a deep, red light, introduced by Theodore H. Maiman in 1959.[8] After the laser was used successfully for medical applications in opthalmology for the first time—"light coagulation" for repair of detached retinas[4]—it caught on very quickly in other medical fields as well. In the early 1960s, Leon Goldman became one of the very first dermatologists to pioneer the use of the ruby laser for treatment of a variety of cutaneous pathologies.[5] Based on Goldman's work and ideas, in 1983 John A. Parrish and R. Rox Anderson presented their concept of selective photothermolysis and showed how to minimize unwanted thermal injury associated with laser treatments on target tissues.[9] Thus was introduced a wide range of therapeutic applications of lasers and new approaches to dermal lesion—including skin resurfacing.

Since the development of the first laser, it has been the object of intense research in Germany for its application in medicine, in particular. In the late 1960s, the laser began to gain prominence there in various medical fields with the help and strong support of the German Federal Ministry of Education and Research, as well as sponsors from industry (interestingly, among others, the Volkswagen Foundation). As early as the 1970s, diverse working groups in urology, gastroenterology, ophthalmology, otolaryngology, and dermatology, among others, were established to enhance laser application in medicine. In 1981, the establishment of the German Society for Laser Medicine (Deutsche Gesellschaft für Laser Medizin e. V. [DGLM]) helped to collect scientific results, expand discussion, and coordinate research activities, including other functions, thereby giving a boost to lasers in medicine.[10] For several national laser societies such as the DGLM, the European Laser Association (ELA) serves as a European umbrella organization. One of these groups, the European Society for Laser Aesthetic Surgery (ESLAS), has since 1997 been a forum for the exchange of knowledge, research, education, and training in aesthetic applications of lasers exclusively.

Today's lasers have become a regular feature of the physician's armamentarium for diagnostics and treatment of diseases, as well as for aesthetic skin rejuvenation.

30.4 Applications in the Face and Neck

From the surgeons' point of view—cosmetic facial plastic surgeons in particular—we have a fairly specific way of looking at things. We examine hanging muscles and excessive skin; we assess the loss of tissue volume and the amount of prolapsing fat, and so forth. Then we consider incisions, excisions, plications, imbrications, and planning the ways of repositioning, tightening, sewing-in-place, and so on. Naturally, a surgeon's attention runs the risk of overlooking both the more superficial alterations of the facial and neck skin that occur during the aging process, and all the dermal pathologies that do not belong

Table 30.1 Laser applications in the face and neck

- **Vascular tumors and malformations**
  - Port-wine stains
    Teleangiektasias / hereditary hemorrhagic teleangiektasias
  - Hemangiomas
    Pyogenic granuloma
  - Venous lake (lips, ears)
- **Pigmented lesions**
  - Hyperpigmentation
  - Lentigines
  - Ephelides
  - Seborrheic keratoses
- **Benign tumors**
  - Seborrheic keratosis
  - Keloids
- **Cutaneous malignancies**
  - Basal cell carcinomas
  - Squamous cell carcinomas
- **Rhinophyma**
- **Hair removal / reduction**
- **Skin resurfacing**
- **Acne scarring**
- **Scar revision**
- **Treatment of tattoos**
- **Skin resurfacing**
- **Photorejuvenation** (nonablative)
- **Photodynamic therapy**
- **Complementary procedure to surgical techniques** (for instance: resurfacing with facelift)
- **Laser assisted surgical procedures** (for instance: blepharoplasty)

to the "true surgeon's classical area of responsibility." But it is exactly these clinical findings that should—especially after having read this book—become the focus of his attention. These data will enable him to enhance both his professional qualifications and patient care by providing more modern, safe, and reliable methods for the treatment of patients who have decided to "trust their faces to a facial plastic surgeon."

▶ Table 30.1 demonstrates that almost all common cutaneous treatments of lasers also apply to the face and neck areas. This is also the case with dermabrasion and chemical peels.

Formerly relegated to a small group of users, primarily dermatologists and a very few cosmetic surgeons, the revolutionary development of injectable treatments for facial aging and contouring has made soft-tissue fillers and neuromodulators the mainstay of cosmetic surgery—in Europe as well as in other parts of the world.[11] To a certain comparable degree, this occurred in the same way with dermabrasion and the use of chemical peels. The evolution of modern laser technology and the use of medical lasers suggest an equal development with cosmetic laser applications also in European facial plastic surgery.

After realizing that we have very good reasons for incorporating lasers and other exfoliant applications into our facial plastic surgery practices, the question that arises should *not* be: "Should we at all?" Because lasers have become a constant part of cosmetic applications, the better question would be: "How can we not?"

30.5 How to Incorporate Lasers into a Facial Plastic Surgery Practice

The following paragraphs should be of interest to those who are considering, or are just about to start, incorporating lasers and exfoliant procedures into their practices. Ideas and suggestions, which may help in developing a sensible plan of action, are presented to think about during the decision-making process.

There are many ways of starting this process. Numerous factors of varying importance and impact influence it, and also vary from country to country and from region to region. The structure of the national health care system, for example, may support the incorporation of lasers into your practice (development and improvement of health care) or make it more difficult (restriction in reimbursement by insurance). Different market situations, competition, structure of the population, and the population's financial health are some of the most crucial factors. The ideas and approaches suggested reflect personal experience and they are recommended because they have been tried and tested by the author in the still-ongoing process of transition from a practice previously based on otolaryngology/head-and-neck surgery to a cosmetically focused facial plastic surgery practice.

Therefore, if you are considering incorporating lasers or other light-deviced or exfoliating procedures into your FPS practice—in Europe or elsewhere, in a highly competitive metropolis, or in a small community—you are advised to always remember and utilize the following four principles in each of your practice decisions and actions.

You need the following:

- *Knowledge* about the role of lasers in medicine, their possible value for your FPS practice, the ways to incorporate them into your practice, and the mechanisms that run the market you will be entering
- *Will* to broaden your professional horizon with laser medicine and to shoulder "whatever it takes" to accomplish your endeavor
- *Ability* and the resources to provide the new service, as well as to rely on a well-prepared business plan and strategy
- *Execution* of your strategy to occur precisely according to your action plan, with undaunted courage and discipline (and patience, in particular)

... in order to be able to incorporate lasers efficiently into your daily work and enhance your FPS practice by producing outstanding results both clinically and economically.

At the beginning of the process, these steps follow each other; however, later they constantly interact with each other in an interdependent and synergistic manner.

30.5.1 Knowledge

This book provides you with a plethora of information about the science, technology, and clinical use of medical lasers in FPS. In what follows, you are given more recommendations and references concerning business development, as well as hints and proposals about getting things started and accomplished.

There are suggestions about issues to be thoroughly considered before making any decisions, to make sure you will feel comfortable and remain successful in this field in the long term.

30.5.2 Will

As noted earlier, there are many good reasons for making lasers, light applications, peels, and abrasions part of your "stock-in-trade." They increase your expertise as a facial plastic surgeon and possibly enhance your ability to achieve previously unattainable results, which may optimize patient care provided by your practice. Because they add new effective and reliable options to those already offered by your practice, at the same time they encourage or, even more, create demand in your regular as well as potential patients.

However, before you begin to integrate these tools into your daily FPS practice, it may be wise to rethink several issues and stay aware of their profiles (▶ Table 30.2). Of course, these "cons" are not insurmountable obstacles and, when viewed with the correct, constructive attitude, they may be turned into "pros"—new opportunities for development (▶ Table 30.3). In any case, you should be aware of the fact that you will probably be changing the "character" of your practice and that these changes are accompanied by logistic and economic challenges, as well as demands on the professional qualifications of yourself and your staff members.

Consequently, if you are aware of these issues and have the *will* to deal with them constructively (as the old adage goes, "Where there's a will, there's a way.") you should start to analyze the prerequisites and requirements that are necessary to strengthen your ability to act efficiently and effectively.

30.5.3 Ability

Even if you already have expertise in FPS or a connected field, there is no doubt that you should become a true expert in lasers, peels, and other abrasion modalities. The same holds true for your staff members—although most likely on a different level—who are or will become involved in the process. Since lasers have become a constant part of medicine, most training programs provide at least the essential basic knowledge about medical lasers, and most of us already have been working with

Table 30.2 Obstacles that may need to be overcome

Changing your practice profile (Risk of losing regular patients?)
Higher grade of diversification (Risk of taking on too much at the same time?)
Need to change setting/location?
Need to train staff. Need to hire additional (qualified) employees.
What about your own qualifications: additional training necessary?
Feelings of apprehension during learning curve?
Coping with side effects (burned or peeling faces)
High investment costs? Added maintenance costs
Additional efforts and costs for acquisition of new patients
New competitive situation (Impact on referrals?)

Table 30.3 Chances for further development and faster growth of your practice

Enhancing your practice profile
Widening the range of treatment options
Improving your office layout
Increasing your expertise and the qualifications of your staff members
Becoming a true expert in new medical fields
Optimizing the care of your facial-aging patients
New options for your regular patients
Acquisition of potential patients for your new service ("supply creates demand")
Generation of additional income (cross-selling, new patients)

at least one of the medical lasers in use today. This is a stable foundation to build on. Everything noted here about lasers is valid for peels and other abrasions to a certain degree.

This textbook can aid a great deal in conveying information and increasing your knowledge. Medical societies such as the EAFPS, DGLM, ESLAS, or the International Federation of Facial Plastic Surgery Societies (IFFPSS) and the AAFPRS offer a wide range of further training, support, and advice. It is definitely worthwhile becoming a member of one of these organizations.

The author cannot emphasize too strongly the importance of joining a social network of highly qualified experts who are willing to share their expertise with you and be of assistance by giving advice. From personal experience, the author strongly recommends visiting senior specialists at their facilities as a type of short-term observational fellowship and, if possible, participating in a fellowship program. These will provide you not only with additional training but will give you deeper insight into how to manage this type of practice. Again, the medical societies may help with this, too.

To be able to offer skin rejuvenation to your patients, you need an appropriate facility and, of course, the right equipment.

Before investing substantial capital, you might consider sharing equipment (and perhaps a facility) with other specialists. This will enable you to provide high-level laser treatment to your patients, while keeping overhead costs low. Possibly there are some options available in the area in which you live. For several years, the author has worked cooperatively with a laser surgery center adjoining a department of dermatology. Here the author has performed almost every type of skin resurfacing and utilized different types of lasers tailored to patient needs.

If you decide to equip your own office with a laser, there are several different issues to consider before making a choice. Chapter 20 provides you with valuable information for your decision making.

This determination should be accompanied by considerations about cash resources and their allocation. At this point, at the latest, the author strongly advises taking time for some essential preparation and developing a thorough, well-considered business plan in which laser application plays a crucial role. If a business plan already exists, it should be adapted according to your latest decisions.

You can do it on your own—there is a great deal of literature available about the business aspects of this type of practice[12,13,14]—but the author urges you to seek professional advice from a consultant company.

A business plan relies on a vision of your professional future and a *written* mission statement that provide you with constant orientation in your daily work.

The results of a crucial and precise analysis (market, environment, competition, financial health of patients, etc.), the definition of goals (short term and long term) and critical success factors, etc., will finally lead into the development of a strategic plan—including effective marketing options. In this process of incorporating lasers into your practice, your business plan and strategy will provide you and your team with a clear understanding of what is going on and will give everyone the ability to do the right things (effectiveness), in the right way (efficiency).[15]

Your business plan as well as your strategy will remain dynamic to some degree; nevertheless, they must be revised periodically to make sure they are current. Experience shows that the better and more accurately the business plan and strategy have been prepared and developed, the less they will need to be changed. Significant changes, however, in the market, the competition, etc., may require appropriate adjustments over time.

If you have created a good strategy and are ready to start, execute it without hesitation precisely according to your action plan.

30.5.4 Execution

The author assumes that you are excellent at winning over patients during consultations, at performing rejuvenation surgery and resurfacing skin, and at providing outstanding patient aftercare—especially after having read this book. And now you want to incorporate or increase the use of lasers, peels, and other abrasion modalities into your practice and translate your decision successfully into daily actions. But did you know the following? "... 70% of strategic failures come from poor execution of leadership... it is rarely for lack of 'smarts' or vision."[16] You may have developed an ingenious strategy with ambitious goals; you may have a very respectable business plan and well-trained staff; and conditions sine qua non for success in your practice; however, you will most likely be successful exactly to the same degree as you are able to let things happen—or more precisely, to make things happen—in your practice according to your action plan. Whether it is a small business office or a huge organization, those who are successful have one thing in common: They keep the gap between decision making and executing as small as possible.[15]

Because this view corresponds with personal experience, the author cannot emphasize strongly enough the importance of courageous and disciplined execution of your plans for the success of your practice.

Some general principles do exist within this problem, but guidelines can be derived from them. The author applies the concept of "4 disciplines of execution."[17] These help in accomplishing the most important goals of the business strategy, without getting bogged down in the pressing urgencies that occur in the day-to-day business of managing a growing facial plastic surgery practice.

There are several ways of coping with this issue. The author recommends taking a good look at them and making sure that during your daily work, in fact, what has been planned according to strategy is being carried out as closely as possible.[18,19,20] Is the strategy to integrate lasers or other new treatments into your practice? By doing so, you will be able to transform all your activities in a more effective and efficient manner. Transform functions into desired or—as your proficiency increases—outstanding outcomes. All of them can become modules of your success.

30.6 Board Certification by the International Federation of Facial Plastic Surgery Societies

Whether you are an experienced and highly qualified facial plastic surgeon or a young and ambitious doctor on your laborious way toward gaining that expertise, you have probably been thinking about the need for valid and reliable credentialing that demonstrates your very special qualifications to both your patients and to the members of your medical community. The IFFPSS has—in alliance with individual academies such as the AAFPRS and the EAFPS—a board certification program that meets the highest standards of our speciality and, thus far, provides the only valid and internationally acknowledged credentials for a qualified facial plastic surgeon. From the European point of view—which is probably similar in other parts of the world—this puts you and your academy in a very exciting, interdependent relationship. Your academy supports you in obtaining the credentials of board certification. As the number of board-certified surgeons increases, both the academies for FPS and the speciality of FPS are enhanced in the views of the public and the medical communities. And this will remarkably benefit your career and your practice!

References

[1] Eco U. Die Geschichte der Schoenheit. Muenchen, Deutschland: DTV. 3. Auflage; 2009

[2] Etcoff N. Survival of the Prettiest – The Science of Beauty. New York, NY: Random House; 1999

[3] Ekman P. Telling Lies. New York, NY: W. W. Norton; 2009

[4] Houk LD, Humphreys T. Masers to magic bullets: an updated history of lasers in dermatology. Clin Dermatol 2007; 25: 434–442

[5] Tanzi EL, Lupton JR, Alster TS. Lasers in dermatology: four decades of progress. J Am Acad Dermatol 2003; 49: 1–31, quiz 31–34

[6] Wheeland RG, McBurney E, Geronemus RG. The role of dermatologists in the evolution of laser surgery. Dermatol Surg 2000; 26: 815–822

[7] Briedigkeit W, Behrbohm H. Jacque J. Ein Pionier der plastischen Gesichtschirurgie. Berlin, Germany: Hentrich & Hentrich; 2006

[8] Maiman T. Stimulated optical radiation in ruby. Nature 1960; 187: 493–494

[9] Anderson RR, Parrish JA. Selective photothermolysis: precise microsurgery by selective absorption of pulsed radiation. Science 1983; 220: 524–527

[10] Deutsche Gesellschaft Für Lasermedizin V. Available at: https://www.dglm.org/. Accessed March 18, 2014

[11] Maas CS, Ed. Neuromodulators and soft tissue fillers. Facial Plast Surg Clin N Am 2007;15(1)

[12] Mendelsohn JE. Developing and maintaining a successful facial cosmetic surgery practice. In: Truswell WH IV, ed. Surgical Facial Rejuvenation. New York, NY: Thieme Medical Publishers; 2009: 177–190

[13] Waldman SR, Ed. Practice management in facial plastic surgery. Facial Plast Surg Clin N Am 2010;18(4)

[14] Williams EF, III. Business aspects of facial plastic surgery. Facial Plast Surg 2010; 26: 1

[15] Drucker PF. The Essential Drucker. New York, NY: HarperCollins; 2001

[16] Bossidy L, Charan R. Execution: The Discipline of Getting Things Done. New York, NY: Crown Business; 2002

[17] McChesney C, Covey S, Huling J. The 4 Disciplines of Execution: Achieving Your Wildly Important Goals. New York, NY: Free Press; 2012

[18] Drucker PF. The Effective Executive. Oxford, UK: Butterworth-Heinemann/Elsevier; 2007

[19] Allan D. Getting Things Done: The Art of Stress-Free Productivity. New York, NY: Penguin Books; 2003

[20] Covey SR, Merrill AR, Merrill RR. First Things First. New York, NY: Free Press; 2003

31 Lasers, Peels, and Abrasion Techniques for East Asian Skin

Philip A. Young

31.1 Historical Perspective

Beauty has been appreciated throughout our evolution and is responsible for the propagation of our species. Perhaps, controversially, it is the most important trait that we have. The appearance of our skin and the presentation of uniformity in color, texture, and the reflection of light in a smooth and non-abrupt manner as it flows from one anatomical location to another play a major role in facial beauty.[1] With the relatively recent explosion of the cosmetic industry and the ease with which our information is being disseminated (i.e., the Internet and computers), our knowledge and options are increasing. These have evolved to the present day where we have multiple methods to choose from: chemical peels (salicylic, Jessner's Solution, trichloroacetic acid [TCA], glycolic, resorcinol, lactic acid, etc.), dermabrasion, dermarolling, dermasanding, laser resurfacing (carbon dioxide [CO_2], erbium:yttrium aluminum garnet [Er:YAG], etc.), the fractional application of laser resurfacing, and nonablative/ablative combinations.

31.2 The East Asian Patient

East Asia is a subregion of Asia that is made up of about 12% of the Asian continent including more than 1.5 billion people and one fifth of the people in the world. They are represented by countries such as China, Japan, Korea, Mongolia, and possibly Vietnam. The characteristics of the East Asian patient from a dermatological standpoint can also include countries normally considered Southeast Asian such as Laos, Malaysia, Singapore, the Philippines, Thailand, and Cambodia. The variation of skin types within these countries is between Fitzpatrick skin types III to V.

In general in the United States, the Asian American population has been listed as 4.8%. Because of this, the frequency of treating the Asian client is relatively low. With the darker skin, the fear of hypopigmentation and hyperpigmentation often leads to a higher anxiety level for the U.S. clinician presented with this clientele base. Generally for hyperpigmentation, the risk increases as the color of the hair darkens and the skin lightens because the contrasting reaction of the skin tends to take on the color of the hair. Hypopigmentation risks increase as the skin darkens for similar reasons.

The Asian patient has a tendency to form pigmentary disorders versus wrinkling. Histologically the skin of the Asian clientele is characterized by larger melanocytes with increased production of melanin and melanosomes. Two groups found that Asians developed wrinkling one to two decades later than age-matched Caucasians.[2,3] Melasma, ephelides, lentigines, and postinflammatory hyperpigmentation (PIH) are the most common conditions.

Because of recovery length and severity with traditional ablative techniques, multiple nonablative options have been popularized in the past several years. Lasers from 500 to 2,000 nm based on selective photothermolysis have avoided epidermal ablation while targeting pigment and blood vessels within the skin at progressively deeper layers. Radiofrequency and ultrasound have been introduced to nonspecifically treat the deeper tissue layers and create nonablative tightening. Although significant results can be achieved through these choices, the greater number of treatments needed, risk of hyperpigmentation, inferior results to ablative techniques, and the decreased effectiveness of treating both wrinkling and pigmentary issues with one modality maintain the utility of ablative methods in the recent trend of nonablative techniques. Ablative methods are indicated when patients want skin tightening for wrinkles, improvement of the uniformity of skin texture/tone, and reduction of pigmentary issues together in one treatment and can accept the more prolonged associated downtime.

31.3 Chemical Peels

Chemical peels can improve skin texture/tone and decrease the presence of active acne, acne scars, actinic keratosis, ephelides, fine and deep lines/wrinkles, melasma, and telangiectasias. Depending on the severity of each condition, one can devise a plan for each person.[4] A full discussion of chemical peels is beyond the scope of this chapter. The author concentrates on the pertinent elements regarding chemical peels in the East Asian patient. A personal perspective is presented along with literature findings[4] to help with the discussion.

In regard to ablative techniques, one can consider an aggressive skin care regimen of alpha hydroxyl acid fruit-acid peels, beta hydroxyl acid peels, Jessner's peels, retinoic acid peels, TCA peels, laser resurfacing, phenol peels, and dermabrasion in that approximate order of increasing strength and depth of treatment. An aggressive skin care regimen starting with topical vitamin A and alpha hydroxy acid peels can be started and this can be done for a period of 4 to 8 weeks to prepare the skin for a deeper treatment. This is not mandatory but is thought to prepare the skin to heal faster (i.e., rapid re-epithelialization) and allow a more even peel when the deeper treatment is applied. It can also serve as an effective skin care maintenance program. What has been a standard for deeper treatments with moderate-depth chemical peels (i.e., Jessner's and TCA 35% combination), laser resurfacing, phenol peels, and dermabrasion techniques is a 2- to 6- week pretreatment of the skin with Retin A, hydroquinone (or other bleaching agent), and hydrocortisone 1 to 2%. Both approaches aim to prepare the skin to be at even levels so that the penetration of the ablative method is uniform and to prevent PIH. Many studies are showing, however, that pretreatment may not benefit either the goal of more rapid epithelialization or the prevention of hyperpigmentation.[5] Although open to debate, if a pretreatment regimen is utilized it should be stopped 6 to 7 days prior to the deeper treatment. For the East Asian patient, 4 to 6 weeks of pretreatment have been historically advised.

Alpha hydroxy acid peels are sometimes referred to as fruit-acid peels and include citric, glycolic, lactic, malic, and tartaric acids, and so forth. They are often used to subtly treat fine wrinkles, patchy dryness, and uneven pigmentation. Glycolic acids are perhaps the most common and range from 10 to 70% concentrations. Beta hydroxy acid peels such as salicylic acid appear to have more penetration into pores than the fruit-acid peels and can decrease sebum production; they are often formulated in skin products to treat acne. Jessner's peels are formulated with 14% weight/volume of salicylic acid, resorcinol, and lactic acid in ethanol; they can be used to achieve a deeper peel than can be accomplished with fruit-acid and beta hydroxy acid peels. Glycolic peels with stronger preparations are preferred in an office setting at 30 to 70%, whereas the 10 to 30% are used at home for continual maintenance. Jessner's peels are used for deeper peels in the office and are employed to prepare the skin to allow a deeper peel using TCA at 30 to 35% strength immediately after. There are many options for chemical peeling. Having a simplified approach can markedly ease patient anxiety during the subsequent discussion of options with patients. In terms of chemical peeling, a complete approach to skin rejuvenation can be accomplished in the office with 30 to 70% glycolic peels, Jessner's peels, and TCA peels (20, 35%).

Preoperatively, along with the pretreatment regimen, there are other precautions that should be followed. The patient should avoid blood thinners 2 weeks before and after ablative resurfacing (mostly moderate-depth peels or ablation techniques) that may have significant risk of causing bleeding. Medical risk assessments, a full history, and physical and other preoperative checks are done as with other measures commonly used for sedation. Specific contraindications are covered in other relevant chapters. Contraindications can include the following:

- A current or history of skin cancer, especially malignant melanoma, or recurrent nonmelanoma skin cancer, or precancerous lesions such as multiple dysplastic nevi
- Any active skin infection
- Disease that may be stimulated by light at 560 to 1,200 nm, such as history of recurrent herpes simplex, systemic lupus erythematosus, or porphyria
- Use of photosensitive medication and/or herbs such as isotretinoin, tetracycline, or St. John's Wort that may cause sensitivity to 560- to 1,200-nm light exposure. Accutane (Roche, Basel, Switzerland) could warrant 1- to 2-years cessation before deep skin-ablation methods.
- Immunosuppressive disease, including acquired immune deficiency syndrome (AIDS) and human immunodeficiency virus (HIV) infection, or use of immunosuppressive medications
- Patient history of hormonal or endocrine disorders, such as polycystic ovary syndrome or diabetes, unless under control
- History of bleeding coagulopathies, or use of anticoagulants
- History of keloid or hypertrophic scarring
- Very dry skin or conditions that would create healing issues in postprocedure phase
- Exposure to sun or artificial tanning during the 3 to 4 weeks prior to treatment. Sunblock should be applied 2 weeks or more before any ablative procedure, using a product that is sensitive for the skin and contains titanium dioxide or zinc oxide.

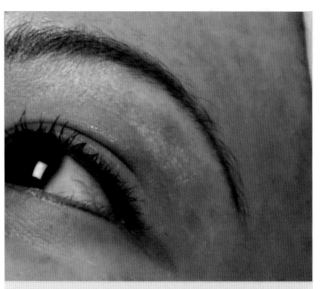

Fig. 31.1 The first level of peeling is shown in pink and red. The upper eyelid is starting to show a slight frost with speckles of white turning into a sheet of translucent white, indicative of the peel penetrating the superficial papillary dermis just beyond the basement membrane.

- Fitzpatrick skin types V and VI
- Pregnancy and nursing
- Ectropion (outward turning of the lower eyelid), excessively dry eyes, and previous lower blepharoplasty
- Koebnerizing diseases (prior radiation therapy leading to a loss of adnexal structures), extensive fibrosis resulting from prior cosmetic treatments (e.g., dermabrasion, deep chemical peels, silicone injections)

Perhaps the most important part of this discussion is about the levels of penetration that are reached through chemical peels and how to discern each level (▶ Fig. 31.1). When doing the Monheit moderate-depth chemical peel this can be paramount to avoid scarring. With this peel, the Jessner's peel is started and two to four passes are done to prepare for the TCA 30-35% peel, which is usually one to two passes but based on the parameters enumerated below:

1. The first level is when the skin turns pink/red. The depth has been thought to reach the basement membrane, with stimulation of the dermal blood vessels leading to the pink/red hue. This is mostly done with the Jessner's peel. Peeling may or may not occur at 1 to 3 days.
2. The second level is when the skin starts to have specks of white, indicating the penetration into the papillary dermis and coagulation of dermal proteins just beyond the basement membrane. This can be achieved with the Jessner's peel as well; however, it is better to stay at the first level with the Jessner's peel prior to the 30-35% TCA. Peeling may or may not occur at 2 to 4 days.
3. As the specks turn into a layer of translucent white with a pink background, you have essentially penetrated the basement membrane and your peel has gone into the superficial papillary dermis. Because the anchoring fibrils are disrupted, the epidermis slides or moves more readily with manipulation. Peeling may or may not occur at 3 to 5 days.

4. When the pink background disappears and a solid layer of white frost is created, the next layer is reached with a moderate-to-deep peel. At this depth, the peel has reached the deeper layers of the papillary dermis because the vessels are constricted (leading to the disappearance of the pink/red) with further coagulation of the dermal proteins. The further coagulation also restricts the movement of the skin and the epidermal sliding disappears. This is the usual goal for the moderate-depth peel. Peeling may or may not occur at 4 to 7 days.

5. A gray background indicates a peel that has gone to the papillary reticular dermis junction depth and this is to be avoided because the risk for scarring increases at this level. Peeling may or may not occur at 6 to 10 days.

Chemical peeling is an "art" and requires experience. The levels described can rapidly progress from one level to the next and one can find oneself with a gray background quickly, especially with the stronger peels. Starting slowly and being conservative is important. The amount of peeling agent left in the cotton ball or other applicator used should be consistent. It has been advocated that 1 to 3 drops of solution should be left in the applicator for each application. This has been detailed as a process where the cotton ball is squeezed until only 1 to 3 drops are left, and this can be tested a few times before the actual application. The thickness of the peel solution on the skin is subjective as well and can require experience. These points help the clinician to advance through the different levels of peeling in a gradual and safe manner.

What can be most important of all is the postprocedure care after chemical peeling and other deep ablative resurfacing (▶ Fig. 31.2). For superficial peels that penetrate to the basement membrane, the use of Vaseline or Aquaphor (Beiersdorf Inc., Wilton, Connecticut) for 1 to 2 days is indicated (with petroleum jelly being preferred). At this depth, the watertight barrier that is created partially by urocanic acid in the middle portion of the epidermis, epidermal lipids, the cell-to-cell tight barrier created by desmosome connections, and the basement membrane itself are compromised—along with the skin barrier protective functions. Applying a proven nonreactive formulation such as Vaseline or other petroleum jelly can prevent unwanted skin reactions that can occur with application of other products with multiple ingredients. The key to faster healing is frequent cleaning. If this is done in the most effective way, peeling is much less of an event because the constant cleaning removes the desquamation. Use 1 teaspoon of over-the-counter white clear vinegar in a quart of distilled water along with a gentle cleanser such as Cetaphil (Galderma Laboratories, Fort Worth, Texas) or an equivalent. The areas treated are first washed with the gentle cleanser by patting and with as little rubbing or massaging as possible. These are then rinsed with the vinegar/water solution for 5 to 10 minutes. This is repeated as frequently as possible to keep the crusting to a minimum. The goal is pink, raw skin. Sometimes, immersing the entire treated area in a bowl of solution is necessary to moisten the crusts and allow them to slough off. The patient is directed to cleanse as frequently as every hour to achieve the goal. Frequent follow-up is mandatory. Pictures sent daily via text, e-mail, or provided in person can help tremendously. Importantly, the faster the healing the less likely scarring,

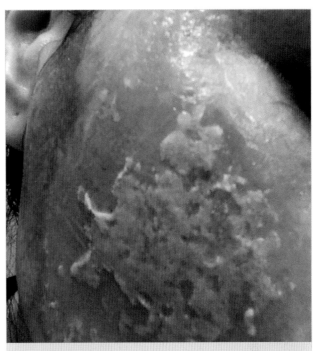

Fig. 31.2 Postprocedure day 3 after ablative resurfacing. This patient has too much crusting and needs to increase the frequency and length of cleaning to remove the crusts. These should be removed after each cleaning session and before Vaseline is applied. Also, the pink/red, raw area is the clinical level reached during the actual procedure.

hyperpigmentation, and hypopigmentation will occur in the East Asian clientele.

The combined use of the moderate-depth chemical peel using Jessner's peel and TCA 30 to 35% peel with dermasanding, can be very effective (▶ Fig. 31.3). As can be seen in the before and after images (▶ Fig. 31.3a, b), the deep wrinkles have been markedly reduced along with the finer wrinkles. The skin, although still erythematous at the 2-month mark, shows a much more uniform tone and is lighter in complexion. The texture is generally smoother in the after photo as well.

31.4 Carbon Dioxide Laser Resurfacing

The CO_2 laser was developed around the 1960s. It was the first laser to be utilized for skin, ophthalmological, and other surgical applications. Originally, the CO_2 laser used continuous applied energy instead of pulses, which often led to adverse outcomes. In the 1980s, Dr. David Lawrence first used the CO_2 laser for cutaneous resurfacing. With the continuous wave approach, extensive thermal injury that led to scarring and prolonged healing times occurred (measured in watts [W] = joules [J]/second [s]). Selective photothermolysis and the understanding of thermal relaxation times for different chromophores in the skin helped scientists develop pulsed lasers that were able to deliver high-energy pulses of short duration that limited the surrounding damage. The thermal relaxation time of skin 20 to 30 µm in thickness is about 1.0 ms, which is the time required for 50% of the heat to diffuse. The threshold for skin

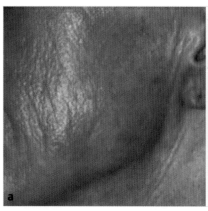
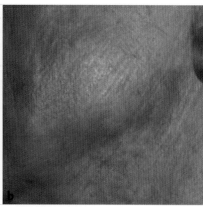

Fig. 31.3 Chemical peeling before (**a**) and after (**b**) the combined use of Jessner's peel and trichloroacetic acid (TCA) 30 to 35% peel, and dermasanding for the lower cheek–jawline area 2 months postoperative.

vaporization is about 5 J/cm^2. With the fluence from 5 to 7 J/cm^2, the CO_2 laser can provide clean and efficient tissue ablation with much of the heat dissipated in the plume/smoke of the tissue (fluence is measured in joules/centimeters squared). This provides approximately 50 to 70 μm of ablation with about 20 μm of surrounding tissue injury.[6] With the knowledge of average skin thicknesses,[7] one can estimate the depth of resurfacing. This depends on the settings of the laser, with which one should be familiar. For example, at 100 mJ (millijoules), density scale 1, and 125-Hz frequency, the ablation depth is 70 μm and the thermal depth is 75 μm.

The preoperative and postoperative regimens for CO_2 laser resurfacing are much the same as for chemical peels. The obvious difference is the mode by which the ablation is carried out. Traditional CO_2 laser resurfacing is totally ablative, removing progressive amounts and layers of skin. The healing time can range from 5 to 10 days depending on the depth and the efficiency of the postoperative care.

Intraoperatively, because of the discomfort of CO_2 laser resurfacing, a certain amount of sedation is needed. Oral sedation is quite commonly used. Intravenous sedation is perhaps more effective. Local and regional anesthesia is also a necessity to decrease the pain of CO_2 laser resurfacing. With oral sedation, diazepam can be used at 5 to 40 mg to reach a level at which the patient is sedated but able to respond to vocal cues. The onset is slow, however, requiring 30 minutes to more than an hour to reach an effective state. Intravenous sedation is faster and potentially safer in some ways. A combination of propofol, ketamine, midazolam, fentanyl, and so forth can be used to reach a level of sedation where the patient is still able to respond to vocal and physical cues, while maintaining oxygen saturation above 95%. Eye shields are strongly recommended. Moistened, sterile towels around the field are necessary as well. Having a basin of saline as well as larger containers with water immediately around the field is useful for potential fires. Again, protective eye shields are needed. A complete CO_2 laser resurfacing protocol for safety should be followed, as well as adherence to Accreditation Association for Ambulatory Health Care (AAAHC) standards or other appropriate credentialing institutions required by your state.

The laser settings used will require some familiarity with the particular CO_2 laser. With the UltraPulse (Lumenis Ltd., Yokneam, Israel), a setting of 100 mJ, 150-Hz frequency, density scale 5, with cool scan is usually used with the first pass for traditional-type resurfacing. As seen in ▶ Fig. 31.4, traditional resurfacing entails the use of densities of 4 to 5, whereas fractional resurfacing utilizes densities of 1 to 3—which will be discussed. The second pass with traditional resurfacing is with 90 mJ, and a density of 4. The end results should show that the epidermis is ablated revealing the dermal layer. Viewing ▶ Fig. 31.2, the pink, raw area is the goal after the second pass and with removal using saline-soaked gauze. During the procedure what appears pink in ▶ Fig. 31.2 can be whiter in the operating room. Since skin thicknesses differ in individuals, one may find that for some patients this level is not reached after the second pass and in some this level may be too deep. In general these settings have been reliable. Of course, others vary these settings and still remain safe. Sasaki et al[7] did an extensive study looking at the skin thickness of different areas of the body. The eyelids and neck are the thinnest areas and should require lower settings; 70 to 90 mJ are often used in these areas for the first pass and 60 to 80 mJ are used for the second pass with densities at 4 and 3, respectively. Some believe that the neck is better treated with fractional CO_2 laser resurfacing, given the higher risk for complications in this part of the body. Nonfacial body parts tolerate CO_2 laser resurfacing much the same as the neck and fractional resurfacing is often preferred as a safer option. The clinical indicators for CO_2 laser resurfacing are:

1. Removal of the epidermis occurs when the pigmented layer and skin texture are removed. This is noted when after the eschar is debrided gently with moistened gauze, the pigmented epidermis is removed revealing the smooth pink background of the superficial papillary dermis.
2. The upper reticular dermis is reached once a gray color is shown after gentle debridement or removal of the eschar.
3. The midreticular dermis reveals a chamois-brown color.

After the first two laser passes, it is prudent to reduce the energy of subsequent laser passes. After the first pass with 100 mJ and then the second pass with 90 mJ, 70 to 80 mJ can be used to slowly reach deeper levels. Others have done the third pass with the same settings used with the second pass. In general, three to four passes are the most that should be done because the penetration depth is limited past three passes.[8] In addition, what previously was thought to be the midreticular dermis and the chamois-brown color that indicated this change, is now believed to be color really due to desiccation and not the actual appearance of the anatomical depth. The other alternative is to mechanically reach the deeper layers

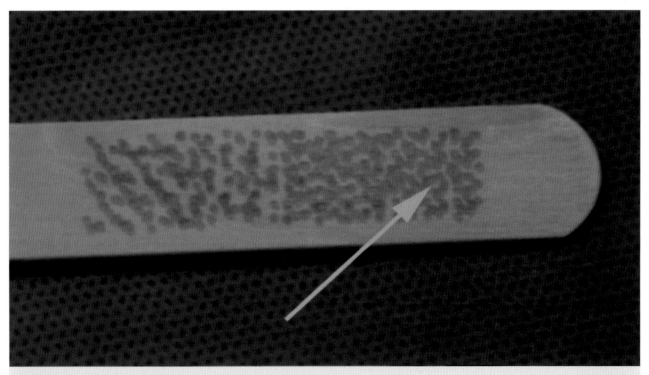

Fig. 31.4 The arrow points to density 5 for the UltraPulse (Lumenis Ltd., Yokneam, Israel) laser. Moving to the left-most spot size, the density becomes 2. This Active FX (Lumenis) handpiece uses a 1.3-mm spot size.

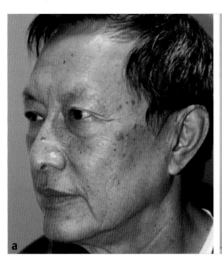
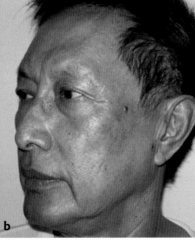

Fig. 31.5 Carbon dioxide (CO_2) laser resurfacing before (**a**) and after (**b**) with traditional methods combined with dermasanding. This patient requested removal of sunspots and improving his skin appearance. Moles were not targeted.

through dermabrasion or dermasanding, as will be described. Other end points are: (1) the elimination of the scar, lesion, or wrinkle, (2) a yellow-brown discoloration (or gray-brown), or (3) no further shrinkage. After CO_2 laser resurfacing, fine and deep wrinkles are improved (▶ Fig. 31.5). The skin's texture is more even and consistent. Lentigines and ephelides are reduced. The skin's tone is more uniform as well as lighter in complexion.

Typically, the fear with the Asian clientele is the appearance of hyperpigmentation or hypopigmentation. Hyperpigmentation may be unavoidable in the East Asian client and a full discussion of this possibility is needed to avoid an unhappy patient. Pretreatment may be necessary as a prophylactic measure. Some believe that in the East Asian patient a full 6 weeks is

necessary before laser resurfacing. Topical medications including Retin A, hydroquinone, azelaic acid, kojic acid, mequinol, an assortment of botanicals, and other agents have been used. Retin A, azelaic acid 15 to 20% (hydroquinone has been standard but may be carcinogenic), and hydrocortisone 1 to 2% are preferred. A test spot is always advocated (pretreatment and posttreatment) and subsequent applications should be done on skin that is not inflamed or still red from the previous application. PIH can be treated with serial chemical peels that can be done with glycolic peels at home[4] and stronger peels in an office setting every 2 to 3 weeks. Jessner's peels are also a good option in the office setting. The key with serial chemical peels is to avoid starting them too early, especially when there is still significant erythema or inflammation. Doing serial chemical peels at this

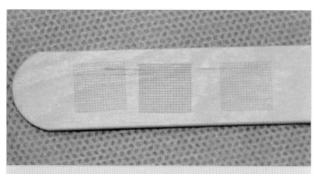

Fig. 31.6 Deep FX (Lumenis) handpiece component that treats the deeper tissue causing skin tightening with thinner cones of carbon dioxide (CO_2) laser energy that penetrate deeper into the tissue. The Deep FX spot size is 0.12 mm, 10 times smaller than the Active FX (Lumenis) superficial component but with penetration approximately 5 times deeper.

premature stage may be too deep and aggressive and can cause hypopigmentation and possibly scarring. Very superficial peels are advocated. One pass with Jessner's Solution getting slight erythema is ideal. Low-percentage glycolic peels are also preferred. Persistent PIH that translates to something long term may need another traditional resurfacing procedure or other laser modality for resolution.

31.5 Fractional Carbon Dioxide Laser Resurfacing

Traditional resurfacing, although effective, can require a lengthy downtime, significant discomfort, and a labor-intensive postprocedure phase for the patient. The risks of scarring and prolonged erythema are some other drawbacks that patients often voice. Fractional CO_2 laser resurfacing was created to bridge the gap between traditional resurfacing and less-invasive methods, achieving better results than you would normally expect from a less-invasive approach. Fractional resurfacing is based on treating a fraction of the skin's surface. As can be seen in ▶ Fig. 31.4, the densities of Active FX (Lumenis) increase from density 2 to density 5 moving from left to right. Traditional resurfacing entails doing two passes with density 5 followed by density 4 (sometimes clinicians prefer a density of 5 and then density 5 again). In contrast, fractional resurfacing ranges from densities 1 through 3, which leaves healthy tissue between the smaller spots to help the skin heal faster. Also in contrast, the surface component (Active FX) is used with one pass and then a deeper piece (Deep FX, Lumenis) is used to create zones of trauma that are also thinner than the surface component (▶ Fig. 31.6). When the Active FX and Deep FX, or superficial and deeper modes, are used together it is referred as Total FX (Lumenis) or the most intense fractional resurfacing treatment. Whereas the Active FX superficial component can treat pigmentation, fine wrinkles, and surface texture/tone, the Deep FX deeper component will tighten the skin, shrink the overall skin surface, and improve larger, deeper wrinkles and deeper scars. Together the two pieces can treat the superficial conditions and also shrink the skin similar to traditional methods, while avoiding the prolonged redness, recovery, and risk of scarring. It has been found that the average depth of the Active FX handpiece with its 1.3-

mm spot size, using 100 and 125 mJ, is about 70 and 100 µm of ablation and 75 and 110 µm of thermal damage, for a total of 145 and 210 µm at a density of 1. The Deep FX, with its 0.12-mm spot size (10 times smaller than Active FX), using 15 and 20 mJ, at a density of 1, showed an ablation depth of 420 and 660 µm and thermal damage of 280 and 440 µm for a total penetration depth of 700 and 1,100 µm, respectively. The depth of Deep FX was about 5 times deeper than Active FX (Lumenis).[7]

The preprocedure and postprocedure regimens are the same as for chemical peeling and CO_2 laser traditional resurfacing. Intraoperatively, some have advocated topical anesthesia using lidocaine/tetracaine 23/7% or benzocaine/lidocaine/tetracaine 20/6/4% as the sole means for anesthesia. The experiences of others have shown the safety of applying coats of topical anesthesia in serial fashion for the face, arms, legs, and so forth.[7] Even with these topical anesthetics, patients still feel the laser to a degree that makes clinicians and patients uncomfortable with this approach. Oral, intravenous, and general anesthesia all have been used to make the procedure more tolerable. Lidocaine toxicity is always a concern especially when doing multiple areas. What is advocated here is intravenous sedation (propofol, ketamine, Versed, and fentanyl) using multiple regional facial nerve blocks with more local anesthesia in the temple, cheeks, and the third division of the trigeminal nerve, which tends to be more difficult to anesthetize. Straight lidocaine 1% and epinephrine 1:100,000 are more effective and the entire face can be treated without violating the 7.5 mg/kg-systemic limit. Although experience, anecdotal reports, and literature point to the body's tolerance of much higher doses (25–50 mg/kg in large liposuction cases), staying close to this limit and trying to inject areas in a serial fashion will avoid unnecessary risk. This applies to traditional resurfacing as well.

Because CO_2 lasers differ in their approach based on different properties of how they deliver the CO_2 laser energy, experience with each particular laser is essential. For the Lumenis Ultra-Pulse, the parameters for facial areas are 12.5 to 20 mJ, density 1 to 2, for the Deep FX handpiece, and 100 to 125 mJ, density 1 to 3 at 125 to 150 Hz for the Active FX handpiece. The periorbital region requires Deep FX 12.5 to 17.5 mJ and Active FX 80 to 90 mJ, density 1 at 125 Hz, respectively. For the neck and nonfacial areas, Deep FX 12.5 to 15 mJ, density 1 and Active FX 80 to 90 mJ, density 1 have been safe. Others suggest that Active FX should only be used in the nonfacial areas and limited to 90 to 100 mJ, density 1 at 125 Hz. With Total FX, the Deep FX handpiece is used first followed by Active FX. Because the Deep FX is hard to follow visually, it is important to know where the previous spots are laid down to avoid excessive overlap. The Active FX char is more visible, so overlap is much more easily avoided. Although Sasaki[7] found that total coverage occurred when densities were above 4 for both Active FX and Deep FX handpieces, there have been reports of complications when the Deep FX is used with densities of 2 or higher. It is thus advocated to keep the Deep FX handpiece at a density of 1 to avoid scarring and adjust the energy used with the Deep FX as the variable to manipulate.

The results one can achieve with fractional resurfacing are significant. There may be some potentiating effect that allows the results to come closer to traditional approaches; however, in general to achieve more dramatic outcomes, traditional resurfacing is preferred as long as the patient accepts the longer

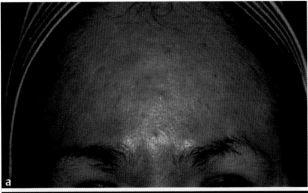
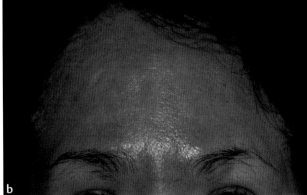

Fig. 31.7 Before (**a**) and after (**b**) carbon dioxide (CO_2) Total FX (Lumenis) fractional resurfacing on the forehead of a person with Fitzpatrick skin type IV with resulting improved texture, more even pigmentation/tone, and reduction of fine lines.

downtime and higher risk. In ▶ Fig. 31.7, obvious improvement can be seen after one treatment with Total FX—using both the Active FX (100 mJ, density 2) and the Deep FX (10 mJ, density 1) handpieces. Texture and tone are better and more uniform. Some of the keratoses, lentigines, and other areas of pigmentary issues are improved. Fine wrinkles have also been improved as well. The downtime compared to more traditional methods is better in many ways.

From a postprocedure standpoint, the care is much the same as it is for traditional laser resurfacing; however, the duration is much shorter and the intensity of the oozing, discomfort, and frequency of cleaning is much less. The areas treated after fractional resurfacing take about 3 to 5 days to heal as compared to 6 to 10 days with traditional resurfacing. Cleaning every hour will speed up the healing time. Typically, the cleaning frequency required for the fractional resurfacing to heal without complications can be much less. Instead of cleaning nearly every hour, a schedule of every 2 to 4 hours can be sufficient to keep the crusting away and the skin pink after fractional resurfacing. Oozing is minimal to none with fractional resurfacing but can be severe with traditional laser methods. The pain is much more severe with traditional resurfacing: sometimes graded as 7 to 10 on a scale of 1 to 10, as compared with 1 to 3 on a scale of 1 to 10 with fractional resurfacing. People often return to work by days 3 to 6 after fractional resurfacing. With traditional resurfacing, people are still anxious about appearing in public sometimes into the later part of the second week posttreatment. What is given up in results is more than made up for with

the other positive factors related to fractional resurfacing. Educating patients on this can be important regarding expectations as well as the positives and negatives with each approach. The clinician who does a better job of this will be more successful.

For the East Asian patient and the risks of hyperpigmentation and hypopigmentation, the hope was that fractional resurfacing might be better able to avoid these issues. Because of the limited depth of fractional resurfacing and decreased healing times, *hypo*pigmentation is avoided more easily than with traditional means. The experience with *hyper*pigmentation, however, has not been the same in all instances. In fact, for example, using Deep FX at 12.5 to 15 mJ, density 1 at 100 to 200 Hz, and Active FX at 125 mJ, density 2 at 100 to 200 Hz, except the eyes at 80 mJ, significant PIH has been noticed even more than with traditional resurfacing using 100, 90 mJ, densities 5, 4, respectively, at 100 to 200 Hz in the East Asian clientele. This paradoxical result may be due to the reactions of the remaining melanocytes that are not removed with fractional approaches, and that become hyperactive leading to hyperpigmentation. PIH may be reduced with traditional means where the melanocytes are actually reduced in number by the shear depth of ablation. In support of these paradoxical findings, studies and anecdotal experience have shown the persistence of melasma with superficial treatment (glycolic peels, Jessner's, microdermabrasions, etc.), but more effective treatment of melasma with deeper ablative resurfacing (Monheit moderate-depth peels, dermabrasion, and deeper CO_2 laser treatments).

31.6 Erbium:Yttrium Aluminum Garnet Laser Resurfacing

Er:YAG laser resurfacing was developed in the 1990s and is another option for laser resurfacing. The 2,940-nm wavelength has a 10- to 16-times greater absorption coefficient for water when compared to the CO_2 laser. The erbium laser is mostly considered for more superficial papillary depth ablation because blood vessels are encountered beyond this. Because Er:YAG lasers show less coagulative effects on vessels, the bleeding encountered at this level interferes with deeper penetration even with multiple passes. The thermal effects of the erbium laser are inferior to those of the CO_2 laser. The CO_2 laser causes a more intense inflammatory response and induces more neocollagenesis compared to short-pulsed Er:YAG laser wounds. Clinically, the limited ablation depth and the decreased collagen production make the erbium laser inferior to the CO_2 laser in treating moderate-to-severe rhytids, photodamage, and acne scarring. The author has limited experience with the Er:YAG laser and prefers the CO_2 laser for ablative resurfacing.

31.7 Dermabrasion, Dermasanding

Dermabrasion has been an effective technique for more than 100 years. Older accounts in ancient Egypt discuss techniques not much different from modern-day dermasanding. The principle of dermabrasion entails the progressive removal of skin using rotary instruments with abrasive elements or nonrotary instruments such as sterilized sandpaper. Dermabrasion techniques have been indicated for acne scarring, photodamage, moderate-to-deep wrinkling, superficial malignancies, rhinophyma, and even to lighten tattoos. Preoperative and postoperative preparation and care are much the same as described earlier. The benefits of dermabrasion are the low cost to introduce this type of resurfacing and the possibly lower risk of damage to melanocytes and subsequent hypopigmentation. The concerns with dermabrasion are the aerosolization of blood and the risk of transmission of infectious agents. During the HIV epidemic that is still live today, this made dermabrasion a very unattractive modality in the eyes of many clinicians. In addition, the technique is very operator-dependent. Variables such as the amount of pressure against the skin, rotation speed of the instrument, coarseness of the tip, and the patient's skin type and texture can all play crucial roles in outcomes.

Intraoperatively, oral or intravenous sedation can be used along with topical and/or local, regional anesthesia, all depending on the size and location of the area to be treated. Cryogen/refrigerant spray, manual methods, and tumescent anesthesia to firm the skin to allow even penetration have been advocated. The clinical end points are:

1. The first level is the removal of pigment located in the epidermis. This will indicate penetration through the basement membrane. Here the pink dermis becomes evident.
2. Very shortly after this penetration, small, pinpoint bleeding (less than 0.2–0.5-mm spots) is seen indicating that the level of superficial papillary dermis is reached. The source is corn-row bleeding of the small vascular loops in the dermal papilla. The pink background starts to take on more of a red appearance.
3. Larger bleeding points/red dots indicate that the reticular dermis is reached. White parallel lines of collagen are seen. Fibrosis of scarring and solar elastosis, not as robust as normal collagen, crumble and disrupt like hard cheese. The pink background has progressed to deeper red.
4. Avoid the yellow globules of the sebaceous glands indicating that the lower dermis is reached.

Dermasanding is a good option for manual abrasive resurfacing. The unfavorable elements of dermabrasion are avoided with this method. Using sterilized sandpaper, the clinical end points can be reached without aerosolized blood products. The drawbacks of dermasanding are the labor-intensive element and the time consumption. Dermasanding is not preferred for full-face or large-region resurfacing; however, it is good for focal targeting of problem areas such as deeper scars, deeper wrinkles, or removal of elevated lesions. ▶ Fig. 31.8 shows a dermasanding procedure on the cheek. The CO_2 laser has been used to reach the superficial papillary dermis, as noted with the epidermis removed and the pink background of this layer. Pinpoint bleeding is seen in the midlower center of the image. ▶ Fig. 31.9 shows before and after images of traditional CO_2 laser resurfacing and dermasanding approximately 2 months postoperative for acne scarring that had left boxcar, ice-pick, and some rolling scars.

Dermabrasion and especially dermasanding are useful modalities to have some control in the resurfacing process. Additional passes with the CO_2 laser and chemical peeling can be risky and unpredictable. The basic traditional treatment with the CO_2 laser with two passes or the Monheit moderate-depth peel to the superficial papillary dermis can then allow the focal use of dermasanding and dermabrasion to safely move into deeper layers to efface scars and deeper wrinkles.

In the East Asian client, to avoid hypopigmentation and scarring, the dermabrasion resurfacing should stay at the level where the smallest pinpoint bleeding is reached. With chemical

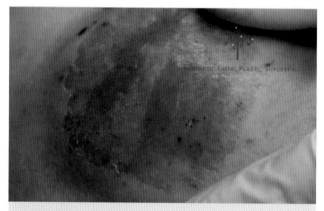

Fig. 31.8 Dermasanding clinical end points. Pinpoint bleeding indicates penetration into the papillary dermis. Progressively larger vessels indicate deeper penetration.

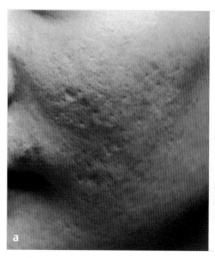
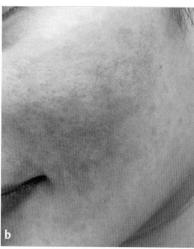

Fig. 31.9 Before (a) and after (b) carbon dioxide (CO_2) laser resurfacing and dermasanding to treat acne scarring that had left ice-pick, boxcar, and rolling scars in this East Asian patient.

peeling and laser resurfacing, the bleeding is attenuated due to the coagulation effects of both methods. Hence one should be patient to see what size the bleeding actually is before progressing to larger vessels and deeper penetration. Manual pressure or compression between the surgeon's fingers should help determine the size of the vessels. The level where larger vessels are seen (>0.25–0.50-mm spots) will be much more likely to have hypopigmentation or noticeably lighter areas of skin. Scarring is also much more likely to happen where larger vessels are seen as well. Hyperpigmentation is always a concern for the East Asian patient and the recommendations set forth in earlier sections also apply here. Again, the surgeon who educates patients the most and establishes the better rapport will have the most success.

31.8 Hyperpigmentation and Hypopigmentation

A discussion of hyperpigmentation was done previously. Again, a lengthy pretreatment period (4–6 wk) before the actual procedure can help avoid hyperpigmentation. Perhaps the use of topical medications preemptively will have more of an effect in determining sensitivities and preparing the patient to use them postoperatively more efficiently. Waiting for most of the inflammation to subside is the key between applications. Postoperatively, topical medications are not started until about 4 weeks after the ablative procedure. Test spots are important to consider. Excessive irritation with the test spot should alert the patient to wait another week. Educating the patient on how to apply the topical medications is more than half the battle. Again, waiting for all redness and irritation to end before the next application will prevent a strong anxiety toward these medications that is often established for many patients who don't heed this "pearl of wisdom." Serial chemical peels at home and in the office for PIH should be started only after all significant irritation and redness are resolved in the postoperative phase. Doing so will avoid the possibility of additional scarring or hypopigmentation. Usually, this is also started at the 4-

week mark at the earliest. Waiting is always prudent despite extreme patient anxiety and pressure.

Hypopigmentation is perhaps most feared due to its relatively permanent nature. Narrowband ultraviolet B (NB-UVB), Fraxel repair, or the 308-nm excimer lasers have been used to address hypopigmentation. The CO_2 laser has also been used to re-pigment the hypopigmented area by stimulating melanocytes to repopulate the area.

Scarring is more likely if the complete epithelialization is longer than 7 to 10 days. Persistent redness greater than in other areas that have healed faster can be a sign. Wounds that start to heap up higher than the surrounding skin areas can be another sign. If concerned, high-dose steroids can be used. Clobetasol (Temovate, Fougera Pharmaceuticals Inc., Melville, New York) applied once or twice a week for 1 to 4 weeks can be considered in the early healing phase around weeks 2 to 6. If scarring is seen, the use of Total FX applied more aggressively, traditional resurfacing, and even incision FX modes (5 W, 10-ms pulse width, 0.1-s repeat) can treat the scarring. With these methods, sometimes complete resolution of scarring is possible.

References

[1] Young PA, Sinha U, Rice DH, Stucker F. Circles of prominence: a new theory on facial aesthetics. Arch Facial Plast Surg 2006; 8: 263–267

[2] Chan HHL, Jackson B. Laser treatment on ethnic skin. In: Lim HW, Honigsmann H, Hawk JLM, eds. Photodermatology. New York, NY: Informa Healthcare; 2007: 417–432

[3] Ho SG, Chan HHL. The Asian dermatologic patient: review of common pigmentary disorders and cutaneous diseases. Am J Clin Dermatol 2009; 10: 153–168

[4] Fulton JE, Porumb S. Chemical peels: their place within the range of resurfacing techniques. Am J Clin Dermatol 2004; 5: 179–187

[5] West TB, Alster TS. Effect of pretreatment on the incidence of hyperpigmentation following cutaneous CO2 laser resurfacing. Dermatol Surg 1999; 25: 15–17

[6] Kauvar AN, Dover JS. Facial skin rejuvenation: laser resurfacing or chemical peel: choose your weapon. Dermatol Surg 2001; 27: 209–212

[7] Sasaki GH, Travis HM, Tucker B. Fractional CO2 laser resurfacing of photoaged facial and non-facial skin: histologic and clinical results and side effects. J Cosmet Laser Ther 2009; 11: 190–201

[8] Burkhardt BR, Maw R. Are more passes better? Safety versus efficacy with the pulsed CO2 laser. Plast Reconstr Surg 1997; 100: 1531–1534

32 Lasers for African Skin

Amy Li Richter, Jose E. Barrera, Ramsey F. Markus, and Anthony E. Brissett

32.1 Introduction

In the last decade there has been a rise in the use of lasers for facial skin rejuvenation. Due to improved technologies, patients are able to confront dermatological concerns in an office-based setting with outpatient procedures. Conditions such as photoaging, acne vulgaris, and dyschromia can be treated with laser therapy, with improved risk profiles and decreased recovery times. Whereas the demand for facial rejuvenation and cosmetic procedures continues to rise among all ethnic populations and skin types, not all patients and skin types are the same and there is no "one size fits all" treatment algorithm. The U.S. Bureau of the Census reports that by 2056 the number of non-Caucasian citizens will rise from 29% to more than 50%.[1] With this epidemiological shift, it is important to remember that different skin types have specific histopathological compositions and react differently to cutaneous diseases and laser therapy. Additionally, the complications of therapy vary among skin types; careful attention must be paid to these reaction patterns and specific treatment options.

Skin types and colors are divided into six phototypes, Fitzpatrick skin types I through VI, with I being the fairest, and VI being the darkest (▶ Table 5.1).[2] Within a single ethnicity, there may be variable phototypes and it is important to tailor the treatment to the patient. The number of melanocytes is consistent throughout all ethnicities. Melanocytes derive from neural crest cells and transfer melanosomes, which contain melanin, into keratinocytes. Melanin functions to protect the skin from ultraviolet radiation. The color of skin is dependent on the density, size, and activity of melanosomes because darker skin has a higher density of larger melanosomes.[3] In addition, darker skin types, Fitzpatrick V and VI, have thicker and more compact skin layers with thicker collagen bundles, which increase the epidermal barrier and reduce skin sensitivity (▶ Fig. 32.1).[4,5] This barrier delays skin damage from the environment and ultraviolet radiation and aging in darker phototypes when compared to lighter skin types. Due to these histological differences, darker skin is at increased risk for injury due to incidental laser absorption by melanin, problems with postinflammatory hyperpigmentation, and decrease of melanin production leading to hypopigmentation.

Although there are many of types of lasers, the fundamental principle is the same: All lasers treat the skin by targeting a specific chromophore. A chromophore is an endogenous molecule that has a unique absorption spectrum and peak absorption wavelength. The main chromophores of the skin are hemoglobin, melanin, and water. In general, resurfacing lasers are designed at specific wavelengths that use water as a chromophore to cause targeted thermal damage in the dermis in order to promote new collagen formation and skin tightening.[6] Other targetable chromophores include melanin, which has a broad, but gradually decreasing, absorption coefficient from 250 to 1,200 nm. The selection of a laser with a longer wavelength can allow for targeting of deep melanin or tattoo pigmentation in darker skin types.[5]

Other variables important to lasers include the thermal relaxation time, pulse duration, and energy fluence (▶ Table 32.1). The thermal relaxation time is the time required for a tissue to cool to one half the temperature to which it was heated. Heating the tissue for time longer than the thermal relaxation time can cause thermal damage to surrounding tissue. In darker skinned individuals, it is important to select a pulse duration longer than the thermal relaxation time of the epidermis but shorter than the target chromophore in order to avoid

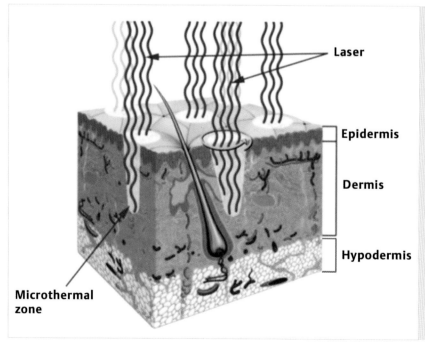

Fig. 32.1 Layers of the skin. The skin is divided into the epidermis, dermis, and hypodermis. Darker skinned individuals have increased density of larger melanocytes, more compact skin layers, and thicker collagen bundles.

Laser

Epidermis

Dermis

Hypodermis

Microthermal zone

Table 32.1 Variables of lasers

Variable	Function	Example
Chromophore	Laser target molecule, unique absorption spectrum and peak absorption wavelength	Hemoglobin, melanin, water
Wavelength	Property of light measured in nanometers (nm) that influences how chromophores are targeted	Hemoglobin (variable absorption from 300 nm–infrared) Melanin (gradually decreasing absorption from 250–1,200 nm) Water (1,000 nm–1 mm)
Thermal relaxation time	Time required for tissue to cool to one half the temperature to which it was heated	Melanosome (250 ns) Vessels (2–10 ms) Hair follicles (100 ms)
Pulse duration	Time to heat tissue to target tissue; choose pulse duration less than or equal to thermal relaxation time of target chromophore to avoid damage to surrounding tissue	Pulse duration 10–100 ns to target melanosome
Energy fluence	Joules per square centimeter (J/cm^2) of energy emitted by a pulsed laser device	25 J/cm^2 used by a 1,064-nm Nd:YAG for laser hair removal; highest tolerated fluences are 100 J/cm^2 (*IV, V*) * and 50 J/cm^2 (*VI*)[3]

Abbreviations: ms, milliseconds; Nd:YAG laser, neodymium:yttrium aluminum garnet laser; ns, nanoseconds.
Note: Lasers perform differently based on variable characteristics, and the understanding of these variables may facilitate the selection of a laser for a specific treatment goal.
*Italic type in parentheses denotes Fitzpatrick skin types.

epidermal blistering, crusting, pigmentation changes, and scarring.[5] The fluence is the joules per square centimeter (J/cm^2) of energy emitted from the laser handpiece. The laser fluence may need to be decreased to protect the epidermis in order to safely treat a patient with darker compared to lighter skin types. Other helpful strategies in safely treating patients of color include longer wavelengths; longer pulse durations; and skin cooling before, during, and/or after the procedure to avoid overheating the epidermis.[5,7]

32.2 Treatment Goals

Lasers may be considered for a variety of indications and the goals of the treatment should reflect the patient presentation.

32.2.1 Skin Laxity

There is an increased desire in all patients to achieve more youthful and refreshed facial skin. Over time, facial skin experiences photodamage, soft-tissue volume loss, rhytids, abnormal pigmentation, and irregular textures. The primary environmental factor that affects aging is ultraviolet radiation; however, given the protective effects of melanin and a thicker epidermis, individuals with darker skin may experience less skin laxity due to gravity and volume loss compared to others with fair skin.[5]

32.2.2 Dyschromia

The primary concerns of patients may vary depending on ethnicity and skin type. Hispanic patients commonly present with complaints of acne vulgaris, eczema, contact dermatitis, photoaging, facial melasma, and hyperpigmentation.[5,8] African American patients frequently complain of acne vulgaris, dyschromia (▶ Fig. 32.2), contact dermatitis, alopecia, and seborrhea

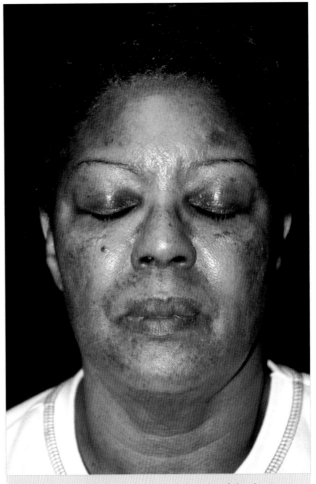

Fig. 32.2 Dyschromia. This alteration of the color of the skin may present as hyperpigmentation or hypopigmentation and is one of the most common treatment goals of laser therapy in ethnic populations.

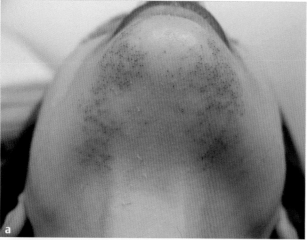

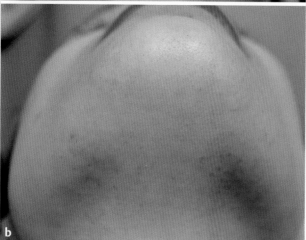

Fig. 32.3 Laser hair removal. Lasers can be used for treatment of hypertrichosis in all skin types by targeting the melanin chromophore in the hair follicle. (a) A patient with Fitzpatrick skin type IV prior to laser hair removal of chin hair. (b) Postprocedure.

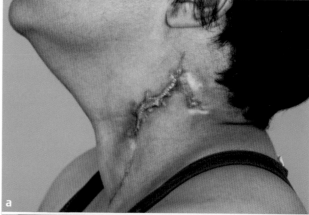

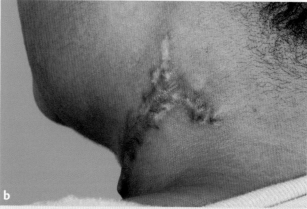

Fig. 32.4 Keloids and hypertrophic scarring. Lasers can be combined with intralesional steroid injection for the treatment of keloids and hypertrophic scarring. (a) Detailing of keloid formation on the neck of a patient with Fitzpatrick skin type V. (b) The same patient is shown with improvement in keloid dyspigmentation and scar thickness following laser treatment.

dermatitis.[3,8] And Asian patients often present with pigmentary disorders, facial melasma, freckles, lentigines, Ota-like macules, acne vulgaris, and hypertrophic scarring.[4,8] Dyschromia is a common presentation of darker skinned patients and it is important to distinguish between melasma and postinflammatory hyperpigmentation when considering laser therapy.[4,7,8,9,10] Options for laser treatment of dyschromia include the neodymium:yttrium aluminum garnet (Nd:YAG; CoolTouch, ICN Pharmaceuticals, Costa Mesa, California) laser and fractional nonablative devices.[9]

32.2.3 Laser Hair Removal

The use of lasers for hair removal (▶ Fig. 32.3) relies on melanin absorption within the hair follicle. Laser hair removal may be complicated in patients with darker skin due to disruption of melanin and subsequent risk for hypopigmentation at the site of hair removal.[5] With this in mind, longer wavelength lasers (1,064-nm Nd:YAG; ICN) with lower fluences and postprocedural cooling may be used successfully in darker skin types for the treatment of hypertrichosis.[3] When choosing a laser for hair removal, the 1,064-nm Nd:YAG is the safest choice in darker

skinned individuals because the wavelength is poorly absorbed by melanin, which reduces the damage to dark epidermal pigmentation.[3] The pulse length can be adjusted to deliver the pulse over a longer time period to facilitate cooling. Other laser choices for hair removal include the alexandrite and diode lasers at lower fluences and wider pulse widths. As with laser treatment of other skin disorders, multiple treatment sessions may be needed to achieve permanent results. Risks of laser hair removal in Fitzpatrick skin types IV through VI include blistering and temporary dyspigmentation with a low risk of permanent hyperpigmentation or hypopigmentation.[3,4]

32.2.4 Keloids and Hypertrophic Scarring

Keloids and hypertrophic scars (▶ Fig. 32.4) occur more commonly in darker skinned individuals. Laser treatment of thickened scars may be considered in combination with intralesional steroid injections.[5] The pulsed dye laser has been shown to decrease erythema, improve pain and pruritus, decrease lesion height, and improve hypertrophic scar pliability. These effects may facilitate intralesional steroid injection. However, the pulsed dye laser can target epidermal pigmentation and must be used with caution in patients with dark skin. Keloids may also be treated with the 1,064-nm Nd:YAG laser with moderate results of mild keloids. The lesion can be injected with intralesional triamcinolone 10 mg mL^{-1} up to 3 mL prior to starting therapy with regular laser treatments (fluence 13–18 J/cm^2, 2,000 pulses) for 6 weeks.[3] After 7 weeks, the lesion may be reevaluated and treatment repeated if necessary.

32.3 Medical Optimization

Before embarking on laser rejuvenation of facial skin, it is important to emphasize routine skin care to patients in order to optimize facial skin health prior to procedures. Sun should be avoided when possible and mechanical and chemical blockade (broad ultraviolet A and B sunscreens) should be used daily. Acne vulgaris can be treated with topical and oral antibiotics, hormonal treatments, and isotretinoin safely in all skin types and should be optimized before starting laser rejuvenation therapy.[11] However, all isotretinoin should be avoided for a year prior to starting laser therapy due to increased risk of dyspigmentation. Furthermore, all herpes simplex virus (HSV) outbreaks should be treated with antivirals, and prophylaxis antivirals should be given to patients with HSV prior to starting laser treatments. Additional topical treatments with melanin suppressors, such as hydroquinone, kojic acid, azelaic acid, or emblica, may be considered for treatment of dyspigmentation and melasma before laser treatments, particularly in darker phototypes where nonablative laser therapies require several treatments with moderate results.[5]

In addition to using lasers with longer pulse duration and longer wavelength to decrease the risk of discoloration or scarring, periprocedural cooling should be considered to decrease thermal damage to surrounding tissues.[4] Contact and noncontact cooling have the added benefit of improving patient comfort during laser therapy while decreasing thermal damage to the epidermis without interfering with laser intensity and direction. Options for contact cooling include skin moistening, application of ice or ice packs, and laser-specific cooling tips.[7]

When considering laser therapy on a patient with darker skin, a test spot adjacent to the intended area of treatment may be performed because individuals of the same ethnicity and phototype will react differently to the laser depending upon variable skin characteristics.[12] Test spots should be started at low density, low fluence, and longer pulse duration settings. Full response and side effects should be observed at 1 month, at which point scarring and pigment changes will likely be evident.

32.4 Classes of Lasers

The major classes of lasers include ablative and nonablative lasers in both nonfractionated and fractionated varieties (▶ Table 32.2). Ablative lasers target water molecules in the epidermis, causing vaporization of skin cells and retraction of the dermis with collagen formation. Ablative lasers are more aggressive and function similarly to a skin peel with prolonged recovery time and a higher adverse-event profile.[8] Nonablative lasers preserve the epidermis and target the dermal tissues to promote collagen formation. These nonablative treatments are milder and reduce the adverse-event profile and recovery time. Fractionated lasers are designed to target microscopic treatment zones (MTZs) to create columns of thermal injury with adjacent normal skin.[5] This promotes healing and improves skin texture compared to nonfractionated lasers, without the high side-effect profile of ablative lasers. There are several options for laser therapy and it is important to consider the

Table 32.2 Classes of lasers and clinical outcomes

Laser	Outcomes	Risks
Ablative nonfractionated 10,600-nm CO_2 2,940-nm Er:YAG Combined CO_2 Er:YAG	Dramatic improvement in wrinkle reduction, alleviate acne and atrophic scars[8]	Oozing, bleeding, and crusting [100%][8]; acne, transient hyperpigmentation and hypopigmentation (IV) [55–68%][8,12]; scarring and poor wound healing; permanent skin hypopigmentation[5,8]
Nonablative nonfractionated 1,319-nm Nd:YAG 1,320-nm Nd:YAG 1,450-nm diode	Improvement in scar severity [29%][4]; improvement in acne scars [10–50%][3,13]; atrophic scarring and acne-induced PIH (III–VI) [51–75%][6]; limited wrinkle improvement[3]	Minimal, few hours of erythema; no scaling or peeling; no abnormal pigmentation[8]
Nonablative fractionated 1,410 nm 1,440-nm Nd:YAG 1,540 nm 1,550-nm erbium 1,927-nm thulium fiber	Moderate improvement in texture and wrinkles[5]; significant improvement in acne scarring [51–75%][4,6]; overall appearance: excellent [30%], significant [59%], moderate [11%][4,13]; safer in darker skin types due to limited tissue damage and melanocyte stimulation[8]	Moderate downtime; moderate pain[6]; PIH (III–V) [3, 12, 33%][6]; acne [2%][12,14]; herpetiform eruptions [2%][12,14]
Ablative fractionated 10,600-nm fractional CO_2 2,940-nm fractional Er:YAG 2,790-nm fractional Er:YSGG	Moderate resurfacing power for mild skin laxity and rhytids[3]; moderate improvement in photodamage, scars [37%], and dyspigmentation[3,8]	Moderate downtime; moderate complications[12]; PIH (III–VI) [44%][4]; use with caution in Fitzpatrick skin type VI[3]

Abbreviations: CO_2, carbon dioxide; Er:YAG laser, erbium:yttrium aluminum garnet laser; Er:YSGG laser, erbium:yttrium scandium gallium garnet laser; Nd:YAG laser, neodymium:yttrium aluminum garnet laser; nm, nanometers; PIH, postinflammatory hyperpigmentation.
Note: The four principal categories of lasers are presented here with examples of each laser and expected clinical outcomes and associated risks based on Fitzpatrick darker skin types (III–VI).

expectations of your patient while balancing the risks and benefits associated with laser therapy in patient-specific phototypes.

32.5 Choosing a Laser

▶ Table 32.2 describes categories of lasers with specific examples of each type of laser.

Ablative nonfractionated lasers include the 10,600-nm carbon dioxide (CO_2) laser, the 2,940-nm erbium:yttrium aluminum garnet (Er:YAG) laser, and the combined CO_2 Er:YAG laser. These lasers target the water molecules in the dermis and vaporize the epidermis. This class of laser has the most significant outcomes with significant improvement of fine wrinkles and acne scars.[13] However, side effects of acne, permanent hypopigmentation, temporary hyperpigmentation, and skin infections are common. For these reasons, ablative nonfractionated lasers should be used with extreme caution in Fitzpatrick skin type IV patients and are contraindicated in phototypes V and VI due to the increased risk of scarring and dyspigmentation.[5]

Because of the high side-effect profile of the ablative nonfractionated lasers, a more gentle approach using nonablative technology was developed. The nonablative nonfractionated lasers include the 1,319-nm Nd:YAG laser, the 1,320-nm Nd:YAG laser, and the 1,450-nm diode laser. These lasers have demonstrated slight improvement with skin resurfacing and good results with acne treatment.[2] There is minimal recovery time required, little erythema, and minimal peeling. The nonablative nonfractionated lasers often require serial treatment sessions (four–six treatments) to obtain improvement; however, they can be used safely in patients with darker skin due to decreased risk of scarring and dyspigmentation.[8]

In order to more effectively treat the skin, nonablative fractionated lasers were developed to combine a more aggressive pulse and the safety of fractionation while still avoiding the epidermal loss incurred with ablative lasers. These include the 1,410-nm laser, the 1,440-nm Nd:YAG laser, the 1,540-nm laser, the 1,550-nm erbium laser, and the 1,927-nm thulium fiber laser. These nonablative fractionated lasers frequently require several treatments (two–six) with moderate improvements in skin tone and texture with moderate downtime.[8] The targeting of tiny diameter and deep dermal penetration of each MTZ allows for stimulation of collagen formation while avoiding disruption of the epidermal barrier function.[13] These lasers can be used safely in darker phototypes with a small risk of temporary hyperpigmentation.

The ablative fractionated lasers are the most recent addition to the laser family. These lasers were developed in an attempt to increase resurfacing effectiveness while still enjoying quicker healing with fewer complications compared to ablative nonfractionated resurfacing. These include the 10,600-nm fractional CO_2 laser, the 2,940-nm fractional Er:YAG laser, and the 2,790-nm fractional erbium:yttrium scandium gallium garnet (Er:YSGG) laser. These lasers target MTZs with ablation and vaporization of dermal and epidermal tissues. A series of sessions may result in resurfacing results nearly comparable to the ablative nonfractionated lasers but with much-improved safety profiles.[8] These lasers can improve skin laxity and mild rhytids; however, due to the violation of the epidermal layer, there is a

risk of infection, scarring, and dyspigmentation and they should be used with caution in patients with Fitzpatrick skin types IV through VI.[8]

Ablative technologies offer the most significant reduction of rhytids and scarring but have the greatest risk of complications and should only be used in lighter phototypes.[13] They can be utilized with extreme caution in Fitzpatrick skin type IV patients but should not be used in Fitzpatrick skin types V and VI because of risks of scarring and dyspigmentation.[5] Nonablative fractionated and nonfractionated lasers may be used in all skin types with modest results for the reduction of fine wrinkles. These lasers may involve several treatments but require little recovery time with minimal erythema and sloughing.[8]

32.6 Postprocedural Care

The importance of postprocedural planning and skin care cannot be overstated when managing patients following laser therapy. Because many of these procedures often entail several sessions, reducing skin damage between treatments can optimize epidermal healing and dermal collagen regeneration. The skin is more sensitive than usual for a short time after laser treatment and sun blockade and cooling agents should be used judiciously. Darker phototypes have more reactive and labile fibroblasts compared to Fitzpatrick skin types I through III and further dermal injury should be avoided.[3] Most laser patients feel a sunburnlike sensation for the rest of the day following laser therapy. Topical skin care, oral analgesics, and cooling agents can all be used to improve patient comfort. Topical cooling agents, such as ice packs, are encouraged postprocedure to enhance patient comfort as well as decrease inflammation. Topical steroids may be considered in patients with persistent erythema.

Depending on the type of laser used, mild erythema, edema, peeling, and flaking may occur and typically resolve over several days.[14] The time period for full recovery depends on the type of laser process, and postoperative care must be tailored to the treatment administered. The postoperative skin care routine should include keeping the skin clean and moist to allow for re-epithelialization and to minimize the potential of scarring. In general, chilled, saline-soaked gauze can be applied intermittently for the first several days. The therapy area should be gently treated with a mild cleanser such as Cetaphil (Galderma Laboratories, Fort Worth, Texas) followed by the application of an oxygen-permeable ointment such as Aquaphor (Beiersdorf Inc., Wilton, Connecticut). Patients should be urged not to pull or pick at their skin as it starts to flake or peel because this may increase the likelihood of scarring. Depending upon the type of laser or resurfacing technique utilized, re-epithelialization typically occurs within a week. Avoidance of sun and the liberal use of sunscreen should be encouraged. Patients should avoid the use of retinoids and other bleaching agents at risk of causing irritation.

32.7 Management of Possible Complications

Careful patient selection combined with conservative and judicious implementation of laser treatments can result in positive

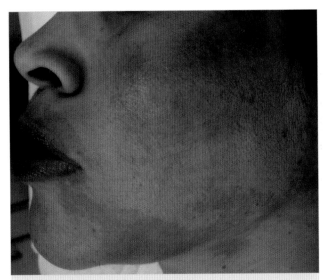

Fig. 32.5 Posttreatment postinflammatory hyperpigmentation. This complication is common with ablative lasers and may be reduced by using nonablative and fractionated techniques.

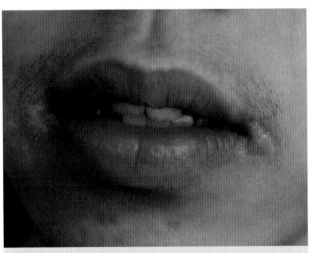

Fig. 32.6 Posttreatment hypopigmentation. Hypopigmentation following laser therapy is a rare complication that may present several months after treatment. This patient demonstrates hypopigmentation of the right anterior commissure and hypertrophic scarring of the left commissure.

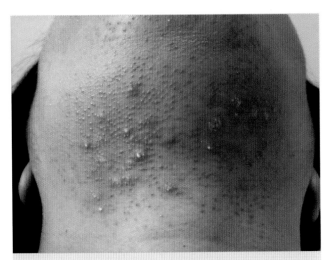

Fig. 32.7 Posttreatment acneiform eruptions. The most common complications following laser therapy are acneiform eruptions and herpes simplex virus (HSV) infections. The risks can be minimized with premedication in select patients with skin types predisposed to such infections.

outcomes, when dealing with patients of color and darker skin types. In this particular subset of patients, the most common postprocedural concerns are related to dyspigmentation and scarring.

Postinflammatory hyperpigmentation is a very bothersome side effect in darker Fitzpatrick phototypes (V and VI) (▶ Fig. 32.5).[3,8] There are several choices for topical therapies when considering the treatment of hyperpigmentation, including hydroquinone, azelaic acid, kojic acid, and emblica. Hydroquinone, a common treatment option, is a plant-derived tyrosinase inhibitor and is often used to treat discrete hyperpigmented patches.[5] Deleterious outcomes related to the use of hydroquinone may include hypopigmentation surrounding the treated area due to adjacent bleaching, in a "halo" effect.[3,14]

Delayed hypopigmentation is a less-common complication usually seen following ablative nonfractionated laser resurfacing several months after treatment (▶ Fig. 32.6). This complication is permanent and a major cause for avoiding ablative nonfractionated resurfacing in dark-skinned patients. This can be confused with hypopigmentation attributed to the use of retinoids and hydroquinone prior to laser treatment that resolves with discontinuation of the medication.[14]

In addition to dyspigmentation following laser treatment, additional complications such as acneiform eruptions and HSV infections may occur in all skin types (▶ Fig. 32.7).[15] Acne eruptions are more common in patients with acne-prone skin and can be minimized by premedicating with oral antibiotics such as tetracycline. In general, prophylactic antivirals are recommended in patients with a history of orofacial HSV. When treating patients with a history of HSV outbreaks with laser exposure, antivirals should be started prior to the initiation of laser therapy and continued up to a week after laser application. Laser rejuvenation should not be performed on patients with active HSV infections.

Although bacterial superinfections are uncommon, they should be treated aggressively to minimize scarring and dyspigmentation.[12,15] Bacterial superinfections typically present with pain, increased erythema, exudates, erosions, and crusting. Infections should be cultured and treated with broad-spectrum oral antibiotics to reduce long-term risk of scarring. When treating patients of darker skin types, the development of acne eruptions, HSV, or bacterial superinfections can intensify the likelihood of pigment issues and discoloring of the soft-tissue envelope. Every effort should be made to prevent these complications or treat them aggressively should they occur.

There are several anatomical sites that have escalated risk for scar formation including the periorbital region, the mandibular area, and the neck (▶ Fig. 32.8).[14] The thin skin of the neck with few pilosebaceous units and poor vasculature make this a high-risk location for scar formation. Topical steroids, silicone gel formulations, and intralesional steroid injections may reduce

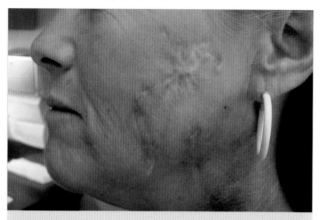

Fig. 32.8 Posttreatment scarring. The use of lasers in the head and neck region has an increased risk for posttreatment scarring compared to other areas of the body, due to the thinner epidermis and fewer dermal structures such as hair follicles, sebaceous glands, and blood vessels.

hypertrophic scarring, particularly in patients with risk of keloid formation.[3] The goal of steroids and efficient epidermal cooling with use of ice packs following the procedure is to decrease the amount of thermal damage to surrounding tissues to avoid scar formation and hypertrophic scarring.

32.8 Conclusions

Ethnic skin presents a unique challenge for laser skin rejuvenation due to higher density of larger melanosomes, thicker collagen bundles, and increased fibroblast responses. Special considerations need to be made when considering laser therapy for ethnic patients for the treatment of skin laxity, dyschromia, hypertrichosis, keloids, and hypertrophic scarring. Lasers may be safely used in patients with darker skin tones by choosing fractional technologies with longer wavelengths, lower fluences, longer pulse durations, and maintaining careful attention to preprocedural and postprocedural management strategies. When considering the use of lasers, the treatment goals should reflect individual patient complaints and the realistic expectations of laser skin rejuvenation. Patients should be counseled on the risks of laser therapy, including scarring, postinflammatory hyperpigmentation, and hypopigmentation. With this in mind and in the hands of an experienced laser surgeon, laser resurfacing in darker Fitzpatrick skin types IV through VI may

eliminate unwanted hair; improve the appearance of fine wrinkles; and even skin tone, texture, and pigmentation.

32.9 Disclosures

Authors Amy Li Richter, MD, Jose Barrera, MD, and Anthony Brissett, MD, have no significant financial or other relationships with commercial companies whose products may be discussed in this article. Ramsey Markus, MD, discloses equipment loans from Lumenis Ltd. and Syneron-Candela Corp.

References

[1] US Bureau of the Census. Projections of the Resident Population by Race, Hispanic Origin, and Nativity: Middle Series, 2006 to 2010. Washington, DC: Populations Projections Program, Population Division, US Bureau of the Census; 2000

[2] Fitzpatrick TB. The validity and practicality of sun-reactive skin types I through VI. Arch Dermatol 1988; 124: 869–871

[3] Woolery-Lloyd H, Viera MH, Valins W. Laser therapy in black skin. Facial Plast Surg Clin North Am 2011; 19: 405–416

[4] Alexis AF. Lasers and light-based therapies in ethnic skin: treatment options and recommendations for Fitzpatrick skin types V and VI. Br J Dermatol 2013; 169 Suppl 3: 91–97

[5] Rossi AM, Perez MI. Laser therapy in Latino skin. Facial Plast Surg Clin North Am 2011; 19: 389–403

[6] Carniol PJ, Woolery-Lloyd H, Zhao AS, Murray K. Laser treatment for ethnic skin. Facial Plast Surg Clin North Am 2010; 18: 105–110

[7] Tierney EP, Hanke CW. The effect of cold-air anesthesia during fractionated carbon-dioxide laser treatment: Prospective study and review of the literature. J Am Acad Dermatol 2012; 67: 436–445

[8] Davis SA, Narahari S, Feldman SR, Huang W, Pichardo-Geisinger RO, McMichael AJ. Top dermatologic conditions in patients of color: an analysis of nationally representative data. J Drugs Dermatol 2012; 11: 466–473

[9] Preissig J, Hamilton K, Markus R. Current laser resurfacing technologies: a review that delves beneath the surface. Semin Plast Surg 2012; 26: 109–116

[10] Ho SG, Chan HH. The Asian dermatologic patient: review of common pigmentary disorders and cutaneous diseases. Am J Clin Dermatol 2009; 10: 153–168

[11] Davis EC, Callender VD. Postinflammatory hyperpigmentation: a review of the epidemiology, clinical features, and treatment options in skin of color. J Clin Aesthet Dermatol 2010; 3: 20–31

[12] Cole PD, Hatef DA, Kaufman Y, Pozner JN. Laser therapy in ethnic populations. Semin Plast Surg 2009; 23: 173–177

[13] Doherty SD, Doherty CB, Markus JS, Markus RF. A paradigm for facial skin rejuvenation. Facial Plast Surg 2009; 25: 245–251

[14] Metelitsa AI, Alster TS. Fractionated laser skin resurfacing treatment complications: a review. Dermatol Surg 2010; 36: 299–306

[15] Graber EM, Tanzi EL, Alster TS. Side effects and complications of fractional laser photothermolysis: experience with 961 treatments. Dermatol Surg 2008; 34: 301–305, discussion 305–307

33 Lasers, Peels, and Abrasion Techniques for Latino Skin

Rafael Espinosa Delgado, Miriam de la Torre Campos, and David Galarza Lozano

33.1 Introduction

In the last 5 years the Latino population seeking cosmetic treatments has substantially increased, and one of the main cosmetic concerns of this group is pigmentary disorders, with melasma being the primary clinical condition. It has been reported that the incidence of facial melasma induced by pregnancy in Mexican women can be as high as 50%.[1] Other common cosmetic concerns are sunspots, acne scars, enlarged pores, and aged skin.

Latinos come from a mix of various cultures and races. In the pre-Hispanic world, from northern Mexico to southern Chile and Argentina, the local population was already diverse in race and culture. Then various European races came to the Americas and started mixing with the local people. The result was the mestizo population from the combination of Spanish, French, German, and African peoples with an already diverse native Central and South American population. "Latino" also defines all Hispanic and Latin American people. According to the last U.S. census, it is the fastest growing minority in the United States. Latinos are a group of many different, rich cultures and strong traditions. In 2013, the Associated Press reported that one half of the population in the United States under age 5 was composed of ethnic minorities. This means that in three decades, one half of the population of the United States will be non-White Americans.

Patient education is a key element in treating Latino patients and dark-skinned patients. It is mandatory that they understand how their skin can react to light-based treatments or chemical peels. They must be made aware of the risks and benefits attendant to each procedure. Latin people have a tendency toward excessive sun exposure without proper sunblock. Many believe that their darker skin will protect them from the sun, and most Latino men do not like to wear creams on their faces, including sunblock. Ethnicity and culture play important roles in how people perceive beauty and how they take care of their skin.

The authors' practice is located in Hermosillo, Sonora, Mexico (northern Mexico, in the Sonoran Desert where the temperature reached 118°F in 2013, the area's hottest day on record). Most, if not all, of the authors' patients are mixed races with Fitzpatrick skin types IV to VI. The main conditions for which they seek cosmetic treatments are melasma, sunspots (▶ Fig. 33.1), acne scars (▶ Fig. 33.2 and ▶ Fig. 33.3), enlarged pores, and aged skin (▶ Fig. 33.4). The authors have been using fractional lasers since 2008. The experience in the practice has been with the Fraxel Restore erbium:yttrium aluminum garnet (Er:YAG) 1,550-nm laser (formerly Reliant; Solta Medical, Hayward, California) and the AcuPulse carbon dioxide (CO_2) fractional laser (Lumenis Inc., Palo Alto, California).

33.1.1 Latino Skin Considerations

The skin has 3 layers: epidermis, dermis, and subcutaneous.[2] The epidermis is composed of the stratum corneum, stratum granulosum, stratum spinosum, and stratum basale. It has four cell types: keratinocytes, melanocytes, Langerhans cells, and Merkel cells. The stratum corneum, the outer layer of the epidermis, contains the nonliving cells (corneocytes) with a bilipid membrane that surrounds them. It is considered the epidermal barrier. This physical barrier maintains skin hydration, prevents evaporation, and is a defense barrier for microorganisms, ultraviolet light trauma, and so forth. The epidermis renews itself every month. During this process, the living keratinocytes migrate from the basal layer of the epidermis to become the corneocytes of the stratum corneum on the surface. They will ultimately desquamate.[2,3] Melanin is mainly found in the epidermis; it can also be found in the dermis in some skin conditions such as melasma.[2,3,4]

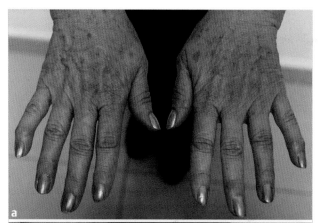
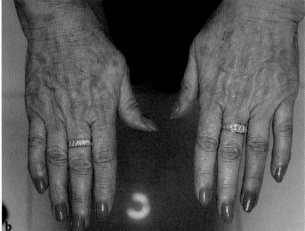

Fig. 33.1 (a) Hands of a 55-year-old patient before carbon dioxide (CO_2) fractional laser treatment for sunspots and wrinkles. (b) Same patient after CO_2 fractional laser treatment with Lumenis AcuPulse (Palo Alto, California) spot treatment on the sunspots' settings doughnut shape in smallest size, energy 17.5 mJ, 5% density; deep fractional full-hand fractional settings 10 mJ, 10% density; and superficial treatment settings 100 mJ, 40% density. Improvement is seen in skin texture and sunspots.

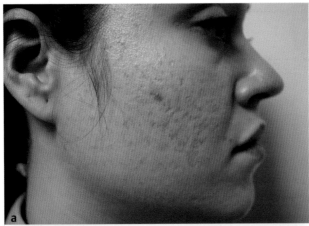

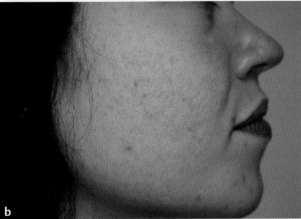

Fig. 33.2 (a) A 25-year-old Fitzpatrick skin type IV patient with deep acne scars before carbon dioxide (CO_2) fractional laser treatment. (b) Same patient after CO_2 fractional laser treatment with Lumenis AcuPulse (Palo Alto, California) spot treatment on the scars' settings doughnut shape in smallest size, energy 22.5 mJ, 5% density; deep full-face fractional settings 12.5 mJ, 10% density. Improvement on acne scars and skin tone can be seen.

33.1.2 Anatomical Differences of Darker Skin

In darker skin types eumelanin is more prominent; this is a darker melanin that goes from brown to black. In lighter skin types pheomelanin, a lighter melanin that goes from yellow to red in color, is more predominant. Melanogenesis occurs in melanocytes in the basal layer of the epidermis; a similar number of melanocytes are found in light and dark skin types. The difference is the type of melanin that predominates. In darker skin types, melanin is stored in large, single melanosomes containing darker melanin, and in light skin types melanin is stored in clustered, small melanosomes containing light-color melanin. Dark skin types have more melanin per square inch of skin.[2,4]

There are other differences between dark and light skin. Dark skin has more cell layers in the stratum corneum with higher lipid content and is more compact than in lighter skin types. Darker skin types also have a more compact and thicker dermis than lighter skin types. The thickness is proportional to the degree of pigment; also, darker skin types have prominent, thicker dilated blood vessels. The fibroblasts are larger in size and number in darker skin. These cells are responsible for synthetizing the main structural elements of the dermis but they also influence how skin scars; therefore, they have an important role in hypertrophic scars and keloid formation in darker skin types.[2,4]

33.2 Fractional Lasers in Latino Skin

The use of fractional lasers in Latino patients has always been a challenge—even with the use of pretreatment regimens with hydroquinone, alone or in combination with retinoids and corticosteroids, to avoid postinflammatory hyperpigmentation (PIH) or worsening of melasma. The first fractional laser that was available was the erbium 1,550 and it promised hope in

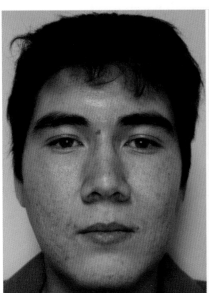

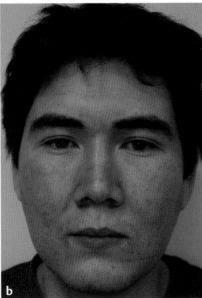

Fig. 33.3 (a) A 23-year-old Fitzpatrick skin type IV patient with deep acne scars and sunspot on the nose before carbon dioxide (CO_2) fractional laser treatment. (b) Same patient after CO_2 fractional laser treatment with Lumenis AcuPulse (Palo Alto, California) spot treatment on the scars' settings doughnut shape in smallest size, energy 22.5 mJ, 5% density; deep full-face fractional settings 12.5 mJ, 10% density; and superficial treatment settings 90 mJ, 40% density. There is improvement in acne scars and skin texture; the sunspot on the nose has almost disappeared.

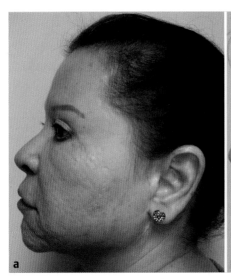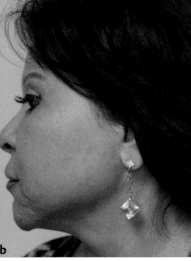

Fig. 33.4 (a) A 55-year-old Fitzpatrick skin type IV patient with photodamage, wrinkles, enlarged pores, acne scars, and sunspots before carbon dioxide (CO_2) fractional laser treatment. (b) Same patient after CO_2 fractional laser treatment with Lumenis AcuPulse (Palo Alto, California) spot treatment on the scars' settings doughnut shape in smallest size, energy 17.5 mJ, 5% density; deep full-face fractional settings 12.5 mJ, 10% density; and superficial treatment settings 90 mJ, 40% density. Improvement shown in acne scars, skin texture, fine wrinkles, photodamage, and skin tone.

the treatment of melasma and hyperpigmentation disorders in darker skin types, and was Food and Drug Administration (FDA)-approved for this purpose.[5,6] Short-term follow-up studies claimed its efficacy, but medium- and long-term follow-ups were disappointing.[7] The fractional ablative CO_2 laser has become the "gold standard" in facial rejuvenation and skin resurfacing.[8,9]

33.2.1 Fractional Laser Concepts

Thermal Relaxation Time of Tissue

The thermal relaxation time of tissue is the time it takes tissue that has received laser energy to lose one half of the generated temperature, 0.8 ms. This means that the laser has to deliver the energy in less than 0.8 ms to avoid thermal damage to surrounding tissue.[10]

Photothermolysis—Nonablative Fractional Resurfacing

The erbium 1,550-nm Fraxel Restore (Solta Medical) is in the near-infrared wavelength. Its chromophore is water.[11] It works by laying abundant microscopic zones of thermal damage in columnar fashion, leaving the surrounding tissue of each column damaged and the stratum corneum intact; the remaining undamaged tissue will migrate to the damaged zones to accelerate healing.[8] This device has the ability to control the diameter and depth of each microthermal zone, as well as the density of each treatment. It covers 15 to 20% of the skin at a time.[6] Following the treatment, microscopic epidermal necrotic debris (MENDs) will form just below each column of coagulated tissue and will be extruded in 5 to 7 days.[6] During each treatment, the handpiece must pass eight times over each area of the face, causing elevation of the skin temperature eight times in a procedure. It requires one session per month for five to seven months, depending on the skin condition to be treated.

Ablative Fractional Resurfacing

The wavelength of the CO_2 laser is 1,064 nm. This wavelength is highly absorbed by water. Human skin is 60 to 70% water. The laser creates small columnar holes of vaporized tissue surrounded by undamaged tissue that will help the healing process.[12] The AcuPulse CO_2 device (Lumenis) has the capability to deliver superficial and deep treatments with a single scanner. The deep treatment has a superpulse mode and a 0.12-mm spot size. For the superficial mode the system takes the 0.12-mm spot size and draws a spiral 1.3-mm superficial spot. Neither in the deep nor the superficial mode does the AcuPulse compromise the thermal relaxation time of tissue as ablation occurs.[9,11] Thus the possibility of thermal damage to the surrounding tissue and the risk of PIH are minimized.

Preparation of Latino Skin Patient for Fractional Laser Treatment

The preparation of the skin takes at least 4 weeks prior to the treatment.[13] In this period of time it is crucial to avoid ultraviolet radiation exposure. The use of sunblock with at least sun protection factor (SPF) 60 every 3 or 4 hours during daylight is advised. The daily, bedtime application of a bleaching cream containing hydroquinone 4%, tretinoin 0.05%, and fluocinolone acetonide 0.01% (Tri-Luma; Galderma Laboratories, Fort Worth, Texas) is encouraged. This triple combination therapy has been the gold standard in the treatment of melasma, and its principles also apply to PIH.[14,15] It is believed that using hydroquinone for a period of 4 weeks will inhibit the melanocyte activity and melanin formation during the inflammatory phase of the laser treatment.[10]

Suggested Pretreatment Regimen

1. Avoid sun exposure 4 weeks before and 6 months after fractional laser treatment.
2. Use sunblock SPF 60 or higher every 3 to 4 hours during daylight, 4 weeks prior to treatment and 4 to 6 months after.
3. Use hydroquinone triple therapy 4 weeks before and 4 months after procedure.[10]

Topical Anesthesia

Cleanse the skin with neutral soap and water, so there are no residual creams and makeup; dry the skin completely to apply topical anesthesia. The authors use a compound pharmacy gel that consists of benzocaine 20%, lidocaine 7%, and tetracaine 7% (BLT). Apply this in a circular fashion giving a gentle massage, so the anesthetic penetrates the skin better. Apply an even coat (as demonstrated in Video 33.1) to the whole area to be treated and let it sit for 1 hour. The authors also give patients 1.5 g of acetaminophen 1 hour before the procedure to reduce discomfort. Side effects of BLT gel can go from allergy to death,[16] and have a direct relation to the size, surface area, body location, the amount of product used, and length of time of skin contact; do not apply BLT to extensive or multiple areas at the same time. Check on the patient every 10 minutes; after an hour remove the BLT gel completely before starting the treatment.[16,17]

Use of Chillers

The authors use a Zimmer (Zimmer Cryo; Zimmer Medizin Systems, Irvine, California) chiller machine routinely. It is used at level 4 or 5 and moved around the treatment area at a distance of 10 cm from the skin to reduce heating and patient discomfort. Do not use the Zimmer at higher settings or too close to the skin because there has been reported PIH due to overcooling.[18]

Use of Smoke Evacuator

The authors use a Buffalo Filter Smoke Evacuation System with a ViraSafe 6 filter (Tekyard, Burnsville, Minnesota) that provides safety to clinical personnel and patients by preventing potential virus particles in the plume from floating around the procedure room.

Treating Latino Skin with Fractional Erbium 1,550-nm Laser

With the erbium 1,550-nm laser, the authors use low energy and low-density settings. The passes are carried out slowly. This ensures minimum heat diffusion to the skin. The Zimmer (Zimmer Medizin) skin chiller is set at low settings to avoid overcooling and subsequent skin damage. On small areas wait for a couple of seconds between each pass; do not perform more than one pass on Fitzpatrick skin types V and VI, and wait at least 6 to 8 weeks between treatments.[10]

Treating Latino Skin with CO_2 Fractional Laser

In the case of a CO_2 fractional laser, do a single pass, do not overlap passes, and use a superpulse or ultrapulse laser that does not compromise the thermal relaxation time.[9] Use low-fluence, low-density settings. Air skin cooling is advised at a low setting because overcooling can also trigger PIH.[18] In Fitzpatrick skin types IV and V with acne scars (▶ Fig. 33.2 and ▶ Fig. 33.3) or sunspots (▶ Fig. 33.1), we tailor the therapy, treating the scars or sunspots directly with the doughnut shape at the smallest size that will fit each acne scar. We spot treat at a higher energy but lower density (17.5–22 millijoules [mJ] and 5% density on the Lumenis AcuPulse), and treat the rest of the face at lower energy and lower density levels (10–12.5 mJ and 5–10% density on the Lumenis AcuPulse). This allows us to address the specific problem with adequate energy and avoid PIH for the rest of the face.

Fractional Laser for Fitzpatrick Skin Type VI

A different approach is used for Fitzpatrick skin type VI patients seeking fractional laser treatments. For scars or pigmentary disorders, the laser settings are below clinically noticeable results and the risk of complications such as PIH is still considerable. The authors prefer a series of superficial peels and topical bleaching treatments in this group of patients. Fillers are used in scars, sometimes combined with subcision, or punch elevation, or resection techniques.[19]

33.3 Chemical Peeling in Latino Skin

The authors always start on the safe side with chemical peels in any skin type. With chemical peels, do superficial peeling first. Once a comfort level has been attained with this type of peeling, advance to the medium chemical peels. When enough experience has been gained, graduate to the deep chemical peels. There will be less complications and better outcomes. The senior author does not recommend deep peels in Fitzpatrick skin types V and VI, as well as in patients with a history of PIH following cosmetic treatments, and hypertrophic or keloid scars. It is better to go slowly toward your clinical goal then to head rapidly into a cosmetic disaster.

Training is key to good outcomes when it comes to facial cosmetic procedures. The best investment you can make is in education and training. There are many organizations including the American Society for Laser Medicine and Surgery, the American Academy of Facial Plastic and Reconstructive Surgery, and the American Academy of Dermatology that offer educational meetings and training. It is critical to have proper training and have someone with experience to rely on when you are first starting.

The most common issue in Latino skin is melasma.[20] This condition is an acquired dysfunction in the pigmentary system characterized by blotchy, brown macules distributed symmetrically on the face; it is most common in Fitzpatrick skin types IV to VI.[20] Its treatment is still a challenge to the dermatologist and the facial plastic surgeon. Sometimes aggressive procedures can make it worse. A multitreatment approach, combining chemical peels, lasers, topical therapies, and photoprotection, has proven to be more promising but not a cure.[20,21]

33.3.1 Pretreatment Regimen

As with lasers, it is important to prepare the skin before a chemical peel. In the case of chemical peels, it is not only to prevent PIH but also to reduce seborrhea and thin the epidermis. This allows a better and more uniform penetration of the peeling agent.[21] Hydroquinone, tretinoin or glycolic acid as a topical depigmenting agent is applied at least 2 weeks before the peeling. In patients with a history of herpes simplex, antiviral prophylaxis is indicated and active acne should be treated prior to the procedure. Antibiotics can be used to prevent a breakout.[21]

33.3.2 Chemical Peeling Agents for Fitzpatrick Skin Types IV to VI

There are a great many chemical peeling agents available, but the choice of these agents in darker skin types is limited due to their depth of penetration. Deep chemical peels are not recommended for Fitzpatrick skin types IV to VI.[20] Medium-depth peels should be used with extreme caution because they can lead to permanent hyperpigmentation and hypertrophic scarring.[2,17,20]

Superficial Chemical Peels

The superficial chemical peels penetrate the epidermis and upper papillary dermis. They renew the epidermal layer of the skin where most of the pigment is found. They help dyschromias and improve sun damage, superficial wrinkles, acne control, and oily skin. They aid in evening out the skin tone, and represent little risk of PIH for the patient. In this category, the traditional glycolic acid peels have proven to be safe and effective. In the authors' practice, superficial peels are the most commonly used peels, particularly glycolic acid peels at a 50% concentration at a 3- to 5-minute end point when used alone.[20,21,22] In combination with microdermabrasion, the authors use the HydraFacial MD System (Edge Systems Corp., Signal Hill, California) (see Video 33.2) and their peeling formulas, which combine glycolic acid with salicylic acid in various concentrations that range from 7.5 to 30% glycolic acid and 2% salicylic acid. The authors like this system because the hydramicrodermabrasion is less irritating than dry microdermabrasion. The skin abrasion and the peeling are not that aggressive; nevertheless, together the desirable results can be achieved with no complications and no discomfort for the patient. It is very safe for dark skin types. The authors have not yet seen any complications with this system because the superficial peels and the HydraFacial treatments must be repeated in a series of sessions 3 weeks apart until the desired outcomes are obtained. The superficial peeling agents that are safe in dark skin types are glycolic acid solution, 30 to 70%; trichloroacetic acid (TCA), 10 to 30%; salicylic acid, 20 to 30%; Jessner's Solution; and tretinoin 1 to 5%.[2,20,23]

Alpha Hydroxy Acid Peels—Glycolic Acid and Lactic Acid

Alpha hydroxy acid (AHA) peels work by producing epidermolysis (corneocyte detachment), dispersing basal cell melanin, thinning the epidermis, and increasing collagen synthesis in the dermis.[21] These peeling agents are very safe to use in Latino skin when applied properly; a clinical end point of 3 to 5 minutes is advised.[2,20,21,24]

Beta Hydroxy Acid Peels—Salicylic Acid

Beta hydroxy acid (BHA) peels are lipophilic compounds that remove intracellular lipids that surround the epithelial cells. Salicylic acid stimulates the basal cells and underlying fibroblasts without directly wounding the dermis or causing inflammation.[20,21,24] That is why all BHAs are safe to use in Fitzpatrick skin types IV to VI. They are used to treat acne, melasma, and PIH.

Trichloroacetic Acid Peel

Low concentrations of TCA (10–35%) can penetrate down to the upper papillary dermis. TCA works as a protein denaturant that precipitates epidermal proteins and produces dermal inflammation. The coagulation of epidermal keratinocyte proteins appears as frosting,[21,24] which is the clinical end point of TCA peels. This is difficult to appreciate in darker skin and can lead to overpeeling that has a high risk of scarring and postpeel dyschromias. Despite these considerations, TCA peels are considered safe to use in darker skin types. They require a longer preconditioning of the skin and the use of low-concentration TCA. As with lasers, spot treatment can be done with TCA peels. For example, they can be applied inside ice-pick acne scars with a toothpick or a small brush to treat just the scars, and the rest of the face can be treated with a superficial peel. This lowers the risk of PIH.[19,24]

Jessner's Peel

The Jessner's Peel is a combination of 14 g resorcinol, 14 g salicylic acid, and 85% lactic acid in a 100-mL ethanol solution. It is used as a superficial peeling agent in all skin types. It is also used in combination with other peeling agents such as TCA peels, allowing a more uniform penetration at a safer, lower concentration of TCA.[20,21,24]

Tretinoin Peel

Also known as retinoic acid (vitamin A), tretinoin peel is available from 1 to 5%, increases the stratum corneum, decreases epidermal thickness, and causes melanin dispersion; it can also be used in combination with other peeling agents.[20,21,24]

33.3.3 Application Technique for Superficial Peels

Clean the skin with neutral soap and water and remove any oil left in the skin with acetone. Then with a piece of soaked gauze or a small brush apply an even coat of the chemical peel. Erythema or frosting will appear on the skin depending on the peeling agent used. That is the clinical end point of the superficial peel. Another clinical end point can be a period of time, for example 3 to 5 minutes. Some superficial peels do not need to be neutralized and others will need to be neutralized with saline, water, or an alkaline substance such as 1% bicarbonate solution. Some erythema and desquamation during the following days can be expected. Sun avoidance and sunblock are recommended. No other extra care is needed. The peel can be repeated every 2 to 3 weeks until the desired result is achieved.[20,21,25]

33.3.4 Superficial and Medium Chemical Peels' Complications

Most of the complications of these types of peels are transitory. The most common is hyperpigmentation, more frequently seen in darker skin types due to a deep peel or improper postpeeling care and poor sun protection. Hyperpigmentation can be managed with hydroquinone, kojic acid, or retinoids alone or in combination with corticosteroids. It usually resolves in 1 to 3 months depending on the severity of the case. The use of intense pulsed light (IPL) is controversial. There are some IPL filters that are pigment-specific, but IPL can also worsen the pigmentation.[17,20,21,23] Persisting itching and burning sensations can be issues. Advise the patient not to scratch or touch the face. Antihistamines and topical creams containing steroids and antibiotics can be used to minimize discomfort. For accidental eye involvement, rinse abundantly with tap water and refer to an ophthalmologist.[17] Prolonged erythema can be managed with topical steroids and proper sunblock applied every 4 hours. Camouflage mineral makeup with sun protection is advised. Systemic steroids may also be used. Exudative lesions, if not treated promptly, may lead to scarring. These can be treated with 3% boric acid solution, topical antibiotics and steroids, and moisturizers; total sun avoidance is also important.[2,17]

Hypopigmentation is a complication most notorious in dark-skinned patients but it can affect any skin type. This condition is usually permanent; camouflage makeup can be used. Sometimes skin needling, micro-grafting, or a tattoo applied to the affected area can help. Hypertrophic scars should be treated immediately. Silicon gel sheets can be applied for 6 months, then intralesional triamcinolone acetonide 10 to 40 mg/mL at 4- to 6-week intervals. Alternatively, in case of hypertrophic scars, wait for 2 months after peeling and treat with fillers or needling. Frequent patient visits for observation are advised when treating darker skin types; early detection of complications and signs that there may be an impending complication are imperative signals to start early treatment. Most complications can be resolved when treated promptly.[2,17]

33.3.5 Laser Complications

As well as with chemical peels, fractional laser treatments have their complications. And, as one can guess, darker skin types are more prone to pigmentary complications.

PIH is an acquired hypermelanosis that occurs after cutaneous inflammation or injury.[14] It is the most common complication of laser treatments. People with darker skin are at greater risk of PIH (▶ Fig. 33.5). It presents as brown macules or patches with poorly defined borders. The severity of the pigmentary response is determined by the degree of inflammation.[26] Transitory pattern hyperpigmentation can occur. It usually resolves in the first 3 months with topical treatments.[10]

After aggressive skin therapy, there is elevated melanocyte activity with increased melanogenesis and transfer of melanin granules to surrounding keratinocytes. An accumulation of melanophages occurs in the upper dermis due to disruption of the basal cell layer. Chemical mediators such as arachidonic acid metabolites, prostaglandin E2, thromboxane B2, leukotriene (LT) C4, and LTD4, increase the inmunoreactive tyrosinase, which is a melanin-forming enzyme.[14,26]

Hypopigmentation has a delayed onset. It can be present 10 months after a laser procedure and can be permanent. It is directly related to the degree of thermal damage (bulk heating) induced in the skin and the depth of the treatment. It is believed that a history of dermabrasion or phenol peeling can predispose to this condition. Camouflage makeup can be used. Sometimes skin needling or micro-grafting may help.[17]

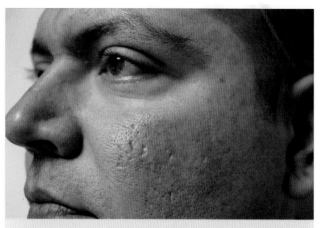

Fig. 33.5 A 31-year-old Fitzpatrick skin type V patient with post-inflammatory hyperpigmentation (PIH) and transitory pattern hyperpigmentation (notice the pigmented dots) treated with Lumenis AcuPulse (Palo Alto, California) carbon dioxide (CO_2) fractional laser—deep fractional settings10 mJ, 10% density; superficial settings 90 mJ, 40% density.

Isotretinoin affects the way re-epithelialization occurs and can lead to scarring. It is advisable to wait for a period of at least 6 months—some advocate up to 2 years—between the end of therapy and laser treatment. Bulk heating from overlapping passes can contribute to scarring. Hypertrophic scars should be treated immediately. Silicon gel sheets can be applied for 6 months. Intralesional triamcinolone acetonide, 10 to 40 mg/mL at 4- to 6-week intervals, may also be effective.[17] After 2 months, hypertrophic scars can be treated with fillers or needling.

33.4 Recommendation

In Latino patients, tailor your treatments to your patients' skin types and problems, either with lasers or chemical peels. Do not treat aggressively. It is better to treat scars or sunspots with a little bit higher energy and lower density, and the rest of the face with lower parameters. Do not treat the entire face as you would a scar or a sunspot. This method will lower the risk of PIH.

The authors do not advise ablative or nonablative fractional lasers for the treatment of melasma because there is a high possibility that the condition will worsen. Several sessions of superficial peels and/or topical bleaching treatment, with proper sun protection, can achieve better results, although it will not be cured.[14]

PIH is the main concern in treating Latino people; to avoid this condition, pretreatment of the skin and sun protection are as important as the posttreatment care.[21]

33.5 Hydramicrodermabrasion in Latino Skin

Microdermabrasion is a minimally invasive procedure that relies on an abrasive component and a vacuum component.[27] Today there are various microdermabrasion systems that differ on the source of the abrasive component. Crystal-free

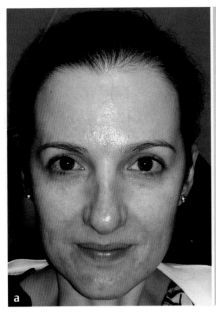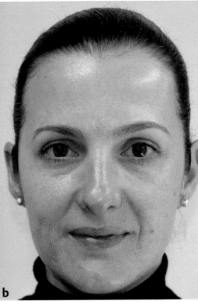

Fig. 33.6 (a) A 38-year-old Fitzpatrick skin type III patient with mild acne, sun damage, light spots, and enlarged pores before treatment. (b) Same patient after six monthly HydraFacials (HydraFacial MD System; Edge Systems Corp., Signal Hill, California). There is improvement in pores, skin texture, acne, sun damage, and skin tone as well.

microdermabrasion was developed to reduce the potential for eye injury.[28] Recently, it has also been used to enhance drug delivery to the skin by removing the stratum corneum. (The stratum corneum provides a barrier to percutaneous absorption of compounds.)[27]

Hydramicrodermabrasion (HydraFacial; Tower System, Edge Systems Corp., California) combines microdermabrasion using a patented abrading tip with pneumatic application of antioxidant-rich serums. It merges multiple therapies to create synergy and optimize results. Therefore, it is considered the next generation of microdermabrasion technology.[28]

The HydraFacial System (Edge Systems) is used to treat a variety of cosmetic maladies of the skin: superficial rhytids, hyperpigmentation, photoaging, lentigines, comedones, acne, acne scars, and enlarged pores.[28] It offers a high safety profile with minimal risk of adverse effects, especially in the Latino population where the majority of skin types are Fitzpatrick III to V.

33.5.1 Risks and Complications

Some patients may have mild erythema. If performed too aggressively, some minor abrasions can occur. Also, some patients may develop petechiae if they have thin and photodamaged skin, especially around the orbit. These complications are short-lived and are operator-dependent.[28,29] Thus hydramicrodermabrasion appears to be a safe procedure in all skin types because no pigmentary changes, focal scarring, or texture abnormalities have been reported following treatment.[28,29]

33.5.2 Results

In various studies, HydraFacial promotes a papillary dermal thickening, increase in fibroblast density, and reorganization of collagen fibers in the papillary dermal matrix. It also augments epidermal thickness and subdermal collagen.[27,28,29,30]

The changes in skin permeability immediately following the initial process of the HydraFacial are responsible for the increased uptake of antioxidants in the skin, which results in changes in skin architecture and elevated protective antioxidants in the skin. The antioxidant levels in the skin increase 32% following HydraFacial treatment, providing skin photoprotection and antiaging properties. However, if antioxidants are applied topically, the antioxidant levels in the skin remain the same as in pretreatment. Hydramicrodermabrasion improves the overall skin quality, texture, and diminishes age-related lesions.[28,29,30] Among clinical results, it is evident that there is decreased pore size, diminished fine lines and rhytids, as well as decreased hyperpigmentation.[28,29,30,31] Therefore, hydramicrodermabrasion is an excellent tool as a nonablative facial rejuvenation treatment with minimal-to-no downtime (▶ Fig. 33.6).

References

[1] Sanchez MR. Cutaneous diseases in Latinos. Dermatol Clin 2003; 21: 689–697

[2] Small R, Hoang D, Linder J. A Practical Guide to Chemical Peels, Microdermabrasion & Topical Products. Los Angeles, CA: Lippincott Williams & Wilkins; 2013

[3] Leu D, Yoo SS. Epidermal and Color Improvement in Ethnic Skin: Microdermabrasion and Superficial Peels. In: Alam M, Bhatia AC, Kundu R, Yoo S, Chan HH, eds. Cosmetic Dermatology for Skin of Color. Chicago, IL: McGraw-Hill; 2009: 29–33

[4] Grimes PE. Aesthetics and Cosmetic Surgery for Darker Skin Types. Los Angeles, CA: Lippincott Williams & Wilkins; 2008

[5] Rahman Z, Alam M, Dover JS. Fractional laser treatment for pigmentation and texture improvement. Skin Therapy Lett 2006; 11: 7–11

[6] Rokhsar CK, Fitzpatrick RE. The treatment of melasma with fractional photothermolysis: a pilot study. Dermatol Surg 2005; 31: 1645–1650

[7] Wind BS, Kroon MW, Meesters AA, et al. Non-ablative 1,550 nm fractional laser therapy versus triple topical therapy for the treatment of melasma: a randomized controlled split-face study. Lasers Surg Med 2010; 42: 607–612

[8] Ancona D, Katz BE. A prospective study of the improvement in periorbital wrinkles and eyebrow elevation with a novel fractional CO2 laser—the fractional eyelift. J Drugs Dermatol 2010; 9: 16–21

[9] Gold M. AcuPulse TM with combo treatment modality: clinical study of patients with skin of color. Gold Skin Care Center and Tennessee Clinical Research Center Inc. 2012;1–3. Available at: http://www.hv.com.br/Medical/Artigos/WHITE_PAPER_AcuPulse_Gold_A4_EXAMPLE.pdf. Accessed June 1, 2012

[10] Delgado RE, Torre MdeL. Use of fractional laser in mixed-race patients. Facial Plast Surg 2013; 29: 161–166

[11] Cassuto DA, Sadick NS, Scrimali L, Siragò P. An innovative device for fractional CO2 laser resurfacing: a preliminary clinical study. Am J Cosmet Surg 2008; 25: 97–101

[12] Reddy UP, Woodward JA. Ablative fractionated CO2 laser resurfacing for the face and neck. Am J Cosmet Surg 2011; 28: 273–275

[13] Bhatt N, Alster TS. Laser surgery in dark skin. Dermatol Surg 2008; 34: 184–194, discussion 194–195

[14] Davis EC, Callender VD. Postinflammatory hyperpigmentation: a review of the epidemiology, clinical features, and treatment options in skin of color. J Clin Aesthet Dermatol 2010; 3: 20–31

[15] Lynde CB, Kraft JN, Lynde CW. Topical treatments for melasma and postinflammatory hyperpigmentation. Skin Therapy Lett 2006; 11: 1–6

[16] Sobanko JF, Miller CJ, Alster TS. Topical anesthetics for dermatologic procedures: a review. Dermatol Surg 2012; 38: 709–721

[17] Tosti A, Beer K, Pia de Padova M. Management of Complications of Cosmetic Procedures. Miami, FL: Springer; 2012

[18] Manuskiatti W, Eimpunth S, Wanitphakdeedecha R. Effect of cold air cooling on the incidence of postinflammatory hyperpigmentation after Q-switched Nd:YAG laser treatment of acquired bilateral nevus of Ota like macules. Arch Dermatol 2007; 143: 1139–1143

[19] Al-Waiz MM, Al-Sharqi AI. Medium-depth chemical peels in the treatment of acne scars in dark-skinned individuals. Dermatol Surg 2002; 28: 383–387

[20] Sarkar R, Bansal S, Garg VK. Chemical peels for melasma in dark-skinned patients. J Cutan Aesthet Surg 2012; 5: 247–253

[21] Rullan P, Karam AM. Chemical peels for darker skin types. Facial Plast Surg Clin North Am 2010; 18: 111–131

[22] Hassan KM, Benedetto AV. Facial skin rejuvenation: ablative laser resurfacing, chemical peels, or photodynamic therapy? Facts and controversies. Clin Dermatol 2013; 31: 737–740

[23] Fedok FG, Carniol PJ. Minimally Invasive and Office-Based Procedures in Facial Plastic Surgery. New York, NY: Thieme Medical Publishers; 2014

[24] Mendelsohn JE. Update on chemical peels. Otolaryngol Clin North Am 2002; 35: 55–72, vi

[25] Joshi SS, Boone SL, Alam M, et al. Effectiveness, safety, and effect on quality of life of topical salicylic acid peels for treatment of postinflammatory hyperpigmentation in dark skin. Dermatol Surg 2009; 35: 638–644, discussion 644

[26] Cayce KA, McMichael AJ, Feldman SR. Hyperpigmentation: an overview of the common afflictions. Dermatol Nurs 2004; 16: 401–406, 413–416, quiz 417

[27] Karimipour DJ, Karimipour G, Orringer JS. Microdermabrasion: an evidence-based review. Plast Reconstr Surg 2010; 125: 372–377

[28] Freedman BM. Hydradermabrasion: an innovative modality for nonablative facial rejuvenation. J Cosmet Dermatol 2008; 7: 275–280

[29] Freedman BM. Topical antioxidant application enhances the effects of facial microdermabrasion. J Dermatolog Treat 2009; 20: 82–87

[30] Freedman BM. Topical antioxidant application augments the effects of intense pulsed light therapy. J Cosmet Dermatol 2009; 8: 254–259

[31] Freedman BM. Topical polyphenolic antioxidants reduce the adverse effects of intense pulsed light therapy. J Cosmet Laser Ther 2009; 11: 142–145

34 Anti-Aging Products and Cosmeceuticals

Jill Lynn Hessler

34.1 Introduction

Cosmeceuticals are a class of topical products used on the skin in an attempt to build collagen and reverse the aging process. The term *cosmeceuticals* was coined by Dr. Albert Kligman approximately 20 years ago at a meeting of cosmetic chemists. This term was created to recognize a class of agents that were more active than a standard cosmetic but that did not have the rigorous, controlled scientific studies associated with them to be considered drugs.

More than 75 years ago, in 1938, the strict distinction between a cosmetic product and a drug was established. The U.S. Congress enacted a statute in response to all of the elixirs that were being promoted at the time claiming to cure all body ailments. In an attempt to protect consumers, this determination was made to allow consumers to know which products had evidence to make medical claims and which did not. A cosmetic was strictly defined as an "article intended for the beautifying and promoting attractiveness." A drug was defined as a substance used in the diagnosis, cure, treatment, or prevention of disease that is intended to affect the structure and function of the body.

A topical preparation is classified not by the ingredients it contains but by the claims made in labeling and advertising. An agent that claims to change the skin and create collagen, under the 1938 statute, would be considered a drug and would need to undergo rigorous testing. Drug development through the Food and Drug Administration (FDA) is slow and expensive for the manufacturer, requiring proof of safety and efficacy. It takes significant time and research to bring a product to market. Cosmetics on the other hand do not require premarketing clearance and can quickly be brought to market. More than $9.7 billion was spent in the United States alone on cosmeceuticals in 2011, with that amount projected to increase to $11.7 billion by 2016.[1]

The United States and Europe continue to have only two class distinctions for topical agents, whereas Japan has added a third category. This third group of "quasi-drugs," available in Japan, consists of cosmetic products with pharmacological action. Most topical agents are found to be somewhere between a cosmetic and a drug. Cosmeceutical aptly describes the products that reside in the space between a cosmetic and a pharmaceutical.

34.2 Photoaging

In order to understand how to treat facial aging, one needs to understand how the skin ages. Skin changes occur as a result of genetic factors (intrinsic aging) and environmental factors (extrinsic aging). Ultraviolet (UV) light has the most significant impact on photoaging, but smoking, medications, and poor nutrition can also influence the skin.

Chronically sun-exposed skin will demonstrate a typical appearance referred to as solar elastosis or dermatoheliosis. When evaluated microscopically, histologically fragmented and disorganized elastic fibers are found in the upper dermis, and collagen degradation is identified. Cellular atypia with varying-sized cells are also present. Clinically aged skin demonstrates both fine and coarse wrinkles as a result of collagen loss. Dryness, rough texture, and sallow complexion are seen on sun-exposed skin, likely due to disorganized collagen and uneven thickness of the skin resulting in poor light reflection off the skin surface. Dyschromias and increased melanogenesis also occur, leading to uneven pigmentation of the skin. Functional abnormalities of the skin occur as well. These include easy dispensability of the skin, uneven tanning due to areas of hypopigmentation, and skin that is easily traumatized with resultant skin sloughing and ecchymosis.

Ideal cosmeceutical products, therefore, are those that increase the amount and quality of collagen in the skin, increase the hydration of the skin, and improve skin texture with the least amount of side effects.

34.3 Retinoids

Retinoids are a diverse class of vitamin A products. Vitamin A is a necessary dietary nutrient involved in bone development, vision, reproduction, and mucosal and epithelial integrity. It is a fat-soluble vitamin found in liver, milk, and eggs. Deficiency of vitamin A manifests as night blindness, exophthalmia, total blindness, hyperkeratosis of the skin, and increased propensity for infections. Retinoids are likely the most studied products in topical antiaging therapy, with more than 12 double-blinded, randomized controlled studies available (▶ Fig. 34.1).

Tretinoin was first used as a topical preparation on the skin in 1983, followed by Kligman's research on the topic a few years later.[2] Retinoic acid is the active form of vitamin A and long believed to exert the most significant effects. New research suggests retinol demonstrates some chemical effects without being converted to retinoid acid.[3] Retinoic acid is available by prescription, whereas all other products are available over the counter.

There are three primary forms of vitamin A: retinol, retinal, and retinoic acid. Retinol is the alcohol form of vitamin A and is involved in differentiation and maintenance of the epithelium. Retinal, the aldehyde form, is involved in vision. Retinoic acid, in the form of all transretinoic acid, is the form responsible for all other biological activities within the body.

Retinoids are absorbed through the skin and primarily converted to retinoic acid in the skin. This retinoic acid is carried by albumin to the cell to be absorbed into the cell and then into the nuclear membrane. Specific nuclear retinoic acid binding proteins, once activated, stimulate gene expression of type I procollagen and type VII procollagen. The result is increased collagen production by augmenting the expression of these procollagen building blocks.

UV exposure is known to increase a family of enzymes known as matrix metalloproteinase (MMP). These enzymes lead to connective tissue damage by degrading collagen and decreasing collagen synthesis. Another way retinoids increase the amount

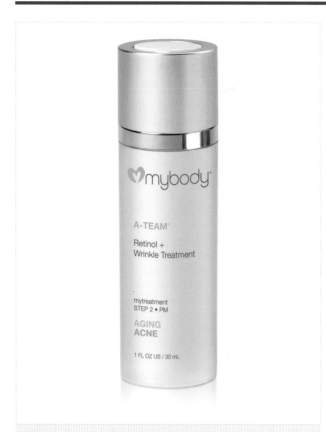

Fig. 34.1 Mybody A-Team. (Courtesy of Mybody Skin Care, Phoenix, Arizona.)

of collagen is by blocking this UV-induced activation of collagen-degrading enzymes to limit the amount of collagen degradation.

Retinoids are very potent products that exert their effects at low concentrations. Duell et al performed a study to assess the skin absorption of the various forms of retinoids. They found a minimum concentration of 0.025% was required for retinol to have an effect.[4] Levels below this did not induce cellular changes but, interestingly, higher levels did not show significantly more benefit. Retinoic acid was found to be more potent and exert its cellular activity in one half the time of retinol.

Multiple studies have demonstrated that topical tretinoin improves the skin at both the dermal and epidermal level.[4,5] The epidermis shows a decrease in epidermal thickness, reduction of corneocyte adhesion, and decreased melanin production. Changes in the dermis include increased collagen production, decreased collagenase, and decreased glycosaminoglycans. These events result in the clinically demonstrable improvement of fine lines and coarse wrinkles, improvement of skin roughness, reduction of sallow coloring, and reduction of pigmentation in the skin.[6] Histological evidence of biopsy specimens also shows increased collagen and elastin deposition.

There are multiple strengths of retinoic acid available: 0.02, 0.025, 0.04, 0.05, and 0.10% are the most commonly prescribed formulations. To evaluate the optimal dosage, a double-blinded, placebo-controlled study was performed researching 0.025% tretinoin versus 0.10% tretinoin versus placebo. A similar statistically significant clinical improvement was seen with both tretinoin dosages compared to placebo. However, there was a greater incidence of adverse effects and skin irritation with the higher dosage.[7] Therefore, there is no rationale for use of the topical tretinoin dosages above 0.025%.

Retinoid products are known to have many local adverse effects referred to as retinoid dermatitis. These side effects include erythema, pruritus, desquamation, and an exaggerated photosensitivity at the beginning of treatment. These sequelae generally begin a few days after starting treatment, peak in the first few weeks, and then wane as tolerance develops. Patients are encouraged to push through these first few weeks if possible; however, these side effects can be diminished by stopping the product for a few days or by changing to alternate-day applications.[8] Avoiding astringents and any other harsh chemicals will also help decrease the associated irritation to the skin. Retinoids will also cause significant dryness to the skin initially. Utilizing a moisturizer or emollients helps with patient tolerance. Any additional moisturizers should be applied at least 30 minutes after the retinoid acid application to allow the greatest absorption of the drug.

There are numerous adverse effects of retinoids to be aware of when recommending these agents to your patients. First, is the most serious concern of teratogenicity. Oral retinoids have been shown to cause limb and craniofacial abnormalities when the fetus is exposed in utero. Cardiovascular and neural abnormalities have also been reported. No cases of fetal harm have been documented with topically applied retinoids. Specifically, Jick et al retrospectively studied a large number of patients exposed to topical tretinoin during pregnancy and no fetal harm was identified.[9] Despite this evidence, given the severity of the potential adverse effects, most dermatologists and plastic surgeons will recommend against tretinoin usage during pregnancy.

Studies in mice have shown increased photocarcinogenicity, but this has not been shown in human studies. Following usage of topical tretinoin, the protective epithelial layer of the skin is diminished, and thus the skin is more susceptible to UV-induced damage. Judicious use of sunscreen is essential for any patient using topical retinoids. Despite these associated adverse effects, retinoids remain the best available and the best-studied topical products with demonstrated effectiveness in the treatment of photoaging.

34.4 Vitamin C

Vitamin C is another well-studied topical vitamin. Vitamin C is an essential water-soluble vitamin. Deficiency of vitamin C leads to scurvy, due to the inability of cross-linking of the procollagen molecules. Because of vitamin C's necessity for collagen production, it was a natural hypothesis that topically applied vitamin C may improve the collagen degradation that occurs with photoaging (▶ Fig. 34.2).

Vitamin C acts as an antioxidant in the skin to neutralize free radicals that can damage elastin and collagen. Vitamin C has also been shown to stimulate collagen synthesis. Human fibroblasts will increase the synthesis of procollagen I and III when exposed to ascorbic acid.[10] Vitamin C also acts a tyrosinase inhibitor, although clinical studies show only mild improvement in pigmentation with topically applied ascorbic acid.

Multiple forms of vitamin C are available. L-ascorbic acid is the biologically active form of vitamin C and the most abundant antioxidant in the skin. L-ascorbic acid is quite unstable and will easily oxidize and turn yellow when exposed to oxygen. The ascorbyl phosphate salts of magnesium and sodium have been shown to be more stable, although these salts impair added thickeners making application challenging. Penetration of vitamin C through the skin is poor, with less than 1% of the topically applied material absorbed.

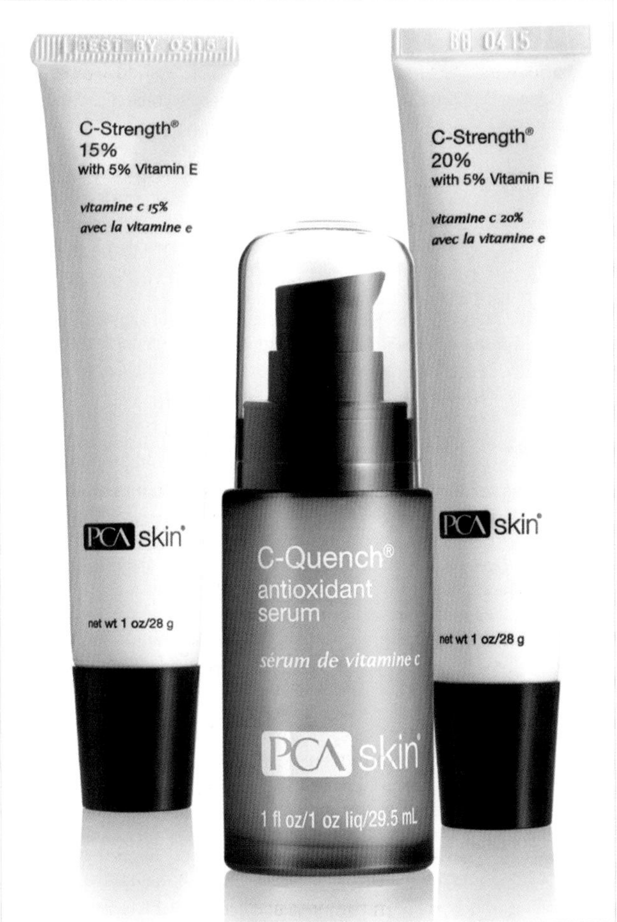

Numerous double-blind studies have demonstrated an improvement in skin texture, fine wrinkling, and skin roughness with concentrations of 5 to 15%. Histologically, Fitzpatrick showed an increase in type I collagen and gene expression of type I collagen in the skin after application of 10% vitamin C to facial skin.[11] Use of vitamin C, with its anti-inflammatory properties, has also demonstrated decreased erythema following laser resurfacing. Vitamin C applied topically is generally well tolerated. Mild stinging can occur with application along with mild skin flaking.

34.5 Vitamin E

Vitamin E comes in many forms, with tocopherol and tocopherol acetate being the most commonly used. Vitamin E is an oil-soluble vitamin, which make formulations for topical preparations less elegant.

Vitamin E is an antioxidant and exerts its effects by harnessing free radicals. The primary benefit studied is in the protection against UV-induced damage. Topical vitamin E can decrease UV-induced redness by 20% with a 2% preparation. Higher dosages provide even greater protection. Some improvement in eye wrinkling has also been demonstrated as well, although more studies are needed to confirm this change.[12]

34.6 Alpha Hydroxy Acids

Numerous compounds fall into the category of alpha hydroxy acids. The most commonly used include glycolic acid, lactic acid, malic acid, and salicylic acid. These chemicals exert their effects by accelerating cell turnover by weakening the cohesion of the stratum corneum. This exfoliation improves both the skin texture and discoloration.

Over-the-counter alpha hydroxy acids are limited to preparations that are at concentrations of 10% or less. Nevertheless, at concentrations above 25%, collagen production and increased epidermal thickness have been shown.[13]

These products can cause skin irritation including dryness, flaking, and redness. Due to the irritation effects, these compounds should generally be avoided with concomitant retinoid usage. These agents can also be used as light facial peels to improve skin texture and coloration (▶ Fig. 34.3).

Fig. 34.2 Physician's Choice of Arizona Inc. (PCA) Vitamin C products. (Courtesy of Physician's Choice of Arizona, Scottsdale, Arizona.)

Fig. 34.3 Mybody product line. (Courtesy of Mybody Skin Care, Phoenix, Arizona.)

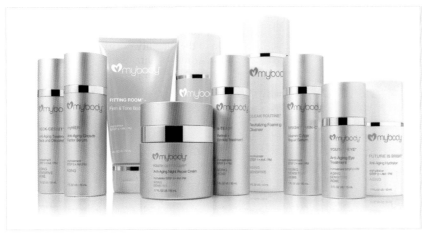

34.7 Peptides

Peptides are macromolecule particles that can be absorbed into the cell and can regulate gene and protein expression. In 1993, fragments of collagen were identified to promote further synthesis of type I collagen by upregulating transforming growth factor-beta (TGF-β).[14] This molecule was refined to allow better absorption resulting in the pentapeptide palmitoyl-lysine-threonine-threonine-lysine-serine (pal-KTTS). This is the predominately studied cosmeceutical peptide in commercial usage as a topical preparation.

At the 2002 World Congress of Dermatology in Paris favorable results were presented on peptides, thus stimulating further research. Subsequently, multiple studies have been conducted to evaluate the efficacy of peptides on photoaged skin, and encouraging results have been demonstrated.

Studies by J. Reagan Thomas et al showed that topical pentapeptides and hexapeptides, when they were applied daily, increased dermal thickness similar to the levels achieved with retinoic acid.[13] Surface roughness was also improved, but not to the same degree. They also identified that use of soy protein, which works as an enzyme inhibitor peptide, results in the improvement of fine lines, wrinkles, and roughness, equivalent to that of retinoic acid. Soy protein also resulted in an increase in the papillae index, the number of papillae per area, which could theoretically improve the fragility of aging skin.[13]

In a double-blinded, placebo-controlled study, Lintner evaluated the effects of peptides on unilateral ocular skin when applied for 28 days. He found objective improvement in wrinkle depth, wrinkle density, and surface roughness.[15] Another double-blinded, placebo-controlled split study evaluated a split-face application of topical palmitoyl peptide to 93 subjects. A significant reduction in wrinkle depth, roughness, and wrinkle volume and density was observed.[16]

Overall, peptides are well-tolerated topical applications that have demonstrated an improvement in photoaging with daily usage. Outcomes approach the results seen with retinoid acid without the adverse effects. Peptides are a relatively newer topical product and contain the theoretical risks of modifying cell regulation and transcription factors. Further studies are needed to reinforce their efficacy and show long-term safety.

34.8 Conclusion

In summary, cosmeceuticals are biologically active agents with significant clinical evidence of efficacy in the improvement of photoaged skin. Over the past 30 years, this class of agents, which exists in the space between cosmetics and tightly regulated drugs, has been rapidly expanding. As this field continues to grow, it will be important for all aesthetic practitioners to educate themselves and understand the biological implications of these agents for their safe use.

References

[1] Bombourg N. Cosmeceuticals in the U.S. 6th ed. 9 July 2012. Available at: http://www.prnewswire.com/news-releases/consumer-products-retail-latest-news/cosmeceuticals-in-the-us-6th-edition-161782015.html

[2] Kligman LH. Effects of all-trans-retinoic acid on the dermis of hairless mice. J Am Acad Dermatol 1986; 15: 779–785, 884–887

[3] Kang S, Duell EA, Fisher GJ, et al. Application of retinol to human skin in vivo induces epidermal hyperplasia and cellular retinoid binding proteins characteristic of retinoic acid but without measurable retinoic acid levels or irritation. J Invest Dermatol 1995; 105: 549–556

[4] Duell EA, Derguini F, Kang S, Elder JT, Voorhees JJ. Extraction of human epidermis treated with retinol yields retro-retinoids in addition to free retinol and retinyl esters. J Invest Dermatol 1996; 107: 178–182

[5] Weiss JS, Ellis CN, Headington JT, et al. Topical tretinoin improves photoaged skin: a double-blind vehicle-controlled study. JAMA 1988; 259: 527–532

[6] Kang S, Voorhees JJ. Photoaging therapy with topical tretinoin: an evidence-based analysis. J Am Acad Dermatol 1998; 39: S55–S61

[7] Nyirady J, Bergfeld W, Ellis C, et al. Tretinoin cream 0.02% for the treatment of photodamaged facial skin: a review of 2 double-blind clinical studies. Cutis 2001; 68: 135–142

[8] Kligman AM, Dogadkina D, Lavker RM. Effects of topical tretinoin on non-sun-exposed protected skin of the elderly. J Am Acad Dermatol 1993; 29: 25–33

[9] Jick SS, Terris BZ, Jick H. First trimester topical tretinoin and congenital disorders. Lancet 1993; 341: 1181–1182

[10] Tajima S, Pinnell SR. Ascorbic acid preferentially enhances type I and III collagen gene transcription in human skin fibroblasts. J Dermatol Sci 1996; 11: 250–253

[11] Fitzpatrick RE, Rostan EF. Double-blind, half-face study comparing topical vitamin C and vehicle for rejuvenation of photodamage. Dermatol Surg 2002; 28: 231–236

[12] Dreher F, Gabard B, Schwindt DA, Maibach HI. Topical melatonin in combination with vitamins E and C protects skin from ultraviolet-induced erythema: a human study in vivo. Br J Dermatol 1998; 139: 332–339

[13] Thomas JR, Jr, Dixon TK, Bhattacharyya TK. Effects of topicals on the aging skin process. Facial Plast Surg Clin North Am 2013; 21: 55–60

[14] Katayama K, Armendariz-Borunda J, Raghow R, Kang AH, Seyer JM. A pentapeptide from type I procollagen promotes extracellular matrix production. J Biol Chem 1993; 268: 9941–9944

[15] Lintner K, inventor. Cosmetic or dermopharmaceutical use of peptides for healing, hydrating and improving skin appearances during natural or induced ageing (heliodermia, pollution). US Patent 6 620 419. September 16, 2003

[16] Robinson LR, Fitzgerald NC, Doughty DG, Dawes NC, Berge CA, Bissett DL. Topical palmitoyl pentapeptide provides improvement in photoaged human facial skin. Int J Cosmet Sci 2005; 27: 155–160

35 The Future of Rejuvenation Techniques for Aging Facial Skin

Donn R. Chatham

35.1 "Prediction Is Very Difficult—Especially if It's About the Future"

In the absence of my trusty but rusty crystal ball, where will the future of skin rejuvenation take us? Just a few short years ago skin rejuvenation seemed limited to lay chemical peels, dermabrasion, "fruit acid" baths, and trauma. Today's landscape is much different.

Let's begin with a review of the physiological changes associated with aging and the multitude of genetic and environmental factors that play key roles in the health and appearance of skin. We focus on the ability of skin to manufacture epidermis, collagen, and elastin; its ability to protect itself from sun and other environmental insults; how well its internal antioxidation processes ("rust") work; the degree of ongoing inflammation in the body; and how well our body processes glycogen (sugars). With aging, the outer skin layer (epidermis) thins, even though the number of cell layers remains unchanged. The number of melanocytes decreases, but the remaining melanocytes increase in size. Aging skin thus appears thinner, more pale, and translucent. Lentigines appear in sun-exposed areas. Connective tissue weakens (elastosis), reducing the skin's strength and elasticity and skin that has received an overdose of irradiation is easily identified. Dermal blood vessels become more fragile, leading to bruising and purpura. Sebaceous glands and sweat glands fail, resulting in increased dryness and itchiness.[1] At a cellular level, cell physiology takes complex pathways. Regeneration and senescence have in common with each other a set of signaling mediators called "cytokines," which include proteins, peptides, and glycoproteins. Cytokines can behave in both positive and negative ways. Bone-marrow–derived mesenchymal stem cells decline with advancing age. Research continues on ways to extract positive cytokines from stem cells and hopefully use them in aging therapy.[2]

Inflammation continues to play a role in cellular, histological, and organ system aging and the role of anti-inflammatory strategies is a growing topic not only in dermatology but in other medical specialties.[3,4]

Therefore, common-sense strategies are directed specifically to preventing, slowing down, and hopefully improving this inevitable process. Young and healthy-looking skin is a feature that is universally admired and considered attractive among humans. People seem obsessed with a youthful and healthy appearance.[5]

35.2 Current Skin Rejuvenation

In order to try to speculate what the future of skin rejuvenation technological advances may bring, it is necessary to examine the current landscape. Topical skin products account for billions of dollars in sales whether they exert any useful biological effect or not and analysis of ingredients taxes the analytical skills of most chemists. Efficacy can also vary from one person to another: one individual's life-saving prescription may be another's poison. How can we know who will benefit from a medication, who will not respond at all, and who will experience adverse drug reactions?[6,7]

One helpful tool is deoxyribonucleic acid (DNA) analysis via a buccal mucosal swab that analyzes genetic neurotransmitter biomarkers. Certain enzymes are necessary for proper drug (and some foods) metabolism and when absent place the patient at increased risk of untoward problems, including ones that could be fatal.[8] DNA analysis is currently available to assist physicians in helping determine which patients are more likely to positively respond to certain classes of psychotropic medications and which patients are at increased risk of adverse reactions. Therefore safety and efficacy of some psychiatric medications can be predicted.[9,10,11]

In addition to epidermal and dermal "wounding procedures" such as chemical peels and dermabrasions, less invasive techniques to stimulate collagen production also include microdermabrasion, microneedling, ultrasonic vibrations, and water jets, and these may be utilized to enhance penetration of topically applied agents.

Lasers including carbon dioxide (CO_2); neodymium:yttrium aluminum garnet (Nd:YAG) 1,064 nm (infrared); erbium (2,940 nm); potassium titanyl phosphate (KTP) 532 (green light); pulsed dye 585 nm (yellow light), 650 nm (red light); and diode lasers hold a ubiquitous position in the medical community and remain heavily marketed (▶ Fig. 35.1).

Intense pulsed light (IPL) and broadband infrared (BBIR) light devices apply very powerful pulses and are effective in targeting skin with excessive red and brown lesions. These may be combined with topical sensitizing agents such as aminolevulinic acid (ALA) in photodynamic therapy (PDT). Light-emitting diodes (LEDs) use visible spectrum, monochromatic light therapy for photoaged skin[12] and are currently offered by both medical and nonmedical businesses. These include light-therapy pods at some fitness centers and spas as a means to "improve skin and slow aging," the only requirement being the consumer's willingness to purchase.[13]

The use of home devices is expanding at lightning speed with P. T. Barnum-like claims of efficacy. Some mechanisms even appear to be based on science and research. Examples of some of today's home-consumer devices are listed in ▶ Table 35.1.

Nonlaser heating devices have also proliferated, attempting to harness various energy technologies to effect desirous changes not only on the outer surface of the skin, but on tissues deep in the skin itself in a hopefully nonablative, nondestructive process. Denaturation of collagen occurs at about 60 to 65°C with ensuing neocollagenesis. The advantages of less downtime, lowered risk, and rapid healing are appealing. Energies include radiofrequency (RF), microwave, infrared (IR), ultrasound (US), LEDs, and combination therapy machines.[14,15]

Some devices first penetrate the skin with microneedles prior to energy delivery, attempting to precisely target and deliver measured RF energy directly into the dermis.[16,17] Other RF skin-tightening devices include those directly contacting the skin surface creating subablative/microablative effects.[18,19] Still other instruments use US waves that induce a molecular vibra-tion in a given tissue creating thermal coagulative focal necrosis.[20]

And yet other tools are contactless ("no-touch") devices with panels that deliver IR thermal energy using frequencies and impedance variances based on tissue levels.[21] Electromagnetic energy is converted to heat and currently targets adipose tissue. And whereas most neuromodulators/neurotoxins are injected subcutaneously to affect muscle function, the use of intra-dermal injections continues to be studied, including measura-ble changes in skin elasticity (D. Ellis, email communication, January 2014). Research also continues in the search for an ideal topical wound-healing accelerator.[22,23] ▶ Fig. 35.2 shows the

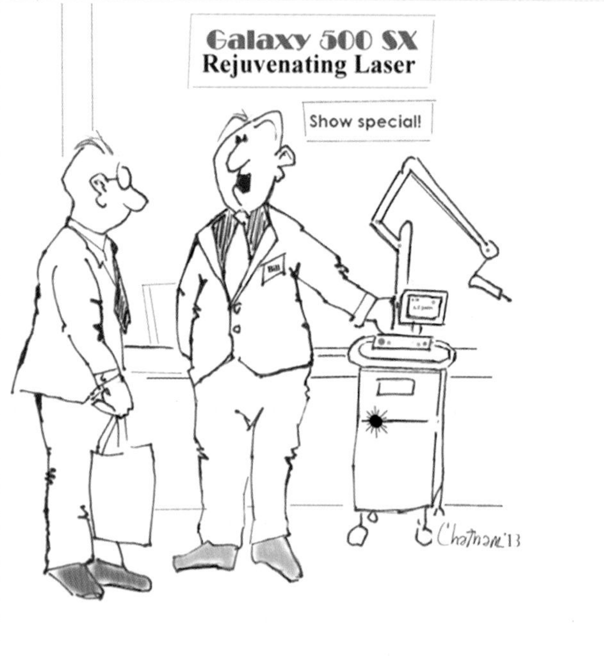

Fig. 35.1 "Doc, you'll double your money before your patients even realize it doesn't do much."

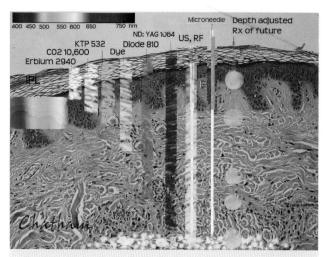

Fig. 35.2 Light spectrum, relative skin penetration of laser wave-lengths, and other energy modalities, including technology of the future.

Table 35.1 Examples of over-the-counter, home-use skin devices

OTC system	Website	Uses
Opal Sonic Infusion System	www.Clarisonic.com	Infuses antiaging serum into epidermis for fine-line and wrinkle reduction
ReFa PRO Platinum Electronic Roller	www.Refusa.com	Uses microcurrent to improve skin tone
Clarisonic Mia2	www.Clarisonic.com	Utilizes sonic frequency to clean pores and deliver topical antibacterials
NuFACE Trinity Facial Toning Device	www.mynuface.com/professionals	Employs microcurrent to stimulate muscles, increase circulation, and stimulate collagen
Tanda Luxe	www.YoungPhar.com	Uses red light and sonic vibration to stimulate collagen and elastic production and increase microcirculation
No!No! Skin	www.my-no-no.com	Utilizes LHE to reduce acne, emitting green and red light and heat to destroy bacteria and reduce inflammation
TRIA Skin Perfecting Blue Light	www.triabeauty.com	Targets *P. acnes* to reduce acne
Claro IPL Acne Clearing Device	www.myclaro.com	Employs blue light to destroy *P. acnes*, red light combined with infrared heat to sooth inflammation
Body Essentials Light & Massage Therapy Brush	www.bodyessentialsforyou.com	Uses red light and LEDs and massage to boost cell energy and increase circulation

Abbreviations: LEDs, light-emitting diodes; LHE, light heat energy; OTC, over the counter; P. acnes, *Propionibacterium acnes*.

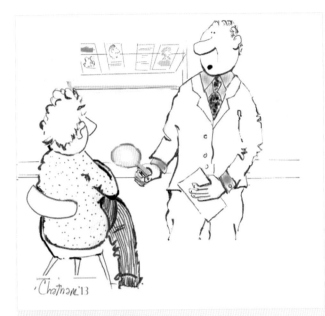

Fig. 35.3 "Well, I could offer you some stem cells. They are fresh and we are offering three for the price of two."

approximate level of skin penetration of laser wavelengths and other energy-producing devices.

35.3 Alternative Therapies: Hope or Hype?

When one peruses some of the seminars and courses offered within the health and beauty industry, one can only marvel at the number of potions, lotions, devices, inventions, techniques, and other gizmos that promise beauty and magic. Here are a few examples:

- Microneedling as a Botox alternative
- Microcurrent therapy to eliminate skin wrinkles and tone skin
- LED therapy for skin suffering from acne and aging
- Infusion therapy using galvanic current and infrared energy
- Stem cells to reprogram skin cell function
- Mesotherapy to awaken stem cells and alter DNA
- Plant stem cells to regulate cellular gene activity
- Growth factor with tetrapeptides to resynchronize cellular rhythm
- Light and sound therapy to oxygenate cells
- Ultrasonic microdermabrasion
- Micronized high-frequency current for photodamage and acne
- Oxygen therapy for skin rejuvenation
- Negative pressure for skin tightening
- Energy-light-sound facial rejuvenation
- Multisensory spa capsules for total body rejuvenation
- Cell-phone apps for treatment of acne from the screen light

35.4 Sexy Topicals

The search for the "Holy Grail" of topical skin rejuvenation magic continues.[24] And the "Sirens' song" of many products

contributes to the cosmeceutical beauty industry growing into sales of $292 billion in 2015, according to one estimate.[25]

One highly marketed cream "merges bio-technology with beauty, ... detects and recruits healthy-looking skin cells to repair and renew the appearance of skin, visibly reversing the look of thin, crepey, aging skin, ... strengthens skin and dramatically increases the appearance of skin density and elasticity, returning fullness, firmness and tone." Another cream claims to contain skin telomerase, an enzyme that creates telomeres capping at the end of chromosomes and "resets your skin's aging clock by minimum of 5 years, converting adult stem cells to newly minted skin cells, results are indelible and life changing." Plant cells from a rare Swiss apple tree "preserves and protects skin stem cells." Another uses tropoelastin secreted from human embryonic stem cells and "enhances the natural formation of collagen and binds with existing protein chains in the skin to make it appear smoother and firmer" (▶ Fig. 35.3). Other creams derived from human skin claim they contain "cell-altering human growth hormones." Yet another uses bovine stem-cell products claiming that "existing cells feel younger, ... older cells act younger and triggers significant increase in cellular growth." A product using tissue from Russian women placenta donors purportedly destroys bacteria and viruses and stimulates regeneration of skin cells. (The U.S. Food and Drug Administration [FDA] bans placenta hormones from use in cosmetics.) Another product claims to contain DNA repair enzymes and technology straight from the sequencing of the human genome.

Wow! Note that the FDA allows the use of "DNA" as a marketing word. Claims are allowed regarding skin appearance. What is *not* allowed is to claim a product affects structure or function. If these claims are made, it is a drug and must be approved as a drug. So, is the claim "revitalizing cells" a medical or marketing term? Certainly the world is a more interesting place with acupuncture, hypnotherapy, homeopathy, herbology, Kirlian photography, aura imaging, gas discharge visualization, and thought-field therapy. But where does fiction end and science begin?[26]

Transdermal administration of drugs such as analgesics and hormones has been successfully used; however, larger molecule or water-soluble drugs such as vaccines, proteins, peptides, and antibodies have difficulty in penetrating the epidermis.

Microneedles, some only 1 mm long,[27] are now used to administer vaccines[28] and other drugs, as a pain-free alternative to traditional needles. Wafer-sized topical patches coated on one side with microscopic needles can facilitate transdermal delivery of a drug that normally cannot pass through the skin. Some are made of hollow steel and others coat the steel with an agent. Yet others are composed of injection-safe soluble polymers whose small protrusions break off when applied to the skin, dissolve, and release the drug. ▶ Fig. 35.4 illustrates three types of microneedle patches and their drug-delivery mechanisms.

35.5 What's in the Future?

When we try to extrapolate from today to tomorrow, I envision continuations and evolutions as a perpetual journey without end. In broad terms, we can expect that the goals of skin rejuvenation will be to protect, maintain, and regenerate. Skin should be as undamaged, healthy, vital, functional, and attractive as

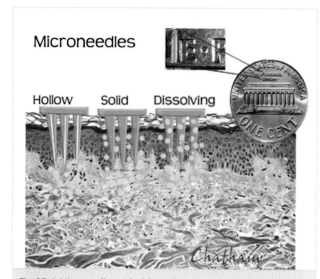

Fig. 35.4 Microneedles with delivered agents.

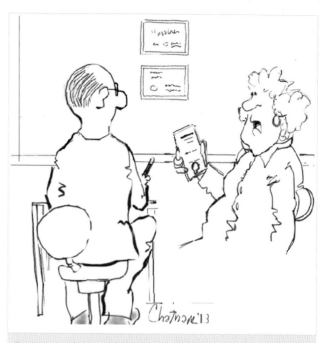

Fig. 35.5 "Is this procedure evidence-based?"

possible. Preventive strategies will always be emphasized. Maintenance will always be important. Regenerative strategies will be necessary when more than maintenance is required. Replacement with new skin will be part of the regenerative process. The message of prevention of skin deterioration will be louder in developed countries and continue to focus on the effects of excessive irradiation, environmental oxidizers, and exposure to tobacco and other ingested and inhaled products. Skin protection will be more greatly valued.

Prediction: One day a vaccine will be administered to help protect the skin at a cellular level from certain external deleterious agents such as ionizing irradiation and pollutant oxidizers. (Zostavax vaccine [Merck & Co., Inc., Whitehouse Station, New Jersey] for herpes zoster already is widely recommended and can help reduce the physical skin and neurological trauma produced by this aggressive virus.[29]) Aging therapies will not be limited to a special few, and will become mainstream. Improving the external visible symptomatic signs of aging will be only one part of a broader strategy of treating the whole body to preserve health and longevity.

35.5.1 Sunshine Act

Topical skin agents applied by the consumer will become more efficacious and ubiquitous because more "regular folks" will adopt use once they are convinced it is in their best interests. Few would argue that today's multibillion-dollar skin lotion and potion business is not a fluffy one, rampant with unsubstantiated claims. Consumers will demand more accountability of promotional claims.

Prediction: Gradually the "hype" associated with this industry will be replaced with science, and grading standards will be applied to skin rejuvenators (much like automobiles and other consumer products are rated today). It is likely that advertising will be more regulated, with unsubstantiated claims tightly curtailed and evidence-based therapies valued (▶ Fig. 35.5). The FDA continues to monitor claims of drug companies and alter food labels[30]; and the U.S. Federal Trade Commission (FTC) now requires more disclosure by medical companies and speakers

than ever before with the Sunshine Act additions.[31] The Sunshine Act requires applicable manufacturers of drugs, devices, biologicals, or medical supplies to report annually to the Secretary of Health and Human Services (HHS) certain payments or other transfers of value to physicians and teaching hospitals. It also requires applicable manufacturers and applicable group purchasing organizations (GPOs) to report certain information regarding the ownership or investment interests held by physicians or the immediate family members of physicians in such entities.

Prediction: As physicians demand more peer-reviewed clinical studies that are not funded and controlled by manufacturers, truthful clinical studies on efficacy of new devices will be the norm rather than the exception.

35.5.2 DNA and RNA

Will it really ever be possible for a topical cream to alter one's DNA or make genes younger? That sounds a bit scary! More likely a product will contain compounds that will assist the body's own natural physiology in its role of protecting and healing the skin. This includes increased use of numerous peptides that act as messengers to a specific cell. The most useful will be those that act to either switch a negative function off or switch a positive function on by increased expression of specific skin biomarkers, thus conferring antiaging skin-care benefits. But since products do not affect all skin cells in an identical manner and may even be toxic to the skin, greater specificity in prescribing will occur.[32]

Pharmacogenomics, the study of how genes affect a person's response to drugs, combines pharmacology (the science of drugs) and genomics (the study of genes and their functions) to develop effective, safe medications and doses that will be tailored to a person's genetic makeup. This will increase. For example, knowledge gained from the Human Genome Project (HGP), completed in 2003,[33] will aid researchers in understanding how inherited differences in genes affect the body's response to medications. The HGP identified nearly 25,000 genes in human DNA and how they are influenced in response to both internal and external stimuli. Many human diseases, including most skin diseases, have origins in the genetic characteristics of the affected individuals.

Prediction: Analyzing the transcriptome (that small percentage of the genetic code that is transcribed into ribonucleic acid [RNA] molecules of a human cell line) using different ingredients will help determine which patients' skin will react positively to prolong cell life and help to avoid prescribing these ingredients to patients whose skin and body react negatively (contact dermatitis as an example). This information will provide answers to the behavior of skin aging that shows an age-dependent increase or decrease of biomarkers and also help validate the efficacy of antiaging compounds formulated into topical solutions.[34]

DNA sequencing, the process of determining the precise order of nucleotides within a DNA molecule, may assist in creating specific treatments for certain genotypes. One method of genetic manipulation of aging genes uses RNA interference (RNAi) technology. RNAi technology provides a potential means for blocking expression of a specific deleterious gene and how a chemical compound might alter it.[35]

Prediction: Specific drugs will be developed to bind with messenger ribonucleic acid (mRNA) molecules and block the production of certain disease-creating proteins, thereby thwarting progression of a specific disease. As overall health is improved, skin health and appearance will also be improved.

35.5.3 Biologics

Human skin surfaces are complex ecosystems for microorganisms, including fungi, bacteria, and viruses, which are known collectively as the skin microbiome. Residing on each square centimeter of skin are approximately 1 million bacteria, and many common skin conditions are associated with both impaired skin-barrier function and increased microbial colonization. Friendly populations of microbiota (naturally occurring commensal bacteria) can be disturbed through harsh soaps and other environmental toxins. The more we learn about the interactions of host gene-microbiota will lead to a better and more individualized treatment and prevention of skin inflammatory diseases. In one study, topical application of 0.2% *Propionibacterium acnes* reduced papules and pustules by 89%.[36] The skin is very closely connected to the gut through the "gut-skin axis."[37] Since many diseases and conditions associated with aging seem tied to inflammation ("inflammaging"), efforts to control inflammation will play a big role in "healthy aging." This inflammation may be seen as acne, eczema, psoriasis, and other types of dermatitis as well as unwanted aging of skin.[3,38,39] Probiotics can reduce gut inflammation, one source of systemic inflammation, and can therefore also improve skin disorders through a similar mechanism.[40,41]

Prediction: New biological therapies will develop to enhance skin function. Topical probiotic formulations will likely assume greater usage, including mimicry of bacterial infection to create an inflammatory response of the skin.[42] Oral nutraceuticals will emerge as adjunctive modifiers of skin biology.

Cultured autologous cells will be reintroduced into the body for a variety of indications and will become predicatively effective in regeneration of healthy tissue, both in the reconstructive and aesthetic arenas, and at an affordable price.[43,44,45] (Offshore labs will have reduced labor costs.) Research will continue in the development of stem cell-derived factors. For example, transforming growth factor-beta (TGF-β3) is the growth factor that distinguishes fetal cell healing from adult cell healing and produces less inflammation while promoting abundant collagen. And if the good anti-inflammatory cytokines dominate, less inflammation means a slower rate of senescence.[46,47]

Prediction: Application of cytokine-related compounds such as growth factors, interleukins, and interferons, including those extracted from stem cells, will increase in use as one means of replacing those cytokines lost through the aging process. Stem cells harvested from stem cell "farms" (labs really) will produce millions of stem cells, with extracted compounds being combined for skin regenerative "cocktails" created for specific skin rejuvenating scenarios.

35.5.4 Telomeres

A telomere is a region of repetitive nucleotide sequences at each end of a chromatid. It protects the end of the chromosome from deterioration or from fusion with neighboring chromosomes (▶ Fig. 35.6). During chromosome replication, the enzymes that duplicate DNA cannot continue their duplication all the way to the end of a chromosome; therefore, in each duplication the end of the chromosome is shortened. This leads to an irreversible state of growth arrest known as cellular senescence or programmed cell self-destruction (apoptosis). Telomere shortening can be hastened by unhealthy factors such as obesity, smoking, and stress.[48] But can telomere degradation be lessened or prevented? Human T cells, which are critical in immunological control over infections and cancer, have the ability to activate the enzyme telomerase that binds and extends the telomeres.[49] Research continues in using cycloastragenol from the Astragalus plant that has been shown in one study to activate telomerase.[50] Telomerase activators have suggested a slowing of aging in mice.[51,52] Other studies on affecting telomeres and increasing protective telomerase continue including lifestyle and dietary factors.[53]

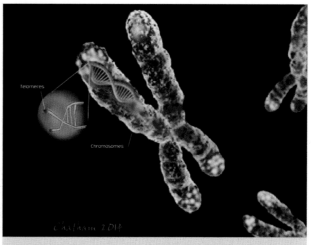

Fig. 35.6 Chromosomes demonstrating end-telomere segment.

Prediction: Pharmacological agents able to stimulate and somewhat activate telomerase and retard the shortening of DNA telomeres will help slow cellular senescence and will one day be available—not to stop aging but to modify its rate. But this will not occur in the near future.

35.5.5 Skin-Penetrating Technologies

Pharmaceuticals that are forced into the skin via fine needles or pressurized energy to induce it to make more elastin will continue to expand. Microchannels induced by various technologies will allow important peptides to more efficiently carry out their mission. More and more combination treatments will emerge and include mixing active ingredients for synergistic effects. Research continues on using microneedles (1 mm in length) to deliver short interfering RNAs (siRNAs) to inhibit gene expression of certain skin diseases.[54] Future applications certainly will expand to help manage not only unwanted dermatological disorders but those associated with deterioration and aging as well.[55,56]

Prediction: Minimally ablative and subablative energies will increasingly be used, with algorithms created specifically based on factors unique to individual patients (age, skin type, skin thickness, photodamage, circulatory integrity, and DNA analysis).[57]

Another step may be topical neuromodulators enhanced with peptide carriers similar to compounds like RT001 (Revance Therapeutics, Inc., Newark, California) to achieve some of the effects of those neurotoxins now injected intradermally.

Prediction: Topically applied patches with very tiny needles will be utilized more frequently as a painless means of introducing cell-altering agents into the dermis.

35.5.6 Medical "Providers"

When we study those modalities that require a "medical provider" (the days when physicians made up the majority of providers appear to be long gone), many of these modalities are being integrated into patient-administered home therapies. It would seem likely that following a provider-administered treatment such as laser therapy, or needling, or peeling that a potent recovery topical will dramatically reduce the morbidity of the procedure by jump-starting the calming and regenerative process of affected skin. For example, if hair transplantation becomes entirely "robotic," it may then be performed in almost any location with a technician, including sites with no physician present.[58] Other computer-programmed devices will proliferate and may be controlled by off-site professionals ("distance medicine").

Prediction: The vast majority of skin rejuvenation consultations and treatments will be managed by nonphysicians. When physicians are involved, it may be from a remote site, including locations from many parts of the globe.

35.5.7 Home Devices

There will be an expanded market of at-home devices for purchase by consumers desirous of reduced costs and fewer on-site visits (▶ Fig. 35.7). In addition to LEDs, blue light, and red light devices, various energy-based heating instruments (at

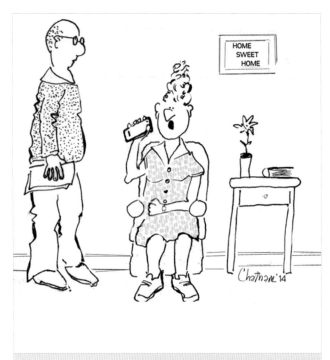

Fig. 35.7 "It's a Smartphone app that stimulates my fibroblasts ... three types of light ... and only $3.99!"

lower fluences), and several fractionated mechanisms will be available with more launching regularly. Closely related will be tools that combine energy technology with cosmeceuticals. Currently the FDA clears only medical devices, not beauty devices, a distinction not always obvious to consumers.

Prediction: Many consumers will oversee their own home-based treatments, including use of Internet-based and offshore consultative services.

35.5.8 Energy-Based Office Devices

First of all, in the not-too-distant future, skin destruction by some of our current ablative methods will be considered archaic. Even liposuction as we know it may be passé.

In-office treatments will be administered not by physicians or nurses, but more frequently by "trained skin-specialty technicians" adhering to their protocols or even computer-generated delivery built into the device itself. (If commercial aircraft can take off and land with computerized systems, shouldn't medical procedures find the same pathways?)

Prediction: The more precise devices will have the capability of measuring the depth of tissue at an anatomical site of an individual patient whose healing factors have been estimated; then determining how much collagen synthesis is needed; adjusting energy settings for age and anatomical region; then delivering the ideal volume of energy to the exact depth while also monitoring peripheral collateral temperatures (▶ Fig. 35.2).

External ("no-touch") mechanisms using electromagnetic energy and US in generating targeted heat at different tissue depths will be more refined, adjusting to specific depths for that individual patient for more enhanced responses.

Prediction: Future energy instruments that do not touch or physically enter the skin will continue to develop and progress and will be preferred by consumers for their seemingly magical rejuvenating energy, especially appealing to those enamored with basking in the radiant energy of sunlike inventions.

35.5.9 New Developments

Every technology has the potential to accomplish two things: (1) become more efficient at what it does, and (2) be utilized for new and different indications. For example, in 1995 the PhotoDerm VL/IPL (515–1,200 nm) (www.Lumenis.com; Lumenis, Inc., Palo Alto, California) laser was introduced for tattoo removal; although it was mediocre for its intended purpose of tattoo removal, it led to the use of IPL for treatment of unwanted hair and later treatment of rosacea and lentigines.[59,60] Treatment of neck laxity with its flimsy tissue will continue to be a challenge; however, newer more precise energy delivery technology designed to precisely stimulate fibroblasts without excess damage will one day be achieved as a viable supplement to surgery.

Prediction: Technologies used today for certain applications will continue to be used for new applications and merge with other energy sources—even three or four simultaneously applied at once, with some surprising results. This will be a marketer's dream.

35.6 Summary

The patient seeking optimal skin rejuvenation in the near future will engage in multimodality strategies. The best results will address biochemical, cellular, histological, and procedural levels simultaneously. Prevention and maintenance will evolve to include dietary nutraceuticals and complex diets along with topical applications including assisted-infusion technologies. Cocoa, pomegranate, and bioavailable superoxide dismutase (SOD) have already been shown to reduce oxidative stress and new food sources will be identified. I predict that saturated fat from animal sources will find a new place at the table! Foods with a low inflammatory index will be the new culinary darlings. Topical biologics that feed friendly bioflora will work synergistically with superpeptide serums and cytokine-compatible balms that reduce cellular misbehavior. At-home devices will become more efficacious and affordable. Therapies designed to alter existing cellular and histological functions will be offered by both professionally educated medical providers and minimally trained technicians relying on computer-assisted programmed tools. Transdermal delivery of selected agents via painless microneedles and coated with or containing very small doses of drugs and RNAi agents will be expanded. Precise energy-producing devices will first measure an individual patient's skin depth, determine the exact level where energy is to be deposited, and measure in real time the energy delivered to that level. More aggressive therapies with potential complications will remain largely under the supervision of physicians but not necessarily those in the specialties we traditionally associate with rejuvenation. The following parable illustrates:

It was a sunny morning when Jane Jetson arose from a deep sleep. Her copper-vanadium–lined pillowcases worked their wrinkle-reducing magic during the night in addition to her bedside oxygenator that upped her room air oxygen (O_2) concentration to 24%. Cells need oxygen, you know. After her probiotic nutrients serum to keep her bioflora fed, she next would apply the cytokine-rich topical microneedle patch containing her own growth factors harvested last year from her skin. The "fibroblast orchard," as she called it, was producing many excellent compounds and her skin looked the best it had in years. Or was it because of the "Longevity Light" she had been using every 3 to 4 days? Utilizing red, green, and LED lights, 15 minutes each session, it stimulated her cells to reduce their senescence activity. At only $999 it paid for itself quickly. Or maybe it was more because of the LifePod sessions she purchased at her health club: she depended on her "certified skin rejuvenation" coach to recommend the settings and frequency of her very relaxing time in the pod. Not only did her entire body receive skin preservation and rejuvenation beams but the aromatherapy, water massage, circulatory enhancement, and gentle suction made her skin feel robust. And just last week her "Health for Life" provider suggested five sessions with the latest noninvasive tissue tightener. Combining IR, RF, US, and BBIR, it was "no-touch" and was actually relaxing. He promised this would delay her face surgery for 10 years or more. She trusted him, because he was board certified by the International Board of Facial and Body Rejuvenation (IBFBR) and had been featured on Dr. Oz, Jr's webcasts. "I want to put off surgery until my 90th," she mused. Going "under the knife," as they used to say back in the old days, was the last resort. These days no one actually used a steel blade; however, it must have been an interesting time during the days of lasers, peeling, sanding, sucking, and cutting. It sounds barbaric! Now, let's get that glass of super antioxidant flavonoids to wash down my capsules of mitochondrial messengers. Must turn off those "grandma genes" and keep the young ones going. "Beauty is as beauty eats," as they say.

35.7 Acknowledgments

I would like to thank these colleagues for their helpful ideas: Kevin Duplechain, MD, Paul Carniol, MD, Mark Hamilton, MD, Jason Pozner, MD, Rich Gentile, MD, Phil Miller, MD, Amir Moradi, MD, Dave Ellis, MD, Mike Persky, MD, Heidi Waldorf, MD, and Jennifer Lindner, MD.

References

[1] Minaker KL. Common clinical sequelae of aging. In: Goldman L, Schafer AI, eds. Cecil Medicine. 24th ed. Philadelphia, PA: Saunders Elsevier; 2011: chap 24

[2] Caplan AI. Adult mesenchymal stem cells for tissue engineering versus regenerative medicine. J Cell Physiol 2007; 213: 341–347

[3] Akbaraly TN, Hamer M, Ferrie JE, et al. Chronic inflammation as a determinant of future aging phenotypes. CMAJ 2013; 185: E763–E770

[4] Gabuzda D, Yankner BA. Physiology: inflammation links ageing to the brain. Nature 2013; 497: 197–198

[5] Matts PJ, Fink B. Chronic sun damage and the perception of age, health and attractiveness. Photochem Photobiol Sci 2010; 9: 421–431

[6] Riedl MA, Casillas AM. Adverse drug reactions: types and treatment options. Am Fam Physician 2003; 68: 1781–1790

[7] What is a serious adverse event? Safety. US Food and Drug Administration. 10 Jan 2014. Available at: http://www.fda.gov/safety/medwatch/howtoreport/ucm053087.html. Accessed March 1, 2014

[8] Sallee FR, DeVane CL, Ferrell RE. Fluoxetine-related death in a child with cyto-chrome P-450 2D6 genetic deficiency. J Child Adolesc Psychopharmacol 2000; 10: 27–34

[9] Mrazek DA, Lerman C. Facilitating clinical implementation of pharmacoge-nomics. JAMA 2011; 306: 304–305

[10] Zineh I, Pacanowski MA. Pharmacogenomics in the assessment of therapeutic risks versus benefits: inside the United States Food and Drug Administration. Pharmacotherapy 2011; 31: 729–735

[11] Mrazek DA. Psychiatric pharmacogenomic testing in clinical practice. Dia-logues Clin Neurosci 2010; 12: 69–76

[12] Weiss RA, McDaniel DH, Geronemus RG, Weiss MA. Clinical trial of a novel non-thermal LED array for reversal of photoaging: clinical, histologic, and surface profilometric results. Lasers Surg Med 2005; 36: 85–91

[13] Leyden J, Stephens TJ, Herndon JH, Jr. Multicenter clinical trial of a home-use nonablative fractional laser device for wrinkle reduction. J Am Acad Dermatol 2012; 67: 975–984

[14] El-Domyati M, El-Ammawi TS, Medhat W, Moawad O, Mahoney MG, Uitto J. Electro-optical synergy technique: a new and effective nonablative approach to skin aging. J Clin Aesthet Dermatol 2010; 3: 22–30

[15] Alexiades-Armenakas M, Rosenberg D, Renton B, Dover J, Arndt K. Blinded, randomized, quantitative grading comparison of minimally invasive, fraction-al radiofrequency and surgical face-lift to treat skin laxity. Arch Dermatol 2010; 146: 396–405

[16] Hantash BM, Ubeid AA, Chang H, Kafi R, Renton B. Bipolar fractional radiofre-quency treatment induces neoelastogenesis and neocollagenesis. Lasers Surg Med 2009; 41: 1–9

[17] Cho SI, Chung BY, Choi MG, et al. Evaluation of the clinical efficacy of fraction-al radiofrequency microneedle treatment in acne scars and large facial pores. Dermatol Surg 2012; 38: 1017–1024

[18] Man J, Goldberg DJ. Safety and efficacy of fractional bipolar radiofrequency treatment in Fitzpatrick skin types V-VI. J Cosmet Laser Ther 2012; 14: 179–183

[19] Berube D, Renton B, Hantash BM. A predictive model of minimally invasive bipolar fractional radiofrequency skin treatment. Lasers Surg Med 2009; 41: 473–478

[20] White WM, Makin IR, Barthe PG, Slayton MH, Gliklich RE. Selective creation of thermal injury zones in the superficial musculoaponeurotic system using intense ultrasound therapy: a new target for noninvasive facial rejuvenation. Arch Facial Plast Surg 2007; 9: 22–29

[21] Fajkošová K, Machovcová A, Onder M, Fritz K. Selective radiofrequency ther-apy as a non-invasive approach for contactless body contouring and circum-ferential reduction. J Drugs Dermatol 2014; 13: 291–296

[22] Hom DB, Linzie BM, Huang TC. The healing effects of autologous platelet gel on acute human skin wounds. Arch Facial Plast Surg 2007; 9: 174–183

[23] Lee JW, Kim BJ, Kim MN, Mun SK. The efficacy of autologous platelet rich plasma combined with ablative carbon dioxide fractional resurfacing for acne scars: a simultaneous split-face trial. Dermatol Surg 2011; 37: 931–938

[24] Crary D. Boomers will be spending billions to counter aging. USA Today. 22 Aug 2011. Available at: http://usatoday30.usatoday.com/news/health/story/health/story/2011/08/Anti-aging-industry-grows-with-boomer-demand/50087672/1. Accessed March 1, 2014

[25] Global anti-aging products market to reach US$291.9 billion by 2015, accord-ing to new report by Global Industry Analysts. MCP-1107: anti-aging products-a global strategic business report. Global Industry Analysts, Inc. 19 Feb 2009. Available at: http://www.strategyr.com/gia_new/strategyr_new/pressMCP-1107.asp. Accessed March 3, 2014

[26] Most SP. Prospective examination of the efficacy of 2 topical over-the-counter cosmeceutical creams for rapid treatment of facial rhytids. Arch Facial Plast Surg 2007; 9: 340–343

[27] Kim YC, Park JH, Prausnitz MR. Microneedles for drug and vaccine delivery. Adv Drug Deliv Rev 2012; 64: 1547–1568

[28] Lambert PH, Laurent PE. Intradermal vaccine delivery: will new delivery sys-tems transform vaccine administration? Vaccine 2008; 26: 3197–3208

[29] Power M, Fell G, Wright M. Principles for high-quality, high-value testing. Evid Based Med 2013; 18: 5–10

[30] NF Label. Proposed changes aim to better inform food choices. US Food and Drug Administration. Feb 2004. Available at: http://www.fda.gov/ForConsum-ers/ConsumerUpdates/ucm387114.htm. Accessed March 3, 2014

[31] Sunshine Act. Physician financial transparency reports. American Medical As-sociation. 18 July 2013. Available at: http://www.ama-assn.org/resources/doc/washington/sunshine-act-physician-financial-transparency-reports.pdf. Accessed March 2, 2014

[32] Geria NM. Genomic-based anti-aging products hope or hype? Household Per-son Products Industry. 27 Sept 2013. Available at: http://www.happi.com/issues/2013-10/view_anti-aging-cosmeceutical-corner/genomic-based-anti-aging-products-hope-or-hype/. Accessed March 4, 2014

[33] National Human Genome Research Institute. National Institutes of Health. Available at: http://www.genome.gov/. Accessed February 28, 2014

[34] Johansson H, Lindstedt M, Albrekt AS, Borrebaeck CA. A genomic biomarker signature can predict skin sensitizers using a cell-based in vitro alternative to animal tests. BMC Genomics 2011; 12: 399

[35] Milhavet O, Gary DS, Mattson MP. RNA interference in biology and medicine. Pharmacol Rev 2003; 55: 629–648

[36] Pavicic T, Wollenweber U, Farwick M, Korting HC. Anti-microbial and -inflammatory activity and efficacy of phytosphingosine: an in vitro and in vivo study addressing acne vulgaris. Int J Cosmet Sci 2007; 29: 181–190

[37] Bowe WP, Logan AC. Acne vulgaris, probiotics and the gut-brain-skin axis - back to the future? Gut Pathog 2011, Jan 31; 3: 1

[38] Meggs WJ. The Inflammation Cure: How to Combat the Hidden Factor Behind Heart Disease, Arthritis, Asthma, Diabetes, Alzheimer's Disease, Osteoporosis, and Other Diseases of Aging. New York, NY: McGraw-Hill; 2004

[39] Singh T, Newman AB. Inflammatory markers in population studies of aging. Ageing Res Rev 2011; 10: 319–329

[40] Akbaraly T, Sabia S, Hagger-Johnson G, et al. Does overall diet in midlife pre-dict future aging phenotypes? A cohort study. Am J Med 2013; 126: 411–419. e3

[41] Albrechts C. Host genome controls skin microbiota and inflammation. Scien-ceDaily. ScienceDaily.com Published 17 September 2013. Accessed 1 June 2015.

[42] Naik S, Bouladoux N, Wilhelm C, et al. Compartmentalized control of skin immunity by resident commensals. Science 2012; 337: 1115–1119

[43] Weiss RA, Weiss MA, Beasley KL, Munavalli G. Autologous cultured fibroblast injection for facial contour deformities: a prospective, placebo-controlled, phase III clinical trial. Dermatol Surg 2007; 33: 263–268

[44] Watson D, Keller GS, Lacombe V, Fodor PB, Rawnsley J, Lask GP. Autologous fibroblasts for treatment of facial rhytids and dermal depressions. A pilot study. Arch Facial Plast Surg 1999; 1: 165–170

[45] Weiss RA. Autologous cell therapy: will it replace dermal fillers? Facial Plast Surg Clin North Am 2013; 21: 299–304

[46] Walter MN, Wright KT, Fuller HR, MacNeil S, Johnson WE. Mesenchymal stem cell-conditioned medium accelerates skin wound healing: an in vitro study of fibroblast and keratinocyte scratch assays. Exp Cell Res 2010; 316: 1271–1281

[47] Wang Y, Wang H, Hegde V, et al. Interplay of pro- and anti-inflammatory cytokines to determine lipid accretion in adipocytes. Int J Obes 2013; 37: 1490–1498

[48] Kong CM, Lee XW, Wang X. Telomere shortening in human diseases. FEBS J 2013; 280: 3180–3193

[49] Harley CB, Liu W, Blasco M, et al. A natural product telomerase activator as part of a health maintenance program. Rejuvenation Res 2011; 14: 45–56

[50] Molgora B, Bateman R, Sweeney G, et al. Functional assessment of pharmaco-logical telomerase activators in human T cells. Cells 2013; 2: 57–66

[51] Bernardes de Jesus B, Schneeberger K, Vera E, Tejera A, Harley CB, Blasco MA. The telomerase activator TA-65 elongates short telomeres and increases health span of adult/old mice without increasing cancer incidence. Aging Cell 2011; 10: 604–621

[52] Bernardes de Jesus B, Vera E, Schneeberger K, et al. Telomerase gene therapy in adult and old mice delays aging and increases longevity without increasing cancer. EMBO Mol Med 2012; 4: 691–704

[53] Ornish D, Lin J, Daubenmier J, et al. Increased telomerase activity and com-prehensive lifestyle changes: a pilot study. Lancet Oncol 2008; 9: 1048–1057

[54] Hickerson RP, Smith FJD, McLean WHI, Landthaler M, Leube RE, Kaspar RL. SiRNA-mediated selective inhibition of mutant keratin mRNAs responsible for the skin disorder pachyonychia congenita. Ann N Y Acad Sci 2006; 1082: 56–61

[55] Wang Q, Ilves H, Chu P, et al. Delivery and inhibition of reporter genes by small interfering RNAs in a mouse skin model. J Invest Dermatol 2007; 127: 2577–2584

[56] Gonzalez-Gonzalez E, Speaker TJ, Hickerson RP, et al. Silencing of reporter gene expression in skin using siRNAs and expression of plasmid DNA delivered by a soluble protrusion array device (PAD). Mol Ther 2010; 18: 1667–1674

[57] Calderhead RG, Goo BL, Lauro F, et al. The clinical efficacy and safety of microneedling fractional radiofrequency in the treatment of facial wrinkles: a multicenter study with the Infini System in 499 patients. Lutronic, Restoration Robotics, San Jose, California. 2013

[58] Hochman M, Adams DM, Reeves TD. Current knowledge and management of vascular anomalies: 1 Hemangiomas. Arch Facial Plast Surg 2011; 13: 145–151

[59] Hellwig S, Schönermark M, Raulin C. [Treatment of vascular malformations and pigment disorders of the face and neck by pulsed dye laser, photoderm VL and Q-switched ruby laser] Laryngorhinootologie 1995; 74: 635–641

[60] Schroeter CA, Neumann HAM. An intense light source. The photoderm VL-flashlamp as a new treatment possibility for vascular skin lesions. Dermatol Surg 1998; 24: 743–748

Index

Note: Page numbers set **bold** or *italic* indicate headings or figures, respectively.